Laparoscopic Surgery

Laparoscopic Surgery

Principles and Procedures
Second Edition, Revised and Expanded

edited by

Daniel B. Jones
Beth Israel Deaconess Medical Center, and
Harvard Medical School
Boston, Massachusetts, U.S.A.

Justin S. Wu
Kaiser Permanente Medical Center, and
University of California
San Diego, U.S.A.

Nathaniel J. Soper
Barnes-Jewish Hospital, and
Washington University School of Medicine
St. Louis, Missouri, U.S.A.

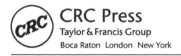

CRC Press
Taylor & Francis Group
Boca Raton London New York

CRC Press is an imprint of the
Taylor & Francis Group, an **informa** business

CRC Press
Taylor & Francis Group
6000 Broken Sound Parkway NW, Suite 300
Boca Raton, FL 33487-2742

First issued in paperback 2019

ISBN-13: 978-0-8247-4622-3 (hbk)
ISBN-13: 978-0-367-39426-4 (pbk)

**Visit the Taylor & Francis Web site at
http://www.taylorandfrancis.com**

**and the CRC Press Web site at
http://www.crcpress.com**

Preface

Nearly two decades after the first laparoscopic cholecystectomy, numerous randomized studies have documented the benefits of less pain, shorter hospitalization, and faster recuperation for many commonly performed operations. Hospitals have redesigned operating rooms with endosuites including monitors hung from the ceiling, voice activated insufflators and tables, and even robotic hands commanded remotely by the surgeon. We no longer hear colleagues heckle the laparoscopic surgeon, "When you have a hammer, the whole world looks like a nail."

Instead, patients come to the office seeking a less invasive approach often after googling the procedure and surgeon on the internet. Whenever we post a case and the word "lap" is missing, medical students, nurses, and colleagues will frequently double-check "What? You're *not* doing it laparoscopically?" While we used to have to justify the rationale for offering a laparoscopic approach, we now must explain why an open approach is preferred for this particular patient and specific problem. This is not a trend, but a quantum change in patient expectation and surgeon practice.

A well-performed open procedure can be better for the patient than a struggle through the scope when exposure is limited, bleeding obscures the camera lens, and multiple adhesions unduly prolong the procedure. As surgeons, the authors still can enjoy the wonderful exposure of mechanical retractors prying apart the abdominal wall, palpation of organs between gloved hands, free range of motion of suturing, and the easy slide of a one-handed knot. Laparoscopy is not for everyone and all diseases, and pneumoperitoneum is not well tolerated by all patients. Readers should glean from this book when to start open or convert as a matter of good judgement.

In *Laparoscopic Surgery: Principles and Procedures*, we acknowledge the "learning curve" to new technology and value the skill set required for advanced laparoscopy. The book is divided into two sections. The first deals with equipment and technology and fundamental principles of laparoscopy. The second section is procedure-specific and provides a comprehensive and yet practical review of commonly performed basic and advanced laparoscopic operations.

The book is geared toward surgical residents in-training, and is ideal reading material for any "call room" bookshelf. Residents can quickly visualize with step-by-step illustrations complex operations and concisely review the key technical aspects of most MIS procedures in minutes. With a more thorough read, residents will learn history, indications, general management, expected outcomes, and potential complications. It is our intent that *Laparoscopic Surgery* will help prepare residents and surgeons in practice to successfully pass the fundamentals of laparoscopy (FLS) examination sponsored by the American Society for Gastrointestinal and Endoscopic Surgeons (SAGES) and the American College of Surgeons (ACS).

The first edition was well received by surgeons and nurses already in practice. The list of equipment for each procedure served as a quick and easy reference to check that instruments and equipment will be available in the operating room and added to the surgeon's procedure preference lists. The "Top Ten" at the end of each procedural chapter offered helpful hints and emphasized technical pitfalls for the surgeon to avoid early in his or her "learning curve."

The second edition updates each chapter with lessons learned over the last decade on controversial operations such as laparoscopic colon resection for malignancy and unilateral hernia repair. Laparoscopic gastric bypass, laparoscopic adjustable band, laparoscopic ventral hernia repair, and laparoscopic esophagectomy are just a few of the operations which have recently gained prominence and are now included in the latest edition. Specialty sections such as endovascular surgery have been totally rewritten. New technologies such as robotic surgery and hand-assisted surgery are thoroughly reviewed. Other chapters survey MIS training modalities using videotrainers, simulators, virtual reality, and teleproctoring.

The authors would like to dedicate this book to our wives, Stephanie, Cindy, and Bernie, and children, Ryan, Cara, Leah, Nick, Robbie, Chris, and Nathaniel. Undertaking this book steals time from family, and we very much appreciate their support.

In addition to our contributors, we are also indebted to Eleanor Goodspeed and to Marcel Dekker, Inc. editors without whose help this book would not have been completed on schedule.

We believe you will find this book up-to-date and a useful quick read on the way to the clinics and operating room. We also welcome your comments and pearls of wisdom for the next edition as the field of minimal access surgery rapidly evolves.

Daniel B. Jones, M.D., FACS
Justin S. Wu, M.D.
Nathaniel J. Soper, M.D., FACS

Contents

PART III APPLICATIONS FOR SURGICAL SUBSPECIALTIES

Contributors

David E. Beck, M.D.   Institute for Minimally Invasive Surgery, Washington University School of Medicine, St. Louis, Missouri, U.S.A.

Matthew G. Blum, M.D.   Northwestern Memorial Hospital, Chicago, Illinois, U.S.A.

Michael J. Bolesta, M.D.   University of Texas Southwestern Medical Center, Dallas, Texas, U.S.A.

William M. Bowling, M.D.   University of Texas Southwestern Medical Center, Dallas, Texas, U.S.A.

Fred Brody, M.D.   Cleveland Clinic Foundation, Cleveland, Ohio, U.S.A.

L. Michael Brunt, M.D.   Institute for Minimally Invasive Surgery, Washington University School of Medicine, St. Louis, Missouri, U.S.A.

Jeffrey A. Cadeddu, M.D.   University of Texas Southwestern Medical Center, Dallas, Texas, U.S.A.

Mark P. Callery, M.D.   Beth Israel Deaconess Medical Center, Harvard Medical School, Boston, Massachusetts, U.S.A.

Jonathan J. Canete, M.D., MPH   University of Massachusetts Medical School, Worcester, Massachusetts, U.S.A.

Stephen L. Carter, M.D.   United Hospital Center, Clarksburg, West Virginia, U.S.A.

Nicole M. Chandler, M.D.   University of Massachusetts Medical School, Worcester, Massachusetts, U.S.A.

Craig G. Chang, M.D.   University of Texas Southwestern Medical School, Dallas, Texas, U.S.A.

Li Ern Chen, B.A.   Washington University School of Medicine, St. Louis, Missouri, U.S.A.

David D. Chi, M.D.   Los Robles Regional Medical Center, Thousand Oaks, California, U.S.A.

Ralph V. Clayman, M.D.   University of California, Irvine Medical Center, Orange, California, U.S.A.

Robert L. Coleman, M.D.   Center for Minimally Invasive Surgery, University of Texas Southwestern Medical Center, Dallas, Texas, U.S.A.

Jonathan F. Critchlow, M.D.   Beth Israel Deaconess Medical Center, Harvard Medical School, Boston, Massachusetts, U.S.A.

Ketan M. Desai, M.D.   Washington University School of Medicine, St. Louis, Missouri, U.S.A.

Sergio Diaz, M.D.   Barnes-Jewish Hospital, Washington University School of Medicine, St. Louis, Missouri, U.S.A.

W. Stephen Eubanks, M.D.   Duke University Medical Center, Durham, North Carolina, U.S.A.

Jason B. Fleming, M.D.   University of Texas Southwestern Medical Center, Dallas, Texas, U.S.A.

James W. Fleshman, M.D.   Institute for Minimally Invasive Surgery, Washington University School of Medicine, St. Louis, Missouri, U.S.A.

Morris E. Franklin, Jr. , M.D.   University Health Science Center, Texas Endosurgery Institute, San Antonio, Texas, U.S.A.

John J. Gonzalez, Jr., M.D.   University Health Science Center, San Antonio, Texas, U.S.A.

Amanda Gosman, M.D.   University of Texas Southwestern Medical Center, Dallas, Texas, U.S.A.

Elizabeth C. Hamilton, M.D.   University of Texas Southwestern Medical Center, Dallas, Texas, U.S.A.

Timothy T. Hamilton, M.D. Southwestern Center for Minimally Invasive Surgery, University of Texas Southwestern Medical Center, Dallas, Texas, U.S.A.

Thomas J. Herzog, M.D. Washington University School of Medicine, St. Louis, Missouri, U.S.A.

Mark R. Jackson, M.D. Greenville, South Carolina, U.S.A.

Daniel B. Jones Beth Israel Deaconess Medical Center, Harvard Medical School, Boston, Massachusetts, U.S.A.

Stephanie B. Jones, M.D. Beth Israel Deaconess Medical Center, Harvard Medical School, Boston, Massachusetts, U.S.A.

Andreas M. Kaiser, M.D. University of Southern California, Los Angeles, California, U.S.A.

Namir Katkhouda, M.D. University of Southern California, Los Angeles, California, U.S.A.

Mary E. Klingensmith, M.D. Washington University School of Medicine, St. Louis, Missouri, U.S.A.

Edward R. Kost, M.D. Brooke Army Medical Center, Ft. Sam, Houston, Texas, U.S.A.

Edward Lin, D.O. Emory University School of Medicine, Atlanta, Georgia, U.S.A.

James D. Luketich, M.D. University of Pittsburgh Medical Center, Pittsburgh, Pennsylvania, U.S.A.

Shishir K. Maithel, M.D. Beth Israel Deaconess Medical Center, Harvard Medical School, Boston, Massachusetts, U.S.A.

Mark V. Mazziotti, M.D. Houston Pediatric Surgeons, Houston, Texas, U.S.A.

W. Scott Melvin, M.D. Ohio State University, Columbus, Ohio, U.S.A.

Robert K. Minkes, M.D., Ph.D. Louisiana State University, New Orleans, Louisiana, U.S.A.

Kenric M. Murayama, M.D. Northwestern University, Feinberg School of Medicine, Chicago, Illinois, U.S.A.

Ninh T. Nguyen, M.D. University of California, Irvine Medical Center, Irvine, California, U.S.A.

John A. Olson, Jr., M.D. Duke University School of Medicine, Durham, North Carolina, U.S.A.

David A. Provost, M.D.   University of Texas Southwestern Medical Center, Dallas, Texas, U.S.A.

Robert V. Rege, M.D.   Southwestern Center for Minimally Invasive Surgery, University of Texas Southwestern Medical Center, Dallas, Texas, U.S.A.

Rod J. Rohrich, M.D.   University of Texas Southwestern Medical Center, Dallas, Texas, U.S.A.

Michael Rosen, M.D.   Cleveland Clinic Foundation, Cleveland, Ohio, U.S.A.

Philip R. Schauer, M.D.   University of Pittsburgh Medical Center, Pittsburgh, Pennsylvania, U.S.A.

Benjamin E. Schneider, M.D.   Beth Israel Deaconess Medical Center, Harvard Medical School, Boston, Massachusetts, U.S.A.

Daniel J. Scott, M.D.   Tulane Center for Minimally Invasive Surgery, Tulane University School of Medicine, New Orleans, Louisiana, U.S.A.

Allan Siperstein, M.D.   Cleveland Clinic Foundation, Cleveland, Ohio, U.S.A.

C. Daniel Smith, M.D.   Emory University School of Medicine, Atlanta, Georgia, U.S.A.

Nathaniel J. Soper, M.D.   Northwestern University, Feinberg School of Medicine, Chicago, Illinois, U.S.A.

Sudhir R. Sundaresan, M.D.   Northwestern Memorial Hospital, Chicago, Illinois, U.S.A.

John F. Sweeney, M.D.   Baylor College of Medicine, Houston, Texas, U.S.A.

James W. Thiele, M.D.   Institute for Minimally Invasive Surgery, Washington University School of Medicine, St. Louis, Missouri, U.S.A.

Robert A. Underwood, M.D.   Surgical Arts, PC, Marietta, Georgia, U.S.A.

Thomas K. Varghese, M.D.   Northwestern University, Feinberg School of Medicine, Chicago, Illinois, U.S.A.

Leonardo Villegas, M.D.   Beth Israel Deaconess Medical Center, Harvard Medical School, Boston, Massachusetts, U.S.A.

Michael D. Williams, M.D.   Baylor College of Medicine, Houston, Texas, U.S.A.

Emily R. Winslow, M.D.   Institute for Minimally Invasive Surgery, Washington University School of Medicine, St. Louis, Missouri, U.S.A.

Andrew Wu, B.S. Northwestern University, Feinberg School of Medicine, Chicago, Illinois, U.S.A.

Justin S. Wu, M.D. Kaiser Permanente Medical Center, University of California, San Diego, California, U.S.A.

Laparoscopic Surgery

1

The Laparoscopic Revolution

ROBERT A. UNDERWOOD

Surgical Arts, PC
Marietta, Georgia, U.S.A.

The rapid acceptance of laparoscopic cholecystectomy as the gold standard for removal of the gallbladder has led general surgeons to embrace minimally invasive surgical procedures, yet laparoscopic techniques have been investigated since the early twentieth century, with early proof of applicability established by gynecologists and urologists. Eventually the drive to adapt the technology to general surgical procedures came not from the academic surgical arena, but from the private sector, spurred by public interest in and demand for its advantages: improved cosmesis, decreased pain, shorter hospital stays, and a quicker return to normal preoperative lifestyle. This rapid and nontraditional developmental pathway has led to questions concerning training requirements, credentialing, and review.

I. HISTORICAL PERSPECTIVE

The use of speculum-type intracorporeal viewing devices dates to the Greco-Roman period, when Hippocrates (c. 460–377 BCE) is known to have performed anoscopy for diagnosis of fistula and hemorrhoids. However, technical limitations of light transmission and optical clarity inhibited use of such devices until the early nineteenth century, when Phillip Bozzini developed the *Lichtleiter* (light conductor) in 1805. This instrument employed a candle, mirrors, and various specula for viewing the rectum, vagina, urethra, and bladder (Fig. 1A). The next major advance came in 1853 when Antonin Desormeaux developed his versatile endoscope that burned *gazogene* (alcohol and turpentine) as a light source and employed a lens system for narrowing and intensifying illumination of the visual field (Fig. 1B). Such scopes led to the development of internal speculum tip–mounted platinum loop light sources, first invented in 1867 by Bruck, a dentist in Breslau, Poland. This device replaced and dramatically improved upon the previous external combustion light sources but was plagued by the inherent problems of the thermal injury and flare, which required angling the viewing lens away from the light source, severely limiting the visual field.

Major breakthroughs during the late nineteenth century included the development of the incandescent bulb by Thomas Edison and the three-lens optical system by Maximillian

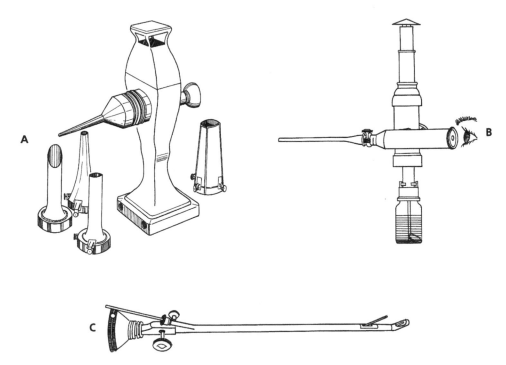

Figure 1   (A) Original *Lichtleiter* with various specula. (B) Desormeaux endoscope. (C) Nitze cystoscope with incandescent globe and instrument channel for ureteral probe.

Nitze and Reinecke, both in 1879. Integration of these two technologies allowed the development of the first viable endoscopes/cystoscopes concomitantly by several individuals, including Newman of Glasgow in 1883, Leiter in 1886, and Nitze in 1887. Nitze's design proved to be the most utilitarian and versatile, particularly with the addition of further improvements such as prismatic lenses for angled viewing and operating channels (Fig. 1C). As a result of this early technology, most open cavity endoscopic procedures (i.e., those with access through natural orifices) had become common clinical practice by the end of the nineteenth century. It was not until the twentieth century, however, that closed-cavity endoscopy was attempted.

II.   DIAGNOSTIC LAPAROSCOPY AND THORACOSCOPY

Laparoscopy (from the Greek *lapro*, the flank, and *skopein*, to examine) was first performed in 1901 by George Kelling of Dresden, Germany, using a Nitze cystoscope in a dog. Kelling named the procedure *Kölioskopie* and described it in a report published in *Münchener Medizinische Wochenschrift* in January 1902. Eight years later in the same publication, Hans Christian Jacobaeus of Stockholm, Sweden, reported the first laparoscopy and thoracoscopy in humans, describing the endoscopic diagnosis of intra-abdominal tuberculosis, cirrhosis, syphilis, and malignancy. Interestingly, as a correlate to current health care motivations, Kelling later reported that his use of the laparoscope had rapidly escalated in the postwar period as a result of the sparse economic resources in Germany. His reasons were basic: smaller incisions, quicker recovery, and shorter, less costly hospital stays. In the United States, Bertram Bernheim was the first to perform laparoscopy in 1911 at Johns Hopkins University using a half-inch proctoscope at a periumbilical site with no pneumoperitoneum.

The first atlas and textbook on laparoscopy and thoracoscopy was written and published by Roger Korbsch of Munich, Germany, in 1927; in this text he expanded the indications for these procedures to include any disorder of these cavities that could not be diagnosed by other methods. Also in 1927, Heinz Kalk of Berlin, a hepatologist, introduced an improved version of the forward-viewing oblique (45°) scope, which improved operator orientation and decreased the operative field blind spot to approximately 10 degrees. The use of CO_2 to create a pneumoperitoneum was first recommended in 1924 by Richard Zollikofer of Switzerland. CO_2 was preferred over air and nitrogen because of its nonflammable nature and rapid reabsorption by the peritoneum. The preferred route of insufflation was the Veress needle, introduced by Janos Veress of Hungary in 1938. This device incorporates a spring-loaded blunt obturator at its tip, which protects the internal viscera from the sharp needle tip once it has penetrated the fascia and peritoneum. This device was originally intended for thoracic use in thoracentesis to produce therapeutic pneumothorax; however, it quickly found favor among laparoscopists and today remains the preferred insufflation needle in many operating suites (Figs. 1, 2).

III. THERAPEUTIC LAPAROSCOPY AND THORACOSCOPY

Therapeutic applications for the endoscope were quickly realized in thoracic surgery as a result of the prevalence of tuberculosis in the early 1900s. The thoracoscope was used to lyse pleural adhesions to produce therapeutic pneumothorax. (Open thoracotomy was not yet an option, since the endotracheal tube for selective ventilation had not yet been developed.)

Therapeutic laparoscopy evolved more slowly, especially in the United States. In 1929 Kalk first described a dual trocar technique that he used for liver biopsy, and in 1933 a German general surgeon, Carl Fervers, was the first to report laparoscopic lysis of abdominal adhesions for bowel obstruction. Since the early 1930s laparoscopic tubal ligations have been performed by gynecologists around the world. Notably, in the United States the preferred abdominal endoscopic procedure through the mid-twentieth century was *culdoscopy*, as developed by American gynecologists Decker and Cherry. In this procedure, performed with the patient under local anesthesia, the patient is positioned prone on knees and elbows, producing gravity-induced negative intra-abdominal pressure and thus a pneumoperitoneum when a needle is passed posterior to the cervix into the cul-de-sac. In Europe, gynecologists preferred the abdominal approach and called it *gynecological celioscopy*. Other gynecological applications of laparoscopy emerged both in the United States and Europe, fostering the development of the requisite instrumentation to perform these procedures (such as the first CO_2 insufflator, developed by Hans

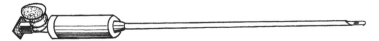

Figure 2 Veress needle.

Frangenheim of Germany in the late 1950s) as well as many general surgical procedures that remain popular today.

The 1960s and 1970s brought two major developments that were essential to the widespread use of laparoscopy. The first was the introduction in 1960 of the rod-lens system by Harold Hopkins of England. This system increased the light transmission of previous scopes by approximately 80-fold. The second, in 1963, was cold light transmission via fiberoptic cables developed by gastroenterologist Hirschowitz in Ann Arbor, Michigan. The combination of these two technologies positioned laparoscopy as a viable therapeutic modality for a variety of problems. Early clinical investigators credited for their pioneering work include Karl Semm of Germany, Patrik Steptoe of England, who published *Laparoscopy in Gynaecology* in 1967, and Melvin Cohen of the United States, who wrote the first American textbook on laparoscopy in 1970.

As the array of clinical indications expanded, the sources of complications such as subcutaneous emphysema, air embolism, visceral perforation, bleeding, burns, hemodynamic and pulmonary compromise, and infection were more clearly delineated and addressed. The automatic gas insufflator and the direct visualization technique of trocar placement were developments that directly addressed many complications in this burgeoning field. The automatic insufflator was designed by gynecologist and engineer Karl Semm in 1966 and greatly reduced the adverse effects of pneumoperitoneum, such as hemodynamic or pulmonary compromise and hypercarbia. The technique of cut-down and direct visualization of the peritoneal cavity before placing a blunt obturated trocar was introduced by Hasson in 1974 and was called *ober laparoscopy* or the *Hasson technique.* This device and technique greatly reduced the incidence of visceral injury sustained from blind peritoneal trocar insertion (Figs. 1–3).

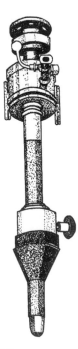

Figure 3   Reusable Hasson trocar.

Semm has played a major role in the development of laparoscopy, or, as he originally called it, operative pelviscopy. He introduced not only the automated insufflation system but also many other devices and techniques, such as the pretied suture endo-loop, the laparoscopic clip applier, the high-flow irrigator, and many operative instruments that serve specific needs in laparoscopy.

IV. LAPAROSCOPY IN GENERAL SURGERY

The link that finally brought laparoscopy into the mainstream of general surgery was the development in 1985 of the charge coupled device (CCD) silicon chip solid state image sensor—the miniature video camera. This technology allowed all members of the operating team to view the operative field simultaneously and from the same video screen orientation, as opposed to the now archaic single-eyepiece viewing of the past.

In 1987 Philippe Mouret performed the first human laparoscopic cholecystectomy in Lyon, France. He was followed within 12 months by other general surgeons around the world, such as Barry McKernan and William Saye from Marietta, Georgia, and Eddic Joc Reddick and Douglas Olsen in Nashville, Tennessee, who were the first to perform this procedure in the United States. Notably, these surgeons were in private practice, community-based hospitals. From 1989 through 1991, it is estimated that approximately 20,000 American general surgeons received training in laparoscopic techniques. Laparoscopic cholecystectomy was quickly accepted as the gold standard for removing a diseased gallbladder. The success with laparoscopic cholecystectomy has had a significant impact on the practice of general surgery and has led to the exponential development of other applications such as laparoscopic appendectomy, adrenalectomy, inguinal herniorrhaphy, colon resection, antireflux procedures, bariatric procedures, hepatobiliary and pancreatic procedures, splenectomy, vascular procedures, and plastic surgery procedures, as well as various intrathoracic pulmonary and cardiac procedures. The current status of each of these will be discussed in subsequent chapters.

SELECTED READINGS

Davis CJ, Filipi CR. A history of endoscopic surgery. In: Arregui ME, Fitzgibbons RJ Jr, Katkhouda N, McKernan JB, Reich, H, eds. Principles of Laparoscopic Surgery: Basic and Advanced Techniques. New York: Springer-Verlag, 1995, pp 3–20.

Fierer AS, Sackier JM. Laparoscopic general surgery: a current state of affairs, parts 1 and 2. Contemp Surg 46(5):239–245, 46(6):297–302, 1995.

Hunter JG, Sackier JM. Minimally invasive high tech surgery: into the 21st century. In Hunter JG, Sackier JM, eds. Minimally Invasive Surgery. New York: MCGraw-Hill, 1993, pp 3–6.

Litynski GS. Highlights in the History of Laparoscopy. Frankfurt am Main, Germany: Barbara Bernert Verlag, 1996.

Mori T, Bhoyrul S, Way LW. History of laparoscopic surgery. In Mori T, Bhoyrul S, Way LW, eds. Fundamentals of Laparoscopic Surgery. New York: Churchill Livingstone, 1995, pp 1–12.

Soper NT, Brunt ML, Kerbl K. Laparoscopic general surgery. N Engl J Med 330:409–419, 1994.

2

Patient Selection and Preparation

EMILY R. WINSLOW and MARY E. KLINGENSMITH

Washington University School of Medicine
St. Louis, Missouri, U.S.A.

JOHN A. OLSON, JR.

Duke University School of Medicine
Durham, North Carolina, U.S.A.

I. INTRODUCTION

No surgical procedure is without risk. Despite the minimally invasive nature of laparoscopic surgery, the potential for adverse outcome is present and should be taken as seriously as in a traditional open procedure. Patients must be carefully evaluated preoperatively to determine their eligibility for a laparoscopic approach. In addition to the patient characteristics and the nature of the disease process that must be considered for open surgery, the surgeon must also consider factors specific to the execution of the procedure laparoscopically. Patient selection and preparation for a laparoscopic procedure is the first step in ensuring a successful outcome.

II. PREOPERATIVE EVALUATION

A careful history and physical examination are the cornerstones of patient selection for surgery. Preexisting conditions that predispose patients to both anesthetic and surgical complications must be identified. Signs and symptoms suggestive of cardiac or pulmonary disease should be specifically sought, even if a previous diagnosis has not been established. Preoperative laboratory evaluation depends on the nature of the surgery, the patient's past medical history, and the preferences of both the surgeon and anesthesiologist. In general, this may include a complete blood cell count, serum electrolyte determination, and urinalysis. In patients older than 40, a screening chest radiograph and an electrocardiogram may be indicated. Coagulation studies are needed in patients with a personal or family history of a bleeding diathesis.

It is important to carefully evaluate the patient with known or suspected pulmonary disease prior to undertaking a laparoscopic procedure, as pneumoperitoneum and hypercarbia may be poorly tolerated. Pulmonary function testing with arterial blood gas determination may be helpful in deciding if the patient can tolerate the planned procedure. It is important to determine the baseline pCO_2 in patients with known pulmonary disease so that the extent of hyperventilation can be better evaluated intraoperatively. Similarly, patients with known or suspected cardiac disease need adequate preoperative risk evaluation because of the effect of pneumoperitoneum on cardiac function (i.e., decreased venous return secondary to inferior vena cava compression with a resulting drop in cardiac output) and the fact that some laparoscopic procedures may take longer than their open counterparts. This evaluation may involve cardiac stress testing and should be done in consultation with a cardiologist.

Several other factors specific to a laparoscopic procedure should be considered preoperatively.

> Prior incisions—The past surgical history and the location of prior incisions should be specifically considered as this will aid in the planning of access method and trocar placement.
>
> Umbilical abnormalities—The patient should be specifically examined for an umbilical hernia or urachal cyst as this may also affect trocar placement.
>
> Positioning limitations—The ability to abduct the arms and hips should be assessed, as many laparoscopic procedures are performed in the lithotomy position.
>
> Presence of ascites—The presence of ascites will complicate abdominal access and may complicate the postoperative course if the fluid becomes infected or leaks from the trocar sites.
>
> History of deep venous thrombosis (DVT)—Patients with a history of a DVT should be carefully evaluated preoperatively, as many laparoscopic procedures are lengthy, require the reverse Trendelenberg position, and can have significant inferior vena cava compression secondary to the pneumoperitoneum. All patients should have compression stockings in place before the induction of general anesthesia; those patients at higher risk (e.g., prior DVT or cancer) may need additional measures including pneumatic compression devices.

III. CONTRAINDICATIONS TO LAPAROSCOPIC SURGERY

As time has passed and experience has accumulated, the contraindications to laparoscopic procedures have been modified. It is important to emphasize that the documented benefits of the laparoscopic approach—a hastened postoperative recovery and improved cosmesis—do not warrant placing the patient at increased risk for adverse surgical outcome. Thus, good judgment must be exercised in any circumstance where a condition exists that may make the laparoscopic procedure more risky than open surgery.

A. Absolute Contraindications

In the following clinical situations, the use of laparoscopy is either prohibitively unsafe for the patient or is almost certain to lead to conversion to laparotomy.

> 1. Hypovolemic shock—Patients showing signs of shock due to hypovolemia are unlikely to tolerate the further decrease in venous return caused by the

pneumoperitoneum. In addition, these patients will benefit from the most expeditious operation, as their end organ perfusion will only be further challenged by a period of general anesthesia. A laparoscopic procedure is contraindicated in patients with significant ongoing abdominal bleeding due to both hypovolemia and technical issues. Significant bleeding makes a laparoscopic procedure difficult to perform because the view is obscured and the surgeon cannot rapidly identify or easily correct the problem.

2.   Hemodynamic instability—Patients with hemodynamic instability for any reason (hypovolemia, depressed cardiac function, sepsis) are poor candidates for laparoscopy. The effects of pneumoperitoneum as well as the extremes in patient position that are sometimes required during laparoscopy will be poorly tolerated by patients already compromised from a cardiovascular standpoint.

3.   Massive abdominal distention—In patients with extremely dilated intestine, it is unsafe to attempt to establish pneumoperitoneum due to the likelihood of bowel puncture. In addition, there will not be sufficient working room in which to operate.

4.   Inability to tolerate a laparotomy—Patients who are not candidates for a laparotomy due to severe systemic disease should not be considered for laparoscopic procedures.

5.   Surgeon inexperience—As with any surgical procedure, if the surgeon is not adequately trained, the procedure should not be attempted. Advanced laparoscopic skills are required to successfully complete many procedures, and without them the procedure should not be done laparoscopically.

B.   Relative Contraindications

In the following clinical situations the use of laparoscopy is not generally advised but may be attempted in specific clinical scenarios by highly trained surgeons.

1.   Generalized peritonitis of unclear origin—Patients with diffuse peritonitis, particularly when the etiology is unclear, are not ideal candidates for a laparoscopic exploration. Because of the difficulty involved with an adequate and expeditious abdominal exploration in this setting, these patients are best approached by laparotomy.

2.   Advanced cardiopulmonary disease—Patients with severe cardiac or pulmonary disease are poor candidates for surgery in general and can be further compromised by a laparoscopic approach. The cardiopulmonary effects of pneumoperitoneum and the duration of the procedure may make an open approach more suitable for these patients.

3.   Advanced pregnancy—Laparoscopic procedures, particularly in the lower abdomen, are particularly difficult in a near-term gravida. The uterus in late pregnancy simply makes access to the appendix or pelvic organs impossible. Laparoscopic procedures in the first and second trimesters have been shown in several series to be safe for both mother and fetus when performed with proper precautions by experienced individuals [1,2].

4.   Uncorrectable coagulopathy—In most cases patients with an uncorrectable coagulopathy are more safely approached through a traditional laparotomy where bleeding complications may be more easily and quickly controlled.

5. Portal hypertension—Patients with portal hypertension may have excessive abdominal wall bleeding from trocar placement. In addition, they tend to have more bleeding during routine abdominal dissections due to collateral blood vessels, which may obscure the field of view and make the procedure unsafe.

IV. CONSIDERATIONS IN SPECIFIC PATIENT POPULATIONS

A. The Pediatric Population

Early in the laparoscopic era, laparoscopic techniques were not used in children because traditional incisions in pediatric patients are relatively small and the instrumentation was not appropriate. However, since that time, laparoscopic procedures in children have become increasingly common, with up to 82% of pediatric surgeons in 1996 performing laparoscopic or thoracoscopic procedures [3]. Recently, it has been recognized that a minimally invasive approach has relatively few complications [4] and benefits even the smallest child [5,6]. In a large Italian multicenter study of all pediatric laparoscopic procedures, conversion occurred in only 1.3% of cases [4]. Although the indications for a laparoscopic approach in children are still evolving and no randomized controlled trials have yet been reported, the laparoscopic approach for some procedures (e.g., cholecystectomy, ovarian cystectomy, and exploration for impalpable testes) has already become the gold standard [7].

B. The Geriatric Population

The geriatric population is the fastest growing segment of our population and presents a challenge to the health care system. Because elderly patients have a higher incidence of cardiopulmonary disease, it was initially presumed that they would not be good candidates for laparoscopic procedures. However, the reported outcomes of the laparoscopic approach for several different procedures have challenged this assumption. The elderly patient population has been most closely examined in the context of laparoscopic cholecystectomy. In a prospective, randomized trial involving 264 patients aged ≥ 65 years, one group found equivalent operative times, a lower incidence of complications, and a shorter length of hospital stay in the laparoscopic compared to the open cholecystectomy group [8]. It has also been noted in a retrospective database review of 18,500 cholecystectomies in patients aged ≥ 80 years that the overall mortality of laparoscopic cholecystectomy was significantly lower than that of open cholecystectomy (1.8% vs. 4.4%, respectively) [9]. Despite the reduction in mortality compared with open cholecystectomy, laparoscopic cholecystectomy in the extremely elderly (≥ 80 years) has been shown to be associated with more complications and a higher rate of conversion when compared to younger patients (65–80 years) [10].

Similarly positive results in elderly patients have been shown in the case of laparoscopic colon resection and laparoscopic antireflux surgery. In a prospective comparative study involving 46 patients aged ≥ 75 years with sigmoid diverticulitis, the laparoscopic group was found to have less pain, fewer complications, a shorter hospital stay, and a shorter duration of stay in a rehabilitation facility when compared to those undergoing open colectomy [11]. In a prospective study of 339 patients undergoing laparoscopic antireflux surgery, patients ≥ 65 years had slightly longer hospital stays and more frequent minor complications than younger patients, but the groups had equivalent rates of major complications and anatomical failure [12].

In summary, although elderly patients may have more complicated perioperative courses when compared to younger patients in some circumstances, they generally tolerate the laparoscopic approach to a procedure better than its open counterpart.

C. The Obese Patient

Obesity is associated with higher rates of complications after many surgical procedures and was initially thought to be a contraindication to laparoscopic procedures. It has become clear with time that although obese patients may have a higher complication rate after laparoscopic procedures when compared to the nonobese, they derive significant benefit from a minimally invasive approach when compared with open surgery. For laparoscopic cholecystectomy, it has been shown that obese patients may have longer operative times when compared to nonobese patients [13], but have similar complications rates and time to recovery [14]. When the results of open cholecystectomy in obese patients are compared with the results of laparoscopic cholecystectomy in obese patients, the laparoscopic approach is associated with fewer complications and faster recovery times [15]. One group has reported high rates of conversion in obese patients undergoing laparoscopic colorectal surgery [16], although another group found equivalent rates in a smaller study [17]. Despite this difference in outcome, both groups recommend a laparoscopic approach in the obese patient, as the complication rates are still lower than those historically associated with open colectomy in this patient population. A small study compared the outcome of obese patients undergoing open appendectomy with that of obese patients undergoing laparoscopic appendectomy and found that although the laparoscopic procedures took slightly longer, the laparoscopic approach was associated with less pain, a faster recovery, and a similarly low complication rate [18].

In summary, there do seem to be some difficulties associated with laparoscopic procedures in the obese patient, as manifested by longer operative times in most series. Despite this, the laparoscopic approach in obese patients has yielded results equivalent to those in nonobese patients in many series. Although there may indeed be a higher complication rate associated with laparoscopic procedures in obese patients compared to nonobese patients, the overall outcome from laparoscopic procedures has still been superior to open procedures in this patient population.

V. PATIENT PREPARATION

As with all surgical procedures, preparation of the patient begins with informed consent. The patient must fully understand the potential benefits, risks, and alternatives to the proposed laparoscopic procedure and should be aware of the possibility of conversion to an open operation. The frequency and circumstances of conversion for the particular procedure should be carefully estimated by the operating surgeon as part of the process of informed consent. Preoperative antibiotics before a laparoscopic procedure should be given before the incision is made in any procedure in which bacterial contamination of the wound or abdomen is possible (i.e., clean contaminated cases). In addition, antibiotics should be given if prosthetic mesh will be placed during the operation. Antibiotics covering skin flora should be given to immunocompromised patients, even in clean surgical procedures. Given the risk of DVT after laparoscopic procedures, many surgeons recommend giving a single dose of subcutaneous heparin several hours prior to surgery and continuing the treatment until the patient is fully ambulatory. Compression stockings and/or intermittent compression devices should be placed on all patients before the induction of anesthesia. Mechanical bowel preparation is not necessary before most routine laparoscopic procedures, but should be given to all patients at high risk of inadvertent intraoperative bowel injury (reoperative ventral hernias, anticipated extensive adhesive disease, etc.) or when bowel manipulation is planned (colorectal surgery).

VI. CONCLUSION

The safety of a laparoscopic procedure relies upon a careful preoperative patient assessment, with recognition of any contraindication to the laparoscopic approach. It must be emphasized that minimally invasive surgery can be major surgery, and concern for patient safety dictates that the patient must be able to tolerate conversion to an open procedure. Finally, if the laparoscopic approach is to be offered responsibly, the surgeon must possess adequate skills in both the laparoscopic and open approach to a given procedure.

REFERENCES

1. Curet M, Allen D, Josloff RK, Pitcher DE, Curet LB, Miscall BG, Zucker K, A. Laparoscopy during pregnancy. Arch Surg 1996; 131:546–551.
2. Reedy MB, Kallen B, Kuehl T. Laparoscopy during pregnancy: A study of five fetal outcome parameters with use of the Swedish health registry. Am J Obstet Gynecol 1997; 177:673–679.
3. Firilas AM, Jackson RJ, Smith SD. Minimally invasive surgery: the pediatric surgery experience. J Am College Surg 1998; 186:542–544.
4. Esposito C, Mattioli G, Monguzzi GL, Montinaro L, Riccipetiotoni G, Aceti R, Messina M, Pintus C, Settimi A, Esposito G, Jassoni V. Complications and conversions of pediatric videosurgery: the Italian multicentric experience on 1689 procedures. Surg Endosc 2002; 16:795–798.
5. Rothenberg SS, Chang JHT, Bealer JF. Experience with minimally invasive surgery in infants. Am J Surg 1998; 176:654–658.
6. Mattioli G, Repetto P, Carlini C, Torre M, PiniPrato A, Mazzola C, Leggio S, Montobbio G, Gandullia P, Barabino A, Cagnazzo A, Sacco O, Jassonni V. Laparoscopic vs open approach for the treatment of gastroesophgeal reflux in children. Surg Endosc 2002; 16:750–752.
7. Tam PKH. Laparoscopic surgery in children. Arch Dis Child 2000; 82:240–243.
8. Lujan JA, Sanchez-Bueno F, Parrilla P, Robles R, Torralba JA, Gonzalez-Costea R. Laparoscopic vs open cholecystectomy in patients aged 65 and older. Surg Laparosc Endosc 1998; 8:208–210.
9. Maxwell jG, Tyler BA, Rutledge R, Brinker CC, Maxwell BG, Covington DL. Cholecystectomy in patients aged 80 and older. Am J Surg 1998; 176:627–631.
10. Brunt LM, Quasebarth ML, Dunnegan DL, Soper NJ. Outcomes analysis of laparoscopic cholecystectomy in the extremely elderly. Surg Endosc 2001; 15:700–705.
11. Tuech JJ, Pesseaux P, Rouge C, Regenet N, Bergamaschi R, Arnaud JP. Laparoscopic vs open colectomy for sigmoid diverticulitis: a prospective comparative study in the elderly. Surg Endosc 2000; 14:1031–1033.
12. Brunt LM, Quasebarth ML, Dunnegan DL, Soper NJ. Is laparoscopic antireflux surgery for gastroesophageal reflux disease in the elderly safe and effective? Surg Endosc 1999; 13:838–842.
13. Angrisana L, Lorenzo M, De Palma G, Sivero L, Catanzano C, Tesauro B, Persico G. Laparoscopic cholecystectomy in obese patients compated with nonobese patients. Surg Laparosc Endosc Percut Techn 1995; 5:197–201.

14. Phillips EH, Carroll BJ, Fallas MJ, Pearlstein AR. Comparison of laparoscopic cholecystectomy in obese and non-obese patients. Am Surg 1994; 60:316–321.
15. Miles RH, Carballo RE, Prinz RA, McMahon M, Pulawski G, Olen RN, Dahlinghaus DL. Laparoscopy: the preferred method of cholecystectomy in the morbidly obese. Surgery 1992; 112:818–822.
16. Pikarsky AJ, Saida Y, Yamaguchi T, Martinez S, Chen W, Weiss EG, Nogueras JJ, Wexner SD. Is obesity a high-risk factor for laparoscopic colorectal surgery? Surg Endosc 2002; online.
17. Tuech J, Regenet N, Hennekinne S, Pessaux P, Duplessis R, Arnaud JP. Impact of obesity on postoperative results of elective laparoscopic colectomy in sigmoid diverticulitis: a prospective study. Ann Chirurg 2001; 126:996–1000.
18. Jitea N, Angelescu N, Burcos T, Cristian D, Voiculescu S, Mircea N. Laparoscopic appendectomy in obese patients. A comparative study with open appendectomy. Chirurgia 1996; 45:203–205.

3

Basic Equipment, Room Setup, and Patient Positioning

JUSTIN S. WU

Kaiser Permanente Medical Center
University of California, San Diego
San Diego, California, U.S.A.

A dedicated "laparoscopic suite" in the operating room is becoming increasingly popular as operating rooms and hospitals are being built or redesigned. Each laparoscopic suite carries the essential basic equipment for laparoscopic surgery, whether they are built into the actual room (suspended from ceilings) or are mounted on mobile carts ("video towers"). In addition to having the basic equipment present and functioning properly before the patient arrives in the operating room, the appropriate room setup and patient positioning are also extremely important prior to starting the actual operation. The entire operating team of nurses, technicians, surgeons, and anesthesiologists must be familiar with the demands of the laparoscopic patient, with the operating room and equipment, as well as with the surgical procedure.

I. BASIC LAPAROSCOPIC EQUIPMENT

The basic laparoscopic equipment includes four essential constituents: the insufflation system, imaging system, irrigation/aspiration unit, and electrocautery unit. Familiarity with the function and use of these systems by the operating team is essential. The presence and functionality of all necessary equipment must be assessed before the patient arrives in the operating room.

A. Insufflation System

The insufflation system allows the surgeon to create a working space in the abdomen in which to see and operate. Pneumoperitoneum is then maintained throughout the procedure, and it should easily be controlled directly by the surgeon as well as the circulating nurse. In most hospitals, a laparoscopy cart is used to house the insufflator system directly below the video monitor. The insufflation system should be continuously in direct view so the surgeon can monitor its minute-to-minute function.

The major components of an insufflation system are the insufflant, the insufflator, and the insufflation needle or trocar. For laparoscopic procedures, the insufflant medium is a gas. Various gases have been evaluated for laparoscopic surgery, including air, oxygen, carbon dioxide (CO_2), nitrous oxide, and inert gases such as xenon, argon, and krypton. Air and inert gases are insoluble in blood and therefore carry a risk of air embolus. Oxygen is flammable and therefore is not used. The preferred agent in the majority of cases is CO_2, because it is not flammable and rapidly dissolves in blood, thus greatly reducing the risk of gas embolus.

The insufflator is a device that allows the flow of gas from the tank into the space being insufflated. Standard functions include adjustable rate of flow (in L/min), an intraperitoneal pressure gauge (in mmHg), display of total amount of gas administered (in L), and the tank pressure of the insufflant. A typical unit is shown in Figure 1. Most units offer variable flow rate settings (low, 1–5 L/min; medium, 6–10 L/min; and high, 11–15 L/min), whereas others have an adjustable range of flow in 0.5 L increments or less. Typically, during initiation of insufflation to obtain a Pneumoperitoneum, low flow rates are used. If initial insufflation pressures are not excessive and a Pneumoperitoneum is being properly attained, the flow rate is then increased. Pressure should be maintained between 10 and 15 mmHg during laparoscopic procedures. At high pressures (> 25 mmHg) the risk of gas absorption and embolism is greatly increased. Furthermore, there is increased risk of decreased venous return resulting from compression of the inferior vena cava, impaired ventilation secondary to pressure on the diaphragm, and the development of systemic acidosis.

B. Imaging System

The quality of the imaging system is extremely important as it functions as the "eyes" of the operating team. Components include the laparoscope, camera, monitor, and light

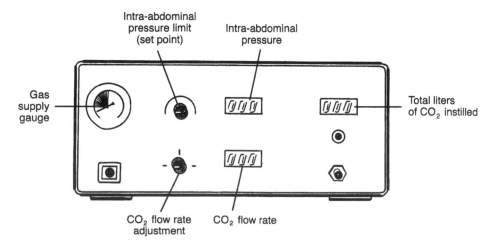

Figure 1 Insufflator unit. The display panel shows important information regarding intraperitoneal pressure and the rate of gas inflow. A gas supply gauge indicates the amount of gas reserve in the gas tank.

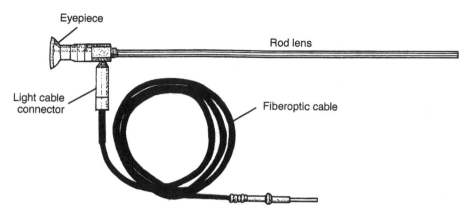

Eyepiece

Rod lens

Light cable connector

Fiberoptic cable

Figure 2 Laparoscope. The rod lens is most often 5 or 10 mm in diameter. An eyepiece for image transmission is the site of attachment of the camera. The flexible fiberoptic light cable is to connect the laparoscope to the light source.

source. The laparoscope allows light transmission into the peritoneal cavity to the surgical field and image transmission out of the peritoneal cavity to the camera. Most laparoscopes consist of a rigid rod-lens imaging system, an eyepiece, and a flexible fiberoptic light-conducting cable (Fig. 2). The most common sizes of laparoscopes used are the 5 and 10 mm scopes; the larger-diameter scopes are capable of transmitting greater amount of light, provide a wider field of vision, and offer better image resolution than do smaller-diameter scopes. Both 5 and 10 mm laparoscopes are available with either straight or angled lenses. The angled scopes enable the surgeon to look around and over tissues. The direction of tilt of the objective lens for an angled scope is usually opposite to the position of the light cable attachment on the circumference of the scope (Fig. 3). There are also multiple angled laparoscopes: 30-degree, 45-degree, and 50-degree scopes.

Direct vision laparoscopy has been replaced by modern camera/video systems. The camera magnifies the endoscopic view 15-fold, allowing high-resolution imaging of anatomical details. The camera attaches to the eyepiece of the laparoscope and transmits digitized optical information from the scope via cable to the video box; the digital image data are then reconstructed and displayed on the monitor. The camera should be focused, and the camera/video system should be white-balanced to optimize image color representation. Insertion of a room-temperature laparoscope into the peritoneum will result in fogging of the lens because of the temperature differential and condensation on the lens. This can be avoided by warming the time of the scope in hot saline solution before it is inserted. Commercially available antifog agents may also be useful to minimize lens fogging problems.

Poor image quality is more commonly the result of malfunction of an instrument or improper assembly of components rather than malfunction of the monitor itself. Frequent causes of poor image quality include inadequate light input from the light source, malfunction of the video or light cable, or incorrect attachment of these components to their respective units. Light sources consist of high-intensity bulbs filled with xenon, mercury, or halogen vapor to provide bright illumination. The output intensity is adjustable and can be controlled at the source. Too much illumination may result in image

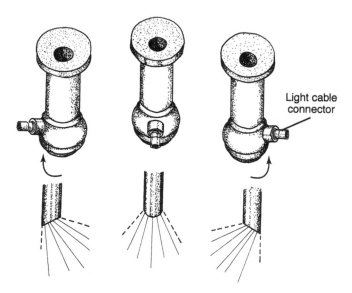

Light cable
connector

Figure 3 Angled laparoscope manipulation. A different viewing angle is obtained by rotating the angled scope using the light source coupler for orientation. The lens is angled for vision in a direction opposite the light cord coupler. Rotation of the scope results in a varying angle of view of the same surgical site.

washout. Some units are equipped with automatic light level adjustment to avoid this problem and optimize illumination. Light is transported from the light source to the laparoscope by a fiberoptic cable. Light cables are flexible and have both laparoscope- and light source–specific couplers. Connections should fit properly and tightly. Rough handling of the light cable may fracture the delicate optical fibers, thus decreasing overall light transmission. The light cord should be checked before the procedure by plugging it into the light source; any dark areas visible in the end of the light cord indicate broken fibers.

C. Irrigation/Aspiration System

In any laparoscopic procedure, a surgeon will benefit by using an irrigation and aspiration device to keep the operating site clean. In most operating rooms, wall suction units with adjustable degrees of suction pressure are used for aspiration. Irrigation units vary, but most hospitals use 1–3 L crystalloid bags, similar to those used for intravenous fluid. The irrigation fluid can flow by gravity, but use of a pressurized bag provides more active flow and is preferred. The most commonly used irrigants are saline solution with 5000 units of heparin added per liter or lactated Ringer's solution. Activation of the suction instrument close to fatty of other mobile tissues may lead to occlusion of the channel. When this occurs the irrigation switch can be briefly depressed to the clear the channel. If the aspirator valve is opened when the instrument tip is not immersed in fluid, the Pneumoperitoneum can be lost quickly. However, this maneuver is sometime deliberately performed to evacuate entrapped electrocautery smoke in the peritoneal cavity when it obscures vision.

D. Electrocautery

Tissue cutting and coagulation is best achieved with an electrocautery unit, which is usually controlled by a foot pedal when used laparoscopically. The most commonly used tip configurations are spatula, J hook, and right-angle (L) hook. Other electrocautery attachable instruments include scissors, dissectors, and graspers, all of which are insulated with a thin nonconductive coating and have an incorporated terminal for the electrosurgical cord so that electrical current can be passed through the instrument and delivered at its tip. The combination of suction/irrigation and electrocautery functions in the same instrument is also commonly used. The cautery instrument should not be activated until the tip is in contact with the tissue. The entire uninsulated tip of the electrode should always be visible during use, because inadvertent injury to surrounding structures can easily occur. Caution should be exercised when using the electrode near metal clips or other uninsulated metal instruments because of the risk of electrical coupling and passage of current through these objects.

II. ROOM SETUP

Different laparoscopic procedures will require slightly different room setups. In general, the surgeon stands on the side of the table opposite the pathological process, whereas the assistant stands on the ipsilateral side. It is common practice for the camera operator to stand close to the surgeon and view the operation on the same monitor. Typically the monitor is placed in a direct line with the surgeon and the surgical field; this has been called the *coaxial setup*. In this arrangement, visualization is maximal and instrument manipulation is easiest. The coaxial alignment can vary during the procedure as the operating site changes. Ideally, the surgeon should change position to keep in the proper line. If the deviation becomes large enough, an adjacent instrument may obstruct the view of the operating site. If this occurs, the surgeon should establish a different viewing axis by moving the laparoscope to a position at which the angle between the camera and the instrument port is wider. Occasionally this may require placement of an additional access port if satisfactory arrangement is not possible using the existing port locations.

When a monitor is used, the video is always opposite the surgeon. In this arrangement, hand-eye coordination is extremely difficult for the assistant, for whom the view is a mirror image. Although not ideal, mirror-image operating skills are readily attainable with advanced training and habituation. If the surgeon and assistant are on opposite sides of the table, typically two monitors are used, one opposite each person. This is the most commonly used monitor arrangement and is preferred by most surgeons for cholecystectomy and other advanced procedures. Both surgeon and assistant have comfortable views directly in front of them. For pelvic operations the video monitor is usually placed at or near the foot of the table. The setup for the more commonly performed procedures is shown in Figure 4.

Once the monitors are positioned, the remaining basic equipment systems are positioned around the operating table at the most convenient sites. A variety of arrangements may be used to suit the particular needs of the procedure. As a general rule,

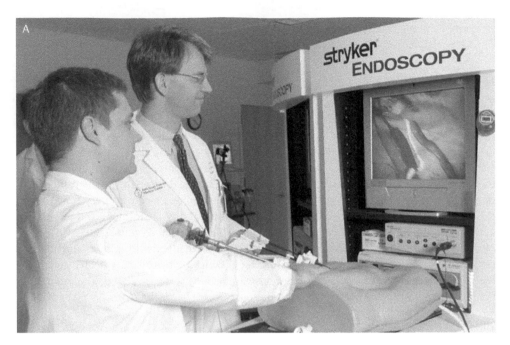

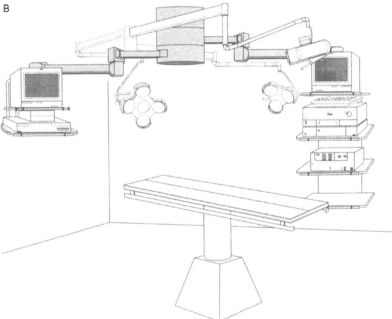

Figure 4   A. Harvard Center for Minimally Invasive Surgery videotrainers (Stryker, CA). Camera and monitors in a classroom setting facilitate for practice and improved task performance. B. Endosuite OR. Monitors and equipment float from booms hanging from the ceiling. Voice recognition controls key systems. Communication systems allow real time input from radiology, pathology or consultation from a surgeon's office. C. Teleproctor station in office at Beth Israel Deaconess Medical Center. Surgeon can consult from the office to the operating endosuite.

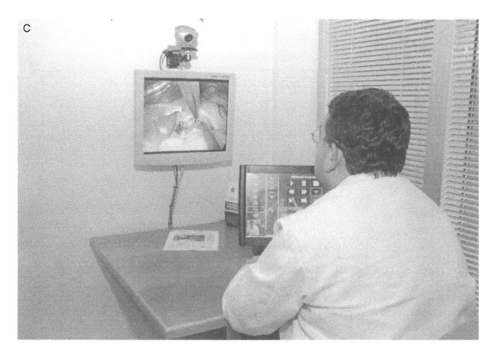

Figure 4 (*Continued*)

the particular piece of equipment and its associated lines coming onto or off of the operating table should be situated on the same side as the person who will be using that equipment. All lines and tubes should be carefully anchored to the surgical drape. In many institutions prefabricated drapes with pockets and/or gutters are used along which lines may be secured; instruments that are not in use can be securely stored in these pockets until needed.

III. PATIENT POSITIONING

Pneumatic sequential compression stockings are placed on the lower extremities before anesthetic is administered after the patient has been placed on the operating table. The patient is also tightly secured to the operating table with a restraint. After induction of anesthesia, an orogastric or nasogastric tube and urethral catheter are routinely placed to decompress the stomach and urinary bladder so that they are not inadvertently injured during trocar insertion or during the operation. The arms may be tucked at the patient's side, depending on the particular procedure being performed.

It is essential that the operating table is readily maneuverable. The patient should be positioned with the target organ elevated so that gravity pulls adjacent organs out of the way. The Trendelenburg position is used for procedures in the pelvis and lower abdomen. The reverse Trendelenburg position if used for procedures on the upper gastrointestinal tract and the biliary tree. The patient should be repositioned often to take advantage of gravity for optimal exposure. In addition, elevation of the operative field also helps to avoid pooling of blood in the surgical site.

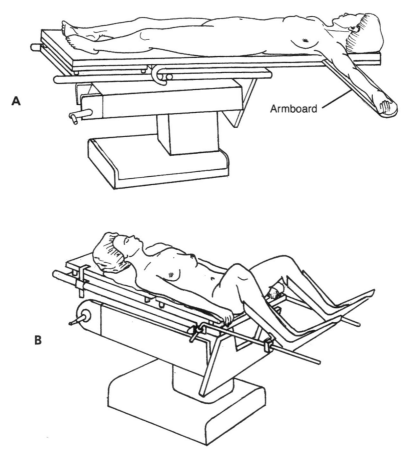

Figure 5 Patient positioning during laparoscopic surgery: (A) the supine position; (B and C) the modified lithotomy position; (D) the lateral decubitus position.

The three most common patient positions are supine, modified lithotomy, and right or left lateral decubitus (Fig. 5). The *supine* position (see Fig. 5A) is used for the majority of laparoscopic procedures, including cholecystectomy, appendectomy, gastric, small bowel, colonic, and vascular procedures. The *modified lithotomy* position (see Fig. 5B,C) is used for procedures in the pelvis. Allen stirrups are used to hold the legs in this position. Padding should be available and nerve injury in the lower extremities avoided by meticulous attention to positioning. The *lateral decubitus* position (see Fig. 5D) is most often used for splenectomy, adrenalectomy, and thoracoscopic procedures. A right or left lateral decubitus position may be used, depending on the side on which the procedure is to be performed. A large vacuum bean bag is very helpful for patient positioning in these cases. The dependent arm is outstretched on an arm board, while the upper arm is supported by a heavily padded Mayo stand or simply several large pillows.

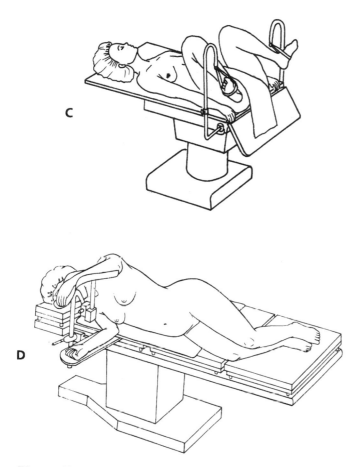

Figure 5 (*continued*)

Endosuites are state-of-the-art operating rooms dedicated to advanced laparoscopy. Monitors may be replaced by HDTV high resolution digital images. Equipment swivels on booms deployed from the ceiling. A workstation manages information. Camera and audio hook-up allow images to be telebroadcast to other locations for consultation or education.

4

Anesthetic Issues

STEPHANIE B. JONES

Beth Israel Deaconess Medical Center
Harvard Medical School
Boston, Massachusetts, U.S.A.

The anesthetic management of laparoscopic surgery has several important goals. The anesthetic technique must maximize patient safety in a patient population that is often much older and more debilitated than the younger gynecological patients in whom the original laparoscopic experience was developed. The complexity of laparoscopic procedures has increased, prolonging operative times, yet length of hospital stay has shortened. Therefore, the anesthesiologist must balance adequate intraoperative amnesia, analgesia, and muscle relaxation with the desire for rapid postoperative recovery and minimal side effects.

I. GENERAL CONSIDERATIONS

Patients scheduled for laparoscopic procedures often come to the hospital for the first time on the morning of surgery. Despite this, a thorough history and physical examination must be performed by the anesthesiologist. Laparoscopic surgery is often recommended for patients with multiple comorbidities, because these procedures have an improved recovery profile compared with that of the comparable open operation. Multiple studies have demonstrated decreased narcotic requirements, shorter hospital stays, and faster return to normal activities with laparoscopy. Laparoscopic cholecystectomy in particular has resulted in improved postoperative pulmonary function when compared with open cholecystectomy. However, laparoscopy can create intraoperative challenges for the anesthesiologist. For example, obstructive pulmonary disease can cause difficulty with elimination of the exogenous carbon dioxide load. Restrictive pulmonary abnormalities may result in prohibitively high peak inspiratory pressures after insufflation. Carbon dioxide is a sympathetic stimulant. When combined with the mechanical effects of the pneumoperitoneum, this may result in tachycardia, increased blood pressure, and increased systemic vascular resistance, which may not be particularly well tolerated in a patient with preexisting cardiovascular disease.

    The pneumoperitoneum is associated with an increased risk of aspiration, because both Trendelenburg positioning and increased intra-abdominal pressure predispose anesthetized patients to silent regurgitation. The risk of aspiration during general anesthesia can be minimized by tracheal intubation. Whenever possible, NPO precautions of at least 6 hours for solid food and 2 hours for clear liquids should be observed. Preoperative administration of an H_2-antagonist (cimetidine, famotidine, or ranitidine) and metoclopramide to increase gastric pH and stimulate gastric emptying, respectively, may be considered. These medications are given either intravenously about 1 hour before or orally 2 hours before induction of anesthesia for optimal benefit.

Preoperative testing should be ordered selectively. Results of tests performed within 6 months prior to surgery are usually adequate, unless there has been a change in the patient's health that might impact a given test. Many healthy patients require no preoperative testing whatsoever, with the possible exception of pregnancy testing in women of childbearing age. The need for other laboratory studies, an electrocardiogram, or chest radiograph depends primarily on the general medical condition of the patient, using the history and physical as the main screening tool:

Preoperative test	Indication
Hemoglobin	Surgical blood loss expected, suspected anemia
Electrolytes, BUN, Cr	Diabetes, liver disease, kidney disease, diuretic use
Liver function tests	Liver disease
PT, PTT	History of abnormal bleeding, liver disease
Pregnancy test	Female of childbearing age
Chest x-ray	Recent respiratory infection, unstable COPD, unstable cardiac disease
EKG	Male > 40 yr, Female > 50 yr, especially if other coronary risk factors present

Not only is nonspecific testing expensive and low-yield, it can result in patient morbidity when false-positive results are evaluated with more invasive testing. Blood typing and screening should be considered for all patients to prepare for the unlikely event of significant hemorrhage. For procedures with anticipated transfusion needs, such as splenectomy or partial nephrectomy, typing and cross-matching for 2 units of allogeneic blood is appropriate.

The possibility of hemorrhage dictates the need for at least one large (18 gauge or larger) intravenous line. In most patients a Foley catheter is placed intraoperatively to decompress the bladder before trocar insertion, although some surgeons will simply have the patient void immediately before a short laparoscopic procedure. An orogastric or nasogastric tube is routinely placed before abdominal insufflation to decompress the stomach. A laparotomy setup, thoracostomy tube tray, and central line kit should always be readily available to expedite the treatment of complications.

Laparoscopic surgery often requires frequent changes in patient position. The patient should be securely fastened to the operating room table and pressure points well padded to help prevent peripheral neuropathies. The lateral, flexed position used for laparoscopic nephrectomies and adrenalectomies can be particularly challenging in this regard. Obese male patients are at an increased risk of ulnar neuropathy, the most commonly cited postoperative neuropathy. The use of shoulder braces in the Trendelenburg position may predispose to brachial plexus neuropathy, especially when combined with abduction of the arms. Fortunately, most postoperative neuropathies resolve within weeks to months.

II. INTRAOPERATIVE MONITORING

Standard intraoperative monitors for any patient undergoing general anesthesia include continuous ECG, a noninvasive blood pressure monitor, a temperature monitor, a precordial or esophageal stethoscope, a pulse oximeter, and capnography equipment. When mechanical ventilation is used, monitoring of airway pressure and tidal volume is also mandatory.

Monitoring with pulse oximetry and capnography is particularly important during laparoscopic procedures because of the intraoperative cardiopulmonary derangements that may occur. Capnography measures exhaled CO_2. In patients with normal pulmonary physiology who are receiving adequate ventilation, end-tidal CO_2 (the exhaled CO_2 measured at the end of a tidal breath) is about 5 mmHg lower than the patient's arterial CO_2 tension ($PaCO_2$). This difference results from dilution of exhaled alveolar gas with dead space gas. In patients with pulmonary disease [e.g., chronic obstructive pulmonary disease (COPD)], this difference between the end-tidal CO_2 and $PaCO_2$ may widen significantly and unpredictably as the amount of dead space increases. When CO_2 is used to create a pneumoperitoneum, it is readily absorbed from the peritoneal space. This can be even more pronounced with preperitoneal or retroperitoneal insufflation. The subsequent rise in $PaCO_2$ (and resulting acidemia) may not be fully appreciated with end-tidal monitoring. Placement of an arterial line for blood gas monitoring should be strongly considered in patients with cardiopulmonary disease, especially when longer procedures (more than 3 hours) are performed.

Invasive monitoring with a central venous pressure (CVP) or pulmonary artery (PA) catheter may also be used for high-risk patients. It must be kept in mind that changes in patient position and abdominal insufflation may make the data obtained from these monitors less useful. Increases in intra-abdominal pressure may be transmitted to the intrathoracic compartment, artificially elevating central venous and pulmonary artery pressure measurements. Therefore, central filling pressures (CVP or pulmonary capillary wedge pressure) can be difficult to interpret under laparoscopic conditions. Transesophageal echocardiography has been shown to be a better measure of left ventricular function during laparoscopy in high-risk patients.

III. ANESTHETIC TECHNIQUES

Although local, regional, and general anesthesia have all been used successfully for laparoscopic surgery, the vast majority of procedures are performed under general anesthesia. Local anesthesia has been used primarily for diagnostic or short therapeutic procedures, such as liver biopsies. Each port site must be infiltrated with local anesthetic. Approximately 5 mL of 0.5% or 1% lidocaine or 0.5% bupivacaine is injected per site, with 1:200,000 epinephrine added to increase the anesthetic duration and decrease systemic absorption. The intra-abdominal structures may also be sprayed with local anesthetic before they are manipulated, keeping in mind the maximal recommended doses of local anesthetic (5 mg/kg for lidocaine, 2.5 mg/kg for bupivacaine).

The use of epidural or spinal anesthesia for laparoscopic surgery has been reported, most frequently for tubal ligation and inguinal hernia repair. A T4 level block is required for adequate peritoneal analgesia and abdominal relaxation, although a lower level can be acceptable for preperitoneal (TEP) hernia repairs. Even with the higher anesthetic level, shoulder pain secondary to subdiaphragmatic irritation by carbonic acid derived from the carbon dioxide may occur. One group reported insufflating with nitrous oxide in order to avoid the shoulder pain issue, but this also required that electrocautery not be used. Neuraxial anesthesia creates a sympathetic blockade that may cause significant hypotension, especially if combined with the reverse Trendelenburg position. Perceived dyspnea is frequently reported in patients undergoing regional anesthesia for laparoscopy, due to blockade of the accessory respiratory muscles. Despite these limitations, regional anesthesia is a viable option if the patient is cooperative, the surgeon skillful, and the procedure short with a minimal degree of manipulation. Local and regional techniques also have the advantage of decreased postoperative nausea and vomiting and the potential for a more rapid recovery.

General endotracheal anesthesia is the most widely used anesthetic technique for laparoscopic surgery. General anesthesia provides complete intraoperative analgesia and anesthesia, a quiet operating field, and optimal muscle relaxation. Relaxed abdominal musculature facilitates insufflation, allowing more working space to be obtained with less increase in intra-abdominal pressure.

Intubation of the trachea with a cuffed endotracheal tube is recommended during laparoscopy under general anesthesia. This reduces the risk of aspiration and allows control of ventilation to compensate for pulmonary alterations resulting from the pneumoperitoneum and positioning. A rapid-sequence induction should be performed in patients undergoing Nissen fundoplication for hiatal hernia, as well as for any patient with a potentially full stomach, to reduce the risk of aspiration. The laryngeal mask airway (LMA) has been used for shorter procedures but does not protect the patient from aspiration of gastric contents. The newer ProSeal™ LMA is designed for positive-pressure ventilation and allows passage of an orogastric tube, which has made some practitioners more amenable to using an LMA during laparoscopy.

No single general anesthetic technique is favored, but one that permits rapid emergence is preferable, since the surgical closures in laparoscopic surgery are of short duration. Total intravenous anesthesia (TIVA) with propofol and short-acting narcotics or use of the short-acting inhalational agents desflurane and sevoflurane improves short-term recovery. The use of nitrous oxide (N_2O) during laparoscopic procedures remains controversial. This agent is often integrated into the anesthetic technique because it reduces the need for longer-acting, more potent inhalational anesthetics. This has become less important with the availability of shorter-acting inhalational agents. Many surgeons believe that N_2O makes operating conditions more difficult by increasing the volume of bowel gas. This was not confirmed in a study that found that the surgeon could not determine when N_2O was used during laparoscopic cholecystectomy. It may, however, make a difference during longer procedures, since bowel gas expansion is a very slow process. N_2O may increase postoperative nausea and vomiting and could cause rapid expansion of a pneumothorax.

IV. POSTOPERATIVE PAIN AND NAUSEA

Laparoscopic procedures are associated with an increased incidence of postoperative nausea and vomiting (PONV). PONV certainly decreases patient satisfaction and can be catastrophic after Nissen fundoplication if retching causes wrap disruption or herniation. A variety of pharmacological agents are available for prophylaxis against and treatment of PONV. Ondansetron and other serotonin receptor antagonists are popular due to their efficacy, lack of sedation, and limited side-effect profile (primarily headache). They are relatively expensive compared to most other antiemetics. Metoclopramide tends to be less effective as an anti-emetic, but does stimulate gastric emptying. Droperidol, a butyrophenone, is nearly as effective as ondansetron, but can occasionally cause extreme dysphoria in awake patients. Administration of small doses (0.625 mg) given during surgery usually avoids this side effect while still providing effective PONV prophylaxis. Its use has more recently been complicated by an FDA black-box warning implicating mostly higher doses of droperidol in cases of torsades-de-pointe arrhythmia. Many now limit droperidol use to patients at very high risk of PONV (e.g., previous history of severe PONV). Dexamethasone has been studied more recently as an antiemetic. Although the mechanism is unclear, a single 5–10 mg dose is very effective, with minimal side effects in otherwise healthy patients. The long half-life also results in prolonged efficacy up to 24 hours postoperatively. This is particularly attractive for outpatients. Timing of administration can also impact the success of antiemetic prophylaxis. Dexamethasone should be dosed at or before anesthetic induction, while ondansetron is best given near the end of the procedure.

Postoperative pain after laparoscopy is less severe than after the analogous open procedure. Pain following laparoscopy arises from multiple sources: incisional, visceral, shoulder pain due to carbon dioxide insufflation, and procedure-specific sources such as bile peritonitis after laparoscopic cholecystectomy or tubal necrosis following tubal ligation. Successful pain management strategies use a variety of modalities to treat the different sources of pain. Injection of the incision sites with local anesthetic (0.25–0.5% bupivacaine plus 1:200,000 epinephrine) may help to minimize postoperative discomfort. There are conflicting reports as to whether intraperitoneally sprayed local anesthetic reduces postoperative pain. Opioids may be used to treat visceral pain, and nonsteroidal anti-inflammatory drugs (NSAIDs) such as ketorolac are useful for visceral pain and inflammation. Selective cyclo-oxygenase 2 (COX-2) inhibitors such as rofecoxib and celecoxib are becoming increasingly popular in the outpatient surgery arena. When compared to nonselective NSAIDs, COX-2 inhibitors are less likely to cause gastric erosion or platelet dysfunction. COX-2 inhibitors administered prior to surgery have been shown to decrease opioid use and postoperative pain scores. Opioid sparing also reduces the incidence of opioid-related side effects such as nausea and ileus.

The concept of preemptive analgesia, although controversial, is important. The theory behind preemptive analgesia is that the presence of analgesia prior to the surgical stimulus prevents "wind-up" or sensitization of nociceptors, reducing overall post-operative pain. Although the strongest evidence for preemptive analgesia exists in animal studies, several human studies do suggest the presence of such an effect. An argument can be made that negative study results might be due to incomplete pain coverage, as studies frequently evaluate only a single modality (e.g., local anesthetic injection at trocar sites).

V. COMPLICATIONS

The complication rates reported for large laparoscopy series range from 0.6 to 2.4%, with approximately one third of these being cardiopulmonary (see Table 1). The anesthesiologist must be particularly vigilant during the creation of the

Table 1 Intraoperative Complications Detected by the Anesthesiologist During Laparoscopic Surgery

Complication	Possible etiological factors
Dysrhythmias	Vagal reflex (peritoneal stretch)
	Inadequate depth of anesthesia
	Gas embolus
	Hypercarbia
	Hypoxemia
Hypertension	Inadequate depth of anesthesia
	Hypercarbia
	Hypoxemia
Hypotension	Excessive intraabdominal pressure
	Hypovolemia
	Patient position (reverse Trendelenburg)
	Gas embolus
	Hemorrhage
	Pneumothorax
	Pneumomediastinum
Hypoxemia	Excessive intraabdominal pressure
	Patient position (Trendelenburg)
	Hypoventilation
	Endobronchial intubation
	Pneumothorax
Hypercarbia	Carbon dioxide pneumoperitoneum
	Hypoventilation
	Pneumothorax
	Subcutaneous emphysema
Venous gas embolus	Insufflation of gas into blood vessel
Pneumothorax	Pulmonary barotrauma
	Extraperitoneal gas migration
Pneumomediastinum	Extraperitoneal gas migration
Subcutaneous emphysema	Extraperitoneal gas migration
Oliguria	Decreased renal vein flow, increased vasopressin release during pneumoperitoneum

pneumoperitoneum and the insertion of the trocars, because many complications occur at these times. Constant communication between the surgeon and anesthesiologist must be maintained to facilitate rapid diagnosis and management of complications as they occur.

Cardiac dysrhythmias are the most common cardiovascular alterations that occur during laparoscopy. Bradycardia is often associated with CO_2 insufflation and the stretching of the peritoneum. Manipulation of intra-abdominal structures may also produce a profound vagal reflex, especially in lightly anesthetized patients. The differential diagnosis of bradycardia during laparoscopy includes hypoxemia, deep anesthesia, and venous gas embolus. The initial treatment of this problem should be directed at eliminating the surgical stimulus and decompression of the pneumoperitoneum. If these maneuvers do not result in an immediate increase in heart rate, glycopyrrolate or atropine should be administered intravenously and cardiopulmonary resuscitation initiated if necessary. Supraventricular tachycardias and/or ventricular ectopy may result if hypercarbia occurs from systemic absorption of CO_2 or hypoventilation. Inadequate depth of anesthesia may also cause sympathetic stimulation and tachydysrhythmias. Most tachydysrhythmias can be prevented by maintaining normocarbia and adequate anesthesia throughout the surgical period.

Hypertension during laparoscopy is frequently the result of the increase in systemic vascular resistance during intra-abdominal insufflation. Other potential causes of hypertension include inadequate depth of anesthesia and analgesia, hypercarbia, or hypoxemia. The initial management of hypertension should be directed toward ensuring adequate oxygenation and ventilation of the patient and increasing the depth of anesthesia.

Hypotension can occur during intra-abdominal insufflation if insufflation pressures exceed 15–20 mmHg and venous return to the heart is decreased. Anesthesia can potentiate hypotension by blunting compensatory autonomic reflexes. Positioning during laparoscopy, especially the reverse Trendelenburg (head-up) position commonly used during upper abdominal procedures, can produce hypotension in anesthetized patients. Hemorrhage and gas embolus must also be considered when hypotension occurs. Retroperitoneal bleeding may not be immediately apparent, as intraperitoneal blood is usually not present. Prophylactic measures for preventing hypotension include gradual intra-abdominal insufflation to pressures of 15 mmHg or less, avoidance of anesthetic overdose, adequate hydration to maintain normal circulating blood volume, and the avoidance of severe head-up positioning. If clinically significant hypotension occurs, treatment should include immediate release of the pneumoperitoneum, decrease in anesthetic depth, administration of intravenous fluid, Trendelenburg positioning, and vasopressor therapy if necessary.

The cause of hypoxemia during laparoscopy may be multifactorial. Ventilation perfusion mismatching may occur if the combination of increased intra-abdominal pressure and positioning (especially the Trendelenburg position) causes pulmonary atelectasis. The Trendelenburg position may displace the lungs and trachea in a cephalad direction while the endotracheal tube remains stationary, thereby creating the potential for an endobronchial intubation. The development of hypoxemia may be rapidly diagnosed by monitoring the patient's oxygen saturation with pulse oximetry. Maneuvers to correct hypoxemia include increasing inspired oxygen concentration, releasing the pneumoperitoneum, and changing the patient from the Trendelenburg to the supine position. The chest should also be auscultated to verify the position of the endotracheal tube and to rule out a pneumothorax.

Hypercarbia represents an imbalance between CO_2 absorption, production, and elimination. During laparoscopy, hypercarbia often results either from systemic absorption of insufflated CO_2 or hypoventilation. Clinical studies suggest that CO_2 absorption is greater during laparoscopic procedures performed through an extraperitoneal route than those performed by an intraperitoneal route. Longer operative times, more port sites, and the Nissen fundoplication procedure also tend to result in higher CO_2 levels. A rapid increase in end-tidal CO_2 may indicate the development of subcutaneous emphysema and/or pneumothorax. Monitoring of end-tidal CO_2 with capnometry allows the anesthesiologist to detect the development of hypercarbia, with some limitations (see Sec. II). Increasing the patient's minute ventilation is usually all that is needed to treat hypercarbia. If necessary, the pneumoperitoneum may be released to decrease absorption of insufflated CO_2.

Venous gas embolus (VGE) is a potential cause of cardiovascular collapse during laparoscopy. This event occurs if a sufficient volume of the insufflation gas is absorbed directly into the circulation, reaches the right side of the heart, and passes into the pulmonary outflow tract. The gas bubbles can impede circulation in the pulmonary artery or cause acute pulmonary vasospasm. VGE produces pulmonary hypertension, the development of acute right-sided heart failure, and a catastrophic drop in cardiac output. Sudden hypotension accompanied by a drop in end-tidal CO_2 alerts the anesthesiologist to a VGE. With CO_2 pneumoperitoneum, the end-tidal CO_2 may transiently increase prior to dropping. A mill-wheel heart murmur, cardiac dysrhythmias, and hypoxemia are common findings. A widened QRS complex and right-sided strain pattern are often seen on the ECG. The initial treatment of VGE consists of ventilating the patient's lungs with 100% oxygen, resuscitative efforts to improve cardiac output and restore circulation, immediately releasing the pneumoperitoneum, discontinuing the anesthetic, and placing the patient in a steep Trendelenburg, left lateral position. This change of position will place the pulmonary outflow tract inferior to the right ventricle and may displace the gas embolus from the pulmonary outflow tract. If a CVP catheter is in place, the anesthesiologist can attempt to aspirate the gas through the catheter. Because CO_2 is highly soluble, small VGE are rarely clinically significant. In fact, transesophageal echocardiography studies show that small emboli occur quite frequently. Inert gases such as helium and argon are alternatives to CO_2 that avoid the hemodynamic changes specific to CO_2 absorption. The insolubility of the inert gases, however, potentially increases the morbidity if a VGE were to occur. This is one reason why CO_2 has maintained its position as the gas of choice for pneumoperitoneum.

Pneumothorax, pneumomediastinum, and subcutaneous emphysema may occur secondary to pulmonary barotrauma or extraperitoneal migration of insufflated gas. Congential or surgically created defects in the diaphragm allow gas under pressure to dissect along tissue planes adjacent to vascular structures and into the mediastinum. Positive end-expiratory pressure (PEEP) may be used in an attempt to decrease the pressure gradient between the intraabdominal and intrathoracic compartments. The insufflation gas may also dissect into the subcutaneous tissues of the thorax, neck, and head, especially during procedures using extraperitoneal insufflation and upper abdominal procedures such as Nissen fundoplication. A diagnosis of pneumothorax is suspected if hypoxemia occurs or peak airway pressures increase during the procedure, often accompanied by increasing end-tidal CO_2 levels. Auscultation of the chest may reveal wheezing and a unilateral decrease in breath sounds, although this could simply be due to endobronchial intubation. Tracheal deviation may be evident. The diagnosis of pneumothorax can be confirmed with a chest radiograph. Pneumothoraces of less than 20% can usually be followed expectantly because a CO_2 pneumothorax resolves rapidly once insufflation is discontinued. A "tension" pneumothorax can occur if the intrapleural gas is under enough pressure to collapse the ipsilateral lung. This event is a potentially life-threatening complication, and a chest tube should be placed immediately. If subcutaneous emphysema occurs, no treatment other than patient reassurance is usually needed because the gas will resorb within hours of termination of insufflation. Patients who may not be able to easily excrete the excess CO_2 (e.g., severe COPD) may require postoperative ventilation. Subcutaneous emphysema may also indicate the presence of pneumothorax or pneumomediastinum.

Prolonged increased intra-abdominal pressure during laparoscopic surgery has been associated with oliguria and even anuria. This decrease in urine output is felt to be secondary to some combination of decreased renal vein flow, increased vasopressin levels, and direct renal parenchymal compression. The anesthesiologist must resist the temptation to administer fluid in an attempt to increase urine output and use other clinical signs of hypovolemia to guide fluid administration. In general, fluid administration at a rate of approximately 5 mL/kg/h will address maintenance and third space needs, and urine output should return to normal postoperatively. A notable exception to this is the laparoscopic roux-en-Y gastric bypass, which requires closer to 10 mL/kg/h (ideal body weight) of crystalloid. This may be due to the extensive bowel manipulation involved in the procedure, resulting in increased third spacing.

Gasless laparoscopy might avoid many of the complications specific to CO_2 pneumoperitoneum. To facilitate surgical exposure, an abdominal lift device is placed inside the peritoneal cavity. Potential drawbacks of this technique include the need for deeper anesthesia to accommodate the increased stimulation by the retraction device, possibly prolonging recovery. Also, some of the advantages of postoperative pain reduction associated with traditional laparoscopy may be lost if abdominal wall pain is increased following surgery with the use of a lift device. The surgical view tends to be inferior to pneumoperitoneum as well, and gasless laparoscopy consequently has not gained favor.

VI. THORACOSCOPY

Thoracoscopy is most often performed for diagnostic purposes, but also includes therapeutic procedures such as pleurodesis and pulmonary wedge resection. This procedure usually does not require CO_2 insufflation, since deflation of the operative lung along with the natural space created by the rib cage provides sufficient visualization. However, some surgeons feel that insufflation further enhances their operative conditions. Thoracoscopy necessitates one-lung ventilation, which can be accomplished by main stem intubation or the use of a bronchial blocker, double lumen tube, or Univent tube. Positioning of the tracheal tube is best confirmed with a fiberoptic bronchoscope. Arterial line placement may be indicated for continuous blood pressure monitoring and assessment of adequacy of oxygenation and ventilation. Dysrhythmias occur frequently, especially if CO_2 insufflation is used, because CO_2 is absorbed more rapidly from the pleural cavity. Mediastinal compression may cause hypotension.

VII. CONCLUSION

A major advantage of laparoscopy is the potential for less postoperative pain and faster recovery. To maximize these benefits and decrease patient risk, the anesthesiologist must understand the physiological changes associated with these procedures and potential complications. Communication between the surgeon and anesthesiologist is essential to maximize patient safety and provide an anesthetic that ensures intraoperative patient comfort and rapid postoperative recovery.

SELECTED READINGS

Alexander JI. Pain after laparoscopy. Br J Anaesth 70:369–378, 1997.
Michaloliakou C, Chung F, Sharma S. Preoperative multimodal analgesia facilitates recovery after ambulatory laparoscopic cholecystectomy. Anesth Analg 82:44–51, 1996.

Murdock CM, Wolff AJ, Van Geem T. Risk factors for hypercarbia, subcutaneous emphysema, pneumothorax, and pneumomediastinum during laparoscopy. Obstet Gynecol 95:704–708, 2000.

Narr BJ, Warner ME, Schroeder DR, Warner MA. Outcomes of patients with no laboratory assessment before anesthesia and a surgical procedure. Mayo Clin Proc 72:505–509, 1997.

Wahba RWM, Tessler MJ, Kleiman SJ. Acute ventilatory complications during laparoscopic upper abdominal surgery. Can J Anaesth 43:7–83, 1996.

Watcha MF. The cost-effective management of postoperative nausea and vomiting. Anesthesiology 92:931–933, 2000.

Wolf JS Jr, Stoller ML. The physiology of laparoscopy: Basic principles, complications and other considerations. J Urol 152:294–302, 1994.

5

Access and Port Placement

SHISHIR K. MAITHEL and DANIEL B. JONES

Beth Israel Deaconess Medical Center
Harvard Medical School
Boston, Massachusetts, U.S.A.

To create a working space in the abdomen, the surgeon distends the patient's peritoneal cavity by insufflating CO_2, a noncombustible, rapidly eliminated gas. The pneumoperitoneum is established through an open or closed technique, and operating ports or trocars are inserted through the abdominal wall to allow access to the abdomen for continuous insufflation and the placement of operating instruments. Correct port placement is vital in facilitating proper retraction and dissection during the operation.

I. TROCARS

The laparoscopic trocar is the means by which abdominal access is secured. All trocars have two common components: an inner obturator to facilitate entry into the abdominal cavity and an outer sheath through which the obturator and operating instruments pass. The sheath contains a valve or membrane through which instruments may be introduced without loss of the pneumoperitoneum. The sheath can also have a side port that can be used for insufflating CO_2 or venting when visibility is impaired by the smoke of electrocautery. A variety of trocar shapes and sizes are available. Trocars for therapeutic laparoscopic procedures vary from 2 to 30 mm in sheath diameter.

Trocars are either reusable or disposable. Reusable trocars are equipped with either a blunt or a pointed obturator for open and closed insertions, respectively, and a "trumpet" or flap type of valve assembly. Before a reusable trocar is inserted, its components should be checked to make certain they are functioning and properly assembled. The Hasson cannula, used in establishing pneumoperitoneum with the open technique, consists of three pieces: a cone-shaped sleeve, a metal sheath with a trumpet or flap valve, and a blunt-tipped obturator. The cone-shaped sleeve can move up or down on the sheath to properly position the sheath tip within the abdomen, and it is then affixed to the sheath with a set screw. The fascial stay sutures are wrapped around the suture wings of the cannula, thus securing the cone against the abdominal musculature. This maintains the trocar in place and preserves pneumoperitoneum during the operation (Fig. 1).

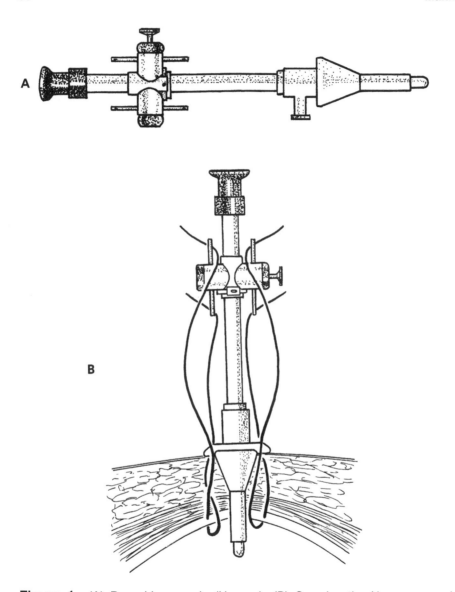

Figure 1 (A) Reusable cannula (Hasson). (B) Securing the Hasson cannula to the abdominal fascia. The fascial stay sutures are tightly wound around the suture wings on the outer sheath securing the sheath in place and sealing the fasciotomy and peritoneotomy.

Disposable trocars usually have a flap valve analogous to those on the reusable trocars and a pyramidal pointed or conical obturator (Fig. 2). A safety shield and a retention mechanism are two other features available on disposable trocars. The safety shield is a spring-loaded, blunt outer covering that retracts as the trocar meets the resistance of the abdominal wall and automatically slides over the sharp tip of the obturator when the trocar meets the resistance-free, gas-filled abdomen. Once released, the safety shield locks in the forward position, covering the tip of the obturator and decreasing the risk of inadvertent injury to underlying structures (Fig. 3). The retention feature on

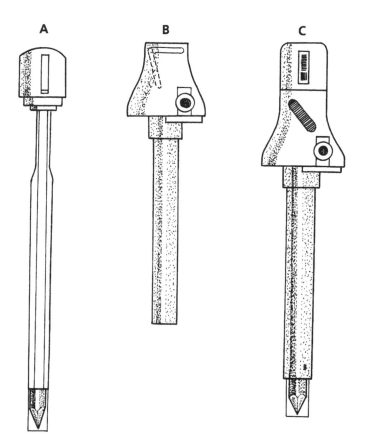

Figure 2 (A) Disposable obturator. (B) Disposable sheath. (C) Disposable trocar, assembled.

some of the disposable trocars consists of a threaded area that is either molded onto the sheath or a collar that attaches separately on the outside of the sheath. The threads are screwed down into the fasciotomy until the sheath or collar traverses the abdominal wall and is then locked onto the sheath assembly.

Disposable trocars come in two major varieties: bladed and bladeless dilating trocars. The bladed trocars are generally accompanied with the safety shield mechanism described above. The dilating trocar has the advantage of creating a smaller fascial defect upon entry into the peritoneal cavity, which contracts upon removal of the trocar. This is intended to reduce the incidence of port site hernias and still eliminate the step of fascial closure, which can be quite an arduous task in the patient with generous subcutaneous tissue.

II. CLOSED TECHNIQUE OF PNEUMOPERITONEUM CREATION

A disposable or reusable Veress needle can be used to deliver CO_2 to the peritoneal cavity using the closed technique. The disposable type is a one-piece plastic design (external diameter, 2 mm; 14-gauge; length, 70 or 120 mm), and the reusable type is made of metal

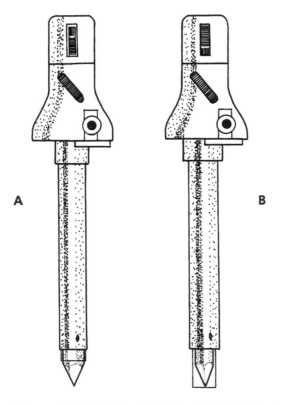

Figure 3   (A) Safety shield retracted. (B) Safety shield extended beyond point of obturator.

and may be disassembled. The needle is checked for patency by flushing saline solution from a syringe with the needle tip open and checked for leaks with the needle tip occluded under moderate injection pressure. If a disposable needle leaks, it should be discarded; if a reusable needle leaks, seals and screws must be appropriately tightened. The retractability of the inner hollow blunt tip of the Veress needle is checked against a hard flat surface. The blunt tip should retract easily as it contacts resistance and spring forward rapidly to extend beyond the sharp edge of the needle when pulled away from the point of resistance, analogous to the safety shield system.

The pneumoperitoneum is established by insufflating CO_2 through a percutaneously inserted Veress needle. In a previously unoperated abdomen, the Veress needle is inserted at the superior aspect (for upper abdominal procedures) or inferior aspect (for lower abdominal or pelvic procedures) of the umbilical ring; this site is next used as the camera port. The abdominal wall at the margin of the umbilicus is immobilized by grasping it between the thumb and forefinger of the nondominant hand or by upward traction on two towel clips. A small stab incision is made with the scalpel in the skin of the midline umbilical margin, and the Veress needle is gently inserted into the wound. The shaft (not the hub) is grasped like a dart, and the needle is inserted at a 45-degree caudal angle to the abdominal wall (or perpendicularly in an obese patient). The insertion should be directed away from the aortic bifurcation and the iliac arteries. Resistance followed by a "give" will be felt at two points. The blunt tip retracts when it encounters the linea alba. After the sharp edge of the needle traverses the fascia, the blunt tip springs forward into the properitoneal space, retracts a second time when it encounters the peritoneum, and springs forward after the needle passes through the peritoneum and enters the abdominal cavity (Fig. 4).

The water drop test is used to confirm the proper position of the Veress needle. A 10 mL syringe containing 5 mL of water is connected to the needle. The syringe is first aspirated to ascertain whether a blood vessel or viscus has been entered. Aspiration of blood, urine, or bowel contents requires removal of the needle, careful reinsertion into the abdomen, and close inspection of the retroperitoneum, bowel, and bladder with the video laparoscope after pneumoperitoneum is achieved. Next, 3–5 mL of normal saline solution is injected through the needle. If any resistance is met, the tip is probably located in the omentum or the abdominal musculature and requires repositioning. The syringe is aspirated again. The plunger of the syringe is removed, and the saline meniscus is observed in the syringe. If the needle is properly situated, the sterile saline solution should flow rapidly by gravity into the peritoneal cavity, and negative intra-abdominal pressure created by respiration or elevating the abdominal wall should enhance the flow of saline solution.

Once the surgeon thinks that the tip of the Veress needle is in the peritoneal cavity, the insufflation line is connected to the inflow port of the needle. CO_2 flow should be set at 1 L/min, and the indicator for total CO_2 is zeroed. The pressure in the abdomen during initial insufflation should always read less than 10 mmHg. If high pressures are noted, the Veress needle is rotated to assess whether the needle tip is resting on the abdominal wall, bowel, or omentum. If the pressure remains high, the Veress needle should be removed and reinserted. Multiple passes may be required to ensure that the needle tip is in proper intraperitoneal position. A sign of proper needle positioning is the loss of the dullness to percussion over the liver after insufflating a small volume of CO_2 An unoperated abdomen should expand symmetrically.

The patient's vital signs are monitored carefully during the initial phase to ensure that a vagal reaction does not occur. If the pulse falls, the CO_2 is allowed to escape, atropine is administered intravenously, and the pneumoperitoneum is reinstituted after the heart rate returns to normal. After 1 L of CO_2 is insufflated, the flow of CO_2 should be increased. (Note: The maximal flow through a 14-gauge Veress needle is 2.5 L/min.) Once the 15 mmHg pressure limit is reached, the flow of CO_2 will cease. At this point, approximately 3–6 L of CO_2 should have been instilled into the abdomen. The abdomen should be symmetrically distended and tympanitic to percussion.

After the pneumoperitoneum is established, the initial trocar is placed. In an unoperated abdomen, the initial trocar is usually inserted at the inferior or superior skinfold of the umbilicus, which corresponds to the point of Veress needle insertion. This location is chosen because the abdominal wall is thinnest at this level, and the postoperative scar is virtually indistinguishable from the umbilicus. Additionally, there are usually no significant blood vessels traversing this area. Relative contraindications to an umbilical entry include a previous midline periumbilical incision, portal hypertension, or a congenital umbilical anomaly.

The skin at the umbilical crease is incised adequately to accept the full circumference of the sheath. The subcutaneous tissue can be dissected with a Kelly clamp to expose the umbilical raphe of the linea alba. The surgeon holds the fully assembled 5 or 10 mm trocar (not the Hasson canula, which is used for open technique) in the dominant hand; the outer aspect of the obturator is secured against the thenar eminence and pushed

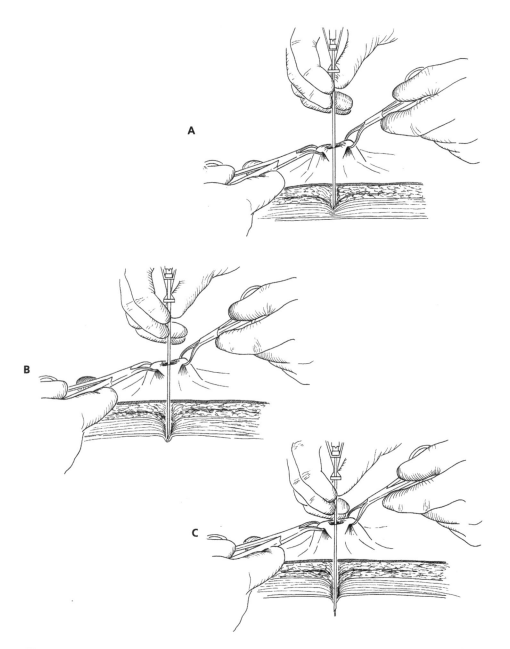

Figure 4   Insertion of the Veress needle through the layers of the abdominal wall. (A) Blunt tip retracts after encountering the fascia of the linea alba. (B) Blunt tip springs forward when it enters the properitoneal space and retracts a second time as it encounters the peritoneum. (C) Blunt tip springs forward on entry into the abdominal cavity.

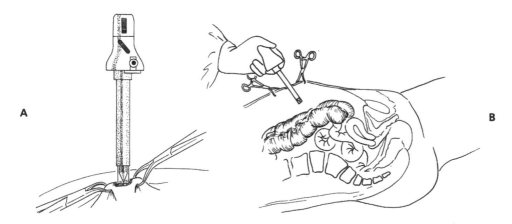

Figure 5 (A) Towel clips placed near the edges of the umbilical incision are used to stabilize the abdominal wall during trocar insertion. (B) Upward traction on the towel clips maintains the distance between the abdominal wall and underlying structures during trocar insertion.

into the sheath. The index or middle finger is extended down the shaft of the sheath and acts as a brake, preventing the trocar from sudden overadvancement into the abdomen. The sidearm of the trocar is in the open position. The nondominant hand elevates the anterior abdominal wall directly beneath the umbilicus. The angle of insertion initially is perpendicular (Fig. 5). A steady, downward, twisting force is applied to the trocar unit. Once the tip of the obturator is through the skin and subcutaneous fat, the trocar may be directed toward the proposed operating field.

The surgeon must not relax the grip on the trocar during insertion, otherwise the obturator will become disengaged from the sheath. Trocars with a safety shield have an indicator on the obturator that clearly shows when the safety shield is activated (locked over the obturator tip) or deactivated (capable of spontaneous retraction during the passage of the trocar into the abdomen). As the peritoneal cavity is entered, the surgeon will hear the escape of CO_2 through a hollow reusable obturator or a click as the safety shield moves forward and blocks the tip of a disposable obturator. As the obturator is withdrawn, the sound of CO_2 escaping through the side port is heard. Next, the side port is closed, the sheath is advanced 1 or 2 cm farther into the abdomen, and the obturator is fully withdrawn. Alternatively, a bladeless dilating trocar can be used as the initial trocar after pneumoperitoneum is achieved, thus minimizing the fascial defect.

III. OPEN TECHNIQUE OF PNEUMOPERITONEUM CREATION

The closed technique is popular because of its perceived speed and simplicity. The main disadvantage of the closed technique is the risk of injury to the bowel, major blood vessels, or bladder resulting from the blind insertion of the Veress needle and initial trocar. Open insertion of the initial trocar decreases this risk by placing the first port under direct vision using a "minilaparotomy." The open technique is especially applicable to patients with previous abdominal surgery, pregnancy, or evidence of bowel distention. Depending on the surgeon's preference, the open technique may be used routinely for umbilical trocar insertion, and in experienced hands it is equally fast or faster than the closed technique.

A vertical or semicircular incision of approximately 1.5 cm length is made in the inferior or superior umbilical skin fold. The subcutaneous tissues are separated by blunt dissection (usually with paired S-retractors) down to the linea alba. Once the fascia is visualized, Kocher clamps are placed on the two lateral edges and retracted anteriorly. A 1 cm vertical incision is made in the linea alba, and a Kelly clamp is used to dilate the fascial defect. Next, stay sutures are usually placed in the superior/inferior aspects of the fasciotomy. The sutures can be placed in such a way as to facilitate fascial closure at the end of the operation. The peritoneum can be entered in one of two ways: blunt or sharp dissection. When using blunt dissection, a Kelly clamp is gently inserted into the properitoneal space, directed toward the operative field and pushed through the peritoneum. Alternatively, the peritoneum can be grasped with two straight snaps and opened sharply with scissors. A finger is then inserted into the incision to confirm entry into the free peritoneal cavity and to sweep away any surrounding adhesions. The Hasson trocar is prepared for insertion by adjusting the set screw of the cone for the abdominal wall thickness. The trocar assembly is placed through the fasciotomy and peritoneotomy so that the cone tip abuts the fascia securely. The fascial stay sutures are secured to the suture wings of the trocar.

In a previously operated abdomen, an open or closed technique may be used. When using the closed technique, the Veress needle is placed in a quadrant of the abdomen farthest away from any previous abdominal scars or in the infraumbilical skinfold if there has been no previous midline abdominal incision. Away from the umbilicus, the properitoneal space is more easily insufflated than at the umbilicus, and the needle may need to be inserted deeper into the abdomen to enter the peritoneal cavity. The positions of the liver, spleen, and bladder relative to the site of insertion must be appreciated to avoid iatrogenic injury to these structures during port placement. The open technique can be used through a previous abdominal incision because it is performed under direct vision. The surgeon can also choose to enter at a different site, depending on preference. If doubt exists about the appropriate insertion site, an open technique of initial cannula insertion is the safest method for entering the abdomen. It should be noted that the peritoneum should be entered using sharp dissection. The rest of the maneuvers are as described above.

There is a third option of initial cannula insertion and pneumoperitoneum creation that is a hybrid of the open and closed technique. It utilizes a specially made bladeless dilating trocar into which the laparoscopic camera is inserted. Thus, after the skin incision is made, the trocar can be used to bluntly dissect through the subcutaneous tissue, through the fascia, and finally into the peritoneal cavity, all under direct video laparoscopic monitoring. After the trocar is in place, pneumoperitoneum is created. This technique is especially useful in bariatric surgery, as the morbidly obese patient has a generous amount of subcutaneous and properitoneal fat that makes the traditional open and closed techniques quite difficult.

Once access to the peritoneum is established, a CO_2 line from the insufflator is attached to the side port of the cannula and the flow rate is set at > 6 L/min. The abdomen should distend symmetrically and become progressively more tympanitic. The pressure during initial insufflation should always read <10 mmHg, and the insufflator flow will stop at the preset pressure limit.

IV. SECONDARY TROCAR PLACEMENT

For therapeutic laparoscopy, additional trocars act as conduits for the surgical instruments. The additional trocars are usually inserted under video laparoscopic monitoring. The location of these additional trocars depends on the procedure to be performed and the anatomy of the patient as viewed from the interior (video laparoscope) and exterior (habitus). The array of the primary and secondary trocars varies between operative procedures; these will be discussed in their respective chapters. Generally, the secondary trocars must be placed so that they are not too close to each other; instruments placed in proximity will have limited ranges of motion because the external handpieces will interfere with each other and the internal working tips will strike on one another ("crossing swords"). If the secondary sheaths are too near the initial laparoscopic sheath, the secondary sheath may ride over the primary sheath, inhibiting visibility and access to the surgical field.

Secondary trocars are used as operating trocars for the surgeon's right and left hands and for assisting instruments (retractors and graspers) that expose the operative field. Operating trocars should form a 30–60 degree angle with the axis line of the video laparoscope port and the operative site, forming an equilateral triangle or diamond array with the operative site as one of the apices. If the angle is too small, the operating instruments may eclipse the operative site. With a larger angle, depth perception is impaired and fine movements become awkward. The ideal angle between two operating ports is 60–120 degrees (the vertex of the angle is the operative site). The distance from the ports to the operative site should be about half of the total length of the instruments that will be used for the dissection, which gives the least distortion of movement at the tip from leverage at the fulcrum (the trocar). Since most laparoscopic instruments are 30–40 cm long, the operating trocars should be about 15 cm from the operative site. To assist in the alignment of the trocars, a marking pen may be used to map out anatomical landmarks and putative sites of secondary trocar introduction after the abdomen has been fully insufflated. During the procedure, the Veress needle can be used to simulate a trocar position before the incision is made.

Assisting instruments are used to retract and expose the operative field and are therefore moved less frequently than the operating instruments. Important considerations for placement of assisting trocars are the direction of retraction and avoiding instrument crossing (sword fighting). The assisting ports should be placed at an angle of 30 degrees or more from either the camera or operating ports. If this cannot be achieved, the assisting ports should be placed much closer to the operating site than the operating ports to create a more vertical angle of approach, decreasing the likelihood of clashing with more horizontally placed operating instruments. Alternatively, if the assisting instrument is to be used for cephalocaudal retraction, the port may be placed farther away from the operating site than the operating ports. Placing a port nearer to the operative site maximizes mediolateral retraction, and placing a port farther away from the operative site allows better cephalocaudal retraction.

In more complex procedures, the roles of the individual ports may switch from operating port, assisting port, and camera port; this should be taken into consideration when planning the original placements. Additional ports may be added during the procedure to facilitate the retraction and/or dissection.

To insert a secondary trocar, the abdominal wall should be indented with a finger to select the precise site of placement in relation to the operative field, other ports, and adjacent viscera. The skin is incised transversely for a distance just sufficient to accommodate the size of the trocar to be inserted. To avoid injury to any superficial abdominal vessels, the proposed trocar sites are transilluminated with the video laparoscope from inside the abdomen, and the incisions can be guided away from these visualized vessels. The trocar is held so that the middle finger of the dominant hand extends down the sheath of the trocar to act as a brake. The sidearm of the trocar is turned to the off position. All trocars should be introduced in a direct line with the planned surgical field so that after introduction, even with the sheath not being held, the sheath will naturally point toward the surgical site. This minimizes the pressure placed on the sheath during the procedure and maximizes the surgeon's deft touch and feel necessary for fine dissection and tissue palpation through the laparoscopic instruments. Under direct video laparoscopic monitoring, the secondary trocar is inserted through the abdominal wall with a slow, continuous, twisting motion with steady pressure. The tip of the obturator and its sheath are observed to enter the peritoneal cavity. If the tip of the trocar has pierced the peritoneum but is dangerously close to underlying viscera, several measures may be undertaken to avoid injury. Towel clips may be placed on either side of the trocar and used to elevate the skin to increase the distance between the abdominal wall and underlying viscera. The pneumoperitoneum may be *temporarily* increased to 25 mmHg. The obturator can be angled away from the underlying viscera so that it lies more parallel to the anterior abdominal wall. To prevent laparoscopic sheaths from slipping out of the abdominal wall during the procedure, an integral or detachable outer retention groove can be helpful. The threads are screwed into the peritoneal cavity to an appropriate point under laparoscopic vision, and with a detachable collar, the sheath is pulled back so that 2 cm of the sheath protrudes into the peritoneum and is secured. Alternatively, a suture can be used to affix the body of the sheath to the abdominal skin.

A continuous stream of blood from one of the sheaths usually indicates an injury to an abdominal wall blood vessel. To stem the flow of blood, the sheath is cantilevered into each of the four quadrants under direct laparoscopic vision, and a transabdominal suture is placed in the quadrant in which the blood flow was noted to cease. A straight (Keith) needle is inserted into the peritoneal cavity, pulled completely through the abdominal wall with a laparoscopic needle holder, transferred to a second needle holder, rotated so that the tip of the needle points anteriorly, passed anteriorly through the abdominal wall, and tied over a rolled cotton gauze buttress (Fig. 6).

V. EXITING THE ABDOMEN

After completing the laparoscopic procedure, a survey of the surgical field is performed for hemorrhage or visceral injuries. The operative site is irrigated and hemostasis is achieved until the absence of bleeding is certain. The peritoneal cavity is scanned from the pelvis to the upper abdominal quadrants to exclude any previously unrecognized injury to the abdominal viscera. Each of the primary and secondary port entry sites is carefully inspected to ensure hemostasis. In the event of continued port site bleeding, an Endoclose needle can be used to pass a suture through the existing skin incision transperitoneally and tied subcutaneously, thus obtaining hemostasis by closing the fascial defect and burying the knot. The valves of the sheaths are opened, and the pneumoperitoneum is evacuated with the aid of several vital capacity breaths of the ventilator. The entry site incisions are irrigated and inspected for hemostasis, as well as to exclude bowel herniation. The subcutaneous and muscular layers of the incisions are infiltrated with 0.25–0.5%

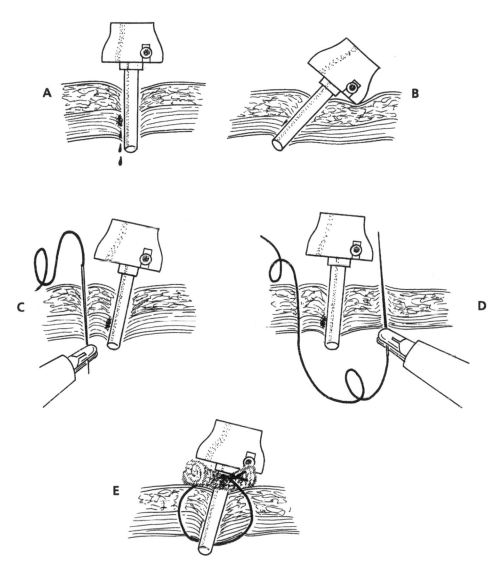

Figure 6 (A) Bleeding from a trocar site. (B) Cantilevering the sheath into each quadrant to find a position that causes the bleeding to stop. (C) Passage of a Keith needle into the abdomen at the inferior border of this quadrant. (D) The needle is reversed inside the abdomen and passed inside out through the abdominal wall at the superior border of this quadrant. (E) The suture is secured over a guaze bolster, thereby stopping the bleeding.

bupivacaine for postoperative pain control. The fascia may be closed by direct placement of sutures after removing the port or by using one of the many new devices that facilitate fascial closure under laparoscopic guidance before port removal for all ports > 5 mm in diameter, such as the Endoclose technique described above. It should be noted that using the bladeless dilating trocars eliminates the step of fascial closure. The skin is closed with subcuticular sutures and Steri-Strips. The 5 mm port sites are closed with a subcuticular horizontal mattress suture and Steri-Strips.

Illustrations in this chapter are from Jones DB, Wu JS, Soper NJ. Laparoscopic Surgery: Principles and Procedures. St. Louis. Quality Medical Publishing, Inc., 1997.

SELECTED READINGS

Patterson-Brown S, Garden J. Principles and Practice of Surgical Laparoscopy. Philadelphia: WB Saunders, 1994.

Soper NJ. Laparoscopic cholecystectomy. Curr Probl Surg 28:585, 1991.

Way, LW, Bhoyrul S, Mori T. Fundamentals of laparoscopic surgery. New York: Churchill Livingstone, 1995.

6

Hand-Assisted Approach

MICHAEL D. WILLIAMS and JOHN F. SWEENEY

Baylor College of Medicine
Houston, Texas, U.S.A.

I. INTRODUCTION

Laparoscopic surgery has afforded significant benefits over conventional open surgery and thus has been incorporated into the surgeons' armamentarium. Laparoscopic techniques progressed from being utilized by a few surgical pioneers to ultimately being established as the gold standard for certain common procedures. Hand-assisted laparoscopic surgery (HALS) has acquired a role in the evolution of laparoscopy. The limitations of laparoscopic surgery such as loss of direct tactile sensation, diminished depth perception, and retrieval of organs are compensated by the insertion of a hand into the laparoscopic field. Leahy et al. first reported the concept of HALS in 1994 [1]. Initially the gloved hand was inserted into the abdomen via a small incision and pneumoperitoneum maintained by apposition of the wound edges [2]. In 1996 Bannenberg and associates reported a hand-assisted laparoscopic nephrectomy in a porcine model using a prototype device [3].

II. DEVICES

There are presently five commercial devices available for the facilitation of HALS. The single piece devices include the Lapdisc (Hakko Medical, Tokyo, Japan) and the Omniport device (Advanced Surgical Concepts Ltd., Dublin, Ireland.) The multipiece devices include the Dexterity device (Dexterity Inc., Roswell, GA) and the Intromit device (Medtech Ltd., Dublin, Ireland), which are both connected to the abdomen by an adhesive flange. An additional multipiece device based on the kissing balloon principle is known as the Handport device (Smith-Nephew PLC, London, England).

A. Ergonomics

Despite the differences in the commercially available devices, several common concepts for performing HALS exist. The ideal location for the hand port is chosen after establishing pneumoperitoneum and laparoscopic visualization of the target organ. An incision on the insufflated abdomen approximately equal (in cm) to the size of the surgeon's glove size is performed. The device is then attached to the abdomen and the nondominant gloved hand inserted into the device. If one chooses to place the gloved hand directly into the abdomen without a device, sutures may be placed in the subcutaneous tissue in order to establish a gas-tight seal [4].

B. Advantages

There are several advantages of having a hand in the laparoscopic field and an abdominal incision that accommodates a surgeon's hand. There are no commercially available laparoscopic instruments that offer the versatility of the human hand [4]. The hand can be used for blunt dissection, palpation of lesions or blood vessels, organ retraction, hemorrhage control, and knot tying [4,5]. Generally the nondominant hand is placed into the abdomen while the dominant hand is reserved for manipulation of the laparoscopic instruments (Fig. 1). Many advanced laparoscopic procedures require a minilaparotomy for specimen retrieval. In HALS the minilaparotomy incision is utilized at the onset of the procedure as a working port and as a retrieval port upon completing the dissection.

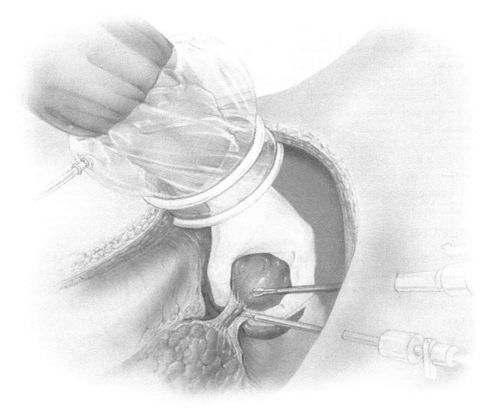

Figure 1   Renal dissection using the Omni device. [Courtesy of Weck (RTP, NC) and Advanced Surgical Concepts (Dublin, Ireland).]

C. Disadvantages

There are a few inherent disadvantages to the various hand-assisted devices. Device malfunction resulting in troublesome air leak may necessitate device replacement or conversion to open procedure [6]. Intra-abdominal hand fatigue and cramping has been reported in about 21% of cases [7]. The hand may limit dissection by obstructing the videoscopic view due to space constraints [8]. A fascial incision large enough to accommodate a surgeon's hand is subjected to the obvious risk of incisional hernia.

III. INDICATIONS

HALS may be indicated in several commonly encountered circumstances. Procedures where conditions generally yield difficult dissection but necessitate enlargement of the trocar site for specimen retrieval at the end of the procedure are ideal cases for hand assistance. Failure to progress with standard laparoscopic dissection is an indication for HALS when the versatility of the hand may obviate conversion to open [9]. Another proposed indication for HALS is the simultaneous resection of multiple organs [9].

IV. REPORTED PROCEDURES

There is a broad spectrum of laparoscopic procedures, which HALS has been reported to facilitate [10–15]. The obvious procedures are those that necessitate a minilaparotomy incision for organ retrieval. HALS techniques significantly reduced the warm ischemia time for living donor nephrectomy [13]. HALS has been reported to be safe and effective for benign and noncurative colorectal resection while maintaining the benefits of minimally invasive surgery [14]. HALS is advocated for super massive spleens while maintaining a minimally invasive approach [15]. Other reported procedures utilizing HALS include esophagectomy [10], aortobifemoral bypass grafting [11], gastric bypass for morbid obesity [12], liver resections [17], and pancreatic resections [18].

V. SUMMARY

HALS is an important adjunct in performing complex operative procedures while providing a compromise between open surgery and standard laparoscopy. Several surgical tasks can be performed with an age-tested tool—the human hand. To efficiently use the technique of hand-assisted laparoscopic surgery, the decision to incorporate hand assistance should be done initially as opposed to as a last resort maneuver.

REFERENCES

1. Leahy PF, Bannenberg JJ, Meijer DW. Laparoscopic colon surgery: a difficult operation made easy. Surg Endosc 1994; 8:992.
2. Boland JP, Kusminsky RE, Tiley EH. Laparoscopic mini-laparotomy with manipulation: the middle path. Min Invas Ther 1993; 2:63–67.
3. Bannenberg JJG, MeijerDW, Bannenberg JH, et al. Hand-assisted laparoscopic nephrectomy in the pig: initial report. Min Invas Ther Allied Technol 1996; 5:483–487.
4. Darzi A. Hand-assisted laparoscopic colorectal surgery. Surg Endosc 2000; 14:999–1004.
5. Cushieri A. Laparoscopic hand-assisted surgery for hepatic and pancreatic disease. Surg Endosc 2000; 14:991–996.

6. Southern Surgeons' Club Study Group. Handoscopic surgery: a prospective multicenter trial of a minimally invasive technique for complex abdominal surgery. Arch Surg 1999; 134:477–486.

7. Litwin DEM, Darzi A, Jakimowicz J, et al. for the HALS Study Group. Hand-assisted laparoscopic surgery (HALS) with the HandPort system: initial experience with 68 patients. Ann of Surg 2000; 231:715–723.

8. Gill I. Hand-assisted laparoscopy: con. Urology 2001; 58:313–317.

9. Troxel S, Das S. Hand-assisted laparoscopic approach to multiple organ removal. J Endourol 2001; 15:895–897.

10. Yoshida T, Inoue H, Iwai T. Hand-assisted laparoscopic surgery for the abdominal phase in endoscopic esophagectomy for esophageal cancer: an alteration on the site of minilaparotomy. Surg Laparosc Endosc Percutan Tech 2000; 6:396–400.

11. Kolvenbach R. Hand-assisted laparoscopic abdominal aortic aneurysm repair. Semin Laparosc Surg 2001; 2:168–177.

12. Sundbom M, Gustavsson S. Hand-assisted laparoscopic bariatric surgery. Semin Laparosc Surg 2001; 2:145–152.

13. Lindstrom P, Haggman M, Wadstrom J. Hand-assisted laparoscopic surgery (HALS) for live donor nephrectomy is more time and cost-effective than standard laparoscopic nephrectomy. Surg Endosc 2002; 3:422–425.

14. Hand-assisted laparoscopic surgery vs standard laparoscopic surgery for colorectal disease: a prospective randomized trial. HALS Study Group. Surg Endosc 2000; 14:896–901.

15. Targarona EM, Balague C, Cerdan G, Espert JJ, Lacy AM, Visa J, Trias M. Hand-assisted laparoscopic splenectomy (HALS) in cases of splenomegaly. Surg Endosc 2002; 3:426–430.

16. Romanelli JR, Kelly JJ, Liwin DE. Hand-assisted laparoscopic surgery in the United States: an overview. Semin Laparosc Surg 2001; 2:96–103.

17. Fong Y, Jarnagin W, Conlon KC, DeMatteo R, Dougherty E, Blumgart LH. Hand-assisted laparoscopic liver resection: lessons from an initial experience. Arch Surg 2000; 7:854–859.

18. Gagner M, Gentileschi P. Hand-assisted laparoscopic pancreatic resection. Semin Laparosc Surg 2001; 2:114–125.

7

Suturing and Knot Tying

SERGIO DIAZ

Barnes–Jewish Hospital
Washington University School of Medicine
St. Louis, Missouri, U.S.A.

NATHANIEL J. SOPER

Northwestern University
Chicago, Illinois, U.S.A.

DANIEL B. JONES

Beth Israel Deaconess Medical Center
Harvard Medical School
Boston, Massachusetts, U.S.A.

Surgeons performing laparoscopic procedures should know several methods for ligating vessels, reapproximating tissue surfaces, and reconstructing organs. Developing suturing skills is no less important simply because stapling devices and clip appliers are available in the operating room. Sometimes the surgeon may want to tie an extracorporeal knot and advance the knot within the abdominal cavity. After suturing on delicate tissue, most surgeons prefer to instrument-tie intracorporeally.

Throwing a square knot after an open incision requires a different set of skills than laparoscopic suturing and knot typing. The difficulty with tying knots arises from various factors. Laparoscopic instruments are long, restrict ease of movement, and diminish tactile feedback when compared to the open counterpart. Furthermore, most video systems currently under use cannot take advantage of the stereoscopic capabilities of human vision. Moreover, the 15-fold magnification requires a proportional adjustment in speed and enhanced efficiency in movement for completion of tasks in a reasonable period of time. However, technology is finding a solution, at least in part, to these difficulties. Robot-assisted laparoscopic surgery using computer-controlled instrument motion and three dimensional (3-D) vision video systems, instead of limiting the surgeon's skills, actually can improve them.

As to the process of learning laparoscopic suturing and knot tying, only a serious dedication to practice will develop the necessary dexterity; fortunately, today residents acquire laparoscopic skills from the beginning of their training along with other surgical skills, making it part of the integral process of becoming a surgeon.

I. PORT PLACEMENT

Port placement will either impede or simplify laparoscopic suturing. Ideally, the shaft of the needle holder should be placed parallel to the line of incision being reapproximated. The tip of the needle driver should easily reach the working area with only half ($\sim$ 15 cm) of the instrument's length within the abdominal cavity. The assisting grasping forceps should also comfortably reach the line of incision from the opposite side, and together the two instruments should form a 60–90 degree angle from the axis of the laparoscope (Fig. 1). At a minimum, three port sites are necessary. The most "natural" video projection occurs with the camera positioned between and behind the grasper and needle driver. This ideal positioning is sometimes impractical, and an acceptable alternative position is for the laparoscope to approach the operative field from one side of the two working instruments. The camera should never approach the operative field opposite the vector of the working instruments, because the video image will be reversed (mirror image), and it becomes virtually impossible to precisely manipulate the instruments. Also, ports inserted too close together (< 7 cm) will result in "sword fighting" of instruments and obscured camera visualization.

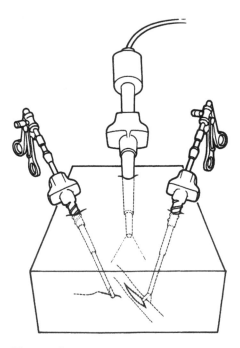

Figure 1   Correct arrangement of laparoscopic ports for suturing. Laparoscope is behind and between suturing instruments, which enter operative field from oblique angles. (From McDougall and Soper, 1994.)

The ideal trocar for laparoscopic suturing must allow the passage of large (10 or 12 mm) as well as small (5 mm) instruments through the same reducer, and it must be sturdy enough to tolerate multiple needle passes without loosening the gas seal. There are many disposable trocars available in the market with these characteristics. In a nondisposable trocar is used, usually the needle must be backloaded into a reducer before insertion into the abdominal cavity.

Suturing requires both hands. Securing working ports with screw threads, balloons, or suture will help prevent the port from becoming accidentally dislodged as the surgeon withdraws instruments from the abdominal cavity during suturing. A skilled first assistant an simplify laparoscopic suturing by presenting tissue to the tip of the needle at right angles whenever possible. Atraumatic instruments should be used to prevent inadvertent tissue injury. If the surgeon is struggling with a particular angle, an additional port may be inserted. Careful port placement at the beginning of the operation is especially important when a considerable amount of suturing is anticipated during a case.

II. MATERIALS

A. Suture

Selection of suture materials (catgut, silk or synthetics, monofilament or braided, permanent or absorbable) is no different from that for open surgery. Catgut suture may catch and get caught up in the port as the surgeon advances a throw. This problem is usually avoided by the use of synthetic sutures (2-0 or 3-0 polydioxanone), which slide easily during knot advancement. Although newer synthetic fibers have greater tensile strength, monofilament sutures may be difficult to manipulate due to the "memory" of the tail hindering effective knotting. Consequently, synthetics require more throws to prevent an individual knot from unraveling. Intracorporeal knotting uses only 8–15 cm of suture material, thereby minimizing the amount of suture dragged through tissues. During extracorporeal knot tying, longer suture lengths (60–90 cm) are required to reach the operative field and return out of the same port.

B. Needle Types

There are three basic types of needle curvatures: straight, ski tip, or curved (Fig. 2). Straight needles are easiest to position and hold within the jaws of the needle driver but are

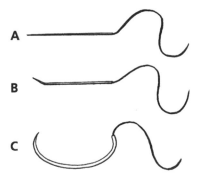

Figure 2 Types of needles: (A) straight; (B) ski tip; (C) curved.

difficult to drive in an arc through tissue. When using a straight needle, the assisting grasper must position adjacent tissue to include an appropriate purchase by the needle. Ski-tip needles (straight in the shaft, curved near the tip) load like straight needles, but with the added advantage of the curve near the tip, allowing it to arc through tissues with minimal damage. The curved needle is the most difficult to position properly within the jaws of the needle driver. The benefit of the curved needle is that the bite of tissue is the same as that the surgeon is accustomed to during open surgery. By supinating the wrist, the needle cleanly passes through tissues without tearing. Thanks to the progressive improvement of laparoscopic instruments, most needle drivers now have an excellent grasping strength comparable to that of those used in open surgery, making the laparoscopic handling of curved needles easier and their use widespread.

Suture and needle may be passed directly through the port or backloaded to ensure that the port's valve is not torn by the needle. To backload suture into a reducing sheath (Fig. 3), the suture should be grasped at least 5 mm behind the needle. Obviously, pop-off needles are avoided for laparoscopic procedures because they may detach prematurely. Large curved needles may not fit through a 10 mm port; if a large needle is necessary, either the port size can be enlarged or the part can be removed temporarily and the needle introduced directly through the skin incision.

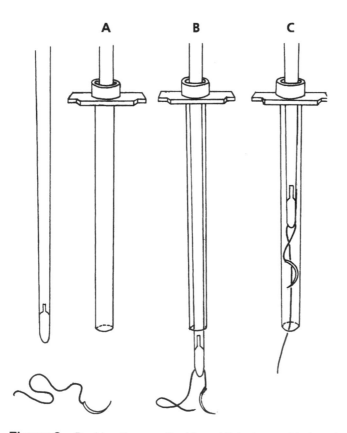

Figure 3   Backloading needle driver. (A) Instrument is inserted in reducer sheath; (B) the suture is held at least 5 mm behind the needle base; (C) the instrument and needle are withdrawn into the sheath.

C. Needle Holders

Surgeons develop their own preferences for needle holders. In general, needle holders should be capable of grasping the needle firmly, positioning the needle at a 90 degree angle, releasing the needle smoothly, and grasping suture without destroying the braid. Pistol grip needle holders allow for a more physiological resting wrist position but at the same time are awkward to manipulate and may cause digital cutaneous nerve injury; therefore, for the most part these have been placed by needle drivers with in-line shafts (coaxial), which rotate easily. The in-line position allows the surgeon to perform precise surgical maneuvers and operate unencumbered. Many surgeons prefer needle holders with two moveable serrated, diamond-shaped jaws that provide more grasping strength. Spring-operated needle holders are available with predetermined angles (45 degrees right, 45 degrees left, or 90 degrees), but fixed angles limit suturing flexibility and are not suited for intracorporeal knot tying.

A well-designed complementary assisting forceps facilitates intracorporeal suturing and knot tying. Assisting instruments with curved tips aid looping the suture and do not obscure vision of the operative field during intracorporeal knot tying. The smooth tapered end of the forceps prevents the loop from catching on the instrument's shaft. A pointed tip warrants caution, though, because it may puncture the liver or spleen, and sharp jaws may fray suture. Control of the instrument tips under constant camera visualization prevents iatrogenic injury.

The surgeon should be relaxed while operating. During laparoscopic suturing the arms will quickly tire if the elbows or shoulders are abducted and neck muscles tensed. Most surgeons will palm their instruments at waist level. For more delicate suturing control, the instruments may be held at shoulder level and manipulated with the fingertips. Operating table height and position is adjusted to keep the surgeon as comfortable as possible. For example, during procedures involving upper abdominal organs it is often convenient for the surgeon to stand or sit between the abducted legs of a patient in the lithotomy position.

III. NEEDLE LOADING

Correct positioning of the needle in the jaws of the needle holder is one of the most difficult actions to perform with monocular vision. When done properly, the surgeon's assisting grasper quickly introduces the needle and hands it off at a perfect 90 degree angle. More often, though, the surgeon should be prepared to adjust the angle after grasping it initially. If the surgeon does not take care and time to position the needle properly, the needle may slip in the jaws or tear tissue.

Several different methods work well for adjusting the needle within the needle holder's jaws. A straight needle that is held loosely at an oblique angle is easily positioned at 90 degrees by slowly withdrawing the needle driver until the needle abuts the edges of the reducer sheath. A curved needle's direction may be changed by gently tugging on the suture tail while the needle driver holds the needle loosely and allows it to swivel (Fig. 4). Grasping the suture too firmly may fray and weaken it. Rather than passing the needle to the needle holder, many surgeons rest the needle on the surface of the liver or stomach and pick up the needle at the intended angle without the need to coordinate the movements of both the needle holder and assisting grasper. One way to quickly locate the needle in space is by opening the needle driver jaws around the shaft of the assisting instrument that holds

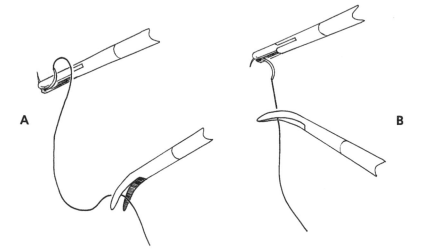

Figure 4   Reversing the needle direction. (A) The assisting grasper pulls the suture while the needle pivots within the needle holder jaws; (B) the needle is loaded in the opposite direction.

the suture. The jaws then slide down the shaft and suture to load the needle. The assisting grasper lightly taps the needle into final position.

IV. EXTRACORPOREAL KNOT TYING

Extracorporeal techniques can be used to ligate vessels, approximate tissue, reconstruct organs, and suture anastomoses. Extracorporeal knot tying refers to knots that are tied outside the abdominal cavity and then advanced into the operative field with a knot pusher. Preformed knots are readily available today, but with practice an extracorporeal knot can be quickly completed by the surgeon. A square knot or sliding loop knot is the most frequently thrown extracorporeal knot.

Several disadvantages of extracorporeal knot tying limit its application. For one, a significant amount of suture is drawn through tissue before being brought back out the port for knot tying. Lengthy suture may saw through tissue as the knot is formed and cinched. Second, an air leak occurs whenever introducing or withdrawing the suture through the reducer sheath. Any ongoing air leak is minimized by an assistant sealing the reducer orifice with a fingertip during extracorporeal knot tying. The sudden loss of pneumoperitoneum is offset somewhat by the use of newer high-flow insufflators that rapidly replace escaping gas. A third common problem is tearing tissues during advancement of the extracorporeal knot with the knot pusher. To avoid disruption, the knot pusher should be envisioned as an extension of the surgeon's finger. As in standard knot tying, the knot is pushed down to the tissue without pulling up on the suture. It may be helpful for the assistant to hold the suture with a forceps near the tissue during knot advancement and in this manner dampen suture tension.

A. Preformed Knots

The Endo Loop (Ethicon, Inc., New Brunswick, NJ) and Surgitie (U.S. Surgical Corp., Norwalk, CT) are performed sliding knots used to tie off a pedicle such as a blood vessel, cystic duct, or appendiceal base. Loop ligatures also close openings in cystic structures and prevent spillage (e.g., from a ruptured gallbladder). The preformed loop is introduced after backloading into a 3 mm reducer sleeve. A grasping forceps is passed through the loop and stabilizes the pedicle of tissue (see Fig. 5). The loop is slid off the grasping instrument and encircles the pedicle. The proximal plastic end of the push-bar apparatus is snapped, the suture pulled, and the loop is closed snugly around the pedicle. Finally, the suture is cut with scissors, leaving a 5 mm tail. The key to proper loop ligature placement is to place the tip of the knot-pusher exactly where the knot should finally rest.

The Pre-Tied Endo Knot (Ethicon, Inc.) is a preformed knot with an attached needle. After passing the suture through tissue, the needle and suture are withdrawn from the abdominal cavity out of the same port. A pretied knot is slipped off a disposable knot pusher and advanced intracorporeally with the knot pusher. The preformed knot is a modified Roeder-type knot, which is secure and reliable, particularly when one is using chromic catgut, which swells after hydration. As laparoscopy became widely used and more complex procedures were undertaken, the expertise of most laparoscopic surgeons made unnecessary the use of pretied knots.

B. The Roeder Knot

With practice a Roeder knot can be thrown quickly and more economically than commercially packaged pretied knots. The Roeder knot was originally used for tonsillectomies in children and now has been adapted for application in laparoscopic surgery. A needle that is attached to a long suture (60–90 cm) is used. After suturing the tissue, the two ends of the suture material are withdrawn from the abdomen through the

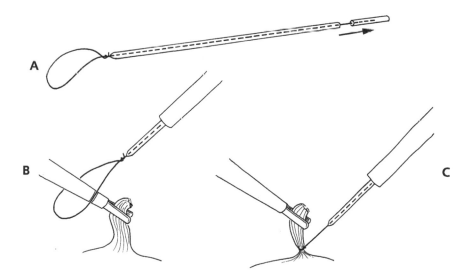

Figure 5 (A) Preformed loop ligature. (B) After lassoing the grasping instruments, the pedicle is isolated. (C) The loop is slid to proper position and tightened.

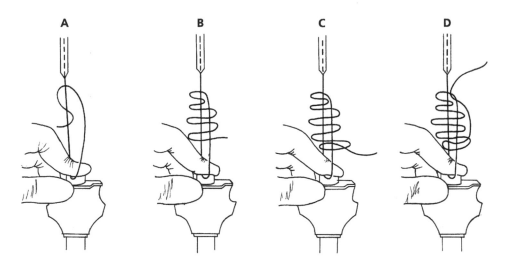

Figure 6 Roeder knot. (A) After suturing, both ends of the suture are withdrawn and separated by an assistant's finger; (B) a half-hitch is formed; (C) three wraps around both suture ends are made before inserting the long end through the last loop; (D) the long end may also be inserted through the initial loops.

same port. An assistant places a finger over the reducer to minimize air leak and separate the suture ends. A half-hitch is thrown and the know may be held in place with the surgeon's thumb and third finger (Fig. 6A). The free end is wrapped three times around both suture strands (Fig. 6B). The tail of the suture is then passed through the last loop (Fig. 6C). A variation of this knot next passes the tail through the loop formed by the initial half-hitch (Fig. 6D). This step is probably advantageous, with newer synthetic suture materials that have a tendency to loosen. Catgut and silk suture swell with hydration and form a strong knot without adding the extra step. Pulling gently on the tail will complete the knot. A 5 mm tail is cut and the knot is advanced with a knot pusher. Most surgeons find the Roeder knot trustworthy, but a metallic or a polydioxanone clip (Lapra-Ty, Ethicon, Inc.) can be applied on the knot edge for added safety.

C. The Square Knot

An extracorporeal square knot is the simplest yet most secure knot to tie through a laparoscope. After suturing the tissue, both ends of suture material are exteriorized through the same port. The square knot is created by separately advancing two half-hitches with a knot pusher (Fig. 7). Care is taken to throw the second half-hitch in the opposite direction to the first half-hitch to create a square knot. If both half-hitches are thrown in the same direction, a slip knot is formed rather than a square knot. To advance the square knot, both half-hitches can be converted first into a sliding slip blot configuration by lightly pulling above and below the knot on the same side (right or left side) (Fig. 8). With the slip knot, the throws are easily advanced with knot pusher to the desired tension. The locking square knot configuration is again formed by pulling the two limbs of suture in opposite directions. As with open surgery, additional half-hitches are formed and advanced to complete the knot. Rapid loss of pneumoperitoneum is frequently a problem during the

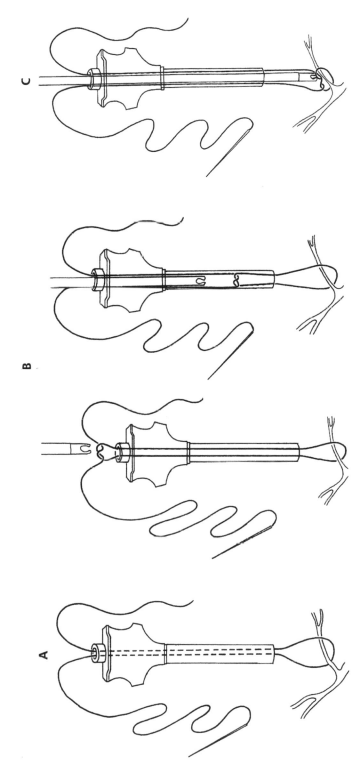

Figure 7 Extracorporeal square knot. (A) The needle end of the suture is withdrawn through the suture introducer; (B) an assistant's finger separates the suture end while the surgeon forms a half-hitch; (C) the first throw is advanced with a knot pusher. A second half-hitch in the same fashion forms a slip knot, while a second half-hitch thrown in the opposite direction creates a square knot.

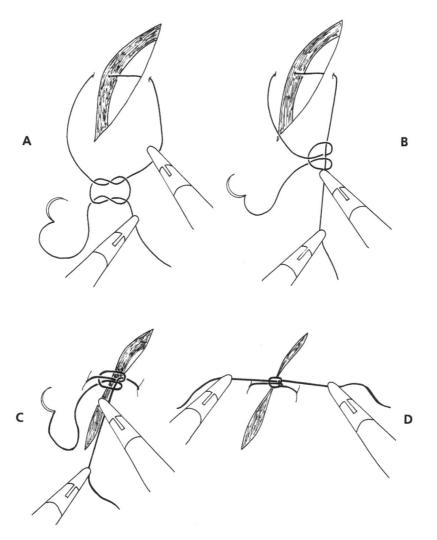

Figure 8 Converting a square knot to a slip knot intracorporeally after introducing an extracorporeally formed knot: (A) square knot; (B) slip knot; (C) advancement of the slip knot; (D) reconverting to a square knot.

period of extracorporeal knot tying. Methods to simplify and speed knot tying will help reduce air leak. For this reason, some surgeons place all individual half-hitches spaced 1 cm apart sequentially before pushing each down with a knot pusher.

The most significant drawback of extracorporeal square knotting is that a long length of suture must be dragged through tissue, and some tension on the tissue is inevitable; thus, this technique should be used with simple sutures placed in resilient tissue, such as the stomach during fundoplication. Many surgeons have found that improper suture selection will hinder knot trying. As previously mentioned, synthetic materials are particularly well suited for extracorporeal suturing, since the knots will slide down easily and cause minimal tissue tearing.

V. INTRACORPOREAL KNOT TYING

Intracorporeal suturing is favored for delicate structures or after completing a running suture line. There are many situations in which intracorporeal suturing is needed, for example, choledochotomy, reinforcement of stapled bowel anastomoses, and closure of gastric seromyotomies. Working within the abdomen avoids the seesaw effect and tugging on tissues that occur during extracorporeal knot tying while carrying long segments of suture material through tissue and out the same port. The major disadvantage to intracorporeal suturing is its degree of difficulty, especially in tight spaces. Under greater than 10-fold magnification, all movements are exaggerated and require the surgeon to be intentional and precise; otherwise, considerable operative time is lost. Although difficult to master, intracorporeal knot tying is an important skill in the laparoscopic surgeon's armamentarium.

A. The Square Knot

The square knot is achieved in a similar fashion to the "instrument tie" done during open surgery (Fig. 9). The suture length should be between 8 and 15 cm; shorter or longer suture will complicate looping suture around the instruments. Needle and suture are inserted through a multisize disposable trocar/reducer or backloaded through a reusable reducer sleeve. After incorporating a bite of tissue, the suture tail is best kept short and strategically placed next to the knot, where it can be readily grasped.

There are several ways to loop a suture around an instrument. To begin, two loops are fashioned around one instrument similar to a traditional twice-thrown surgeon's knot. Double winding for the first half-knot enables a certain amount of locking. Whether the suture is looped once or twice, the wrapped instrument holds the short end of the suture and carries it through the loop. Grasping the tail as near to the tip as possible will facilitate passing the suture through the loop. The second half-hitch is begun by looping the long end about the instrument, but in this instance the wrap is in the opposite direction to square the knot. As before, the instrument wrapped with suture grasps the short end of the suture and pulls it through the loop. Alternating the direction of further loops ensures that the knots will be squared.

When attempted laparoscopically, the loops are frequently difficult to throw because of the angle at which the instruments enter the abdomen. Holding the tip of the curved needle perpendicular to the needle driver's shaft will improve the angle and facilitate loop placements. Inserting additional trocars or placing the camera in a different port may also be helpful. Angled scopes and three-dimensional video laparoscopic technology may improve visualization and orientation. Remember, altering the suture length, using curved assisting grasper instruments, and effectively planning trocar placement is sometimes all that is necessary to make intracorporeal instrument tying manageable.

An alternative method to forming loops is the triple-twist knot. With the needle held at its tip, the needle holder is rotated 360 degrees four times as the suture wraps around the instrument's shaft. The needle is then dropped. Next, the needle holder grasps the tail of the suture and passes it through the loops. The throw is completed in the usual fashion by pulling the ends of the suture apart to form a surgeon's knot. Additional ties are thrown for greater knot security. Sometimes it is difficult to maneuver instruments within a given port angle. In this situation, the suture may be positioned to form a loop upon itself while lying on adjacent tissue (Fig. 10). A grasping instrument is then used to pick up the suture where

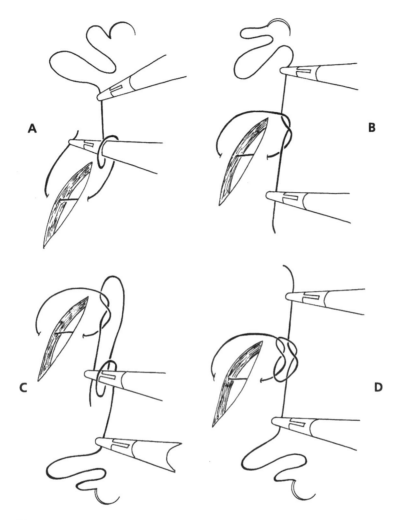

Figure 9 Intracorporeal instrument tie: (A) initial loop; (B) first half-hitch; (C) second loop in opposite direction; (D) square knot.

it crosses itself, or the loop may remain lying on the tissue surface. A second instrument is inserted through the loop and grasps the short tail of the suture to complete the throw. The second half-hitch is similarly formed, but in the opposite direction. This technique is particularly easy with the depth perception gained from three-dimensional laparoscopes.

Instruments have been developed specifically for the purpose of intracorporeal suturing and knot tying. The semi-automatic suturing device, the Endo Stitch (U.S. Surgical Corp., Norwalk, CT), allows suturing without the use of a second instrument for receiving the needle after it passes through the tissue. Since there is no need to manually position the needle in the instrument, its use is readily learned even by surgeons without large laparoscopic experience (Fig. 11). It has been used in urological, gynecological, and general laparoscopic procedures, and it is especially useful for areas of difficult access.

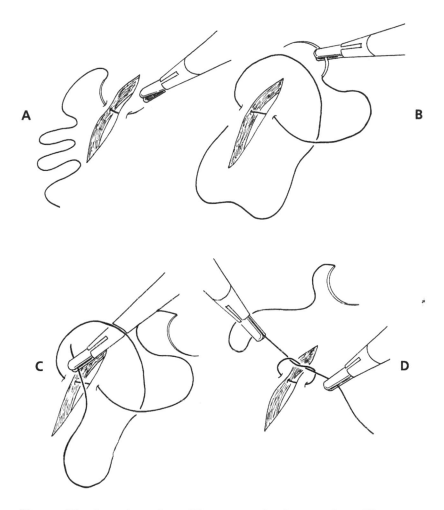

Figure 10 Jones insert knot: (A) suture on the tissue surface; (B) suture crossed; (C) an instrument is inserted through the loop and grasps the suture tail; (D) the first half-hitch is tightened. Subsequent half-hitches are formed in a similar fashion, alternating the direction of crisscrossing suture.

The disadvantage of the Endo Stitch is that it utilizes a short, straight needle, making it difficult to ascertain the depth of needle bite.

B. The Dundee Jamming Knot

An externally formed slip knot at the end of a suture can be used to initiate a running suture line without an intracorporeal knot. By crossing over and then under itself, a double loop is formed, resembling a figure of eight (Fig. 12). The suture is passed in and out through both loops. Leaving a 1.5 cm tail, the knot is introduced through a reducer to the operative field. After running the first stitch, the needle and suture are passed through the loop of the slip knot. The suture is pulled until the loop impinges on the tissue. The Dundee knot is

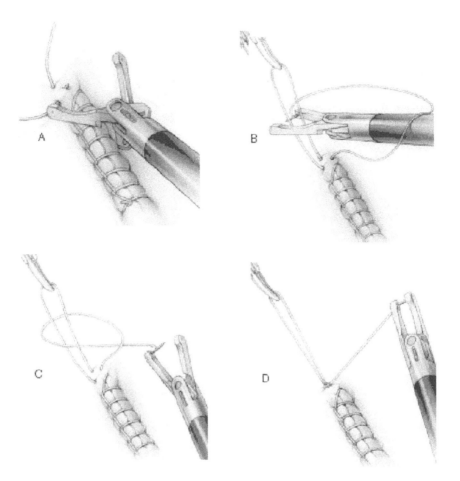

Figure 11   Knot tying with the Endo Stitch device (A) The suture line is finished, leaving a final loop; (B) the loop is placed between the open jaws and the needle is passed from the right to the left jaw; (C) the first half-hitch is completed; (D) tightening is done while keeping the instrument jaws closed. Subsequent half-hitches in alternating directions create a square knot.

tightened by pulling the tail in the opposite direction to the suture, thereby jamming the knot. The suture line can then be completed in the standard fashion.

C.   The Aberdeen Knot

The Aberdeen knot may be used to complete a running suture line (Fig. 13). An initial loop is brought beneath the previous throw. A second loop is passed through the initial loop and tightened. The tail of the suture is inserted through the second loop to clinch the knot. The assistant should keep tension on the suture and prevent gaps in the suture line. This may require rubber-shod atraumatic instruments to avoid damage to the suture.

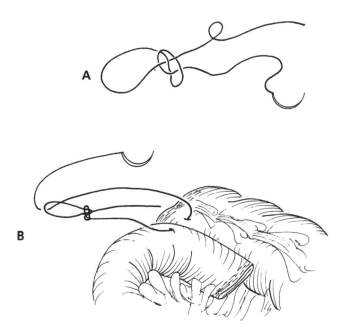

Figure 12 The Dundee jamming knot may be used to start a running suture line: (A) external component of knot; (B) adjusting the loop size by pulling on the tail; (C) the needle is passed through the loop.

VI. TOP TEN SURGICAL TIPS

Know your tissue; choose the appropriate needle, suture, and technique.
Anticipate suturing when deciding on port placement.
Needle holder and assisting grasper should form a 60–90 degree angle.
Suture length should be 8–12 cm (intracorporeal).
Suture length should be > 30 cm (exracorporeal).
Never grasp suture tightly, because it will fray and lose tensile strength.
"Square" knots—do not accept "air knots."
Angled lens laparoscopes are preferable.
Practice techniques in a pelvic trainer before going to the operating room.
Relax; body positioning should be comfortable, not awkward.

VII. CURRENT STATUS AND FUTURE INVESTIGATION

New devices for laparoscopic suturing are continuously being developed, but only a few of these are accepted and incorporated into surgical practice. Surgeons must realize that both extracorporeal and intracorporeal laparoscopic suturing is a necessary and essential skill to the practice of advanced laparoscopy. The changing world economics requires physicians to make effective use of available resources. For laparoscopic surgeons, this translates into being able to use the appropriate technique for each individual case.

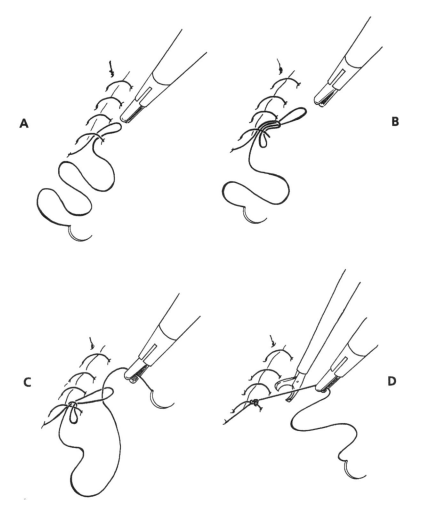

Figure 13 The Aberdeen knot is used to finish a running suture line: (A) initial loop; (B) second loop; (C) tightened loop; (D) completed knot.

The possibility of performing very fine sutures in areas of difficult access using minimally invasive techniques has now become a reality with the help of computer-assisted robotic devices. However, the use of this developing technology is limited by high costs at present time.

SELECTED READINGS

Fergany AF, Novick AC, Gill IS. Laparoscopic urinary diversion. World J Urol 18:345–348, 2000.
Gill F, Enzelsberger H. The Endo-Stitch needle. A disposable instrument for Burch's pelviscopic preperitioneal incontinence. Gynaecol Endosc 6 (suppl 1); 19, 1997.
Jones DB, Soper NJ. Suturing and knot-tying technique. In: MacFadyen BV, Ponsky JL, eds. Operative Laparoscopy and Thoracoscopy. Philadelphia: Lippincott-Raven Publishers, 1125–1143, 1996.

Laws HL. Credentialing residents for laparoscopic surgery: a matter of opinion. Curr Surg 48:684–686, 1991.

McDougall DM, Soper NJ. Laparoscopic suturing and knot-tying. In Soper NJ, Odem RR, Clayman RV, McDougall EM, eds. Essentials of Laparoscopy. St. Louis: Quality Medical Publishing, 148–183, 1994.

Murphy DL, Endoscopic suturing and knot tying: theory into practice. Ann Surg 234:607–612, 2001.

Rogers A, Barker G, Viggers J, Mason T, Swam J, Mayall P. A review of 165 cases of transvaginal sacrospinous colpopexy performed by the Endo Stitch(TM) technique. Aust NZ J Obstet Gynaecol 41:61–64, 2001.

8

Instruments for Ligating, Tissue Approximation, Gluing, and Coagulation

NAMIR KATKHOUDA and ANDREAS M. KAISER

University of Southern California
Los Angeles, California, U.S.A.

I. INTRODUCTION

Laparoscopic surgery has caused a major revolution in surgery. Contributors to this success story were the surgeons' pursuance, on the one hand, and the continued technical and instrumental advancements, on the other. The importance of laparoscopic equipment and instruments is evidenced by the constant drive to perform safer surgery. Inability to prevent and control intraoperative bleeding, to visualize the anatomy, or to approximate tissues (e.g., anastomosis) accounted for the majority of conversions in the early days of laparoscopy. Lacking the advantages of tactile sensation, the ability to perform bloodless surgery is essential to maintaining a good view and exposure to the site of dissection. A number of tools and techniques have evolved that will be outlined in this chapter. It is advisable to learn the features of and become familiar with each instrument or technique prior to using them during a procedure. Many devices are secured with a special handle or mechanism that should not be released before proper positioning of the instrument has been assured.

II. LIGATURES

Unlike in open surgery, where ligatures are the mainstay of surgical hemostasis, their use in laparoscopic surgery is more difficult and therefore limited, even though not impossible. Nonetheless, the endo-loop (Fig. 1) is still a very useful tool to ligate structures such as the appendix or an enlarged cystic duct or to temporarily close a gallbladder leak that occurs during the dissection. It requires some skills to introduce the premanufactured preknotted loop with its applicator, to grasp the structure to be ligated through the loop, and to tie it down at the desired tissue level by means of simple traction.

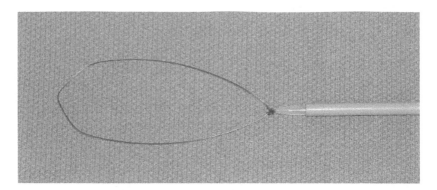

Figure 1 Laparoscopic endo-loop.

III. CLIPS

Clips of different sizes and materials (titanium, PDS, polymer) are used to secure and ligate vessels and to close luminal structures such as ducts, ureters, etc. They essentially serve the same purpose as suture ligatures, but the tissue is mechanically compressed and occluded by the clips branches. Ideally, the clip ends are approximated first, i.e., before the body of the clip is closed, in order to assure that the tissue does not slide away (Fig. 2). The length of the clip should be at least 1.8 times the diameter of the structure to be clipped. Various products have emerged that facilitate the application of clips, e.g., by pulling the tissue into the applicator before firing. Newer generations of polymer clips may even be locked (and reopened if necessary) to achieve a higher level of security during minimally invasive surgery. Even though most clip appliers still require at least a 10 mm port, 5 mm clip, applicators have recently come out.

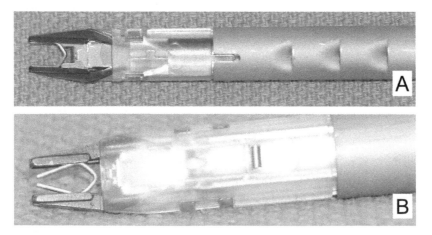

Figure 2 Laparoscopic clip applier: (A) clip in firing position; (B) the clip ends approximate before the body of the clip is closed, thus preventing the tissue from sliding away.

Clips are also being used in open surgery, although at a lesser degree and often by means of manual clip applicators, which need to be loaded from a clip rack. The reason that the use of clips has expanded in laparoscopic surgery is that they are applied with one hand only and much faster than suture ligatures. In addition, the development of instruments with 360° rotation knobs, articulating features, and multifire capabilities has facilitated (at higher cost) their application during laparoscopic procedures because these new devices obviate the distraction of taking out and bringing back the instrument for reloading every single clip. Instead, the preloaded clips individually advance after each clip application. Therefore, a series of clips can be applied consecutively without a change of instruments or exposure. For incidental need of a clip, the use of a manual clip applicator may still be sufficient, but care should be taken not to lose the clips on the way through the port into the peritoneal cavity and to the operative site.

IV. STAPLES

Staplers are instruments that deliver several rows of staples in a prearranged fashion. Depending on the purpose of the device, the staples are deployed either in linear geometry over a distance of 30–60 mm (linear staplers) or as concentric rings (circular staplers). Delivery of three rows of staples without cutting the tissue is used to close defects such as an enterotomy. Combined with a cutting knife in between two to three stapler rows, the staplers allow one to cut and close off the tissue on both cutting edges at the same time (Fig. 3). Spillage of luminal contents (blood, stool, etc.) can therefore be avoided. The staples come in different sizes and are preloaded into the stapling device itself and the reload cartridges (Fig. 3B). Different cartridge colors are used by the manufacturers to highlight different indications, e.g., white cartridge for vascular, blue cartridge for bowel.

The optimal staple size and depth vary according to the tissue that it is being used for. Vascular staplers have a tighter design and exert more hemostatic compression on the vascular structures in order to prevent bleeding. Staplers for hollow viscous organs (bowel, stomach, etc.), on the other hand, are designed to avoid ischemia at the cut edge and thus at the site of the anastomosis. The stapling procedure for both situations is the same. However, the impact of a potential stapling failure is much higher for high-flow vascular pedicles than for low-pressure bowels. In order to develop safe habits for vascular stapling, it therefore seems advisable to (1) keep the staple closed after firing for a few minutes to allow for intrinsic hemostasis to take effect and (2) maintain at the stapling site control on both vascular ends by means of instruments. This prevents the vessels from retracting and permits one to easily reapply another staple row or to use clips to control a bleeding, should it occur. The risk of creating arterio-venous fistulae after mass occlusion of vascular pedicles is anecdotal.

While linear stapling devices have been adapted for use in laparoscopic surgery, circular staplers (21–33 mm diameter) are essentially the same as those used during open surgery. Their standard application is the creation of a safe intestinal anastomosis in the pelvis after recto-sigmoid resection. The long and curved stapler body is inserted transanally, and the anvil is centrally deployed under direct vision, next to the staple line on the rectal stump. The stapler head, on the other hand, is inserted into the proximal bowel end after resection of the specimen; the bowel is subsequently returned into the peritoneal cavity, where the anvils of the stapler head and body are connected with an audible click either in hand-assisted or in purely laparoscopic technique after reestablishing the pneumoperitoneum. Firing the stapler results in an inverting

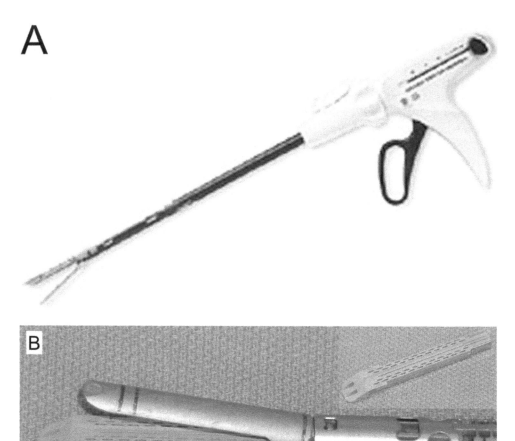

Figure 3 Stapling devices. (A) Linear stapler (United States Surgical-TYCO, Norwalk, CT). Sequential firing allows this device to staple and divide more tissue. (B) Stapling in two rows with simultaneous cutting in-between (inset: reload cartridge) (Ethicon, Cincinnati, OH).

anastomosis and should result in two intact tissue rings ("doughnuts") and an air-tight anastomosis.

V. ELECTROCAUTERY

Bipolar and monopolar electrocautery equipment is universally available in all operating rooms. Most of the reusable and one-way laparoscopic instruments may be connected to the cautery, allowing one to apply the electric current to the tissue during the dissection. In contrast to the harmonic scalpel, which will be discussed in the next section, electrosurgery (and lasers) coagulates the tissue by burning at relatively high temperatures (150–400°C). Blood and tissues are desiccated and charred, forming an eschar that covers and seals the bleeding area. Disadvantages of electrocautery, apart from generating smoke, are largely related to collateral damage when other than the target tissues are affected by side currents, damaged insulation, or excessive heat development.

VI. ULTRASONIC SHEARS

The development of ultrasonic technology for cutting and coagulation has proved to be of enormous value for laparoscopic surgery. Its routine use since 1996 has profoundly changed laparoscopic surgery for solid organ surgery and laparoscopic Nissen fundoplication. Before that time, all vessels had to be tediously clipped, resulting in increased operative time and unsatisfactory operations because surgeons were cutting corners, especially during Nissen fundoplication, resulting in tight wraps and increased intraoperative bleeding.

All this changed with the introduction of harmonic shears, which have become the standard of care in advanced laparoscopic surgery. Use of the harmonic shears (5 or 10 mm, Ethicon Endosurgery, Cincinnati, OH) with its grasping ability (Fig. 4) allows one to perform a virtually bloodless and smoke-free surgical dissection during laparoscopy and to proceed with greater precision and improved visibility near important structures in the surgical field. A generator, which provides the mechanical energy to blades oscillating at 55,000 cycles/s, activates this instrument. Hemostasis is achieved when it generates

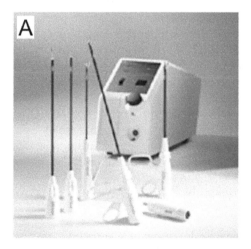

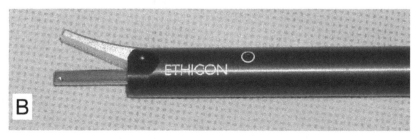

Figure 4 Harmonic shears come in 5 mm or 10 mm. A. 5 mm autosonic coagulator (United States Surgical – TYCO, Norwalk, CT). Pointed tip allows pinpoint enterotomy during stapled anastomosis. B. 10 mm (Ethicon, Cincinnati, OH).

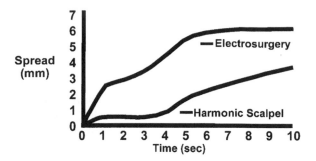

Figure 5   Compared with electrosurgery, ultrasonic shears limit the lateral thermal spread to < 2 mm.

localized heat in the range of 50–100°C, which seals blood vessels by inducing focal coagulation and denaturation of vascular proteins. Limitation of lateral thermal spread to less than 2 mm (Fig. 5) allows one to use the instrument next to the bowel, stomach, or spleen. Two different oscillating modes permit coagulation with cutting (higher frequency) or coagulation with less cutting effect (lower frequency). Rotation of the blade allows fast cutting (sharp edge), hemostatic cutting (blunt edge), or maximal coagulation (flat edge). The use of harmonic shears has reduced operative time and bleeding complications and has made it possible to reproducibly perform many complex operations even in a teaching environment. Several studies have demonstrated a dramatic reduction in operative time for laparoscopic Nissen fundoplication. More recently, the use of the harmonic shears was proven to be safe and effective in laparoscopic liver resection as it seals not only blood vessels but also bile ducts. Laparoscopic liver surgery will become more widely used with the assistance of the harmonic shears.

It should be noted that the harmonic shears may not be sufficient for transsection of major vascular stalks. Securing these major "named" vessels (> 5 mm), such as the splenic vessels, hepatic artery or vein, left gastric artery, or colic arteries, with clips or a vascular staple is advisable. The autosonic shears (Ossa, Norwalk, CT) offer the advantage of a pointed tip to add in precise application of energy to tissue.

VII.   LASERS

Several types of laser (CO_2, KrP, Nd:YAG) are available for use in laparoscopic surgery. These devices have been advertised as being more precise and safe for cutting. However, lasers have not proved to be of any benefit, particularly since poor tissue penetrance makes them ineffective for cauterizing bleeding vessels. Together with the exorbitant purchase and maintenance costs, their role during laparoscopic surgery has become increasingly marginalized.

VIII.   ARGON BEAM COAGULATOR

The argon beam coagulator is a device commonly used for hemostasis after surgery on solid organs. It was initially used primarily in open surgery, but it has recently been adapted for laparoscopic cases. The technique requires a flow of inert and inflammable argon gas to conduct radiofrequency current to the tissue. The motion of current through the gas beam ionizes the argon gas, giving it a blue color. It is the arcing of the current into the tissue that causes coagulation. Argon beam coagulation has several advantages over conventional electrocoagulation. The depth and lateral extent of the coagulation are relatively fixed. Because the argon gas is at room temperature, the thermal build-up is limited and the tissue is comparatively cooler. The temperature of the eschar does not rise above 125°C, whereas it can reach up to 270°C with conventional electrocoagulation. Finally, the gas flow generated by the argon beam clears blood away from the tissues, thereby allowing better coagulation. This property has been the cause of several accidents, including deaths from argon gas emboli. Following argon beam coagulation, five deaths were reported (two following open procedures and three after laparoscopic resection of liver tumors); one 18-month-old child sustained serious neurological sequelae. All these accidents occurred following the resection of the tumor and during the application of the argon beam. In all cases, aspiration of gas through the central venous catheter confirmed the diagnosis of gas embolism.

IX. FIBRIN GLUE

Fibrin sealant reproduces the last stages of the natural hemostasis cascade (Fig. 6), i.e., the conversion of fibrinogen into fibrin monomers and the cross-linking of these into an insoluble fibrin matrix. This hemostatic agent is widely used in Europe and Asia, e.g., on the raw surface of the liver after a resection in order to control oozing and bile leaks. Commercial fibrin sealant (Fig. 5), examined under the optical microscope, is indistinguishable from native fibrin, which stabilizes the platelet clot during wound healing. It appears as a three-dimensional mesh that entraps red cells, thus achieving hemostasis. Under the chemotactic influence of thrombin, fibroblastic growth will replace the fibrin mesh that acts as scaffolding. This usually occurs 10–12 days following the application. The benefits of the use of fibrin sealant in liver surgery have been well documented.

During laparoscopic surgery, the use of two-component fibrin glue (e.g., Tisseel VH fibrin sealant, Baxter Healthcare Corporation, Deerfield, IL) may have an even wider range of indications (Fig. 7). In the absence of a tactile sensation, covering a newly created intestinal anastomosis or a hernia mesh with fibrin sealant may secure the surgical site. Yet, it should be noted that the fibrin sealant fails and should therefore not be used to compensate for suboptimal anastomotic technique. Long applicators (Fig. 7), which can be

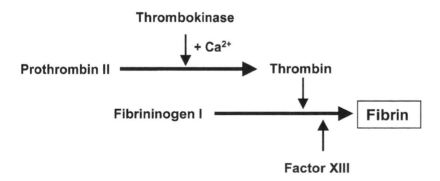

Figure 6 Coagulation cascade.

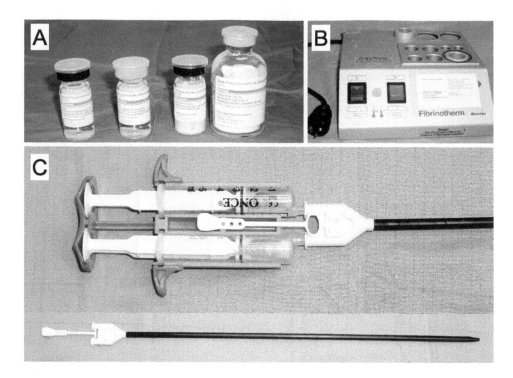

Figure 7 Two-component fibrin glue (Tisseel VH fibrin sealant, Baxter Healthcare Corporation, Deerfield, IL) in ready-to-mix vials (A), with heater/stirrer (B), and applicator with laparoscopic extension (C).

inserted through a 5 mm port, have facilitated the application of the sealant, but there is an increased loss within the tubing's deadspace.

X. CONCLUSION

Several new technologies have provided a wide spectrum of approaches to prevent surgical complications or to deal with them without conversion to open surgery. More inventions are simply a question of time, and it will be necessary for surgeons and hospitals to assess the benefits and costs of such developments.

SELECTED READINGS

Bhoyrul S, Mori T, Way LW. Principles of Instrumentation. In Way LW, Bhoyrul S, Mori T, eds. Fundamentals of Laparoscopic Surgery. New York: Churchill Livingstone, 1995, pp 100–120.

Goldstein DS, Chandhoke PS, Kavoussi LR, Odem RR. Laparoscopic equipment. In Soper NJ, Odem RR, Clayman RV, McDougall EM, eds. Essentials of Laparoscopy. St. Louis: Quality Medical Publishing, 1994, pp 104–147.

McDougall EM, Clayman RV, Soper NJ. Laparoscopic clips and staples. In Soper NJ, Odem RR, Clayman RV, McDougall EM, eds. Essentials of Laparoscopy. St. Louis: Quality Medical Publishing, 1994, pp 184–203.

Swanstrom LL, Pennings JL. Laparoscopic control of short gastric vessels. J. Am Coll Surg 181:347–351, 1995.

9

Ultrasonography

JONATHAN J. CANETE AND NICOLE M. CHANDLER

University of Massachusetts Medical School
Worcester, Massachusetts, U.S.A.

MARK P. CALLERY

Beth Israel Deaconess Medical Center
Harvard Medical School
Boston, Massachusetts, U.S.A.

I. INTRODUCTION

Laparoscopic ultrasonography (LUS) has evolved as an accurate diagnostic tool to substitute for the ability to perform manual palpation during minimal access surgery. Learning proper techniques and interpreting images can be challenging. However, as surgeons apply LUS to various clinical situations, their ability to perform a thorough intracorporeal ultrasound examination can quickly improve. To begin, a laparoscopist must first have an understanding of basic ultrasound principles and an appreciation for the technology available.

II. ULTRASOUND TECHNOLOGY

Ultrasound is a longitudinal wave that transmits mechanical energy through a medium at a frequency of 2–20 MHz. The frequency, which is the number of complete ultrasound waves emitted per second, remains unchanged as it traverses different media. However, the velocity of an ultrasound wave may be altered, depending on the medium through which it is traveling. Since velocity is directly related to wavelength, any change in wavelength causes a proportional change in the velocity. The wavelength for ultrasound in turn depends on its propagation medium: long wavelengths occur in solids and short wavelengths occur in gases. Therefore, the velocity of ultrasound through solids is faster than through gases.

Ultrasound waves are generated by a transducer, which converts one form of energy into another. For medical applications, ultrasonographic equipment consists of a transducer probe and a digital electronic scanner. The scanner supplies the electric current that stimulates a piezoelectric crystal in the transducer probe. This crystal then vibrates and changes shape to create a sound pulse. The frequency of the ultrasound wave that is produced is determined by the thickness of the piezoelectric crystal. Most laparoscopic ultrasound transducers typically generate frequencies between 6.5 and 10 MHz. Acoustic coupling of the probe to an anatomical structure may be enhanced by using a gel, liquid, or special solid acoustic interface. However, in laparoscopic ultrasonography, examination of structures is most often accomplished by direct contact of the transducer probe with actual tissues.

Once ultrasound waves are emitted from a transducer, they enter tissue to a depth of penetration in centimeters, estimated by dividing the frequency into 40 (e.g., a 5 MHz probe divided into 40 = 8 cm of tissue penetration). These waves are then either reflected, refracted, or absorbed by tissue or tissue interfaces. Reflected waves are those that get redirected back toward their source (i.e., the transducer). The percentage of the sound beam that is reflected depends on that beam's angle of incidence and a tissue's acoustic impedance, as approximated by the tissue's density. At a tissue interface, the magnitude of the difference in density between the adjacent tissues is directly proportional to the percentage of reflected ultrasound. In contrast, when an ultrasound beam is bent so that it travels in a direction different from its original path, the beam is refracted. Refraction occurs when the ultrasound waves traverse two different tissues with different densities, such as bone and fat. Absorption, on the other hand, results when the mechanical energy of the ultrasound wave is converted to heat. The amount of mechanical energy lost to absorption increases as the frequency of the ultrasound wave increases.

As ultrasound waves traverse a given medium and absorption occurs, these waves lose intensity. Intensity is the amount of energy flowing per unit of time through a unit cross-sectional area (W/cm^2). A loss of intensity in an ultrasound wave becomes important when trying to image structures deep within tissue. For example, an ultrasound wave generated with an incident intensity equal to 10 is transmitted through the liver. If this wave is reflected off a mass such as a tumor and returns to the transducer with an intensity of 0.001, then intensity of the ultrasound wave is lost.

The ultrasound image is formed only from reflected sound waves called echoes. These echoes are detected by the transducer by means of the mechanical energy applied to the crystal being converted to electrical energy. The magnitude of the electrical potential produced is proportional to the amplitude of the echo and is represented on a video monitor as shades of gray. Large reflectors within the body produce large-amplitude echoes called specular echoes. By contrast, small point reflectors send low-amplitude diffuse echoes back to the transducer, because much of the incident ultrasound pulse is lost to absorption and refraction. In the case mentioned previously, if a wave is reflected with low intensity (i.e., low energy), the piezoelectric crystal will then produce a small electric potential. This small electric potential then translates into a faint image on the gray scale.

The clarity of ultrasound images is described by two variables: lateral (horizontal) resolution and axial resolution. Lateral resolution is the ability to distinguish two structures that are perpendicular to the longitudinal axis of the sound beam and equidistant from the transducer. The beam width must be narrower than the space that separates the adjacent structures to recognize two distinct images. Crystal size, ultrasound frequency, and beam focusing determine lateral resolution. Conversely, axial resolution is the ability of the sound beam to distinguish two structures located along its longitudinal axis (i.e., structures that overlie one another). As the transducer frequency is increased, the axial resolution is improved, but this sharper image is obtained at the cost of decreased tissue penetration. Many ultrasound machines allow the operator to adjust the transducer frequency to 5.0, 6.5, or 7.5 MHz. The 5.0 MHz setting provides a penetration depth of

130 mm and an axial resolution of 0.6 mm. By contrast, the 7.5 MHz setting gives a penetration depth of only 90 mm, but the axial resolution is improved to 0.4 mm.

Several ultrasound transducers are available that produce real-time images, which are possible only if a minimum of 30 frames (images) per second are created. Linear array, convex, and sector transducer probes are most commonly used for LUS. The mechanical sector scanner contains a single crystal element that oscillates. This type of transducer in a laparoscopic instrument allows for either forward viewing when the crystal is positioned in the instrument's distal tip or side viewing when the crystal is oriented perpendicular to the axis of the instrument (Fig. 1A, B). The field of view created by this transducer is sector (pie) shaped and is therefore limiting when examining a structure by direct contact. Some laparoscopists consider this limitation important for laparoscopic ultrasound applications. Linear array transducers are composed of multiple small rectangular crystals arranged in a

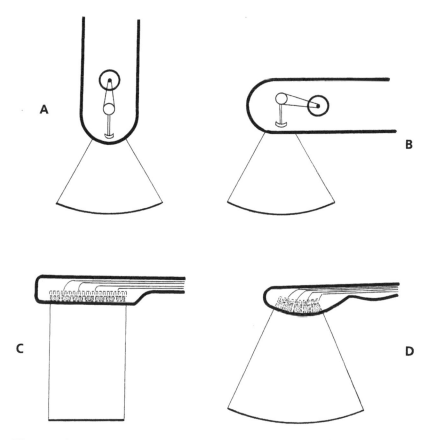

Figure 1 Commonly used laparoscopic intracorporeal ultrasound transducers. (A) Mechanical sector scanner with the piezoelectric crystal positioned in the distal tip of the probe for forward viewing. (B) Mechanical sector scanner with the crystal oriented perpendicular to the instrument's axis for side viewing. Note the sector (pie)-shaped field of view created by this crystal. (C) Linear array transducer comprising multiple small rectangular crystals arranged in a row. The field of view created by this crystal configuration is square. (D) Convex array transducer, which contains multiple crystals aligned in a curvilinear conformation to give a trapezoidal field of view. (From Ref. 11.)

row (Fig. 1C). The net frequency of the transducer depends on the frequency of each crystal. This transducer produces a square field of view, which is optimal for laparoscopic ultrasonography done by direct contact. Similarly, the convex array transducer contains multiple crystals, but these piezoelectric elements are aligned in a curvilinear conformation, which forms a trapezoidal field of view (Fig. 1D). This transducer is also suitable for direct-contact ultrasound examinations. A phase-delay feature is available for those transducers that contain multiple crystals positioned side by side. Sequentially delaying activation of the crystals produces time delays or phase differences in the ultrasound beam, which then changes the direction of that beam. This feature enables the examiner to avoid anatomical structures that obstruct the path of the ultrasound waves. We prefer linear array laparoscopic ultrasound probes because of their ease of use and versatility when performing direct-contact ultrasonography.

Although a variety of applications for LUS have been described, evaluation of the extrahepatic biliary tree during laparoscopic cholecystectomy and staging of intra-abdominal malignancies are currently the two most common clinical indications for use of this diagnostic modality.

III. APPLICATIONS

Recently, surgeons have reported novel uses for laparoscopic ultrasound to directly guide the drainage of hepatic cysts [1] and laparoscopic radiofrequency ablation of hepatic malignancy [2]. However, the indications that have received the most scrutiny are the evalution of common bile duct stones and the staging of hepatobiliary and pancreatic malignancy.

A. Evaluation of Choledocholithiasis

Imaging the common bile duct by laparoscopic ultrasonography to screen for choledocholithiasis is becoming more widely performed. Numerous prospective studies have compared LUS to laparoscopic cholangiography (LC), which is the gold standard for detecting biliary stones. These studies varied in the types of ultrasound probes used and in the techniques used for both sonography and cholangiography. LUS has been shown to be as accurate as LC in detecting bile duct stones. The reported sensitivities and specificities for LUS in detecting common bile duct stones range from 71 to 100% and 96 to 100%, respectively. By comparison, LC has demonstrated a sensitivity of 59–100% and a specificity of 95–100% for identifying biliary stones [3].

Several laparoscopic ultrasound probes are available. The rigid or inflexible 7.5 MHz linear array transducer has been widely used in most series to date. This transducer produces real-time images, and some models are equipped with color Doppler capability that enables the surgeon to distinguish blood vessels from duct structures. The ultrasound waves generated by the 7.5 MHz transducer penetrate to a depth up to 5.3 cm and create a high-resolution image. To enhance acoustic coupling between the tissue and the transducer, some investigators have submerged the hepatoduodenal ligament in saline solution; others rely solely on direct-contact ultrasonography to provide quality images.

Once the equipment is selected, a method for performing the ultrasound study must be adopted. First, the port through which the ultrasound probe will be passed into the abdomen must be chosen. There are several options. One popular choice is the epigastric port. From this position the transducer can be placed on the anterior surface of the hepatoduodenal ligament. The probe is then swept caudally where one can observe the cystic duct confluence with the common bile duct proximally and the terminal portion of the bile duct, including the intrapancreatic segment, distally (Fig. 2). We find this approach to be very effective in evaluating for choledocholithiasis during laparoscopic cholecystectomy. If the probe cannot be positioned correctly from this port or the anatomy is unclear from the initial scan, then the umbilical cannula may be used. From this orientation, the common bile duct can be nicely imaged in a longitudinal direction anterior to the portal vein. As the distal bile duct turns laterally within the head of the pancreas, the bile duct is imaged obliquely from this port. Many investigators obtain both transverse and longitudinal images using both the epigastric and umbilical ports for a thorough and complete evaluation of the entire extrahepatic biliary system.

Many studies have delineated the advantages and disadvantages of LUS over LC in studying the common bile duct. The principal advantages of LUS include safety, relative noninvasiveness, speed, repeated use, and additional anatomical imaging. In LC, detailed dissection and cannulation of the common duct, injection of contrast material, and use of ionizing radiation is required. LUS requires minimal dissection and can be used in pregnancy and those with contrast allergies. LUS is relatively noninvasive. No additional access ports need to be introduced, and cannulation of the common duct is not required to

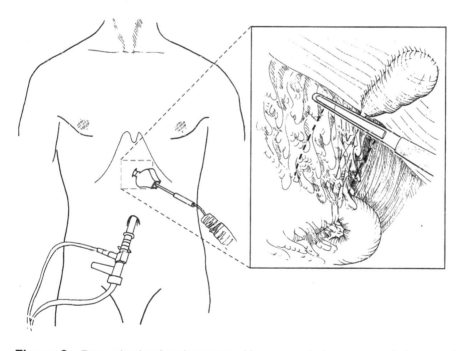

Figure 2 Port selection for placement of laparoscopic intracorporeal ultrasound probes during laparoscopic cholecystectomy. Camera is preferentially introduced through the umbilical port, and the ultrasound probe is passed through the epigastric port. Alternatively, placement of the ultrasound probe and camera may be reversed to optimize the ultrasound examination. (Inset) Intra-abdominal view of region within the dashed lines. Ultrasound probe is positioned on the anterior surface of the hepatoduodenal ligament and swept inferiorly from the liver edge to the duodenum.

perform the study. LUS may be performed at any time and can be easily repeated during the procedure. LUS is more technically demanding, but after an initial learning curve it can be performed more quickly than LC. The time required to perform LUS is about half that to perform LC. Most studies report a time of 4–10 minutes for LUS compared with 10–17 for LC [3]. The speed of LUS can be attributed to real-time imaging and no need for additional dissection or cannulation of the biliary duct. Use of an ultrasound probe with Doppler capability allows for additional images of the arterial and venous anatomy as well as the portal vein and other organs such as the duodenum and pancreas.

Although LUS is valuable in detecting common bile duct stones, it certainly has disadvantages. Surgeon familiarity with the techniques is lacking, and the technology is changing rapidly. Consequently, for surgeons, the interpretation of ultrasound images is more difficult compared with that of cholangiograms, with which they have had much experience. However, John et al. [4] showed that proficiency in correctly identifying structures within the hepatoduodenal ligament can be achieved after performing 40–60 LUS examinations unaided by a radiologist. Despite this success, we emphasize that formal training in LUS techniques and interpretation of images is required to begin using this diagnostic modality in clinical practice. Although there is a need for proper training, many surgeons face a dilemma in that there are limited training opportunities available. Few centers in the United States have the resources not only to perform LUS but also to educate surgeons in this diagnostic method. For most surgeons who do not have access to such a facility, the dilemma remains to be solved. Most studies have concluded that LC provides the most precise and comprehensive images of the biliary system. This superiority of LC is especially true for supracystic duct biliary anatomy, where most anomalies occur. Iatrogenic injuries to the bile ducts are more clearly recognized by LC than by LUS.

Machi et al. [3] performed a prospective study comparing LUS and LC in 100 patients undergoing laparoscopic cholecystectomy. The success of completing the examination was 95% for LUS and 92% for LC. Incomplete visualization of the distal common bile duct was the main reason for an incomplete study by LUS. LUS was also shown to have a better positive predictive value when compared to LC, 100% and 77.8%, respectively. In their review of 12 studies comparing LUS with LC, the time required to perform LUS was shorter by 50%, the positive predictive value and specificity of LUS was better, and the sensitivity and negative predictive values were comparable between LUS and LC. However, LC was able to detect anatomical anomalies of the biliary duct with more precision than LUS.

Laparoscopic ultrasonography during laparoscopic cholecystectomy is currently considered by most laparoscopic surgeons to be a useful screening study in the evaluation of choledocholithiasis. In the hands of experienced surgeons it is often the first-line choice in evaluation of the biliary tree for stones and can be the definitive examination in many cases. However, in cases of undefined anatomy or an equivocal exam, LC should also be performed.

B. Staging of Intra-Abdominal Malignancy

Cancer staging includes determining the extent of tumor spread into contiguous structures or to distant sites. Traditionally, imaging studies such as transabdominal ultrasound and computed tomography with or without angiography have been used preoperatively to determine the stage and resectability of a tumor. These tests are costly and still lack the sensitivity to detect occult lesions which, when later found at laparotomy, preclude resection. However, several authors have shown that laparoscopy is effective in staging esophageal, gastric, pancreatic, gallbladder, liver, colon, and ovarian carcinomas. More recently, laparoscopic ultrasonography has been shown to further improve the accuracy of cancer staging by demonstrating previously unrecognized intraparenchymal tumors or vascular involvement.

As with laparoscopic ultrasonography of the biliary tree during cholecystectomy, we use a 7.5 MHz linear array transducer for tumor staging. After placing the umbilical port and surveying the abdomen laparoscopically for occult tumor deposits, a second port is placed to accommodate the ultrasound probe. For hepatobiliary and pancreatic (HBP) tumors, the second port is often positioned in the right anterior axillary line at the umbilical level. Using direct contact ultrasonography, the liver, biliary tree, pancreas, and surrounding lymph node beds can be thoroughly scanned for the presence of tumor or related vascular pathology. Several small studies have been done that show very promising results for staging intra-abdominal malignancy with remarkable accuracy.

In Europe, John et al. [5] reported results of staging laparoscopy with laparoscopic ultrasonography in 40 patients with periampullary carcinoma. Metastases that were not recognized preoperatively were discovered at laparoscopy alone in 14 patients. Additionally, hepatic metastases or vascular invasion was found in 10 other patients by laparoscopic ultrasonography. This same group has also reported on 50 patients with liver cancer who underwent similar laparoscopic tumor staging. Laparoscopy alone revealed disease that precluded curative resection in 23 patients. Moreover, laparoscopic ultrasonography was performed in 43 of these patients, 14 of whom were found to have parenchymal liver tumors not identified by laparoscopy alone. Information about tumor resectability that supplemented the laparoscopic findings was found in a total of 18 patients.

John and colleagues [6] reported in 1995 their results of a prospective study of 40 patients with pancreatic malignancy deemed unresectable by radiological staging in whom laparoscopic staging (LS) with laparoscopic ultrasound was performed. Laparoscopic staging discovered additional metastatic lesions in 35% of patients. Laparoscopic ultrasound confirmed respectability in 53% of patients, resulting in a change of management in 25% of patients. The addition of LUS to LS improved sensitivity and accuracy from 50% to 85% and from 60% to 89%, respectively.

In the United States, Callery et al. [7] performed staging laparoscopy with laparoscopic ultrasonography in 50 consecutive patients with HBP malignancy. All patients were judged preoperatively by traditional imaging studies to have resectable tumors. However, staging laparoscopy with laparoscopic ultrasonography predicted only 28 patients to have resectable tumors. At laparotomy 26 of these 28 patients were deemed to have tumors that could be resected, indicating a 4 false-negative rate for the combined techniques. Of the 22 patients found to have unresectable tumors, 11 were discovered by laparoscopy alone. The remaining 11 patients had the unresectable tumor diagnosed solely by laparoscopic ultrasonography. Of these 11 patients, 5 were found to have vascular invasion, 5 had lymph node metastases, and one had intraparenchymal metastatic liver tumor. Overall, laparoscopic staging plus laparoscopic ultrasound provided a sensitivity of 96%, a specificity of 92%, and obviated the need for laparotomy in 34% of patients.

In 1999, John et al. [8] again provided insight by prospectively comparing the abilities of laparoscopic ultrasound, transabdominal ultrasound, computed tomography

(CT), and visceral angiography to assess resectability of pancreatic cancer in a cohort of 50 patients in whom resectability was defined by TNM stage. Although no modality made an accurate assessment of nodal status (N stage) and LUS did not improve assessments of metastatic disease (M stage), laparoscopic ultrasound was more specific (100%) than transabdominal ultrasound (64%) or CT (47%) in defining level of invasion (T stage) and, overall, was more predictive than computed tomography (97% vs. 79%).

In the field of laparoscopic colorectal surgery, a group from Cleveland Clinic Foundation prospectively and blindly compared laparoscopic ultrasound versus computerized tomography for liver assessment in 77 consecutive patients undergoing colorectal cancer surgery. Milsom et al. found that laparoscopic ultrasonography of the liver at the time of primary resection of colorectal cancer yielded more liver lesions (95%) than preoperative contrast-enhanced computerized tomography (78%) and should be considered for routine use during laparoscopic oncological colorectal surgery [9]. The median procedure time for the laparoscopic ultrasound evaluation of the liver was 10 minutes (range 5–15).

Accurate staging of intra-abdominal malignancy has important practical value. Patients with advanced disease detected with minimally invasive techniques may be spared unnecessary laparotomies that could otherwise impair both the quality and quantity of remaining life. In addition, a cost savings from avoiding major operations and long hospitalizations is economically appealing. Indeed, McMahon and colleagues' [10] cost-effectiveness analysis of various imaging modalities for assessing pancreatic cancer resectability concluded that laparoscopy with laparoscopic ultrasound was significantly less expensive over a broad range of modality scenarios. If minimally invasive or nonoperative strategies for palliation are to be offered, then accurate staging is necessary. Therefore, the improved accuracy of laparoscopy and laparoscopic ultrasonography in tumor staging shows promise for better management of patients with intra-abdominal malignancy.

REFERENCES

1. Schachter P, Sorin V, Avni Y, Shimonov M, Friedman V, Rosen A, et al. The role of laparoscopic ultrasound in the minimally invasive management of symptomatic hepatic cysts. Surg Endosc 2001; 15(4):364–367.
2. Chung MH, Wood TF, Tsioulias GJ, Rose DM, Bilchik AJ. Laparoscopic radiofrequency ablation of unresectable hepatic malignancies. Surg Endosc 2001; 15(9):1020–1026.
3. Machi J, Tateishi T, Oishi AJ, Furumoto NL, Oishi RH, Uchida S, et al. Laparoscopic ultrasonography versus operative cholangiography during laparoscopic cholecystectomy: review of the literature and a comparison with open intraoperative ultrasonography. J Am Coll Surg 1999; 188(4):360–367.
4. John TG, Banting SW, Pye S, Paterson-Brown S, Garden OJ. Preliminary experience with intracorporeal laparoscopic ultrasonography using a sector scanning probe. A prospective comparison with intraoperative cholangiography in the detection of choledocholithiasis. Surg Endosc 1994; 8(10):1176–1180.
5. John TG, Greig JD, Crosbie JL, Miles WF, Garden OJ. Superior staging of liver tumors with laparoscopy and laparoscopic ultrasound. Ann Surg 1994; 220(6):711–719.
6. John TG, Greig JD, Carter DC, Garden OJ. Carcinoma of the pancreatic head and periampullary region. Tumor staging with laparoscopy and laparoscopic ultrasonography. Ann Surg 1995; 221(2):156–164.

7. Callery MP, Strasberg SM, Doherty GM, Soper NJ, Norton JA. Staging laparoscopy with laparoscopic ultrasonography: optimizing resectability in hepatobiliary and pancreatic malignancy. J Am Coll Surg 1997; 185(1):33–39.
8. John TG, Wright A, Allan PL, Redhead DN, Paterson-Brown S, Carter DC, et al. Laparoscopy with laparoscopic ultrasonography in the TNM staging of pancreatic carcinoma. World J Surg 1999; 23(9):870–881.
9. Milsom JW, Jerby BL, Kessler H, Hale JC, Herts BR, O'Malley CM. Prospective, blinded comparison of laparoscopic ultrasonography vs. contrast-enhanced computerized tomography for liver assessment in patients undergoing colorectal carcinoma surgery. Dis Colon Rectum 2000; 43:44–49.
10. McMahon PM, Halpern EF, Fernandez-del Castillo C, Clark JW, Gazelle GS. Pancreatic cancer: cost-effectiveness of imaging technologies for assessing resectability. Radiology 2001; 221(1):93–106.
11. Jakimowicz J. Laparoscopic intraoperative ultrasonography, equipment, and technique. Semin Laparosc Surg 1994; 1:52–61.

10

Complications of Laparoscopic Surgery

STEPHEN L. CARTER

United Hospital Center
Clarksburg, West Virginia, U.S.A.

JONATHAN F. CRITCHLOW and DANIEL B. JONES

Beth Israel Deaconess Medical Center
Harvard Medical School
Boston, Massachusetts, U.S.A.

Although recent advances in technology have made the use of laparoscopic procedures more widely practicable, the benefits of these minimally invasive operations must be weighed against the unique complications associated with laparoscopic instrumentation and techniques. Surgeons must be familiar with these complications and assess their personal experience and skill levels when considering the risks and benefits of a laparoscopic procedure as an alternative to an open operation. Complications of laparoscopic surgery may be classified as intraoperative and postoperative.

General complications encountered during diagnostic and therapeutic laparoscopy will be discussed in this chapter; complications specific to certain procedures will be covered elsewhere.

I. INTRAOPERATIVE COMPLICATIONS

Intraoperative complications include those unique to laparoscopy—problems related to the pneumoperitoneum, to patient positioning, and to instrumentation. Procedure-specific complications, common to both the laparoscopic and open approaches to an operative procedure, can also occur.

A. Anesthesia

Although some diagnostic laparoscopic procedures can be performed with the use of local anesthesia, therapeutic laparoscopic procedures require the use of general or regional anesthesia, because manipulation of the parietal peritoneum and mesentery cause pain that cannot be controlled by local anesthesia and can cause nausea and bradycardia. A regional anesthetic technique such as spinal or epidural can be used in gynecological or pelvic operations; however, shoulder pain is a common side effect. Nausea and vomiting can occur, but with less frequency than that seen after general anesthesia. Antiemetics can be used to prevent the nausea, but they can cause sedation, dry mouth, and α-adrenergic blockade.

Arrhythmias can occur with all types of anesthesia but have been reported to occur in 25–47% of patients during laparoscopic surgery, typically occurring when the pneumoperitoneum is created and ending with desufflation. This can be seen both in local and general anesthesia cases. Bradyarrhythmias, the most common type, are seen on induction of a pneumoperitoneum. The use of atropine as a premedication can help to prevent a vagally induced cardiac response. Sinus tachycardia and premature ventricular contractions can be caused by hypercarbia produced from systemic absorption of CO_2 or by venous gas embolus or hypoxia. Monitoring the patient's ECG will help to detect arrhythmias. Desufflation, hyperventilation, and release of intra-abdominal pressure are the initial treatment for arrhythmias. Persistent arrhythmias may be treated with appropriate medications (atropine for bradycardia and lidocaine for ventricular arrhythmias).

B. Pneumoperitoneum

1. Extraperitoneal Insufflation

Subcutaneous or properitoneal insufflation occurs in approximately 0.5% of cases and results from incorrect positioning of the Veress needle or cannula or leakage of CO_2 around trocars. CO_2 then accumulates in the subcutaneous tissue or between the fascia and peritoneum. When gas is introduced into the properitoneal space, malposition is detected when high insufflating pressures are registered on initiation of insufflation and by the difficulty in creating a pneumoperitoneum. This may cause significant stretching of the peritoneum and subsequent vasovagal reaction.

Insufflation into the omentum, mesentery, or retroperitoneum can result in cephalad dissection, which results in a pneumomediastinum, pneumopericardium, or pneumo-thorax. A pneumothorax is usually seen on the left side but can be bilateral; subcutaneous emphysema is often seen without an associated pneumothorax. These are most often seen during procedures around the esophageal hiatus and mediastinum (fundoplication, esophageal myotomy, paraesophageal hernia repair). Subcutaneous emphysema is usually a minor problem, which will resolve after desufflation. Severe emphysema may require more prolonged intubation with high FIO_2 until resolution to diminish the risk of airway compromise. A pneumothorax should be considered in situations of increased airway pressures, hypoxemia, or desaturation. An intraoperative chest x-ray is diagnostic. A small intraoperative pneumothorax is treated with lower insufflation pressures and increased positive end expiratory pressures (PEEP). A more symptomatic pneumothorax may require a small chest tube, which can usually be removed after desufflation.

Complications associated with insufflation are much less common when an open insertion technique is used, because the trocar can be placed under direct visualization into the peritoneal space. However, if a closed technique is used, correct placement of the Veress needle is essential. The needle should be held at right angles to the skin and the abdominal wall. Before insufflation, a "drop test" is performed to confirm proper placement of the needle: a small amount of saline solution in the needle hub is allowed to enter rapidly into the abdominal cavity to determine whether the needle is truly positioned intra-abdominally. An aspiration and saline injection test can also be performed to confirm Veress needle placement: after the Veress needle has been inserted, it is connected to a 10 mL syringe, and suction is applied. The return of fluid on aspiration suggests placement of the needle into a viscus or vascular structure. If no fluid can be aspirated, several milliliters of saline solution should be injected through the needle. The saline solution should flow easily into the abdomen, and if the needle lies in the peritoneal space, the saline solution cannot be reaspirated. Removing the plunger should allow saline solution to flow into the peritoneal cavity by gravity alone if the needle is positioned correctly.

2. Cardiovascular Effects

CO_2 gas is most commonly used for insufflation because it is highly soluble in blood and is nonflammable. It can be rapidly absorbed into the bloodstream and eliminated through exhalation. Peritoneal absorption of CO_2 can lead to hypercarbia and acidosis, which can result in ventricular arrhythmias. Hypercarbia stimulates the sympathetic nervous system and can cause tachycardia, increased contractility, and hypertension. In most patients mild acidosis is well tolerated, and hypercapnia can be corrected by increasing the patient's minute ventilation. Intra-abdominal pressure should be kept at or below 15 mmHg to prevent hypercarbia. Careful monitoring of the patient's ventilation and oxygenation is essential, and the use of an end-tidal CO_2 monitor is helpful. In hypovolemic patients, acidosis may be significant, and arterial pH and pCO_2 should be carefully monitored so that necessary, timely ventilatory changes can be made.

Although insufflation to intra-abdominal pressures of 20 mmHg is generally well tolerated, higher pressures can lead to hypotension by producing compression of the vena cava, thereby decreasing venous return and causing a diminished cardiac output. Other less common causes of hypotension include that caused by bradycardia, which can be caused by abdominal wall distention, peritoneal irritation, and a vasovagal response. In addition, these hemodynamic changes can be worsened by the patient's position during the procedure. Treatment of hypotensive episodes includes desufflation, administration of intravenous fluids, and decreasing the anesthetic concentration. The patient may be placed in the Trendelenburg position to increase venous return.

3. Pulmonary Effects

Displacement of the diaphragm by the pneumoperitoneum can decrease total lung capacity and functional residual capacity and cause CO_2 retention and atelectasis. The alveolar dead space can be increased and cause ventilation-perfusion mismatching, leading to elevated airway pressures, decreased pulmonary compliance, and hypoxemia. The Trendelenburg position can worsen the diaphragmatic displacement and may cause further ventilation-perfusion mismatch by causing pooling of blood in dependent portions of the lung. Mechanical ventilation PEEP, increased minute ventilation, and an intra-abdominal pressure of 15 mmHg or less help to counteract these pulmonary changes.

4. Gas Embolism

Despite the high solubility of CO_2 in blood, a CO_2 embolism may cause acute hypotension and significant cardiovascular compromise. The usual cause of a gas embolism is inadvertent placement of a Veress needle into a major vessel and insufflation with CO_2. Intraoperative injury to a large vein during pneumoperitoneum may also lead to embolism.

A substantial amount of CO_2 must enter the vein at a rapid rate (>1 L/min) before a significant gas embolism can occur. A characteristic millwheel murmur can be heard on auscultation. Diagnosis can be confirmed by demonstration of air bubbles in the heart by transesophageal echocardiography (TEE). Treatment includes desufflation and placing the patient in Trendelenburg position in a left lateral decubitus rotation. Placement of a central venous catheter facilitates aspiration of the gas from the right side of the heart.

Because of the adverse effects of the CO_2, the use of alternative gases such as nitrous oxide and helium is being studied for use in creation of the pneumoperitoneum. Neither of these gases causes hypercarbia or acidosis; however, both are less soluble in blood than CO_2 and theoretically have increased risk of causing a gas embolism. Further studies are required, however, before these gases can be used routinely.

C. Instrumentation

1. Vascular Injuries

In the closed insertion technique, the Veress needle and first trocar are inserted blindly. Although many precautions are taken in both technique and instrumentation, serious and even fatal complications can occur. Blood vessels or viscera can occasionally be penetrated. Visceral injuries have been reported to occur in 0.025–0.2% of patients, and the incidence of vascular injuries is 0.017–0.05%, with a mortality rate of 8.8–13%. Because the aortic bifurcation lies below the umbilicus, it, the vena cava, and the iliac vessels are susceptible to injury. If the Veress needle is inserted into a major vessel, it is usually noticed by aspiration with a syringe. Although it may be a small puncture, it should not be assumed that it will be self-sealing, and it is often difficult to accurately assess a retroperitoneal hematoma laparoscopically. If the Veress needle has punctured a major vessel, the abdomen should be opened and the area inspected for any injuries that need to be exposed and repaired. Delay increases the risk of death. A major vessel injury from a trocar presents with visible hemorrhage and hypotension. These injuries are often fatal, and immediate action to open the abdomen (without removing the trocar) to gain control of the vessel is mandatory. Although less likely to occur with open insertion or direct-view trocars, vascular injuries have been reported with these techniques.

2. Bowel Injuries

Bowel injuries are often caused by Veress needle puncture, but most of these cause no sequelae and need no repair; the needle is simply removed. The incidence of bowel injury is 0.06–0.14%, with a mortality rate of approximately 5%, but many of these injuries probably go unrecognized or unreported. Trocar injuries, on the other hand, mandate immediate repair. The injury is usually diagnosed when bowel contents are seen with the laparoscope or coming through the trocar. Because more than one injury or enterotomy may have occurred, careful examination of all nearby structures should be performed, because subtle enterotomies may be overlooked. Risk factors for bowel injury include previous abdominal surgery, metastatic disease, and abdominal distention. When any of these are present, an open insertion technique for laparoscopy is the safest approach. A nasogastric tube is inserted and a Foley catheter placed to decompress the stomach and bladder, respectively, to decrease the incidence of injury to these organs by Veress needles or trocars.

3. Solid Organ Injury

Solid organ injuries may also occur, but this is rare because the initial Veress needle and trocar are most often inserted at a midline umbilical site. Secondary trocars should be placed under direct laparoscopic vision, and injury should be rare. At the time of insertion of the Veress needle, a solid organ injury may be suspected if insufflation pressures are high and blood or blood-tinged saline solution is aspirated. If an injury does occur from a Veress needle, it can be directly coagulated with electrocautery or argon beam coagulator, or a hemostatic agent such as Gelfoam, Surgicel, or Avitene can be placed over the injury site. If a significant injury has occurred, an open repair will probably be required.

4. Abdominal Wall Bleeding

Injury to an abdominal wall vessel by a trocar can cause bleeding and is noticed by blood dripping from the trocar into the abdomen or bleeding around the trocar site during the procedure or, more often, after trocar removal. These can be prevented by identifying the epigastric vessels through transillumination of the abdominal wall with the laparoscope and placing the trocars so that the vessels are missed. Most trocar site bleeding resolves without intervention, but if bleeding persists, hemostasis can be achieved with sutures or ligation. Extracorporeal through and through sutures placed with a modified Veress or Gracie needle are very useful in deep wounds. Removing the trocar and placing the Foley catheter balloon through the tract and tamponading the vessel for up to 30 minutes may be effective in difficult cases. Use of radially expanding large trocars can diminish the incidence of this problem.

5. Nerve Damage

Abnormal stretching or compression of a nerve may cause peripheral nerve damage during a laparoscopic procedure. Brachial plexus injuries are the most common and may relate to improper positioning of the patient, especially in patients who are in the Trendelenburg position or whose arms are abducted beyond 90 degrees. Care should be taken to ensure that the patient is properly positioned and bony prominences are padded. The use of a beanbag for patients requiring steep positional changes can help to prevent nerve damage.

6. Thermal Injuries

Electrocautery and lasers may cause thermal damage to viscera and abdominal vessels. One common cause of thermal injury is a failure to have the patient properly grounded when using a unipolar device. Unipolar cautery requires a ground path between its point and the patient's grounding pad, and if the ground is inadequate, a high-resistance pathway and subsequent thermal damage can result. Current may arc from a trocar or poorly insulated instrument, causing injury at a site away from the area of dissection. Injuries to the common bile duct, gallbladder, duodenum, ureters, bladder, and the colon have all been reported. Many of these thermal injuries heal without operative management. For ureteral injuries, most heal with such nonoperative management as ureteral stenting and administration of antibiotics.

The extent of thermal injury depends on the type of current. With bipolar current, the injury is limited to the tissue that lies between the forceps' prongs, whereas in monopolar current injuries, damage may be more extensive, and the onset of symptoms may be delayed as much as 2 weeks. Usually thermal injuries to the bowel result in fever and abdominal pain. The extent of injury also depends on the magnitude of the current, with higher currents producing more extensive injury.

Complication rates are not significantly different when one compares procedures performed with lasers with those in which monopolar electrocautery is used. A laser coagulates or vaporizes tissue by converting photon energy to kinetic energy. Its advantage over monopolar cautery is that tissue damage is restricted to a small area, because no flow of current goes through the patient. However, the laser beam can damage tissue beyond what is intended by overshooting, which can result in vascular, biliary, or intestinal injuries, especially around the hepatoduodenal ligament.

II. POSTOPERATIVE COMPLICATIONS

A. Peritonitis/Wound Infection

Infections in the wound are rare and may be caused by skin organisms or by bacteria that have spread from the peritoneal cavity. The incidence of wound infections is not increased with spillage of gallstones, although abscesses may form. The risk of abscess formation can be decreased with irrigation of the area after spillage. Risk factors for infectious complications include advanced age, obesity, and diabetes mellitus. Necrotizing fasciitis rarely occurs but has been reported after laparoscopic procedures; it requires surgical debridement and administration of broad-spectrum antibiotics.

A postoperative fever or abdominal tenderness may be the first sign of a bowel perforation from a trocar, Veress needle, or thermal injury. Signs and symptoms of perforation may take up to 2 weeks to be manifested. The diagnosis is made by clinical examination and an obstructive series (chest x-ray and abdominal films), though free air may be expected for several days following uncomplicated laparoscopy. A computed tomography (CT) scan of the abdomen with an oral contrast medium may be helpful for showing extravasation of the contrast medium from the bowel. Surgical exploration and possibly a diverting enterostomy are required if a bowel perforation has occurred.

B. Delayed Hemorrhage

Ongoing blood loss from the operative field will result in hemodynamic instability. However, this must be differentiated from other causes such as myocardial infarction, pulmonary embolism, sepsis, or hypovolemia. The diagnosis of ongoing bleeding is suggested by prolonged or redeveloping abdominal pain, abdominal distention, a falling hematocrit level, tachycardia, oliguria, and hemodynamic changes. Its management depends on its source and the hemodynamic changes it produces. Bleeding may occur from a trocar site in the abdominal wall, an injured intra-abdominal vessel, or the operative field. If immediate surgical exploration is not required, observation with a CT scan of the abdomen may be useful to identify the size of the hematoma. A radiolabeled red blood cell study can also be done to identify the presence or absence of ongoing bleeding. Prevention includes meticulous attention to hemostasis at the end of the procedure. The pneumoperitoneum should be decreased and a thorough inspection performed for bleeding in the abdomen and on the abdominal wall.

C. Incisional Hernia

An incisional hernia that develops at a trocar site may be caused by infection, inadequate reapproximation of the fascial edges, or premature suture disruption. Trocar sites that are 5 mm in diameter or less have a very low risk of developing late incisional hernias, but trocar sites of 10 mm or greater may herniate if the fascia is not closed at the end of the procedure. The diagnosis is usually made on physical examination when a bulge can be palpated at a previous port site. Alternatively, an ultrasound or abdominal CT scan may help to diagnose a fascial defect with herniation in obese patients in whom a diagnostic physical examination may be difficult or in patients with persistent pain around a trocar site. The patient may present with localized abdominal discomfort or a mass at the site that may be tender, depending on its entrapment. Patients presenting with small bowel obstruction after laparoscopy must be suspected of having an incarcerated Richter's hernia at a port site. The hernia can be repaired laparoscopically or with an open procedure. Failure to diagnose an incisional hernia may lead to bowel incarceration or strangulation, causing further morbidity and the need for an open procedure. Prevention consists of closure of the fascia for any trocar site that is 10 mm or greater or the use of nonbladed or radially expanding trocars.

D. Tumor Metastases

A rare complication of laparoscopy is malignant dissemination at a trocar site. Seeding along the tracts of an instrument has been reported with primary cancers of the stomach, ovary, and biliary tract, although most cases occurred when the primary tumor was adenocarcinoma of the colon. In a hamster model, a pneumoperitoneum of 10 mmHg for 10 minutes more than doubled tumor cell implantation at trocar sites, suggesting that the pneumoperitoneum may contribute to the seeding of the trocar sites. The use of laparoscopic procedures for resections of cancers remains a controversial issue, even though the incidence of this phenomenon is no higher with laparoscopy than that of wound implantation following open surgery in large areas.

E. Azotemia

An unrecognized bladder perforation may lead to azotemia, especially when it is associated with ascites and hyponatremia. Hematuria or pneumaturia can suggest a bladder injury, and a rising creatinine level with hyperkalemia and hyponatremia is consistent with a bladder perforation. A cystogram is necessary to confirm the diagnosis; cystoscopy can determine the location and extent of the injury. If the injury is small, it usually resolves with continuous bladder drainage. If it is large, surgical repair is needed. Prevention consists of emptying the bladder or decompression with a Foley catheter before any instruments are placed, especially if closed techniques are used.

III. CONCLUSION

Although laparoscopic procedures have been shown to have beneficial outcomes, they can be associated with unique complications that must be considered before a decision is made to perform a minimally invasive procedure. Familiarity and training can help to prevent technical complications resulting from two-dimensional imaging, limited hand and instrument motion, and unusual operative views. Such complications as those related to creating and maintaining a pneumoperitoneum or those caused by the insertion of a Veress needle or trocar can often be prevented by understanding the physiology, being familiar with the instrumentation, and paying meticulous attention to detail. Early identification and management of complications are necessary to limit the occurrence of further potentially devastating complications. Long-term complications from laparoscopy, such as adhesions, hernias, and tumor seeding of trocar sites, are still being evaluated, and further recommendations will likely be developed.

SELECTED READINGS

Bhoyrul S, Payne J, Steffes B, Swanstrom L, Way LW. A randomized prospective study of radially expanding trocars in laparoscopy surgery. J Gastrointest Surg 2000; 4(4):392–397.

Bhoyrul S, Vierra MA, Nezhat CR, Krummel TM, Way LW. Trocar injuries in laparoscopic surgery. J Am Coll Surg 2001; 192(6):677–683.

Bongard F, Dubecz S, Klein S. Complications of therapeutic laparoscopy. Curr Probl Surg 1994; 31:857–932.

Harkki-Siren P, Kurki T. A nationwide analysis of laparoscopic complications. Obstet Gynecol 1997; 89(1):108–112.

Jones DB, Callery MP, Soper NJ. Strangulated incisional hernia at trocar site. Surg Laparosc Endosc 1996; 6:152–154.

Jones DB, Guo L, Reinhard MK, Soper NJ, Philpott GW, Connett J, Fleshman JW. Impact of pneumoperitoneum on trocar site implantation of colon cancer in hamster model. Dis Colon Rectum 1995; 38:1182–1188.

Jones DB, Soper NJ. Complications of laparoscopic cholecystectomy. Ann Rev Med 1996; 47:31–44.

Nordestgaard AG, Bodily KC, Osborne RW, Buttorff, JD. Major vascular injuries during laparoscopic procedures. Am J Surg 1995; 169(5):543–545.

See WA, Monk TG, Weldon BC. Complications of laparoscopy. In Soper NJ, Odem RR, Clayman RV, McDougall EM, eds. Essentials of Laparoscopy. St. Louis: Quality Medical Publishing, 1994, pp 215–240.

11

General Postoperative Care

DAVID D. CHI

Los Robles Regional Medical Center
Thousand Oaks, California, U.S.A.

I. INTRODUCTION

Over the past few decades, laparoscopic surgery has become more commonplace among all surgical disciplines. Reduced trauma to the patient, less morbidity, and faster recovery are considered to be the main motivating reasons for patients and physicians to opt for these less invasive procedures. The overall postoperative benefits of certain laparoscopic operations, such as laparoscopic-assisted colon resection for cancer, may not be as great as most others, and further studies are needed to establish its role.

Factors such as cost containment and patient preference have allowed many laparoscopic operations to be performed on an outpatient basis. Even when patients require admission to the hospital postoperatively, length of stay is typically significantly reduced. Nonetheless, it is important to realize that although the incisions may be smaller, most procedures remain major operations and therefore general postoperative principles still apply.

II. GENERAL CONSIDERATIONS

As with any operation requiring general or regional anesthesia, patients need to be closely monitored in the postoperative period. Frequent vital signs and close cardiopulmonary monitoring are essential. In general, patients may resume preoperative diets and medications once they are fully awake and tolerating oral intake. If the intestinal tract has not been violated or manipulated, clear liquids are typically initiated immediately and diets are appropriately advanced. In most cases, patients undergoing laparoscopic procedures resume regular diets faster compared to the open procedures. Once the patient is mobile and ambulating, antithrombotic measures such as compression stockings and sequential pneumatic leggings, and medications such as subcutaneous minidose heparin or enoxaparin (Lovenox) may be discontinued.

III. MEDICATIONS

Most patients are restarted on their preoperative medications. In addition, analgesics and antibiotics are used as indicated by the specific procedure. Narcotics may be given immediately postoperatively, although many patients may not need them after 24–48 hours. At the extremes, some patients may not require any narcotic analgesia, whereas others will be narcotic dependent for more extended periods. Oral analgesic preparations such as acetaminophen-codeine, acetaminophen-oxycodone, and acetaminophen-proxyphene usually suffice, especially if local anesthesia (such as lidocaine or bupivacaine) is infiltrated into the incision perioperatively.

In the absence of active infection, antibiotics have been shown to be effective only during the perioperative period. Furthermore, other studies have shown no difference in rates of infection with the routine use of perioperative antibiotics. In general, there is no apparent need for extended oral antibiotics unless the operation was a clean-contaminated or contaminated case (e.g., gangrenous or ruptured appendicitis) or if the patient had special considerations (e.g., cardiac valvular disorders or prosthetics).

Antiemetics are also occasionally needed postoperatively. These are especially important in esophageal reflux disease, because the fundoplication or hiatal hernia repair can be disrupted with retching or vomiting. Antiemetics typically used include prochlorperazine (Compazine), trimethobenzamide (Tigan), thiethylperazine (Norzine), and ondansetron (Zofran). Ondansetron is most effective if a dose is given before induction of anesthesia and postoperatively (for adults: 4 mg intravenously over 2–5 min preoperatively and then every 4 h postoperatively), but it is also the most costly option.

IV. OUTPATIENT LAPAROSCOPY

Outpatient laparoscopic surgery has increasingly been shown to be safe, cost-effective, and preferable to patients. Procedures such as laparoscopic cholecystectomy, laparoscopic antireflux surgery, and even bowel resections have been performed on an outpatient basis. Since these patients may not necessarily be followed as closely, it is imperative that they are well instructed prior to discharge.

Since most intra-abdominal and many extra-abdominal laparoscopic operations require general anesthesia, these patients should be appropriately instructed prior to discharge. Driving should be prohibited for at least 24 hours. Patients should also be aware of other common symptoms associated with general anesthesia, such as headache, fatigue, nausea, vomiting, and throat irritation from endotracheal intubation. Fortunately, these problems resolve spontaneously with expectant and symptomatic management.

When the patient is fully awake, alert, and can tolerate oral intake, the IV line may be removed and the patient discharged to home. The bandages should be left in place for 1–2 days, after which they may be removed and left off. Typically, patients may shower 48–72 hours after the procedure. Likewise, tolerated activities may resume in 2–3 days.

Patients should be informed of possible symptoms they may experience after they go home. In addition to the residual effects of anesthesia, patients and their families should look for other surgery-related issues, including chest and shoulder pain. The shoulder or chest pain may occur in the first 3–4 hours after surgery and is often attributed to diaphragmatic irritation from the CO_2 pneumoperitoneum. However, the clinician must maintain a high degree of suspicion to rule out other causes, including cardiopulmonary complications (such as myocardial infarction or pulmonary embolism).

Patients must call their surgeon if they become febrile [temperature greater than 100°F (38°C)], develop progressive abdominal distention, intense or increasing abdominal pain, bleeding or drainage from the incision, dyspnea, or pleuritic or substernal chest pain.

V. SPECIAL POSTOPERATIVE CONSIDERATIONS

The specific details of postoperative care for the surgical patient is beyond the scope of this chapter. However, the physician caring for the patient who has undergone laparoscopic surgery needs to realize that the basic principles remain applicable. There are, however, considerations particular to laparoscopy that warrant attention.

A. Incisional Pain

Although the amount of pain associated with smaller incisions is less than that of traditional open operations, the patient and physician need to expect a certain amount of pain. The amount of pain depends upon certain factors, including the type of surgery, size of the incision, amount of dissection required, and the individual patient's tolerance and perception of pain. Often patients will have a preconceived idea that with smaller incisions, the pain will be negligible. Therefore, during the preoperative consultation, the patient must understand that incisional pain is only a component of the postoperative pain. For example, while the incisions associated with laparoscopic hernia repairs are small, the inguinal floors usually require extensive dissection. As a result, although most patients have less incisional pain, the pain in the inguinal regions may be great enough to delay immediate return to normal activity.

Incisional pain that develops after the immediate postoperative period or persists for more than a few days need to be evaluated further. In these situations, the physician must consider infection or an incisional hernia. Wound infections are treated with incision, drainage, and antibiotics if there is associated cellulitis. Although uncommon, incisional hernias may be present in the larger port sites, particularly in those greater than 10 mm in the lower abdomen or umbilicus. Hernias can be reduced and repaired in the operating room by making an incision over the post site, resecting the hernia sac, and closing the fascial defect (usually with mesh). Alternatively, the hernia can be repaired laparoscopically, which may be preferable in certain individuals, such as the obese patient.

Diffuse abdominal pain may indicate a bowel obstruction from adhesions, an unrecognized bowel injury, intra-abdominal abscess, or incarcerated hernia with obstruction, ischemia, or perforation. Expedient evaluation and surgical intervention are paramount in such situations.

B. Shoulder Pain

At the conclusion of a laparoscopic surgery, the CO_2 gas is released from the peritoneal cavity. However, it is not possible to remove all of the gas. The trapped gas will rise to the upper region of the peritoneal cavity as the patient begins to assume upright positions. The gas irritates the diaphragm, which is felt by they patient as shoulder pain. The referred pain is known as "Kerr's sign." The retained gas is eventually completely resorbed by the peritoneal cavity, but may take several days or even weeks to occur.

C. Subcutaneous Emphysema

Laparoscopic surgery usually requires creating a space by insufflating CO_2. Pressures up to 15 mmHg or more may be required to maintain an adequate working space. The gas is pumped into the operative space through a trocar, which usually seals off the body wall.

Occasionally, however, the CO_2 gas will escape into the subcutaneous planes, creating subcutaneous emphysema. The trapped CO_2 gas is manifested by crepitus. The amount of crepitus is dependent upon the quality of the tocar seal, the pressure used to create the working space, and the location of the trocar.

The crepitus is rarely life threatening, unless the upper airway becomes compromised. The CO_2 gas typically resolves in several hours. Supportive care and reassurance for the patient are all that are typically necessary.

D. Postoperative Hydrocele

Hydroceles may occasionally develop in male patients, particularly after laparoscopic procedures of the pelvis. Examples of procedures where this is commonly seen are in laparoscopic hernia repairs and pelvic lymph node dissections.

These are scrotal accumulations of irrigating fluid and hematoma from the procedure and may not be noticeable until the patient is ambulatory. Typically, ecchymosis and swelling may be seen in the scrotum and base of the penis on the second postoperative day. If the scrotal swelling and ecchymosis is massive, or if it develops a few hours after surgery, the patient needs to be evaluated immediately to rule out active hemorrhage.

The hydroceles rarely cause significant pain, but are usually quite uncomfortable. Occasionally additional bedrest with scrotal elevation and scrotal support may be necessary. Otherwise, reassurance and supportive care are sufficient since the symptoms resolve spontaneously in 1–2 weeks.

E. Lower Extremity Edema

In the patient who has undergone laparoscopic pelvic surgery (such as laparoscopic hernia repairs or laparoscopic pelvic lymph node dissections) and presents with lower extremity edema, immediate evaluation is mandatory. Etiologies to consider include lower extremity deep vein thrombosis, congestive heart failure, pelvic lymphoceles, pelvic hematomas, and fluid overload. Lower extremity doppler studies, EKGs, chest radiographs, complete blood counts, serum chemistries, arterial blood gases, atrial naturetic factor levels, and troponin levels may be helpful. CT scans of the pelvis should also be obtained to rule out lymphoceles, hematomas, or abscess.

Lower extremity deep vein thrombosis (DVT) requires immediate and aggressive treatment to avoid potential lethal complications such as pulmonary embolisms and postphlebitic venous insufficiency. Although not all calf DVTs require treatment, they must be taken seriously since up to 30% will continue to extend proximally. If anticoagulation therapy is withheld in such cases, close monitoring is needed. Otherwise, DVTs are generally treated with anticoagulation with intravenous heparin or subcutaneous enoxaparin, followed by warfarin (Coumadin) therapy for at least 1–6 months. In the patient with contraindications to anticoagulation therapy (upper or lower GI bleeding, dysmenorrhagia, patients prone to falling) or patients with pulmonary embolisms while on anticoagulation therapy, placement of an inferior vena cava filter may be necessary.

Pelvic lymphoceles and hematomas large enough to cause lower extremity edema require aggressive intervention. Often CT-guided percutaneous aspiration or drainage will alleviate the symptoms. Small lymphoceles or hematomas which are asymptomatic or cause minimal symptoms can be treated conservatively with bedrest, elevation of the lower extremities, and close monitoring to rule out developing DVTs.

Congestive heart failure, fluid overload, and myocardial infarction require immediate admission to the intensive care unit and aggressive therapy, depending upon the underlying cause. Mechanical ventilation, central venous monitoring, and diuresis may be necessary. Myocardial ischemia or infarction may require angiography, thrombolytic therapy, stent placement, anticoagulation, or coronary artery bypass grafting.

12

Skills Training

DANIEL J. SCOTT

Tulane Center for Minimally Invasive Surgery
Tulane University School of Medicine
New Orleans, Louisiana, U.S.A.

DANIEL B. JONES

Beth Israel Deaconess Medical Center
Harvard Medical School
Boston, Massachusetts, U.S.A.

I. BACKGROUND AND PREMISE

Laparoscopy has undoubtedly advanced the field of surgery beyond the wildest dreams of the early pioneers. However, these advancements have not come without a price. It is clear that laparoscopy requires additional surgical skills that are not routinely used during conventional open operations and specialized training is required. Early in the advent of laparoscopic cholecystectomy, many surgeons were less than adequately trained, and the result was a high rate of ductal injuries. Efforts today are aimed at effectively training surgeons before they perform a new procedure so that complications may be minimized or avoided altogether. Although the surgeon must know the principles governing a specific disease process, the relevant anatomy, and the details of an operation, pivotal to the successful completion of a laparoscopic operation is having sufficient technical skill to perform the procedure. Therefore, in addition to traditional cognitive teaching, a major focus is now centered on laparoscopic skills training.

Laparoscopic procedures impose a unique set of constraints on the surgeon that open operations do not. First, visualization is altered and the surgeon is required to use a two-dimensional video monitor to see the operative field. With loss of depth perception, new visual cues must be learned in order to judge three-dimensional spacial relationships on a two-dimensional monitor. Second, the instrumentation is very different from conventional open surgery. Laparoscopic instruments are long and substantially diminish tactile feedback. The surgeon must therefore rely more heavily on visual cues to prevent traumatic tissue handling. Ports, which act as fixed pivot points in the abdominal wall, limit the range of motion of instruments and require the surgeon to move an instrument handle in the direction opposite to the desired motion of the instrument tip. This "fulcrum" effect, as it is known, is far from intuitive and must be learned with practice.

As is commonly seen with junior residents, a surgeon's first encounter with laparoscopic surgery can be awkward, frustrating, and potentially hazardous. The premise behind laparoscopic skills training is that surgeons should first be taught outside of the operating room and acquire the necessary skills prior to performing an operation. With better skills, the risks to patients may be minimized. Similarly, frustration to both the trainee and the instructor may be alleviated. Instead of using valuable operative time to acquire basic skills, the trainee can focus on anatomical details and learn the nuances of the procedure, resulting in a more meaningful learning experience. Costs may also be minimized. It has been estimated that training residents in the operating room cost $48,000 per graduating resident or $53 million annually. Teaching residents outside of the operating room may be not only safer and more efficient, but also more cost effective. Furthermore, most residents are currently graduating from training programs in the United States with inadequate laparoscopic experience. There are simply not enough experienced instructors, and residents are not achieving competency based on operative experience alone. Since operative experience is inadequate in most residency programs at this time, alternate training modalities are needed.

Options for training include cadavers, animals, inanimate models, and simulators. Although cadavers provide actual human anatomy, drawbacks include noncompliant and nonperfused tissue, potential disease transmission, high costs, and limited supplies. Animals provide well-perfused and compliant tissue, but often are limited by anatomical differences from humans, ethical concerns, costs, and the need for housing facilities and handling personnel. Despite their limitations, both cadavers and animal models may be very useful for specific training needs.

For broad-scale applications, skills laboratories that use inanimate models and simulators may be ideal. Skills laboratories offer surgeons unlimited practice in a safe environment. Few resources are required compared to an animal or cadaver laboratory. Models and simulators are reproducible, and standardized curricula may be offered. Often very little supervision is required and trainees can participate according to their own schedules. Skills laboratories have become very popular among training institutions and will be the focus of this chapter.

II. BASIC SKILLS TRAINING

One of the most basic requirements of laparoscopic surgery is the ability to handle the instruments. As mentioned previously, the fulcrum effect and alterations in depth perception and tactile feedback make simple movements quite difficult for the novice. Laparoscopic dexterity is far from an innate ability. Instead, video-eye-hand coordination must be learned. With practice, movements become refined and performance improves.

A. Videotrainer

Several platforms have been developed to teach basic video-eye-hand coordination. One of these is known as a videotrainer (GEM, Karl Storz Endoscopy, Culver City, CA). The videotrainer (Fig. 1) consists of laparoscopic equipment combined with inanimate bench models. The laparoscopic equipment, including the instruments, the laparoscope, and the

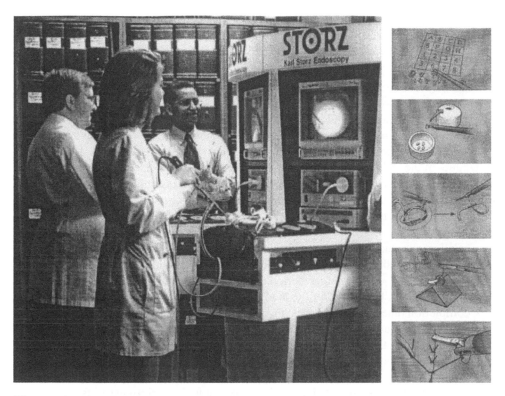

Figure 1 Southwestern Center for Minimally Invasive Surgery Guided Endoscopic Module (GEM). The videotrainer (GEM, Karl Storz Endoscopy, Culver City, CA) has six stations and may be used with the five tasks as shown. (From Scott et al., 2000a.)

imaging system, is identical to that used in the operating room. The bench models are usually basic dexterity drills, but can be based on organ models or specific operative procedures, as discussed below.

At the Southwestern Center for Minimally Invasive Surgery (SCMIS) at the University of Texas Southwestern Medical Center in Dallas, the curriculum has included five videotrainer tasks (Fig. 1). Some of these are modifications of tasks developed at Yale University by Rosser and at Washington University by Jones. The Checkerboard drill involves arranging 16 metal letters and numbers in the appropriate squares on a flat surface. The Bean Drop drill consists of individually grasping five beans and moving the beans 15 cm to place them in a 1 cm hole at the top of an elevated cup. The dominant hand is used to grasp the beans while the nondominant hand moves the laparoscope to provide adequate visualization during the procedure. The Running String drill mimics running bowel; two graspers are used to run a 140 cm string from one end to the other, grasping the string only at colored sections marked at 12 cm intervals. The Block Move drill consists of individually lifting four blocks using a curved needle (held in a grasper) to hook a metal loop on the top of each block. The dominant hand manipulates the grasper to move the blocks 15 cm and to lower them onto a designated space on a flat surface. The nondominant hand moves the laparoscope to provide adequate visualization during the procedure. The Suture Foam drill consists of using an Endostitch device (United States Surgical Corporation, Norwalk, CT) to suture two foam organs together and tie a single intracorporeal square knot. Tasks are scored on the basis of completion time, and a stopwatch is used.

Using these five videotrainer tasks, SCMIS designed a curriculum and performed a prospective randomized controlled trial to prove that basic skills training improved performance during actual operations. Residents trained for 30 minutes per day for 10 sessions over a 2-week period were compared to a control group, which consisted of residents who did not receive any training outside of the operating room. All residents were tested in the operating room during a laparoscopic cholecystectomy and were rated by blinded evaluators who used a global rating scale (developed by Reznick and colleagues at the University of Toronto). Data confirmed that residents who received basic skills training performed significantly better in the operating room than did the control group. This study validated the videotrainer curriculum as beneficial and worthwhile and definitively established the transferability link between the skills laboratory and the operating room.

Follow-up studies looked at the learning curve for the videotrainer tasks. The performance of second year medical students with second and third year residents were compared over a 2-week training period. Although the medical students had the worst initial performance, by the end of the study they outperformed the residents according to task completion times. In other words, the medical students seemed to gain the most from training. Medical students possibly were the most eager learners and had the most positive reinforcement, and therefore benefited the most from the same amount of training. An analysis of the learning curves revealed information about task repetitions and plateaus in performance. Generally, trainees reached a plateau in performance over the 2-week period and 32 repetitions corresponded to a 90th percentile in performance. Based on this information, SCMIS recommends practicing each of the five tasks at least 35 times and initiating skills training as early in residency as possible.

B. Virtual Reality Simulation

Similar to videotrainers, computer-based virtual reality simulators may be used for basic skill acquisition. The system most widely used at this time is the Minimally Invasive Surgical Trainer—Virtual Reality, or MIST VR system (Mentice, Inc., San Diego, CA). The MIST VR (Fig. 2) uses special software to create a virtual laparoscopic trainer on a personal computer. Laparoscopic instrument handles activate virtual instrument tips within the computer, and the trainee can play a laparoscopic "videogame." Six different tasks may be performed and include transferring, traversing, positioning, and cauterizing various targets in one-handed and two-handed configurations. According to the manufacturer, the tasks are based on coordinated movements required during laparoscopic cholecystectomy and are designed to provide the trainee with basic video-eye-hand coordination. The computer is programmed to alternate between dominant and nondominant hands and automatically records task completion time, errors, economy of motion, and economy of cautery. Thus, compared to the videotrainer, complete ambidexterity is required and additional measures of performance are generated. Also, the tasks are computer standardized, with exact start and stop endpoints and complete reproducibility. However, one of the major drawbacks of the current system is the total lack of tactile or haptic feedback. The system operates solely based on visual cues and does not provide any sense of "touch" or manual resistance. Further versions are planned to include computer-generated haptic feedback to overcome this shortcoming.

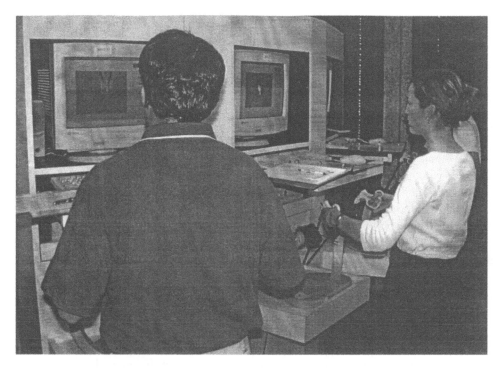

Figure 2 The MIST VR system uses a computer-based virtual reality platform to teach and test basic skills (Mentice, Inc., San Diego, CA).

Data generated from our laboratory as well as others indicate that the MIST VR effectively provides skills that translate to the operating room. At SCMIS, residents practiced on the MIST VR for 30 minutes per day for 10 days over at 2-week period. After training, a significant improvement in operative performance was detected during a laparoscopic cholecystectomy according to global rating scale data. Despite its effectiveness, residents seemed to prefer training on the videotrainer over the MIST VR during a head-to-head comparison. Reasons cited included that the videotrainer provided more realistic laparoscopic visualization, better depth perception, and better tactile feedback compared to the MIST VR. Technological improvements will undoubtedly improve these limitations. Furthermore, because MIST VR generates numerous objective performance measures, it may be well suited for testing purposes in addition to its role in training. Ultimately, there will likely be a role for both virtual and videotrainer-based formats; skills acquired on the two modalities seem complementary.

III. ADVANCED SKILLS TRAINING

Advanced skills are generally taught to midlevel and senior residents who have already mastered basic video-eye-hand coordination. Advanced skills include suturing, ultrasound, and specific operations. It may be very useful to combine skills training in advanced techniques with CD-ROMs, videotapes, lectures, and reading assignments so that cognitive components are taught simultaneously.

A. Suturing

Laparoscopic suturing is much more difficult than suturing during open operations, and the skills laboratory is well suited for acquisition of the necessary skills. A variety of techniques exist, including the use of a laparoscopic needle driver combined with a conventional suture using extracorporeal and intracorporeal knot-tying. Alternatively devices designed to make suturing easier, such as the Endostitch device (United States Surgical Corporation, Norwalk, CT) or the Suture Assistant device (Ethicon Endo-surgery, Cincinnati, OH), may be used. To facilitate practice, the videotrainer may be set up with foam or other props. Initial instruction may be given either by one-on-one tutorials, CD-ROM, or videotape. Significant practice is required to master the techniques, and trainees usually must spend a large amount of self-study time on the videotrainer before competency is achieved. In the very near future, virtual reality trainers will also have training modules for suturing.

B. Ultrasound

Surgeon-performed ultrasound, and specifically, laparoscopic ultrasound may be quite difficult for novices to learn. Curricula include ultrasound physics, orientation to instrumentation, and hands-on practice. Courses are routinely taught through the American College of Surgeons and may be quite useful as an introduction. To become proficient, time-consuming hands-on practice is essential. The skills laboratory can easily be set up to allow trainees to practice. An ultrasound system is required, and hands-on practice may be afforded by commercially available ultrasound phantoms. Such phantoms are the most popular choice, since they are reproducible and clean. Alternatively, animal organs may be used. The phantom can be placed within a videotrainer so that the laparoscopic ultrasound probe may be used. A picture-in-picture setup allows simultaneous viewing of the laparoscopic and ultrasound images. Trainees become familiar with scanning techniques and with recognition of abnormalities. Additionally, core needle biopsies may be performed and freehand biopsy techniques may be practiced. Ultrasound training curricula have been successfully introduced at the medical student level.

C. Specific Operations

One operation that has proven difficult to learn and amenable to simulation on the videotrainer is laparoscopic common bile duct exploration (Fig. 3). Trainees become familiar with the instrumentation and can practice stone retrieval using baskets, balloons, and a choledochoscope. Again, a picture-in-picture setup is useful. CD-ROM tutorials can be quite valuable in covering the indications and the technique.

Totally extraperitoneal (TEP) hernia repair has been effectively taught on a rubber simulator (Fig. 4), combined with a multimodality curriculum. The model consists of a removable insert, which represents the preperitoneal anatomy, including the iliac vessels, the inferior epigastric vessels, the gonadal vessels, and the vas deferens. There are three hernia defects demonstrated, including an indirect, a direct, and a femoral hernia. Trainees practice mesh insertion, positioning, and fixation using helical fasteners, and an adequate repair is verified. Once the repair is completed, the insert is removed and the helical fasteners are unscrewed to remove the mesh and allow for additional practice. We found that the simulator was durable and afforded excellent practice. In a prospective

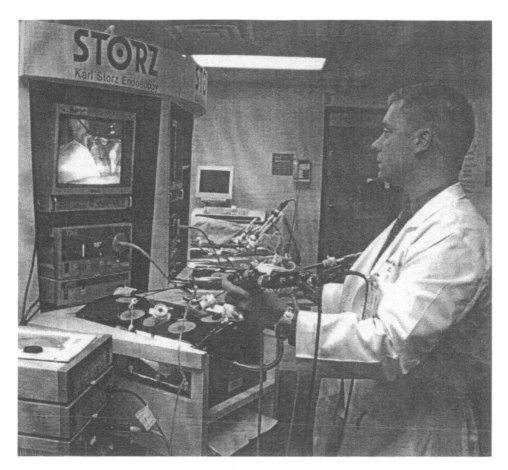

Figure 3 Common bile duct simulation using a rubber model (Cook Surgical, Bloomington, IN), a choledochoscope (Karl Storz Endoscopy, Culver City, CA), and the videotrainer (GEM, Karl Storz Endoscopy, Culver City, CA).

randomized controlled blinded trial, we demonstrated that the multimodality curriculum resulted in significant improvement in operative performance during an actual TEP procedure. Moreover, residents gained confidence in the operation and were much more likely to offer the procedure to their patients.

Other curricula have been described to teach advanced procedures using models. Most of these center around Nissen fundoplication, using anatomical rubber models for suturing practice. Intestinal anastamoses may also be practiced using models.

Although rubber models are useful and seem to be a valid teaching method, they inevitably require setup time and can be expensive. They are also limited in scope to a single procedure. A tremendous amount of space and resources would be required to establish a laboratory equipped to teach all advanced laparoscopic procedures using physical models. Virtual reality simulators are much more malleable and may be ideal for advanced training in specific procedures. Ideally, a single simulator could be programmed to replicate a wide range of anatomical models to allow practicing a variety of operations. Additionally, variations in anatomy and pathology could be incorporated into the models

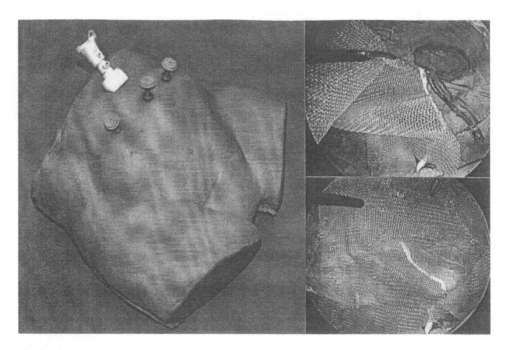

Figure 4   Totally extraperitoneal (TEP) laparoscopic hernia simulator (GSI, Cupertino, CA), which allows practice of mesh positioning and fixation. (From Hamilton et al., 2001.)

to simulate the variability encountered in real-life conditions. Similar to flight simulators for pilots, surgeons could be trained to overcome adversity in a variety of situations and to accomplish their mission safely. Such virtual surgical simulators are on the horizon, and in the very near future the skills laboratory will afford trainees the opportunity to practice numerous basic and advanced laparoscopic operations.

D.   Robotics

Computer-enhanced or robotic surgery is gaining tremendous popularity as the systems technologically evolve. Robotic surgery offers the advantages of tremor-free movement, motion scaling, surgeon comfort, and the potential for telesurgery. Moreover, by incorporating articulating effectors at the instrument tip, robotic systems currently offer two additional degrees of freedom compared to traditional laparoscopic instruments. Thus, surgeon performance may be enhanced by robotic systems, and operations that might not have been previously feasible using a minimally invasive approach may now be performed. Like any new system, additional training is required. Inanimate tasks in the skills laboratory may be easily set up to afford practice using the robotic systems. In the future, robotic systems or simulators to teach robotic surgery may be part of the skills laboratory. However, while an enabling technology, robotics does not ameliorate the importance of mastering advanced laparoscopic skills.

IV.   CURRENT STATUS AND FUTURE INVESTIGATION

Although technology is quite advanced compared to the early 1990s, when laparoscopy was initially gaining momentum, there is still considerable room for improvement in the simulation arena. One serious limitation is the lack of haptic (tactile) feedback in virtual reality trainers. Also, anatomical modeling seems rudimentary. Especially compared to commercially available videogames, the graphics on surgical simulators is lacking. As new technologies are introduced, simulators will rapidly improve. In the very near future, simulators will be available with high fidelity modeling, haptic feedback, and software to replicate numerous operations with scenario exercises.

As simulators become more widespread, cost will decrease and most residency programs will incorporate them as a routine part of training. Thus, residents will be afforded with much-needed additional practice in laparoscopic surgery. Similarly, community surgeons can stay up to date with new procedures by practicing them in the safe environment of the skills laboratory.

To realize these goals, curricula must be validated, means of assessment must be improved, and standards must be set. There is a national focus to ensure that surgeons in training and in practice are competent. The skills laboratory and surgical simulation will play a major role in assuring surgeon competency and reducing surgeon error.

V. TOP TEN TRAINING TIPS

1. Visit an established skills laboratory before getting started.
2. Start with the basics and work your way up.
3. Design a structured training curriculum.
4. Obtain support from your chairman and residency coordinator to endorse the curriculum and the concept of required training.
5. Allocate protected time for training.
6. Enlist help and make it a group effort.
7. Work with industry on helping to equip your laboratory.
8. Measure your results by performing assessments before and after training.
9. Publish your results—this is a relatively new field that needs ongoing validation.
10. Incorporate multiple modes of training, including CD-ROM, DVD, and videotapes, to augment skills training.

SELECTED READINGS

Bridges M, Diamond D. The financial impact of teaching surgical residents in the operating room. Am J Surg 1999; 177:28–32.

Derossis AM, Bothwell J, Sigman HH, Fried GM. The effect of practice on performance in a laparoscopic simulator. Surg Endosc 1998; 12:1117–1120.

Hamilton EC, Scott DJ, Kapoor A, Nwariaku F, Bergen PC, Rege RV, et al. Improving operative performance using a laparoscopic hernia simulator. Am J Surg 2001; 182:725–728.

Jones DB, Brewer JD, Soper NJ. The influence of three-dimensional video systems on laparoscopic task performance. Surg Laparosc Endosc 1996; 6:191–197.

Reznick R, Regehr G, MacRae H, Martin J. Testing technical skill via an innovative "bench station" examination. Am J Surg 1996; 173:226–230.

Rosser JC, Rosser LE, and Salvalgi RS. Skill acquisition and assessment for laparoscopic surgery. Arch Surg 1997; 132:200–204.

Scott DJ, Bergen PC, Rege RV, Laycock R, Tesfay ST, Valentine RJ, et al. Laparoscopic training on
    bench models: better and more cost effective than operating room experience? J Am Coll Surg
    2000a; 191:272–283.
Scott DJ, Valentine RJ, Bergen PC, Rege RV, Laycock R, Tesfay ST, et al. Evaluating surgical
    competency using ABSITE, skill testing, and intra-operative assessment. Surgery 2000b;
    128:613–622.
Scott DJ, Young WN, Tesfay ST, Frawley WH, Rege RV, Jones DB. Laparoscopic skills training.
    Am J Surg 2001; 182:137–142.

13

Surgical Robots, Telesurgery, and Future Technologies

CRAIG G. CHANG

University of Texas Southwestern Medical School
Dallas, Texas, U.S.A.

W. SCOTT MELVIN

Ohio State University
Columbus, Ohio, U.S.A.

I. INTRODUCTION

The last two decades have seen an exponential explosion in medical technology. In the early 1980s, laparoscopic cholecystectomy became widespread secondary to the advances in fiber optics and lens technology. New tools like the harmonic scalpel and endoscopic staplers allowed surgeons to perform increasingly complex procedures laparoscopically. Prior to 1990, Nissen fundoplications and gastric bypasses were not performed laparoscopically, whereas today, approximately 90% of Nissen fundoplications and 40% of gastric bypass are performed laparoscopically. In spite of these advances, the fundamental relationship between the surgeon and his or her tools did not change—the surgeon directly manipulated an instrument to effect a change in the patient's tissues. During the 1990's, this relationship changed dramatically on an experimental basis. Advances in robotics, communication, and computer software allowed surgeons to perform procedures without directly touching the patient. Today it is possible for a surgeon to perform a procedure halfway around the world with robotic assistance. Potential applications include performing procedures on patients in space (where the cost of return to earth would be prohibitive) and on wounded soldiers (where surgery on the battlefield might endanger the entire operating staff). This technology would also allow centralization—experts in certain disciplines could care for patients across the globe.

In order to better understand current advances in robotic surgery, one must understand the basic definitions. *Webster's Ninth New Collegiate Dictionary* defines a *robot* as "an automatic apparatus or device that performs functions ordinarily ascribed to human beings or operates with what appears to be almost human intelligence." With this definition, very few of the instruments used today would be classified as robots. Virtually all require some degree of programming and input by the operating surgeon. They lack the implied degree of automation. A better definition of a *surgical robot* would be a combined mechanical, electric, and computer system capable of performing complex operative tasks. Any robot will be comprised of multiple parts. The *manipulator* is the arm-like part that moves or holds another tool. The *end-effector* is the last link of the robot, which performs the desired task such as grasping or cutting. *Actuators* are the mechanical motors that move robotic joints or effectors. The *working envelope* is the range of motion of the manipulator.

Any complex robotic movement may be simplified to two elementary motions: rotational and translational. There is only one rotational movement—rotation on the axis, as in rotating a laparoscope (Fig. 1). The translational movements are pitch (superior-inferior), yaw (side-to-side), and insertion. The summation of these elementary motions is defined as the *degree of freedom* (dof). For example, the piston of a syringe has one dof (insertion/withdrawal) and the laparoscope has four dof (rotation, pitch, yaw, and insertion). The human arm has seven dof; the shoulder has three dof, the elbow has two dof, and the wrist has two dof. At least six dof are required for complete freedom of motion. A robot may acquire one more dof when the end-effector is included (e.g., grasping).

Surgical robots can assist the surgeon in a variety of tasks. They can perform repetitive motions automatically, thus relieving the surgeon of a tiring task (e.g., making

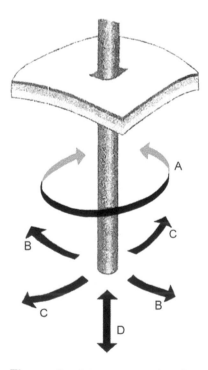

Figure 1   A laparoscope has four degrees of freedom: (A) rotation; (B) pitch; (C) yaw; (D) insertion. (Modified from Rassweiler et al., 2001.)

small increments of motion for diathermy of a region). They can position tools at a predefined location or move them through a complex trajectory. This requires accurate imaging of the target tissue and integrating this information with the robot. This process is called *registration*. Typically, computed tomography (CT) or magnetic resonance (MR) is used for imaging. The robot is then positioned around the patient according to external landmarks. If none exist, artificial markers such as small metal screws (*fiducials*) may be placed at the time of imaging.

Robotic procedures have the highest degree of precision and accuracy because they constrain the end effector to a preset path. However, they may limit the user's ability to modify the course of the task or procedure. Therefore, most "robots" in clinical practice fall under *computer-assisted surgery* (CAS). Here, the surgeon manipulates tools on a control unit, which converts the motion to a digital or electric signal. It then sends the signal to the surgical robot, which converts it back to a physical movement on the patient in real time. This is the basic principle of the master-slave manipulator.

II. INDIVIDUAL ROBOTS

A number of robotic systems are in use for other disciplines like neurosurgery, orthopedics, and urology. Most of these are highly specialized and limited to a single task. Therefore, they will not be discussed here. Instead, the "general purpose" robots that have been used across the surgical specialties will be discussed. These robots can be grouped as laparoscope holders and telesurgical systems.

A. Laparoscope Holders

Several FDA-approved passive mechanical devices have been developed for positioning of the endoscope (e.g., Leonard Arm, Leonard Medical, Inc., Huntington Valley, PA). The main benefit of these devices is that they reduce distractions to the operating surgeon by eliminating inadvertent and disorienting movements of a human assistant. While they are simple and cost-effective, they require the surgeon to manually reposition the instruments. As an alternative, Taylor et al. developed the LARS robot, a seven-dof device that holds and pivots the laparoscope about the point where it enters the abdominal wall. Though used in experimental settings, it has not gained significant clinical use. Begin and colleagues subsequently modified a commercially available A460 industrial robotic arm (CRS Plus Company, Toronto, Canada) to maneuver the laparoscope during cholecystectomies. Although the system was successful, it was limited by safety concerns.

AESOP (Automated Endoscopic System for Optimal Positioning, Computer Motion, Santa Barbara, CA) was the first robot to receive FDA approval for active control of the laparoscope. It is a seven-dof laparoscope holder which attaches to the OR table. It can be controlled with either a hand controller or voice commands. Typically it holds the laparoscope steadier than a human counterpart and reduces lens smearings. In addition, it restores complete control of the view to the surgeon. The latest version, AESOP-HR, allows the surgeon to define preset positions of the laparoscope. This allows the surgeon to move the scope between areas of interest quickly. AESOP-HR also has three speed settings enabling a surgeon to speed up or slow down the robot's movements dependent on the surgical application. It is compatible with most brands of endoscopes. It can accommodate rigid scope sizes from 2.9 to 11 mm in diameter with any angulation. There are two important safety features: two passive joints that prevent lateral forces from being applied to the abdominal wall and a magnetic collar that automatically uncouples the laparoscope if the applied force is greater than 4 lb. Previous concerns that AESOP would increase operating room setup time and expenses were addressed by Kavoussi et al., who determined that neither was increased. In contrast, robotic surgical assistants may be more economical for busy laparoscopic surgeons. The U.S. list price of AESOP is $80,000.

B. Telesurgical Systems

These are generally modular commercial systems that allow the surgeon to perform computer-assisted surgery. These are master-slave manipulators. The surgeon works at a console that is physically removed from the patient. Most clinical descriptions have placed the surgeon's console in the operating room with the patient (remote presence surgery), but the capability exists to place the console in another room or another country (*telepresence surgery*—see below). These telesurgical systems have several advantages. They facilitate a minimally invasive approach to cardiac, thoracic, abdominal, gynecological and urological procedures by magnifying the surgeon's view (as much as 15×). They can be scaled; a relatively large movement of the surgeon's hand is translated to a very small movement of the instrument within the patient. They tend to dampen out inadvertent hand tremors and thus allow more precise suture placement. They allow a single surgeon to manipulate multiple instruments. However, a well-trained surgical assistant is still needed to change the instruments on the robot and to assist if complications arise or mechanical malfunctions occur. The commercially available telesurgical systems are ZEUS and da Vinci.

The ZEUS Surgical System (Computer Motion, Santa Barbara, CA) consists of a surgeon control console and three table-mounted robotic arms (Fig. 2). The surgeon is seated in a high-backed chair and interfaces with two MicroWrists^{TM}. These devices are about the same size as standard Jackson Pratt suction bulbs. The surgeon has his primary viewing monitor directly in front. This monitor can provide a two- or three-dimensional view depending on the surgeon's preference. Secondary monitors provide vital signs/ telemetry readings and an alternate camera view. Finally, a touchscreen monitor allows the surgeon to modify settings such as movement response, wrist rotation, and yaw.

The right and left arms of ZEUS are intended to replicate the two arms of the surgeon by allowing independent operation of two surgical instruments. They provide five dof. The third arm manipulates the endoscope and is based on AESOP technology (see above). The instruments range in diameter from 3.5 to 5 mm. Many are articulated for greater freedom. All instruments are reusable. This system does not incorporate haptic technology (force feedback—see below).

ZEUS has already been used for cardiac, gynecological, urological, general surgical, and pediatric surgical procedures. The ZEUS system has received FDA clearance for the control of blunt dissectors, retractors, atraumatic graspers, and stabilizers during laparoscopic and thorascopic surgery. There are ongoing trials with general surgery procedures, coronary artery bypass, and thoracic procedures. The U.S. list price of ZEUS is $750,000.

The da Vinci Surgical System (Intuitive Surgical, Sunnyvale, CA) is composed of the surgeon control console and three cart-mounted arms (Fig. 3). The video images are gathered by an endoscope that contains two three-chip cameras and transmitted to separate monitors in the viewing section of the surgeon console. This restores a three-dimensional view of the field. The surgeon interfaces with Intuitive$^{®}$ master controls which are

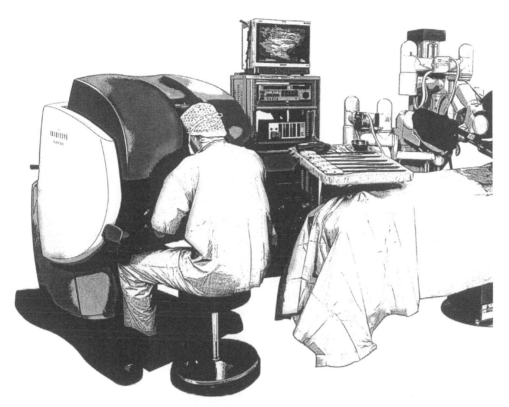

Figure 2   da Vinci telesurgical system.

ring-like devices through which the surgeon inserts his fingers. They are positioned below the viewing ports to minimize fatigue. The system has four foot pedals for actuation of instruments, camera manipulation, and focus control.

Two of the three robotic arms are designed for surgical manipulation. The third arm is used for camera control. The surgical arms provide three dof (pitch, yaw, and insertion). The end-effector at the tip of the instruments is a cable-driven mechanical wrist (EndoWrist™ Instrument), which adds three more dof plus actuation of the tool. The grip torque of the end-effector (i.e., needle-holder, DeBakey forceps) is programmed to 1.0 N. Monopolar and bipolar cautery can be applied to different tools with actuation by the foot pedal. All instruments are 10 mm in diameter.

Both da Vinci and ZEUS allow the user to scale the master-slave motion relationship. A motion scale of 3:1 would require 3 mm of movement at the master control to produce 1 mm of movement of the end effector. In addition, 6 Hz motion filters reduce unintended movements caused by human tremor. Finally, it is possible to disconnect the end-effectors from the manipulators while the position of the surgeons instruments remain unchanged (clutch function). This always allows an ergonomically optimized position for the surgeon.

The da Vinci system is FDA-cleared for laparoscopic, thoracoscopic, and prostate surgery. There are three ongoing cardiac trials: mitral valve repair, atrial septal defect repair, and coronary artery bypass graft. The retail cost of da Vinci is $1,000,000.

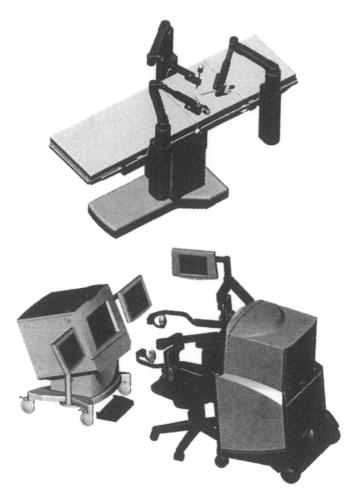

Figure 3 ZEUS telesurgical system.

III. TELESURGERY APPLICATIONS

Under the heading of telesurgery, there are several components (listed in increasing order of complexity and technical demands). *Teleconsultation* may involve transmission of still or video images for review by a remote specialist who then communicates his or her findings to the local surgeon (i.e., by telephone). This can be done with most internet connections. *Teleproctoring* utilizes a one-directional video and audio from the local operating room to the remote specialist. Its primary value lies in observing and evaluating another surgeon's performance. *Teleconferencing* requires uni- or bidirectional video and bidirectional audio communication. This requires a much higher rate of information transfer (bandwidth—discussed below). *Telementoring* involves active real-time teaching in addition to teleconferencing. Often the remote surgeon has control of the laparoscope and can guide the local surgeon to the area of interest. This interaction depends largely on the bidirectional, simultaneous transmission of video and audio signals and a frame rate high enough to allow a smooth picture. *Telepresence* surgery utilizes telecommunication lines or a satellite link to allow the surgeon to actually perform a procedure from a location physically removed from the operating theater.

Several significant technical barriers prevent broad application of these technologies. The greatest barrier is *bandwidth*, which is the amount of data that can be transmitted over a telecommunication line or satellite link. This is measured in bits per second (bps), kilobits per second (Kbps; 10^3 bps), or megabits per second (Mbps; 10^6 bps). Bandwidth varies among the different communication channels. An integrated services digital network (ISDN) line or standard phone line provides a bandwidth of 128 Kbps. A hardwired Trunk-1 (T1) line is a specialized internet connection that provides 1.544 Mbps. A cable modem potentially provides 2 Mbps. As an example of current bandwidth demands, it takes four ISDN lines to provide bidirectional teleconferencing with 300×300 pixel resolution and a standard 30 frames per second.

The data transferred for telepresence surgery include the video and audio signals in addition to the digital signals representing the surgeon's movements. Each signal will consume bandwidth, and thus, as one signal becomes more complex, there will be less "space" left on the communication line for others. For example, if the resolution of a monitor is increased, it will use a greater percent of the communication line and may delay the transfer audio and motion signals.

Another significant limitation is *latency* or *lag time*. This is the time difference from when an action occurs till the surgeon perceives it. For instance, when the Johns Hopkins group performed telementoring procedures between Baltimore and Singapore (9636 miles), there was an approximately 1 second time lag. As time lag increases toward one second, there is degradation in operator performance and increased operator frustration. Although lag time increases with distance, it is largely a function of the *compression-decompression* (CODEC) process. This is the process by which video, audio, and motion signals are converted to digital signals, compressed, and subsequently decompressed and converted back to their respective qualities. As the CODEC hardware and software improve, lag time can be expected to decrease. Lastly, lag time will be affected by bandwidth, as mentioned above.

Finally, *reliability* and *security* may limit telesurgical applications. There are multiple hardware and software components that must function seamlessly in addition to the communications link. Reliability of these components is critical for safe telepresence surgery. Security implies that the data transmission is not subject to tampering or interception. Medical confidentiality is dependent on security. Financial institutions have used encryption to solve this problem. However, encryption adds another layer of data processing, which may increase lag time.

Recently, some of these technical barriers have been overcome. In 1998, a team at Johns Hopkins performed a percutaneous nephrostomy on a patient in Rome, Italy (4500 miles from Baltimore). They utilized a single-purpose surgical robot known as PAKY (percutaneous access to the kidney). In September 2001, a French team of surgeons traveled to New York and utilized ZEUS to complete a laparoscopic cholecystectomy in Strasbourg, France (4000 miles). This became known as Operation Lindbergh. This procedure was notable for several reasons. It utilized much more sophisticated surgical equipment and thus required significant bandwidth. The connection was a fiberoptic link with a bandwidth of 10 Mbps. The CODEC process was optimized resulting in lag time of 150 ms, which represented a significant breakthrough.

IV. FUTURE TECHNOLOGIES

A. Haptic Feedback

This advanced technique involves transmitting force from the robot back to the surgeon's hands, allowing a simulated sense of touch or resistance. Several experimental devices are being refined. DAUM GhbH, Germany, has developed a three-fingered, wrist-articulated, seven-dof miniature laparoscopic hand (Endohand) to improve surgical dexterity. One version of this device allows the surgeon to manipulate a data glove, which transmits resistance back to the surgeon. Although this device falls short of natural tactile sensation, it holds promise in its ability to perform sophisticated maneuvers. The Stanford Research Institute has developed a two-arm, five-dof (four dof with actuation of the end effector) robot with force reflective manipulators and stereoscopic video. The resistance that the surgeon perceives is proportional to the force applied and the characteristics of the tissue. Investigators found that force feedback resulted in more rapid and accurate task completion and decreased operator fatigue. As these technologies are perfected, the remote surgeon will increasingly feel that he or she is encountering the patient directly. This sensation is called *surgical immersion.*

B. Deployable Robots

Experimental deployable devices are being evaluated that communicate with the master unit by radio frequency alone. One example is the colonic "inchworm" robot. This robot is used to inspect and sample the colon for disease. It advances up the colon like an inchworm—the proximal segment attaches to the colon and the distal segment then advances up to the proximal segment and anchors itself. The proximal segment then detaches and advances and the process repeats itself. One could envision this technology being applied to vascular disorders—the robot might perform a localized angioplasty or atherectomy.

C. Completely Robotic Surgery

Currently, all robotic systems require some degree of input or programming. When this registration process (see above) incorporates radiological images, it becomes significantly more complicated. In addition, registration requires "orienting" the robot to specific anatomical landmarks. Bone tends to be the best reference point as it is generally immobile. One example is the "Robodoc" hip surgery robot, which more accurately reams the femoral cavity for implantation of a hip prosthesis. A pin in the femoral head allows the robot to sense motion relative to the robot. Movement greater than 2 mm automatically halts the reaming process. Robodoc has shown improved prosthesis-to-bone contact. It is unclear at present whether this will translate into improved long-term prosthesis performance.

Robotic surgery of the soft tissues tends to be more difficult in that the soft tissues deform with manipulation. This would create error in the previous registration. As software becomes more sophisticated, it may become possible to "teach" the robot to adjust its course. Certainly, artificial intelligence will revolutionize all aspects of robotics and allow robots to function independently. They could then select the best treatment based on an analysis of current data.

D. Personal Status Monitors and Vehicle Status Monitors

In 1993 a consortium of industrial and academic institutions under the direction of the Department of Defense began structuring an optimized trauma system. This system utilized personal status monitors (PSMs) inconspicuously worn like a wristwatch to monitor variables such as heart rate, blood pressure, arterial oxygen saturation, and location (based on the global positioning system). PSMs would automatically report the individual's current data to the local EMS center by wireless radio-frequency communication (wireless LAN) if physiological deterioration were sensed. In addition, a vehicle status monitor (VSM) was constructed to sense vehicle deformation incurred during a collision. It would then relay this information and exact time and location of the accident to an EMS base station. Although these devices are not robotic, they utilize much of the same technology and rely heavily on high-speed communication. They hold promise for advancing surgical care.

E. Bandwidth Developments

Today, increasing numbers of options are available to private citizens and institutions to alleviate bandwidth limitations. Many individuals utilize digital subscriber lines (DSL), which allows simultaneous phone and internet usage. DSL is generally limited to a 14,000 ft radius from a substation because of degradation of the digital signal. Although asymmetrical DSL may download at speeds of 1.5 Mbps, upload may be limited to 384 Kbps. Newer options for institutional use include Trunk-3 (T3) lines with speeds of 44.75 Mbps. High cost makes individual use impractical. Fiberoptic technology holds promise for eliminating bandwidth and lag time problems. One strand of fiber may provide 1.1 Terabytes per second (1.1×10^9 bps). Fiberoptic communication could potentially eliminate most latency from CODEC (see above) as the optical signals do not require compression.

V. CONCLUSIONS

A recent review of robotic cardiac surgery quoted Mark Twain: "The man with a new idea is a crank until the idea succeeds." Twenty years ago, those who performed laparoscopic cholecystectomies were dismissed by the surgical community. Then those who performed laparoscopic Nissen fundoplications and gastric bypass were treated similarly. Now many regard robotic surgery as too complex or expensive. Even experts within the field are skeptical. Bowersox stated that "on the basis of our experiences with telesurgery, and a critical assessment of the clinical, technical, and logistical elements involved in trauma care, we believe that it is highly unlikely that remote surgery will be of value in future battlefields." Ultimately, the future will define whether today's researchers in robotics will be regarded as cranks or innovators.

ACKNOWLEDGMENT

Thanks to the staff at Computer Motion, Intuitive Surgical, and Electra Technologies (San Antonio, TX) for their technical review of this manuscript.

SELECTED READINGS

Cadeddu JA, Stoianovici D, Kavoussi LR. Robotic surgery in urology. Urol Clin North Am 1998; 25:75–85.

Davies B. A review of robotics in surgery. Proceedings of the Institution of Mechanical Engineers. Part H. J Eng Med 2000; 214(1): 129–140.

Lee B, Cadeddu JA, Stoianovici D, et al. Telemedicine and surgical robotics: urologic applications. Rev Urol 1999; 1:104–110.

Link RE, Schulam PG, Kavoussi LR. Telesurgery. Remote monitoring and assistance during laparoscopy. Urol Clin North Am 2000; 28(1):177–188.

Maniscalgo-Theberge ME, Elliott DC. Trauma care in the new millennium. Surg Clin North Am 1999; 79:1241–1248.

Rassweiler J, Binder J, Frede T. Robotic and telesurgery: will they change our future?. Curr Opin Urol 2001; 11(3):309–320.

14

Diagnostic Laparoscopy

LI ERN CHEN

Washington University School of Medicine
St. Louis, Missouri, U.S.A.

ROBERT K. MINKES

Louisiana State University
New Orleans, Louisiana, U.S.A.

For centuries, examination of the abdominal cavity and pelvis for diagnostic purposes has played an important role in medicine. Before the development of radiographic imaging techniques and laparoscopy, laparotomy provided the only means by which the abdominal and pelvic viscera could be inspected. In the early 1900s, George Kelling and Hans Jacobaeus successfully used endoscopes to diagnose diverse intra-abdominal pathology. Gynecologists recognized the utility of laparoscopy for diagnostic and therapeutic purposes in the 1960s and 1970s, but the use of diagnostic laparoscopy in the general surgery community began only after surgeons in France (1987) and the United States (1988) reported on the benefits of laparoscopic cholecystectomy.

I. INDICATIONS FOR DIAGNOSTIC LAPAROSCOPY

Diagnostic laparoscopy is being used with greater frequency in both elective and emergent settings and should be performed only if it is likely to affect patient management. Indications for diagnostic laparoscopy include the following:

Elective	*Emergent*
Assessment of chronic pain	Evaluation of acute abdominal pain/peritonitis
Evaluation of focal liver disease	
Evaluation of ascites of unknown cause	Blunt and penetrating trauma
Staging of malignancy	Evaluation of ICU patients
Workup for fever of unknown origin	
As a second-look procedure	
Evaluation for inguinal or ventral hernia	

The value of laparoscopy in the staging of malignancy has been well documented and is reviewed in a later chapter. Diagnostic laparoscopy is most commonly performed for inspection of the liver. Laparoscopy with guided needle biopsy is superior to blind percutaneous biopsy in the diagnosis of cirrhosis and may be performed under local anesthesia. Blind biopsy may cause injury to the liver and miss focal disease such as small metastases. Laparoscopy is indicated in the evaluation of ascites if radiographic evaluation and paracentesis fail to determine its cause. In many instances laparoscopy in patients with chronic pain syndromes may demonstrate an underlying cause (adhesions or malignancy).

Emergent laparoscopy can help to rule out an operable cause for acute abdominal pain or peritonitis. Use of laparoscopy can decrease the rate of negative laparotomy for questionable appendicitis. The use of laparoscopy is especially beneficial in young women who experience gynecological problems that may mimic appendicitis. In children with ill-defined abdominal pain, laparoscopy can be used to diagnose conditions such as appendicitis, cysts, Meckel's diverticula, or unappreciated hernias. In the intensive care unit (ICU), laparoscopy can prevent nontherapeutic operations in patients with a suspected abdominal catastrophe. Many centers use diagnostic laparoscopy for select patients to assist in the evaluation of blunt and penetrating trauma (see Chapter 13).

II. SURGICAL THERAPY

The preoperative preparation for diagnostic laparoscopy depends on the urgency of the procedure and follows principles outlined in other chapters. Diagnostic laparoscopy can be performed with local or general anesthesia using standard operating room set-up, patient set-up, port placement, and laparoscopic equipment. General anesthesia allows pain-free manipulation of inflamed tissues, biopsy of peritoneal lesions, and, if needed, rapid conversion to an open procedure. The following additional instruments may be needed to aid in exploration and tissue sampling and should be available:

    Angled laparoscope (30-degree)
    Scissors
    Grasping devices
    Liver retractor
    Blunt probe
    Babcock clamp
    Hook cautery
    Cupped forceps
    Biopsy forceps
    Uterine retractor
    Hollow suction/irrigation probe

III. TISSUE SAMPLING

Tissue sampling is an important aspect of diagnostic laparoscopy. For solid hepatic tumors, a Tru-cut biopsy usually provides sufficient tissue samples for diagnosis. Bleeding is controlled with direct pressure. Biopsy instruments can be passed under laparoscopic guidance percutaneously or through an accessory port. Small exophytic lesions can be sampled with punch forceps, an instrument with a cup-shaped blade that will biopsy a small tissue sample without tearing adjacent structures. Incisional biopsy may be needed for larger tissue samples. Hemostatic agents, electrocautery, and occasionally sutures may be required to control hemorrhage. Cysts may be aspirated with a needle, but at the risk that uncontrollable hemorrhage may result if the lesion is a hemangioma or is vascular in nature.

IV. SURGICAL TECHNIQUE

As with an open abdominal diagnostic procedure, a thorough and systematic laparoscopic exploration should be performed to evaluate the abdominal cavity and pelvis. A 5 mm laparoscope placed through a periumbilical port is sufficient for diagnostic purposes; a 10 mm laparoscope is used for therapeutic intervention. A second trocar can be inserted in the flank for adhesiolysis to facilitate a thorough exploration. A third port may be necessary if a second working instrument is needed to retract, palpate, or perform a biopsy. Gentle palpation with a blunt instrument can be valuable during exploration.

A. Pelvis

The pelvic viscera should be examined first. A Trendelenburg position of 30 or 40 degrees may aid in visualization of pelvic structures. In women, the ovaries, fallopian tubes, and uterus are inspected. A uterine manipulator can be used to elevate the uterus and improve access to the adnexa, cul-de-sac, and bladder. Normal ovaries are white, almond shaped, and measure $2 \times 3 \times 3$ cm. Ovaries should be inspected for torsion. Ovarian cysts may be identified. Large cysts may be decompressed with a needle prior to excision. If an ovarian malignancy is suspected, peritoneal washings should be obtained for cytological examination, and the contralateral ovary should be inspected. Salpingitis and early ectopic pregnancy may produce erythema and inflammation of the fallopian tubes. Depending on the stage, endometriosis may appear as red petechial lesions or have a cystic, dark brown, dark blue-black appearance. Uterine leiomyomata are firm gray masses that may be microscopic or may fill the abdominal cavity.

The pelvic floor should be inspected for hernias (see Chapter 21). An indirect hernia appears as a peritoneal defect lateral to the inferior epigastric vessels, whereas a direct defect is located medial to the inferior epigastric vessels. Bowel or bladder adjacent to the defect may represent incarceration. The bladder should be inspected for abnormalities and the sigmoid colon evaluated for diverticular disease, abscess, or tumor. Diverticuli appear as colonic outpouchings between the mesenteric and antimesenteric taeniae.

B. Midabdomen

With the patient in the neutral position, the anterior surface of the intestine, omentum, and stomach should then be examined. The appendix is located by following the taenia of the cecum proximally. In early appendicitis, the appendix may appear erythematous with engorged vessels or be covered by a fibrinopurulent exudate. A green-black focus of necrosis suggests a gangrenous appendix and impending perforation. Search for a Meckel's diverticulum warrants an inspection of the entire length of the small bowel since the diverticulum may occur 150 cm or more beyond the ileocecal valve.

Crohn's disease occurs in demarcated segments of bowel with skip areas and may produce mesenteric fat wrapping. The duodenum should be inspected for masses or perforation. A perforated duodenal ulcer may be covered with omentum and be overlooked. Intestinal ischemia produces a blue, dusky appearance of the bowel. An obstructing lesion of the small or large bowel can act as a transition point producing marked dilation of bowel proximal to the lesion and decompression of bowel distal to the lesion. A clear transition may be less evident if the lesion is only partially obstructing.

The small bowel mesentery should be inspected for defects that allow for a hernia. The mesentery should have a sufficiently broad base. A narrow base, as seen with intestinal rotation abnormalities, puts the patient at risk for a midgut volvulus.

C. Right Upper Quadrant

To examine the right upper quadrant the patient is placed in 30–40 degrees of reverse Trendelenburg position with rotation of the table to the patient's left. This maneuver allows the colon and duodenum to fall away from the edge of the liver. Normal liver appears reddish-brown with a smooth surface. Both lobes of the liver should be carefully examined and the falciform ligament inspected for pathology. Adhesions on the anterior liver surface may be caused by inflammation from Fitz-Hugh-Curtis syndrome. Fatty degeneration makes the liver appear yellow, whereas nodularity suggests cirrhosis. The size and pattern of regenerating nodules can help to determine the prognosis. Primary carcinoma of the liver may appear as single or multiple small nodular lesions and may be associated with widespread peritoneal metastases. Metastatic lesions typically appear as yellow, gray, or white nodules that feel solid. Palpation with a blunt instrument can demonstrate lesions within the liver parenchyma deep to the surface. For solid lesions either a biopsy should be performed with a cutting needle, cupped forceps, or cautery scissors or a needle aspiration should be performed to determine histology and cytology. Hemangiomas appear as bluish cystic lesions; a biopsy of these should never be performed because severe bleeding may ensue. Hepatic, pancreatic, and other lesions may be further evaluated by laparoscopic ultrasonography.

The gallbladder is located on the inferior surface of the liver and may be seen protruding beyond the edge; however, elevation of the liver and lysis of adhesions may be needed if it is not visible. The normal gallbladder has a shiny blue-green color. In acute cholecystitis the gallbladder can become tense, edematous, erythematous, and covered with a fibrinosuppurative exudate. The presence of adhesions surrounding a thickened, gray-white, tough gallbladder wall suggests chronic inflammation. Distal extrahepatic obstruction may cause a dilated gallbladder. A pale or opaque gallbladder may indicate chronic cholecystitis or a tumor. If indicated, laparoscopic cholecystostomy or cholecystectomy may be performed under the same anesthetic.

D. Left Upper Quadrant

The normal spleen is usually not seen and if it is visible, splenomegaly is often present. Inspection is improved with the patient in reverse Trendelenburg position and the table rotated to the right. Splenic biopsy is associated with increased risk of severe hemorrhage and warrants caution. The left hemidiaphragm can be inspected for hiatal hernia and esophageal varices. Inward bowing of the diaphragm may indicate a pneumothorax.

V. POSTOPERATIVE CARE

Postoperative care depends on the extent of the procedure performed. For uncomplicated procedures the patient can be observed overnight or discharged the same day. Common problems in the immediate postoperative period include urinary retention and nausea.

Antiemetics and analgesics can be used liberally. Patients can be given a clear liquid diet in the immediate postoperative period and resume a regular diet the following morning. Patients are not restricted physically and usually may resume normal activity within one week.

VI. DIAGNOSTIC LAPAROSCOPY IN THE INTENSIVE CARE UNIT

It is not unusual for critically ill patients to develop an intra-abdominal source of sepsis or an acute intra-abdominal process for which a general surgeon is consulted. Physical examination findings in this patient population are often equivocal and other techniques are required to evaluate the patient. ICU patients are frequently too unstable for transport and imaging cannot always be obtained. Furthermore, noninvasive imaging modalities are often nondiagnostic. Diagnostic laparoscopy may be useful in this setting.

Diagnostic laparoscopy may be performed at the bedside under local anesthesia. Sedation may be accomplished via an intravenous route. Close monitoring of cardiac and pulmonary status is mandatory. In a patient with adequate pulmonary function, intubation for laparoscopy alone is not a requirement.

Surgical technique does not differ in the ICU setting. Peritoneal fluid may be sent for cell count, gram stain and culture, and amylase levels. Abdominal processes that lend themselves to laparoscopic intervention can be managed at time of laparoscopy or a decision to undergo laparotomy may be made. In addition to avoiding unnecessary laparotomy, the advantages of diagnostic laparoscopy in this patient population include expedited diagnosis, minimization of patient transport, and obviating costs associated with operating room and anesthetic use.

VII. COMPLICATIONS

Intraoperative problems with diagnostic laparoscopy include complications of anesthesia or inadvertent perforation of a viscus or uncontrolled hemorrhage, either of which may require formal laparotomy. Cardiac or pulmonary complications can result from pneumoperitoneum. Nausea and shoulder pain can be encountered in the postoperative period.

VIII. OUTCOMES AND COSTS

A recent review suggests that the diagnostic success rate of laparoscopic examination for acute abdominal pain is 99%, chronic pain syndromes 70%, focal liver disease 95%, abdominal masses 95%, ascites 97%, and retroperitoneal disease 80%. Operative time and hospital stay depend on the underlying disease and need for therapeutic intervention.

IX. CURRENT STATUS AND FUTURE INVESTIGATION

While the value of laparoscopy for diagnosing intra-abdominal pathology in a variety of clinical settings is recognized, the current indications for laparoscopy in management algorithms are still evolving. Current patterns of use show the increasing role of diagnostic laparoscopy. As technology advances and the indications broaden, diagnostic laparoscopy can be expected to be used with greater frequency in the future.

X.　TOP TEN SURGICAL TIPS

1.　Develop a systematic approach to ensure a thorough laparoscopic abdominal exploration.
2.　Adjust the patient and table positions (head up, head down, left and right lateral rotation) to improve access to the area of interest.
3.　Skill at advanced laparoscopic techniques is essential when complications are encountered.
4.　Advance preparation for possible laparoscopic intervention or conversion to an open procedure is essential.
5.　An intraoperative consultation from a gynecologist should be considered if the ovary, fallopian tube, or uterus is abnormal at laparoscopy.
6.　Biopsy should be performed for most suspicious lesions.
7.　Avoid biopsy of vascular structures such as hemangiomas.
8.　Hemostatic agents such as Surgicel and thrombin should be available in the operating room.
9.　Nondiagnostic laparoscopic examinations can be expected.
10.　Laparoscopy should not be performed if open intervention is indicated for definitive treatment.

SELECTED READINGS

Boyce HW. Diagnostic laparoscopy in liver and biliary disease. Endoscopy 1992; 24:676–681.

Brandt CP, Priebe PP, Eckhauser ML. Diagnostic laparoscopy in the intensive care patient. Surg Endosc 1993; 7:168–172.

Easter DW, Cuschieri A, Nathanson LK, Lavelle-Jones M. The utility of diagnostic laparoscopy for abdominal disorders: audit of 120 patients. Arch Surg 1992; 127:379–383.

Kelly JJ, Puyana JC, Callery MP, Yood SM, Sandor A, Litwin DEM. The feasibility and accuracy of diagnostic laparoscopy in the septic ICU patient. Surg Endosc 2000; 14:617–621.

Nord HI, Boyd WP. Diagnostic laparoscopy. Endoscopy 1994; 26:26–133.

Pecoraro AP, Cacchione RN, Sayad P, Williams ME, Ferzli GS. The routine use of laparoscopy in the intensive care unit. Surg Endosc 2001; 15:638–641.

Salky B. Diagnostic laparoscopy. Surg Laparosc Endosc 1994; 3:132–134.

Sozuer EM, Bedirli A, Ulusal M, Kayhan E, Yilmaz Z. Laparoscopy for diagnosis and treatment of acute abdominal pain. J Laparoendosc Adv Surg Tech 2000; 10:203–207.

Walsh RM, Popovich MJ, Hoadly J. Bedside diagnostic laparoscopy and peritoneal lavage in the intensive care unit. Surg Endosc 1998; 12:1405–1409.

15

Laparoscopy in the Evaluation of Patients with Upper Gastrointestinal Malignancies

JASON B. FLEMING

University of Texas Southwestern Medical Center
Dallas, Texas, U.S.A.

Laparoscopy represents a valuable staging modality in many intra-abdominal malignancies. The primary advantage of laparoscopic staging is prevention of non-therapeutic laparotomy as most patients with intra-abdominal metastases do not benefit from resection, and the identification of metastases by laparoscopy can spare these patients the morbidity of laparotomy. However, the place of laparoscopy in the staging algorithm for patients with upper gastrointestinal malignancies is still evolving. This chapter proposes that staging laparoscopy is best applied to patients with upper gastrointestinal malignancies after conventional staging (imaging) has failed to identify distant metastasis and prior to the attempted resection of the primary tumor. This approach is supported by the fact that most esophageal, gastric, hepatobiliary, and pancreatic malignancies present at an advanced stage and the incidence of "occult" intra-abdominal metastases is high. Additionally, postoperative pain is minimized after diagnostic laparoscopy and time to additional therapy for these patients with advanced malignancy is less than after laparotomy. Lastly, therapeutic maneuvers including placement of vascular or enteral access devices can be performed at the time of staging examination. This chapter will outline the technique and application of laparoscopy in the staging of esophageal, gastric, pancreatic, and hepatobiliary malignancies as practiced at our institution and reported by others.

I. INDICATIONS AND CONTRAINDICATIONS

Specific indications for staging laparoscopy of upper gastrointestinal malignancies are currently not defined. The general purpose of staging laparoscopy in patients with upper gastrointestinal malignancies is to simulate the staging that is usually performed during laparotomy prior to resection of the tumor. When used in this manner, staging laparoscopy is best performed in those patients deemed to have resectable tumors by preoperative imaging criteria. This group benefits the most by the identification of previously unknown metastastic disease. The use of staging laparoscopy as a separate procedure or in conjunction with a planned open resection has not been clearly established. Our practice is to perform laparoscopy as a separate procedure for patients being enrolled in preoperative (neoadjuvant) treatment protocols, because pretreatment staging is critical. For example, patients with stage IV esophageal carcinoma would receive definitive external beam radiation (higher dose) for palliative control and not preoperative doses. On the other hand, patients for whom surgery is the first therapy receive laparoscopy after induction of anesthesia and prior to laparotomy. Others use laparoscopy as a separate procedure in all patients.

It is generally agreed that this procedure should not be used in place of standard noninvasive imaging procedures used for staging cancers in each disease site. The routine use of laparoscopy for all upper gastrointestinal malignancies is unproven and should not be performed outside of a trial setting. Similarly, staging laparoscopy should not be used in patients who could not undergo formal laparotomy, possess uncorrectable coagulopathies, or hemodynamic instability. Relative contraindications such as prior intra-abdominal surgery and cardiopulmonary comorbidities should be managed on an individual basis.

II. PATIENT PREPARATION AND OPERATING ROOM SETUP

Patients with upper gastrointestinal malignancies in which a resection of the primary tumor is planned are counseled regarding the potential risks and benefits of staging laparoscopy. Patients are informed that staging laparoscopy will be performed prior to laparotomy for resection of the tumor and that lesions suspicious for metastases found at laparoscopy will be biopsied and pathological examination performed. If metastasis is confirmed, a curative resection will likely not be performed, but palliative procedures will be carried out as indicated. These procedures may include placement of vascular or enteral access devices, gastrointestinal or biliary bypass procedures, or palliative tumor resection. It is important to note that patients and family are informed and consent obtained for *all* of these possibilities prior to the procedure. This allows the surgeon to use the information gathered at the time of laparoscopy to the patient's full advantage.

After induction of general endotracheal anesthesia, a Foley urinary catheter and orogastric tube is placed. Preoperative antibiotics are administered and sequential compression devices placed. The patient is placed in the supine position with arms at the side. The entire abdomen is prepped and draped as for a laparotomy. The operating table is equipped for multiplanar movement, and two monitors are positioned on swinging booms near the head of the table. If needed, the ultrasound monitor is placed across the table from the examiner. The light source, fiber optic videoscopic cable, and insufflation tubing are draped off the right side of the patient with electrocautery and suction/irrigation tubing off the left side.

A. Technique

At our institution the abdomen is accessed via the open Hasson cannula technique in the infra-umbilical position; using this technique, our injury rate is less than 1%. After documentation of intra-abdominal placement of the cannula by visual inspection with the camera, the abdomen is insufflated with CO_2 to 14–15 mmHg at a flow rate of 4–6 L/min. We use a 30 degree angled laparoscope as this affords improved visualization of the diaphragm and lesser omental bursa. Identified intraperitoneal adhesions are divided sharply under direct vision to allow access throughout the upper abdomen.

After pneumoperitoneum is established, a thorough examination of the abdominal cavity is conducted. The peritoneal surfaces are carefully inspected for any evidence of tumor implants, which often appear as dense white nodules distinct from the translucent shiny peritoneum. A distinctive feature of peritoneal metastases is a desmoplaastic reaction of surrounding tissues, which can assist in identification of metastatic deposits. Examination of the undersurfaces of the diaphragm is especially important and is best performed with the patient in the Trendelenburg position. Likewise, reverse Trendelenburg positioning is used for examination of the pelvis. Any ascetic fluid is collected by aspiration and submitted for cytological analysis. Access for abdominal exploration is achieved through two 10 mm ports placed in the left and right upper quadrant at sites two fingerbreadths below the costal margin as marked prior to insufflation. The 10 mm size allows for movement of the camera to separate sites and use of larger, less traumatic Endo-Babcock clamps. Any nodules identified are biopsied and submitted to the pathologist directly for frozen section analysis. The pathologist is instructed to determine if the nodules represent "cancer" or a benign process. The biopsies are submitted as they are removed to limit the amount of "downtime" during tissue processing.

B. Equipment

Necessary equipment includes:

> 0 and 30-degree angled laparoscope
> Cupped biopsy forceps
> 10/12 mm Babcock clamps
> Scissors
> 5 mm grasping devices
> Liver/uterine retractor
> Blunt probe
> 5 mm suction/irrigation probe
> 7.5 MHz laparoscopic ultrasound

III. SPECIFIC APPROACHES

A. Distal Esophageal Adenocarcinoma

Squamous esophageal carcinomas appear to have an almost negligible incidence of peritoneal metastases; this, of course, is in contrast to those tumors with adenocarcinoma histology, in which hepatic and peritoneal metastases occur in up to 40% of cases. The need for accurate staging of distal esophageal adenocarcinomas has arisen out of progress in curative and palliative care for this disease. Attempts at curative resection are reserved for patients without evidence of distant metastases, and selection of these patients for radical surgical resection can be enhanced with staging that is more accurate. Although laparoscopy does not replace preoperative imaging, the ability of computerized tomography (CT), magnetic resonance imaging (MRI), and endoscopic ultrasound (EUS) to assess locoregional and distant disease in esophageal tumors is limited and can be augmented by laparoscopy. Bonavina and colleagues report a sensitivity of 14% for ultrasound and 14% for CT in detecting peritoneal metastases compared to 71% for laparoscopy. False-negative rates for laparoscopy are reportedly in the 3–5% range. Several investigators have reported on the ability of laparoscopy to change the stage of disease, avoid nontherapeutic thoraco-abdominal explorations, and appropriately select patients for neoadjuvant treatment protocols and palliative therapy regimens.

Laparoscopic exploration of the abdomen is begun as described above to visualize any peritoneal or omental deposits and obtain biopsy specimens. In addition, evaluation of the liver and celiac nodal basin is important for staging lower esophageal adenocarcinoma. For examination of the liver, a laparoscopic ultrasound probe is inserted and the anterior liver parenchyma inspected for occult metastases. Using the ultrasound, each segment of the liver is identified by its associated vascular anatomy so that findings are well documented. Masses identified are biopsied with a transcutaneously placed Tru-cut biopsy needle under ultrasound guidance. For inspection of the caudate lobe of the liver, the left lobe of the liver is retracted anteriorly and the ultrasound probe placed in position. If necessary, the hepatogastric ligament is transected to allow greater exposure to the caudate lobe. For inspection of the upper lesser omental bursa, the left lobe of the liver is elevated and the stomach retracted caudally to expose the celiac region and the pancreas. Suspicious nodes encountered in this location should be biopsied as positive nodes in this region are considered distant metastases (stage IVA).

B. Gastric Cancer

Metastases are frequent in those patients who are unfortunate enough to develop gastric carcinoma, and potentially curative resection is possible in less than 50% of cases. Contrast upper gastrointestinal radiography (UGI) or upper endoscopy (EGD) is the usual method of diagnosing gastric cancer. After biopsy confirmation, EUS and CT scanning are used to provide staging information. Although accurate at determining tumor depth (T stage), the sensitivity of EUS in distant regional disease (N2 nodes) is limited. The ability of CT to detect hepatic metastases is well known; however, the ability of CT to detect N2 nodes (25–70%) and peritoneal carcinomatosis is less certain. Laparoscopy as an additive study in the evaluation and accurate staging of gastric cancer patients has been reported to result in a 90% or greater resectability rate for those patients who ultimately undergo laparotomy.

The techniques are similar to those for staging of distal esophageal adenocarcinoma with emphasis on examination of the celiac nodal basin and liver parenchyma. However, local peritoneal metastasis is the most common reason for falsely negative laparoscopy, and lesser sac visualization has been recommended to reduce the reported 4–6% false-negative rate. For examination of the lesser sac, the stomach is retracted anteriorly and the lesser sac entered through avascular portions of the greater omentum. A harmonic scalpel can assist in this approach but is not required. Once the space is entered, inspection of the pancreas and posterior serosal surface of stomach will allow for identification of otherwise occult local peritoneal metastases.

C. Pancreatic/Peripancreatic Malignancies

The terms peripancreatic and periampullary describe cancers arising within or adjacent to the pancreas and presenting with similar symptoms. Included are the distal common bile duct, duodenal, and pancreatic head lesions. Even when completely resected, peripancreatic tumors carry a poor overall prognosis, and the risks associated with surgical resection are high. However, the only known cure for these diseases is complete resection. Therefore, identifying patients with lesions that are resectable and derive the greatest survival benefit from surgery has remained a cornerstone of patient management. Improvements in CT technology have occurred simultaneously with the emergence of laparoscopy as a staging tool in pancreatic cancer. When high-quality CT is performed, the accuracy of radiographic prediction of pancreatic tumor resectability ranges from 75 to 89%, so that up to 25% of patients undergo a laparotomy for an unresectable pancreatic or peripancreatic neoplasm. The initial reports of laparoscopy in this setting resulted in resectability rates of greater than 90%. The improvement is largely due to the detection of small-volume peritoneal carcinomatosis missed by tomographic imaging.

Periampullary malignancies often extend locally along the superior mesenteric artery and vein, and this region is often difficult to image. In addition to the techniques described for other malignancies, inspection of the root of the small bowel mesentery and laparoscopic ultrasound examination of the pancreas should be performed during staging laparoscopy for pancreatic and peripancreatic neoplasms. To inspect the root of the small bowel mesentery, the greater omentum is retracted cranially; this will also retract the transverse colon and its mesentery. Using endo-Babcocks, the proximal jejunum is identified and retracted so as to identify the ligament of Treitz. This will allow visual inspection for tissue retraction or mass effect associated with tumor involvement at the root of the mesentery. Ultrasound examination can be a sensitive method to identify occult tumor invasion into the superior mesenteric or portal vein. Ultrasound examination of the pancreas is performed using a probe introduced through the right-sided 10 mm port. The probe can be placed on the stomach to provide a window to the head of the pancreas where the portal vessels can be evaluated by Doppler ultrasound. Alternatively, the lesser sac can be entered through the greater omentum and the ultrasound placed directly on the pancreatic neck over the superior mesenteric-portal vein confluence.

D. Hepatobiliary Malignancies

As with other upper gastrointestinal malignancies, surgical resection of malignancies affecting the liver is the only effective treatment with potential for definitive cure. The staging before laparotomy, however, is not completely accurate, and 20–50% patients with liver tumors assessed as potentially resectable by preoperative imaging staging are found to have advanced unresectable disease at laparotomy. The main findings resulting in tumor unresectability include extrahepatic disease (peritoneal and lymph node metastases), extensive liver involvement that prohibits resection (insufficient liver remnant), portal vein or inferior vena cava tumor thrombus, or invasion into adjacent organs. Primary liver lesions such as hepatocellular carcinoma frequently arise in a cirrhotic liver with diminished function and reserve. In these cases laparoscopy allows for accurate staging and biopsy examination of the proposed remnant liver if needed. In secondary (metastastic) liver lesions the aim of surgery is to completely excise the implants and preserve uninvolved parenchyma. Laparoscopy with ultrasound will define the extent of disease within the liver and throughout the abdomen. When used in primary and secondary hepatic lesions, laparoscopy determined unresectability in 48% of cases, and when combined with laparoscopic ultrasound, laparoscopy accurately predicted resectability in 93% of cases versus 58% when it was not used.

When laparoscopy is used in patients with secondary hepatic malignancies, nearly all these patients have had prior open abdominal procedures. Therefore, entering the abdomen via the classic infra-umbilical approach may not be possible. If so, the Hasson port may be placed at one of the lateral 10 mm port sites. An additional lateral port is then placed after insufflation, and the midline adhesions are carefully and sharply dissected so that a midline port can be placed. After inspection of the peritoneal surfaces, an additional right lateral port is placed for mobilization of the liver and hepatic ultrasound examination. First, the ultrasound is used to inspect the hepatoduodenal and hepatogastric ligament for suspicious lymph nodes, and these should be biopsied if found. Next, the portal vein should be examined with Doppler for evidence of thrombosis or tumor involvement. If no evidence of extrahepatic or vascular involvement is identified, the hepatic parenchyma is examined by ultrasound for the extent of disease. Using a fan retractor, the right lobe of the liver is retracted medially and the triangular ligament sharply incised; similarly, the falciform and left triangular ligaments are incised. This mobilization of the liver will greatly assist in ultrasound examination of the parenchyma without impacting open resection techniques.

IV. SUMMARY

This chapter has outlined the indications, timing, and methods for use of staging laparoscopy in the care of patients with upper gastrointestinal malignancies. The techniques described are not difficult to perform but, when applied systematically, can contribute much useful information. Using the approaches outlined here, our group has performed staging laparoscopy in over 150 patients with upper gastrointestinal cancer, and nearly all (97%) of these were successfully evaluated by laparoscopy. Of these patients, 19–36% were upstaged by laparoscopic identification of metastatic disease. This approach is well supported by many institutions and adds much to the selection of patients best suited for surgical resection of upper gastrointestinal malignancies.

SELECTED READINGS

Bonavina L, Incarbone R, Lattuada E, Segalin A, Cesana B, Peracchia A. Preoperative laparoscopy in management of patients with carcinoma of the esophagus and of the esophagogastric junction. J Surg Oncol 1997;65(3):171–174.

Burke EC, Karpeh MS, Conlon KC, Brennan MF. Laparoscopy in the management of gastric adenocarcinoma. Ann Surg 1997;225(3):262–267.

Conlon KC, Dougherty E, Klimstra DS, Coit DG, Turnbull AD, Brennan MF. The value of minimal access surgery in the staging of patients with potentially resectable peripancreatic malignancy. Ann Surg 1996;223(2):134–140.

Jarnagin WR, Bodniewicz J, Dougherty E, Conlon K, Blumgart LH, Fong Y. A prospective analysis of staging laparoscopy in patients with primary and secondary hepatobiliary malignancies. J Gastrointest Surg 2000;4(1):34–43.

John TG, Greig JD, Crosbie JL, Miles WF, Garden OJ. Superior staging of liver tumors with laparoscopy and laparoscopic ultrasound. Ann Surg 1994;226(6):711–719.

Stell DA, Carter CR, Stewart I, Anderson JR. Prospective comparison of laparoscopy, ultrasonography and computed tomography in the staging of gastric cancer. Br J Surg 1996;83(9):1260–1262.

16

Liver Surgery

JUSTIN S. WU

University of California, San Diego
San Diego, California, U.S.A.

JOHN J. GONZALEZ, JR.

University Health Science Center
San Antonio, Texas, U.S.A.

MORRIS E. FRANKLIN, JR.

University Health Science Center, Texas Endosurgery Institute
San Antonio, Texas, U.S.A.

ALLAN SIPERSTEIN

Cleveland Clinic Foundation
Cleveland, Ohio, U.S.A.

I. BRIEF HISTORY

Advances in laparoscopic abdominal surgery during the past decade have broadened its applications to include surgery of the liver. Most clinical laparoscopic hepatic procedures have been limited to diagnostic procedures such as laparoscopic-guided liver biopsies and small hepatic wedge resections. Recently, therapeutic laparoscopic liver operations have been performed with reports of treatment of biliary cysts (excision, evacuation, or marsupialization), hydatid cysts, cavernous hemangioma, and wedge resections of small primary or metastatic neoplastic lesions. With the innovations of laparoscopic cavitron ultrasonic surgical aspirator (CUSA) (Valleylab, Boulder, CO) and argon beam coagulator (ABC) (ConMed, Utica, NY), formal laparoscopic hepatic segmentectomies and lobectomies have now become feasible.

In 1992, Gagner et al. reported the first complex laparoscopic liver resection—hemisegmentectomy VI for a 6 cm focal nodular hyperplasia using an ultrasonic dissector, monopolar cautery, and clip appliers. Ferzli et al. in 1995 reported excision of an 8×9 cm segment IV hepatic adenoma using a CUSA and endoscopic vascular staplers. The first successful laparoscopic "anatomical" hepatectomy was reported in 1996 by Azagra et al. from Belgium, in which a left lateral "segmentectomy" (segments II and III) was performed in a woman with a benign adenoma. During the same year, three patients underwent attempted laparoscopic left lateral segmentectomies in Japan, one of which was converted to laparotomy due to uncontrollable bleeding. This group used both a laparoscopic CUSA and a microwave tissue coagulator and an ABC to achieve hemostasis.

We have tried using an abdominal lift device instead of creating a pneumo-peritoneum with CO_2 for two reasons: (1) to avoid rapid changes in pressure and visualization in a closed abdomen due to suction applied by the CUSA and the flow of argon gas by the ABC, and (2) to minimize the possibility of gas embolism. Ambient air pressures should lessen this latter risk if a hepatic vein is lacerated intraoperatively. The CUSA is a useful instrument when performing hepatic resections due to its tissue-selective feature, allowing fragmentation and aspiration of collagen-sparse tissues. The constant suctioning, however, may interfere with maintenance of a pneumoperitoneum and thus the surgeon's visibility during the operation. The ABC is also useful for hepatic resections, primarily for superficial hemostasis. However, the argon gas flows at the rate of 4 L/min into the peritoneal cavity, and thus can dangerously increase intra-abdominal pressures and potentially cause hemodynamic instability when CO_2 pneumoperitoneum is used. Nevertheless, a significant disadvantage of the abdominal lift device is that it creates a tent-shaped working cavity, rather than a dome-shaped cavity. The intra-abdominal organs are thus closer to laterally based port sites and may pose a slightly greater risk for iatrogenic injuries from laparoscopic instruments. More importantly, visibility and accessibility to liver segments can be impaired with the abdominal lift device. Furthermore, a recent report from Meyers et al. at the University of Massachusetts showed that the risk of significant embolus under conventional pneumoperitoneum is minimal during laparoscopic liver resections. Therefore, we use insufflation in all patients.

Simple hepatic cysts are amenable to laparoscopic cyst fenestration ("deroofing" or "unroofing"). These cysts usually contain clear serous fluid, since they do not communicate with the biliary tract. If the liver is polycystic, a hereditary autosomal-dominant disorder, multiple cyst fenestrations as initially proposed by Lin et al. in 1968 can also be performed laparoscopically. The risk of recurrence remains, as in open surgery, but reoperation would seem to be easier because of the presence of fewer intra-abdominal postoperative adhesions, compared to open hepatic cyst fenestrations.

The rationale for treatment of colorectal liver metastases with hepatic artery infusion chemotherapy is that hepatic metastases derive approximately 95% of their blood supply from the hepatic artery, instead of primarily from the portal vein as do normal hepatocytes. Therefore, a high concentration of drug, such as floxuridine (FUDR) or 5-fluorouracil (5-FU), can be delivered directly to the liver bed with maximal effect on the hepatic metastasis. Because of its first-pass hepatic extraction, systemic toxicity is minimized. The success of this route for delivering chemotherapy is dependent on complete perfusion of the liver while avoiding extrahepatic visceral perfusion. The laparoscopic approach provides an alternative to obtain this access and minimize the morbidity and mortality associated with standard laparotomy. Laparoscopic intra-arterial catheter placement is applicable to both metachronous lesions, avoiding a second laparotomy, and synchronous metastases during laparoscopic colorectal resection of the primary tumor.

Radiofrequency ablation (RFA) is becoming increasingly recognized as a new modality for the local control of primary and metastatic liver tumors. Radiofrequency electrical energy refers to an alternating electric current at a frequency of 400 MHz, which is the type used in conventional electrosurgical units. Conventional monopolar electrocautery units rely upon focal contact between the handpiece and tissues. Thermal ablation catheter acts more as an antenna to deliver the electrical energy to the surrounding tissues. When the tissue temperature rises above $45-50°C$, there is protein coagulation necrosis with resultant cell death. The first-generation thermal ablation technology (4- or 7-prong catheter, 50 W maximum power) allowed the ablation of 3.5–4 cm diameter spherical tumor tissue per cycle. The second-generation thermal ablation catheter deploys curved prongs into the tissue to deliver the electrical energy to a spherical volume of tissue with 5 cm diameter. The current generation thermal ablation catheter deploys prongs to incorporate a spherical volume of tissue with 7 cm diameter.

RFA was initiated in Europe in 1994, both in open surgical and percutaneous procedures. In 1994, Allan Siperstein at the University of California–San Francisco (UCSF) described the initial studies in the porcine model that led to the development of techniques for performing laparoscopic ultrasound-guided RFA in patients. Following FDA approval, Siperstein performed the first laparoscopic RFA in patients using a 3 cm probe in January 1996. Over a span of 44 months, a total of 88 cases were performed at UCSF. Since his arrival at Cleveland Clinic Foundation (CCF) in October 1999, Siperstein has treated over 200 cases in 3 years. A second clinical trial was initiated in January 2000 utilizing an improved 5 cm catheter. A third clinical trial utilizing the new 7 cm ablation catheter with the Starburst XLi RITA system (RITA Medical Systems, Inc., Mountain View, CA) was begun in October 2001. The RFA patient population at CCF include colorectal metastases (70%), neuroendocrine tumors (15%), hepatocellular carcinoma (10%), and miscellaneous tumors such as sarcomas, breast cancers, and melanoma.

II. CLINICAL PRESENTATION

The clinical presentation of patients with liver tumors or cysts is dependent on the underlying disease. Many patients are in fact asymptomatic, and liver tumors are discovered incidently during workup of gallbladder disease with an ultrasound, during surveillance abdominal computed tomography (CT) scans in patients with history of colon cancer, or during a CT scan or laparotomy for other reasons. Benign tumors of the liver make up only 5% of all tumors involving the liver (Table 1). In the unusual situation when the patient does present with symptoms, these are usually secondary to an abdominal mass, encroachment on adjacent structures (e.g., jaundice, gastric outlet obstruction), or abdominal pain as a result of stretching of Glisson's capsule. Patients with symptomatic liver malignancies such as hepatocellular carcinoma may have ascites and other manifestations of cirrhosis or chronic hepatitis. Patients with neuroendocrine metastases to the liver can present with symptoms of flushing, diaphoresis, palpitations, and diarrhea. Nonspecific symptoms due to malignant liver tumors include abdominal pain, weight loss, malaise, early satiety, jaundice, and anorexia.

III. DIAGNOSTIC TESTS

The tests required are those for the patient's underlying symptoms and disease. Laboratory data, specifically liver function tests, are usually within normal limits for most benign hepatic tumors. Tumor markers commonly associated with hepatic neoplasms, including carcinoembryonic antigen (CEA) for colorectal metastases and α-fetoprotein (AFP) levels for hepatocellular carcinoma, are usually elevated in the presence of malignancy. Almost

Table 1   Benign Tumors of the Liver

Epithelial tumors
  Hepatocellular
    Nodular transformation
    Focal nodular hyperplasia
    Hepatocellular adenoma
  Cholangiocellular
    Bile duct adenoma
    Biliary cystadenoma
Mesenchymal tumors
  Adipose tissue
    Lipoma
    Myelolipoma
  Muscle tissue
    Leiomyoma
  Blood vessels
    Infantile hemangioendothelioma
    Hemangioma

all patients will require a liver CT scan, triple phase (no contrast, arterial phase contrast, and venous phase contrast) with 7 mm slices. Ultrasonography may be of some utility in differentiating cysts from hemangiomas or more solid neoplasms. Magnetic resonance imaging (MRI) is also very sensitive for differentiating among adenomas, focal nodular hyperplasia, hemangiomas, and malignant neoplasms. ^{99m}Tc-labeled red blood cell flow studies and scintigrams are characteristic for hemangiomas. Ultrasound-guided or CT-guided biopsies are performed if diagnosis remains a question. The goal of these tests is to determine which tumors are benign versus malignant and also to determine which benign tumors have malignant potential that needs to be addressed. For laparoscopic hepatic arterial catheter placement, the authors' (J.G. and M.F.) first experience in 1993 was to obtain a preoperative arteriogram on these patients; since then, we have gained more experience with advanced laparoscopic techniques and are able to assess any abnormalities of the hepatic vasculature intraoperatively and have abandoned preoperative angiography.

IV.   MEDICAL THERAPY

Only a minority of patients with hepatic tumors are candidates for surgical therapy due to multifocal or extrahepatic disease or the patient's underlying medical condition. Chemotherapy remains the mainstay of treatment in patients with colorectal cancer metastatic to the liver, although few patients have significant palliative results. Hepatic artery infusion pumps and chemoembolization are also used in selected patients with colorectal metastases to the liver. In patients with hepatocellular carcinoma, the ability to perform surgical resection or deliver effective chemotherapy is often limited by the underlying cirrhosis. Patients with neuroendocrine tumors metastatic to the liver, from pancreatic islet cell cancer, carcinoid, or medullary thyroid cancer, typically have symptoms from hormone secretion rather than from mass effect of the tumors. Due to the multifocal nature of these metastases, few patients are candidates for resectional therapy. Somatostatin analogues may offer significant symptomatic benefit with little, if any, effect on tumor growth. Due to the slow-growing nature of these tumors, chemotherapy is rarely used, although their highly vascular nature offers a good response to hepatic artery embolization in many patients.

V. SURGICAL THERAPY

Complete surgical resection remains the standard of care in treating liver tumors. Liver surgery in general is considered to be technically difficult and tedious even if performed conventionally. The technical complexity of liver surgery, the risk of life-threatening bleeding, and the fear of gas embolism have prevented many surgeons from attempting laparoscopic liver surgery. However, a number of hepatic lesions do not require large and complex resections, but can be treated with relatively simple surgical interventions.

Not all patients are candidates for resection due to either advanced age, comorbid disease, compromised liver due to cirrhosis, hepatitis, or portal hypertension, postresection recurrence with decreased liver reserve, or extent of liver tumors (excessive number of hepatic tumors or hepatic tumors involving major blood vessels or bile duct bifurcation). Other surgical but less invasive procedures include cryoablation and RFA. Cryoablation may become obsolete secondary to RFA due to several reasons: it is more expensive, is more cumbersome to use, takes longer operative time to ablate tumors, has the potential for cracking the liver, and ablates normal liver tissue as well as tumors. In a comparison between cryoablation and RFA by Bilchik et al., cryoablation resulted in 800 mL of blood loss compared to 40 mL in the RFA group, and mean length of hospital stay for the cryoablation group was 8 days (including 2 days in the intensive care unit) versus 2 days for the RFA group. Furthermore, potential complications associated with cryoablation include coagulopathy (including DIC), thrombocytopenia, bile leak and fistulas, pleural effusions, hepatic abscess, and renal failure from myoglobinuria. Radiofrequency ablation can be performed percutaneously or surgically (either via a laparotomy or laparoscopically). Currently, laparoscopic RFA is becoming increasingly popular, with patients discharged after less than 24 hours.

VI. PREOPERATIVE PREPARATION

The benefits and risks of laparoscopic liver operation are discussed with the patient. As with other laparoscopic procedures, it is made clear that if at any point a laparoscopic operation cannot be continued safely, the operation will be converted to an open approach. Prophylactic antibiotics (second-generation cephalosporin and metronidazole) are administered preoperatively. Anesthesiologists must be aware of potential blood loss and the need for central monitoring and continuous blood pressure monitoring with central venous access and arterial line. Continuous electrocardiogram, pulse-oximetry, and end-tidal carbon dioxide monitoring are established as well. Patients should have blood available for transfusion during the liver resection, but not necessarily for the RFAs. The surgical team should always be prepared to convert to open laparotomy, especially in liver resections where hemorrhage remains a significant and potential complication. A nasogastric tube and a urinary catheter are inserted.

VII. OPERATING ROOM AND PATIENT SETUP

The surgeon stands at the patient's right side, and the assistant and the scrub nurse stand opposite the surgeon. Another option is to spread the legs of the patient apart and for the surgeon to stand between the legs, similar to the position for a Nissen fundoplication. Video monitors placed at either side of the head of the table are viewed easily by all members of the operating team. Special instruments include an angled (30° or 45°) telescope, atraumatic grasping forceps, atraumatic liver retracter, linear cutter/stapler, clips, and a suction/aspirator device. For resections, the laparoscopic CUSA and ABC are extremely important. For RFAs, temperature monitoring of the electrocautery pads is advocated to minimize the chance of a thermal injury at the grounding pad. With either procedure, laparoscopic ultrasound is absolutely required to fully assess the liver lesion, to assess the rest of the liver for additional lesions, and to assess the nearby vascular and biliary structures.

VIII. SURGICAL TECHNIQUE

A. Liver Resection

1. Port Placement and Exposure

Adequate pneumoperitoneum is achieved with either a closed or an open technique in the periumbilical location using CO_2 at 8–12 mmHg pressure. A minimum of four trocars is used, one at the umbilicus for the camera, two others right and left midabdomen (midclavicular line) as working ports for the surgeon, and another in the left upper quadrant for the assistant (irrigation, suction). A fifth trocar is optional in the epigastrium for the assistant to provide additional retraction. A sixth trocar is placed in the right upper quadrant for possible Pringle maneuver if bleeding becomes a problem during the liver resection. Trocars can be 5 or 10 mm in size; 10 mm trocars allow repositioning of the 10 mm laparoscopic ultrasound probe and the CUSA device.

The ligamentum teres and falciform ligament should be transected with the ultrasonic coagulating sheers (e.g., harmonic scalpel, Ethicon endo-surgery) to allow adequate exposure. Liver mobilization is key to any hepatic resection. The lesser omentum is incised with electrocautery or ultrasonic coagulating sheers. Division of the left triangular ligament is performed for lesions in the left lobe, and partial division of the right triangular ligament is for lesions in the right hepatic lobe. In the event of a major resection, it is necessary to be able to approach the side of the suprahepatic vena cava and the trifurcation of the hepatic veins, in particular the left hepatic vein.

2. Dissection and Resection: General Overview

Once the liver is completely mobilized, an ultrasound probe coupled with color Doppler will help define the anatomy and the relationship of the lesion to the surrounding vascular and biliary structures before an incision is made in Glisson's capsule. The planned resection is then demarcated on the liver surface with electrocautery. A 10 mm CUSA is convenient at this point, enabling parenchymatous pulverization while preserving the vasculo-biliary elements. Small intraparenchymal vessels up to 3 mm are easily coagulated and transected with this device. Larger vascular and biliary radicles must be clipped and transected with scissors. In the case of major vessels or biliary ducts, surgeons must not hesitate to resort to using extracorporeal ligatures or linear endostaplers. Finally, at the end of the operation the resected specimen should be removed in a bag that allows extraction without spillage.

3. Wedge Resections and Nonanatomical Resections

These resections are begun by incising Glisson's capsule 2 cm from the tumor. To evacuate the smoke for visibility, intermittent suctioning or slow continuous venting from one of the ports is necessary. The liver parenchyma is slowly dissected, with the edges of the liver being retracted by the assistant. This will create a groove in which coagulating scissors or the CUSA can be used in the working space. In the case of larger vessels, clips must be used. A double-clipping technique is recommended to avoid inadvertent avulsion of a single clip from the vascular pedicle. It is important to constantly have the assistant irrigate and aspirate in the deep groove of the liver to keep the operating field dry. Alternatively, the ultrasonic coagulating sheers can be used for hepatic parenchymal dissection. Once the dissection is complete, hemostasis is achieved with the ABC. Fibrin glue may also be placed on the transected surface of the liver. In cases of small tumor wedge resections, drainage is not necessary. In cases of larger wedge resections, routine cholangiography is recommended to identify possible biliary leaks. Small bile leaks from the transected surface of the liver can be oversewn. A drain is placed through one of the lateral port site as the trocar is subsequently removed.

4. Left Lateral Segmentectomy and Left Hepatic Lobectomy

The porta hepatis is dissected to allow a vessel loop or a laparoscopic clamp across the structure for possible Pringle maneuver in case of hemorrhage during the liver resection. Intermittent clamping (10-minute clamping with 5-minute release periods can limit the ischemia to the liver). Suprahepatic inferior vena cava and the left hepatic vein are bluntly dissected; a clamp or a vessel loop through the epigastric port can provide temporary occlusion during the parenchyma dissection to minimize backbleeding. For the left lateral segmentectomy, instead of a Pringle maneuver, specific inflow occlusion can be provided through the umbilical portion of the Glisson's capsule; the bridge of the parenchyma between segments III and IV is fractured so that the umbilical fissure is exposed. The branches of the arteries and portal vein as well as the biliary radicles feeding the left lateral segment (segments II and III) are divided between clips or ties. For a formal left hepatic lobectomy, specific inflow occlusion is provided by dissecting and ligating left portal vein and left hepatic artery, as well as ligating the left hepatic duct. Intracorporeal or extracorporeal ties are recommended, although a vascular stapler can be used for the left portal vein transection. Prior to the porta hepatis dissection, a cholecystectomy is performed in case of a formal left hepatic lobectomy. The dissection of the left lateral segment or left hepatic lobe is then carried out with the CUSA, clips, scissors, electrocautery, and ultrasonic coagulating sheers described previously. The main left hepatic vein (or left hepatic vein and middle hepatic vein confluence) is divided with a vascular stapler. The raw hepatic surface is inspected, and hemostasis is achieved with the ABC and/or fibrin glue. The greater omentum can also be used to cover the raw surface of the liver. A cholangiogram is performed selectively after left hepatic lobectomy or left lateral segmentectomy. One or two suction drains are placed near the edge of the transected liver. The resected specimen should be removed through a plastic bag for oncological purposes; this can be performed by extending the umbilical port site to 6–8 cm. If the lesion is benign, then morcellation of the specimen in the plastic bag allows extraction through a smaller abdominal incision.

5.   Right Hepatic Lobectomy

Once mobilization of the liver is provided by taking down the round, falciform, right triangular and coronary ligaments, the right liver is further mobilized by dissecting into the bare space between the diaphragm and the posterior aspect of the liver. This maneuver can be helped by prior positioning of the patient slightly in a left lateral decubitus position rather than completely supine. The suprahepatic inferior vena cava and the right hepatic vein are dissected bluntly. A vessel loop or a clamp through the epigastric port can provide temporary occlusion during the parenchyma dissection to minimize backbleeding. Inflow occlusion is provided by a Pringle clamp described previously. Selective inflow occlusion can be performed by dissecting the porta hepatis and selectively ligating and dividing the right hepatic artery and right portal vein. The right hepatic duct is then ligated and divided in a similar fashion. Prior to the porta hepatis dissection, the gallbladder should be removed and the Calot's triangle dissection performed, following the course of the cystic duct and artery to the common bile duct and the hepatic artery. After this stage, many authors convert the procedure to a laparoscopic-assisted procedure, using a 6 cm upper midline minilaparotomy to avoid the danger of gas embolism, although some authors have performed this procedure completely laparoscopically without complications. The line of transection is scored on the Glisson's capsule with electrocautery. The dissection of the liver parenchyma is then performed using the CUSA, clips, scissors, electrocautery, and ultrasonic coagulating shears described previously. The main right hepatic vein is divided with a vascular stapler either prior to liver parenchyma transection or at the end of the liver transection. The raw hepatic surface is inspected and hemostasis is achieved with the ABC and/or fibrin glue. The greater omentum can be used to cover the raw surface of the liver. A cholangiogram should be performed routinely to assess the intact left biliary system and to assure there are no bile leaks. One or two suction drains are placed adjacent to the transected liver. The resected specimen should be removed through a plastic bag for oncological purposes; this can be performed by extending the umbilical port site to 8 cm. If the lesion is benign, then morcellation of the specimen in the plastic bag allows extraction through a smaller abdominal incision.

B.   Hepatic Cyst Fenestration

1.   Port Placement and Exposure

Adequate pneumoperitoneum is achieved with either a closed or open technique in the periumbilical region using CO_2 at 15 mmHg pressure; a 5 mm trocar is placed to allow a 5 mm laparoscope. Two working trocars, both 5 mm, are placed in the right and left midabdomen, in the midclavicular line. A fourth trocar is optional; this is a 5 mm port in the left upper quadrant for the assistant to provide irrigation, aspiration, or retraction if necessary.

2.   Liver Cyst Unroofing

Hepatic cysts are easily identified laparoscopically; these are usually simple thin cysts protruding at the surface of the liver containing serous fluid, thus giving it a mild bluish hue appearance. For cysts on the right lateral aspect of the liver, the patient should be placed in a slight left lateral decubitous position and the surgeon can mobilize the right hepatic lobe to aid in visualizing the cysts. Laparoscopic ultrasound can be used to define the extent of the cyst involving the liver, to detect any additional cysts not easily seen on the surface, and to identify and avoid adjacent vascular or biliary structures. One of the

5 mm trocar must be replaced by a 10 mm trocar in order to accommodate the laparoscopic ultrasound probe.

The thin convex cyst wall is opened with electrocautery, curved scissors or hook. The ultrasonic coagulating shears may be used as well, especially if the excision extends through the liver parenchyma. A suction device is used to aspirate the serous fluid from within the cyst cavity. Once the cyst collapses, the wall of the cyst is grasped and excised. It is essential that as much of the exposed cyst wall as possible be excised to prevent resealing of the wall and hence recurrence of the cyst. For very large cysts, recurrence may be lessened by using clips to fix a pedicle of omentum with the cyst. The cyst wall should be sent to pathology for frozen section examination. If a cystic neoplasm is encountered, then excision of the entire cyst wall, not fenestration, is indicated. For deep intra-parenchymal cysts, one can often gain access through a previously fenestrated cyst cavity, i.e., "transcystic fenestration." This maneuver can be repeated for multiple cysts until all are opened, drained, and excised as much as possible.

C. Hepatic Artery Catheter

1. Port Placement and Exposure

The abdomen is insufflated by a Veress needle to 14 mmHg, followed by placement of a 5 mm trocar in the left midabdomen. Subsequent trocars are placed under direct vision (Fig. 1). A thorough inspection of the peritoneal cavity is performed. Biopsy of any

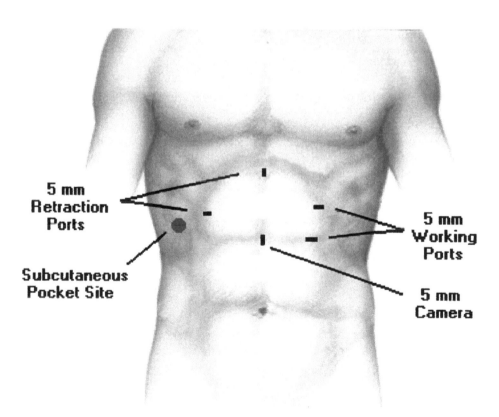

Figure 1 Trocar placement for laparoscopic hepatic artery catheter placement.

suspicious tissue or confirmation of liver metastases is performed and sent for frozen section pathological examination if indicated. The patient is then put in reverse Trendelenburg to improve exposure to the right upper quadrant.

2. Localization of Gastroduodenal Artery

Localization of the gastroduodenal artery is best accomplished at the hepatoduodenal ligament. Caudal traction at the pylorus with countertraction towards the right shoulder using the gallbladder facilitates this maneuver. Sharp and blunt dissection through the peritoneum usually produces the gastroduodenal artery as it runs behind the first portion of the duodenum. The artery is isolated distally, where it disappears behind the duodenal wall. Further dissection is made cephalad until the right-angle junction of the gastroduodenal artery with the common hepatic artery is identified. All collateral vessels to the duodenum and pancreas branching off the gastroduodenal artery in the isolated segment are identified and divided between clips or electrocoagulated. This step is crucial so as to avoid chemical inflammation of these organs during perfusion of the chemotherapeutic agent. The gastroduodenal artery is then ligated with a 2-0 silk tie or clipped distally while double-looping a silk tie around the proximal portion of the vessel to provide physical countertraction and to act as a tourniquet. This suture is also used to anchor the inserted catheter at the conclusion of the procedure. Laparoscopic vascular bulldog clamps are then applied to the most proximal visualized portion of the proper hepatic artery and the most distal visualized portion of the common hepatic artery to prevent bleeding from the gastroduodenal artery at the time of arteriotomy or insertion of the catheter.

3. Catheter Placement

Once the gastroduodenal artery has been isolated, an arterial access system with pre-attached 7 French beaded silicone catheter (Macroport Arterial Access System, Horizon Medical Products, Inc., Manchester, GA) is flushed with heparinized saline and introduced into the abdomen through a predetermined site in the right flank. Gentle upward traction is applied to the double-looped silk tie to expose the gastroduodenal artery. A small transverse arteriotomy is made in the artery approximately 1 cm distal to its junction with the common hepatic artery. The arterial catheter is then directed into the arteriotomy and gingerly advanced towards the common hepatic artery as the retraction on the double-looped silk tie is relaxed to ease its passage. The previously tailored catheter tip should lie below the junction of the gastroduodenal and hepatic arteries without extending into the lumen of the hepatic artery. The catheter is then secured by tying the previously placed sutures below the silicone bead to prevent retrograde catheter displacement. One additional suture is placed and secured intracorporeally to the duodenal serosa as an anchoring stitch. The reservoir end of the system is brought out through the previously selected point of the anterior abdominal wall where a subcutaneous pocket is fashioned. The Macroport is placed within the pocket and sutured securely in place. The laparoscopic bulldog clamps are then removed and the area inspected for bleeding.

Correct placement is then evaluated by slowly infusing 5 cc of methylene blue through the catheter. It is important not to infuse with too much pressure so as to avoid retrograde perfusion of the methylene blue. If placement is correct and there are no aberrant or replaced hepatic arteries, the liver should appear homogeneously stained blue in both lobes. If other organs such as the stomach or duodenum stain blue, visceral branches off the proper hepatic artery require ligation. If only one lobe of the liver is stained blue, there is an aberrant or replaced hepatic artery to the unstained lobe that must be identified and ligated.

Once the hepatic artery catheter is placed, we routinely perform a standard laparoscopic cholecystectomy with intraoperative cholangiogram to avoid the potential risk of hepatic artery chemotherapy-induced cholecystitis, which has been reported in 20–30% of patients. Finally, the omentum is brought up and securely interpositioned between the catheter and the duodenum to help protect against erosion of the catheter into the duodenum.

D. Radiofrequency Ablation

1. Port Placement and Exposure

Most patients are positioned in the supine position; however, selected patients with disease limited to the right posterior segments of the liver are treated in the left decubitus position with the table slightly flexed. Two right subcostal 10 mm ports are placed; occasionally additional trocars are necessary to be able to mobilize the liver adequately in patient with adhesions. The 10 mm ports allow the 10 mm laparoscope and the laparoscopic ultrasound probe to be used interchangeably between the ports. Placement of an umbilical trocar is not useful, as the camera or the laparoscopic ultrasound transducer cannot reach the dome of the liver. The anterior and lateral aspects of the liver are mobilized. It is rarely necessary to take down the falciform ligament or triangular ligaments. Viscera within 2 cm of an intended ablation zone require mobilization from the liver if they are adherent because of prior surgical procedures. Similarly, if lesions encroach upon the gallbladder fossa, laparoscopic cholecystectomy is warranted to avoid thermal ablation of the wall of the gallbladder with delayed bile leakage.

Laparoscopic ultrasound examination is performed of the entire liver parenchyma using a 7.5 MHz rigid ultrasound transducer. The portal and hepatic vein branches can be traced easily to assign a liver segment to each of the lesions treated. Occasional patients will require the use of a flexible ultrasound transducer to image the most cephalad portion of segments 4, 7, and 8. In order to coordinate the movement of the laparoscopic ultrasound transducer with the laparoscopic image, it is found most convenient to use a picture-in-picture box to superimpose a quarter-sized laparoscopic image over the full-sized ultrasound image, making it much easier to coordinate the movement of the instruments. Once all the hepatic lesions are identified and their size measured, color-flow Doppler is performed to assess tumor vascularity. With some tumors, discrete feeding vessels can be identified and this region should be ablated first to facilitate subsequent ablations.

Under ultrasound guidance, 18-gauge core biopsies are performed with a spring-loaded biopsy gun. The biopsy needle is placed into the abdominal cavity through a percutaneous approach and does not require the placement of an additional trocar. The path of the needle is parallel to the plane of the ultrasound so that the entire path can be seen on the ultrasound image as it traverses the liver parenchyma. The tip of the biopsy needle is then positioned at the periphery of the tumor and the trigger is fired. Care is taken to study the 2 cm throw length of the biopsy device before firing to ensure that major hepatic vasculature or extrahepatic structures are not injured. The ablation catheter is then passed using an identical technique. Using the new-generation RITA Starburst XL or XLi catheter (RITA Medical Systems, Inc., Mountain View, CA), a single cycle of ablation can be performed achieving an ablation diameter of 5 or 7 cm in diameter, respectively.

2. Liver Tumor Ablation

With the current RITA Starburst XL 9 prong, 5 cm diameter ablation catheter (Fig. 2) and the RITA model 1500 generator (Fig. 3), a maximum of 150 W of power is delivered until thermocouple temperature at the tip of the prongs equals 105°C. For a 5 cm ablation zone, the power is automatically regulated to maintain this temperature for 20–25 minutes in various deployment lengths. It generally takes a few minutes to reach the target temperature, so the actual ablation cycle takes a little longer than 20–25 minutes. As the metal electrode is 20–30°C hotter than the surrounding tissue, a 30-second cooling-down time after ablation is used to measure the actual tissue temperature at the periphery of the ablated zone. The formation of the lesions is monitored by laparoscopic ultrasound. The lesions are visible on ultrasound due to microbubble formation in the heated tissue and closely correlate to the zone of kill. A 1 cm margin of normal tissue surrounding the tumor is ablated as well, which is the accepted margin for all lesions. Great care is required to position the tip of the ablation catheter precisely in the geometric center of the tumor so that the ablated zone completely encompasses the tumor. With the 5 cm diameter catheter, for lesions larger than 4 cm in diameter, overlapping thermal ablations zones are required to ensure an adequate volume of ablation.

To create a 5 cm zone of ablation, the prongs from the ablation catheters are initially deployed to 2 cm and the device is activated. Once the target temperature of 105°C is reached, which takes approximately 2–3 minutes, the prongs are deployed to 3 cm. Again, once the target temperature is reached, the prongs are deployed to 4 cm, whereupon the

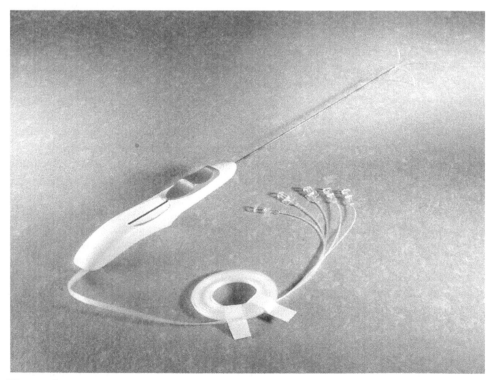

Figure 2   RITA Starburst XLi 9 prong 7 cm ablation catheter.

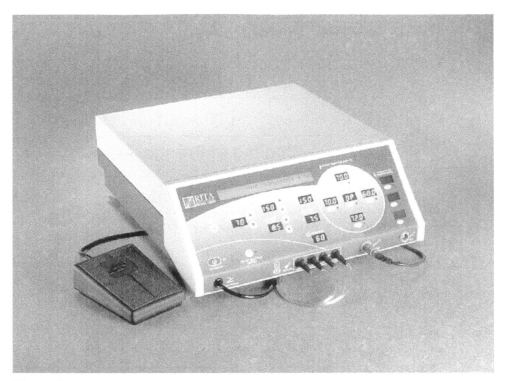

Figure 3 RITA 1500 model generator.

ablation occurs for 7 minutes at target temperature. The prongs are then deployed to 5 cm and the lesion is ablated for another 7 minutes at target temperature (Fig. 4). Thus, the overall process for ablating a 5 cm lesion takes about 20 minutes. Once the delivery of power is stopped, the monitoring of the thermocouple temperatures is continued. These are seen to drop rapidly over the first 10–20 seconds as the temperature of the metal prongs decrease by 20–30°C to equilibrate within the surrounding tissue. The temperatures then decrease at a slower rate as heat is dissipated from the zone of ablation. Thermocouple

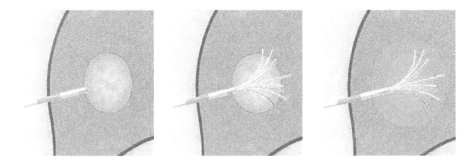

Figure 4 Deployment of radiofrequency ablation catheter into liver tumor with zone of ablation.

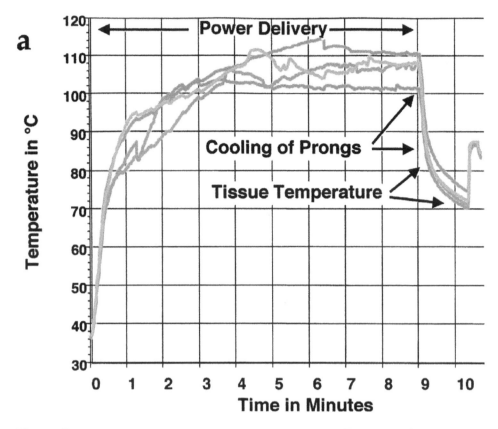

Figure 5 Temperature profile during the ablation process. Thermocouple temperatures increase over 1–2 minutes to an average target temperature of 105°C. This is held for 5–7 minutes to complete the ablation cycle. Once the power is turned off, temperature in the thermocouples cools rapidly to equilibrate with the surrounding tissues. Tissue temperatures of 60–70°C 1 minute after ablation indicate that lethal tissue temperatures have been achieved.

temperatures in the 60–70°C range 30 seconds after the ablation process has ceased indicates that a successful ablation has been performed (Fig. 5). If there are any questions as to the technical adequacy of the ablation, the prongs can be pulled back into the catheter, the catheter is rotated 45°, and the prongs are then redeployed into what had previously been determined in animal studies to be the coolest point of the ablated zone. If thermocouple temperatures at this location are above 60°C, this is interpreted as an adequate ablation. If not, an additional cycle is to be performed with the catheter in this position.

For 7 cm lesions using the XLi catheter, similar technique is applied, except that a continuous 5% hypertonic saline infusion using the Harvard 5-syringe pump is incorporated to the RITA Starburst XLi ablation catheter system (RITA Medical Systems, Inc., Mountain View, CA). This device uses five prongs that deliver the electrical energy and hypertonic saline (that prevents overheating of the electrodes and acts as a conductor to increase their effective size). Four additional prongs are used for temperature monitoring of the periphery of the ablation zone. The prongs are deployed 2 cm into the tumor and ablated until target temperature of 100°C is reached, then deployed to 4 cm until the temperature reaches 90°C, then 5 cm until the temperature is 80°C, then 6 cm until the temperature is 70°C, and finally 7 cm until the temperature is 60°C. During these ablations, the 5% hypertonic saline should be infusing at 0.1 mL/min through five of the nine prongs. When the ablation catheter is introduced into the liver prior to deployment of the prongs, the saline should be infusing at 0.075 mL/min. Due to the increased conductivity provided by the hypertonic saline drip, the ablation grows very quickly at the infusion sites, creating five ablation "balls" that eventually coalesce, grow out toward the passive thermocouples, and fill the targeted site on the liver. All saline infusion should be stopped during track ablation as the catheter is withdrawn from the liver lesion.

Assessment of the ablation process in the operating room is performed in three ways. The first and most crucial is monitoring of the thermocouple temperatures during and after the ablation process. The second is the observed phenomenon of outgassing of dissolved nitrogen into the heating tissues. As the tissues are heated, the solubility of dissolved nitrogen decreases, resulting in microbubble formation within the tissue. This appears as an echogenic blush, seen in most but not all tumors, that enlarges to encompass the zone of ablation. The third method to assess successful ablation is with the use of Doppler ultrasound. In those preablation tumors that demonstrates color flow Doppler signals, this is measured postablation to make sure that no blood flow is present within the ablated zones.

After ablation there usually is no dramatic change in the echogenicity of the tumor or the normal liver. Some patients demonstrate a slight hypoechoic characteristic in the ablated areas, and needle tracks or small amounts of gas often can be observed in the ablated zones. On withdrawal of the needle, bleeding from the needle track is rarely a problem. In some patients, particularly those with cirrhosis, application of 15–30 W of power as the needle is withdrawn through the tissues will serve to coagulate the needle track and minimize bleeding.

IX. POSTOPERATIVE CARE

After laparoscopic liver resection, postoperative management is almost the same as that for conventional surgery. Oral intake is permitted from the second day after major liver resection. Liver function tests, coagulation profile, serum electrolytes, and complete blood counts are monitored. The liver function tests help evaluate the efficiency of the remnant parenchyma and the possible damage after prolonged Pringle maneuver. Most patients are discharged one week after hepatic segmentectomies or lobectomies. Drains that do not show evidence of bile leaks are removed within 2–3 days postoperatively.

Patients with laparoscopically placed hepatic artery catheters are allowed to drink liquids 6 hours after surgery and are advanced to a regular diet as tolerated. We generally initiate chemotherapy in the recovery room and are satisfied with the intraoperative infusion of methylene blue as an indicator of proper perfusion. The patients are discharged home when they are tolerating a regular diet, have return of normal bowel function, are able to ambulate, and have adequate pain control on oral medication. Follow-up CT scans and blood CEA levels are obtained at 2, 4, and 6 months to evaluate for progression of disease.

Postoperative management for patients undergoing lap RFA is more straightforward. These patients are admitted overnight and discharged to home the following morning. Pain is well controlled with just oral pain medications. Many patients may have low-grade fever immediately postoperative, but this is transient without any sequelae. Patients are returned to clinic one week postoperative and receive a new "baseline" CT scan, with subsequent follow-up CT scans at 3, 6, and 12 months and every 6 months afterwards (Fig. 6). Hounsfield unit (HU) measurements on CT scans demonstrate a progressive increase with contrast injection in normal liver tissue, both pre- and post–tumor ablation, and in liver tumor preablation. HU densities of the liver tumor after ablation, however, show a minimal increase with administration of intravenous contrast. The failure of the lesion to increase in Hounsfield unit density in the portovenous phase compared to the noncontrast phase indicates lack of perfusion and thus coagulative necrosis or a successful ablation (Figs. 7 and 8).

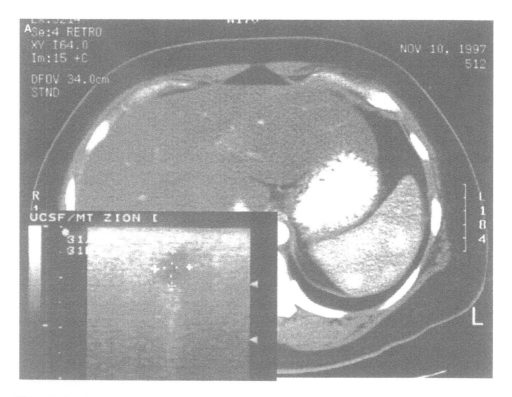

Figure 6   Representative triphasic CT scans from a patient with successful ablation. (**a**) Preop CT scan did not show lesion in segment 3, but was seen on intraoperative laparoscopic ultrasound. (**b**) 1 week postop CT scan showing zone of ablation. (**c**) 3 months postop CT scan showing decrease in lesion size. (**d**) 6 months postop CT scan showing further decrease in lesion size. This lesion also did not enhance significantly with the administration of intravenous contrast, which indicates a lack of perfusion within the ablated lesion.

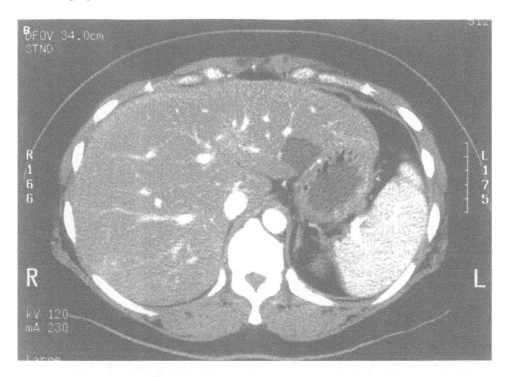

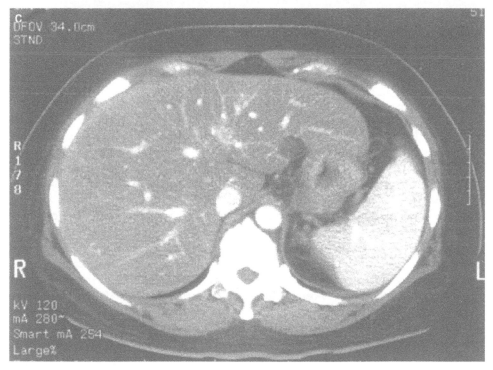

Figure 6 (continued)

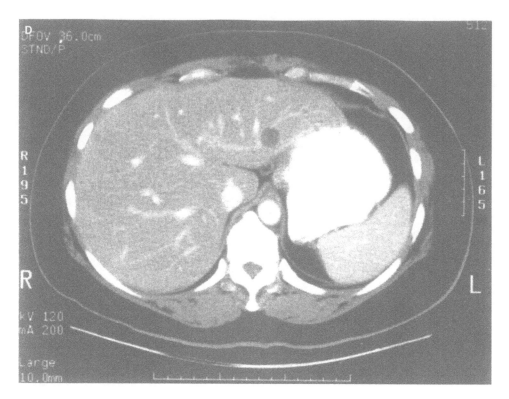

Figure 6   (continued)

X. OUTCOMES

There have been mostly case reports and a few small series (10–20 patients) of laparoscopic liver resections. Most of these are wedge resections, rather than segmentectomies or formal hepatic lobectomies. In a recent review of 70 resections, 47 (67%) of the procedures were attempted for malignancies, including colon cancer metastases, breast cancer metastases, and hepatocellular carcinoma. There were no intraoperative deaths, but one patient died on postoperative day 1 because of liver failure and severe coagulopathy. Postoperatively, one of 70 patients had a biliary fistula. The operative times in general are longer in the laparoscopic groups compared to the open groups, mainly due to the inherent technical challenges, but also due to the learning curve. In several studies the operative times were even longer in patients with cirrhosis due to the fibrotic liver. The duration of hospital stay in many series has been shorter (5–7 days), with quicker postoperative recovery than in the conventional open liver resection group.

Most series of patients undergoing laparoscopic management of nonparasitic hepatic cysts show recurrent disease in 0–18%, with a mean follow-up of 3 years. Recurrent, symptomatic disease is usually evaluated for hepatic resections or open hepatic cystectomies. In contrast, multiple series of patients undergoing laparoscopic management of polycystic liver disease show recurrence rates of 11–75% by 5 years. Most authors agree that laparoscopic management of polycystic liver disease should be reserved for patients with a limited number of dominant, large anteriorly located cysts. Otherwise, these symptomatic patients should be evaluated for liver transplantation rather than cyst fenestration or even liver resections; the recurrence rate for all series of transplanted patients is 0%. One third of these transplanted patients in all series also underwent simultaneous kidney transplants for polycystic kidney disease.

Due to the recent introduction of laparoscopic RFAs, long-term data are not available. In most published reports, median follow-ups have been 12–24 months, with the rate of local recurrence in the 4–19% range. Definition of failure or recurrence is any increase in lesion size after the first week postoperative CT scan and perfused tumors at periphery of ablated zone. In the senior author's (A.S.) series, 14 of 181 lesions (8%) were definite local recurrences and 8 of 181 lesions (4%) were suspected failures, given the multifocal nature of new lesions (Fig. 7). Thus, the overall "failure" rate was 12%. Most (77%) of the recurrences occurred by the 6-month CT scan. Predictors of failure include lack of increase in lesion size at 1-week postoperative CT scan, larger tumors, and vascular invasion on laparoscopic ultrasound. Patients with adenocarcinoma or sarcoma were more likely to recur than those with hepatocellular carcinoma or neuroendocrine tumors.

Radiofrequency ablations performed laparoscopically have several advantages over those performed percutaneously or via laparotomy. Several studies have shown that laparoscopic ultrasound of the liver can detect 19–55% more primary hepatic malignancies or metastatic lesions in the liver compared to abdominal CT scans or transabdominal ultrasounds. The senior author examined 55 patients with 201 lesions on CT scans; laparoscopic ultrasound was able to detect 21 additional tumors (10%) in 11

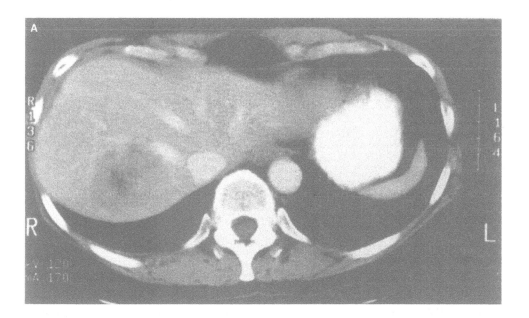

Figure 7 Representative triphasic CT scans from patients with recurrent tumor. (**a**) Preop CT scan. (**b**) 1 week postop CT scan. (**c**) 3 months postop CT scan showing definite recurrence. There is an interval increase in the size of the lesion and there is some tissue at the periphery of the lesion that enhances with the administration of intravenous contrast.

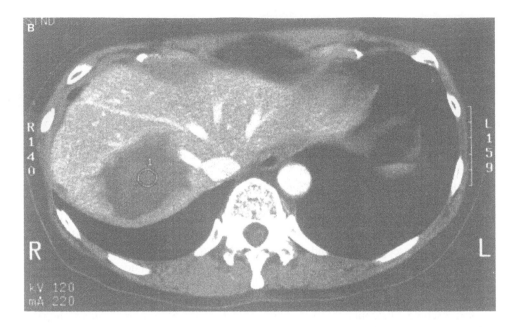

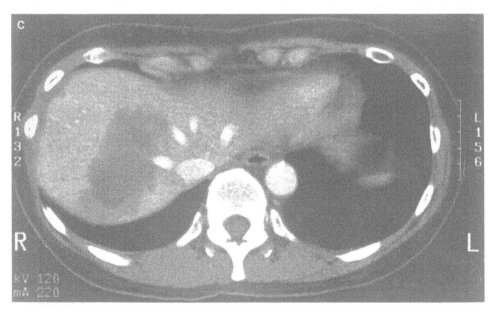

Figure 7   (continued)

patients (20%). In addition, laparoscopy can evaluate metastatic disease throughout the
entire abdominal cavity, unlike the percutaneous RFAs. More importantly, laparoscopic
RFAs pose less danger to diaphragm or adjacent viscera compared to the percutaneous
route. Combination procedures such as laparoscopic colon resections or colostomy
takedowns can be performed at the same time as the laparoscopic RFAs. Finally, it is
minimally invasive, making the laparotomy route the least favorite of the three methods.

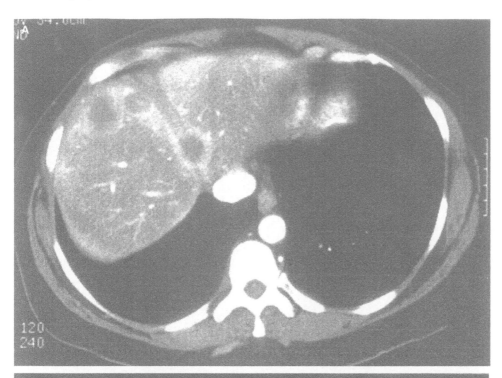

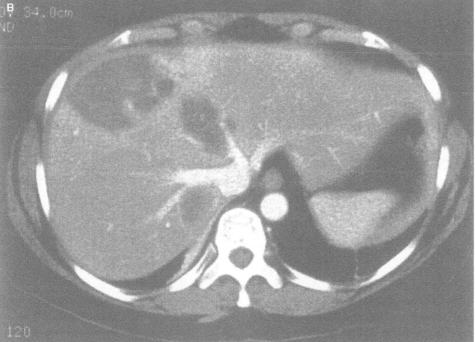

Figure 8 Representative triphasic CT scans from patients with recurrent tumor. (**a**) Preop CT scan. (**b**) 1 week postop CT scan. (**c**) 3 months postop CT scan showing development of multifocal disease. The lesions that abut the ablated lesions could be a result of residual viable tumor cells in the ablated foci or independent lesions that simply abut the ablated foci. (**d**) 6 months postop CT scan.

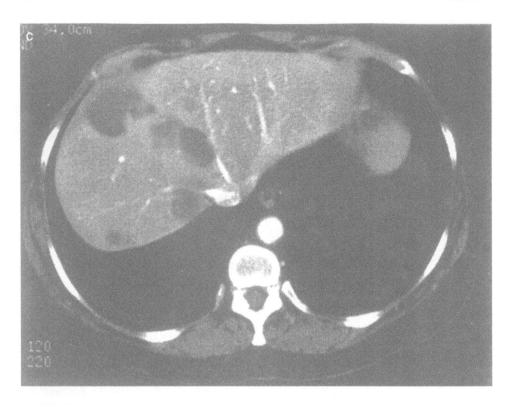

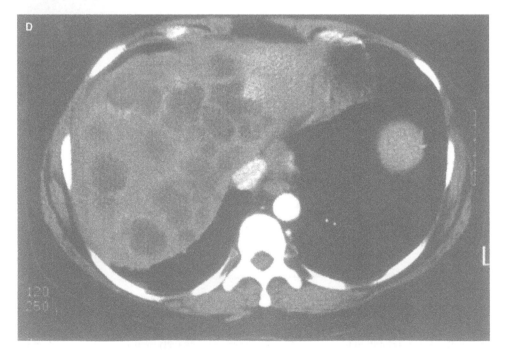

Figure 8   (continued)

XI. COMPLICATIONS AND THEIR MANAGEMENT

Some potential complications include the usual risks of laparoscopy: local wound infection and injury to the abdominal organs, which can be repaired by laparoscopic or open suturing. A major intraoperative complication is hemorrhage. Minimal to moderate oozing can be controlled with electrocautery, clips, or the ABC. Significant bleeding should be controlled with a suture ligature, during which a pringle maneuver and/or temporary clamping of the hepatic vein is provided. If the venous injury is more extensive, such as in a hepatic vein or a branch of the portal vein, one must not hesitate to convert and perform a subcostal incision; conversion is not an admission of failure, but good surgical judgment. One complication specifically related to liver surgery is that of bile leakage. Percutaneous drainage is usually adequate, as most small bile leakage will resolve spontaneously. Major bile leakage is rare, but must be dealt with either endoscopically (decompressing the bile duct with stents or sphincterotomy), percutaneously (transhepatic catheter placement), or surgically (repair or oversew bile duct injuries). Another potential complication specific to liver surgery is carbon dioxide gas embolism. Air and argon gas can also be sucked into the liver veins or arteries. High-pressure pneumoperitoneum or the use of an argon coagulator may add to this risk. Therefore, many authors advocate a low-pressure pneumoperitoneum or a "gasless" environment during the actual parenchymatous resection phase, using an abdominal wall-lifting device.

Reported procedure-related complications of hepatic artery catheter placement include catheter dislodgement, hepatic artery or catheter thrombosis, hepatic artery pseudoaneurysm, infection of the subcutaneous pocket, or erosion of the catheter into adjacent structures. Complications secondary to the chemotherapy include biliary sclerosis, cholangitis, gastritis, hepatitis, gastroduodenal ulceration, and cholecystitis if the gallbladder is not removed during the initial procedure. Technical advances in port/pump placement, as well as the use of 5-FU in place of FUDR, have decreased the severity and/or incidence of many of these complications.

Laparoscopic RFA has its own potential complications: bile duct injury and stricture, hepatic abscess, hemorrhage, liver insufficiency, liver failure, ascites, pleural effusion, and portal vein thrombosis have been reported. In the author's (A.S.) series of 150 consecutive patients, there was only one hepatic abscess, no bile duct injuries or stricture, and no conversions to laparotomies; only three patients were readmitted for pain control.

XII. CURRENT STATUS AND FUTURE INVESTIGATION

Revolutionary techniques have entered the field of general surgery. Virtual-reality imaging of liver disease, computer-guided surgery, and telesurgery are rapidly evolving techniques that hold promise for future liver surgery and are easily made compatible with a laparoscopic approach. New instruments such as the Ligasure (Tyco International Inc., Exeter, NH) that literally seal off blood vessels (perhaps diminishing the chance of gas embolism) may further bring laparoscopic liver surgery within reach.

With the new laparoscopic RFA, there are many unanswered questions. Currently, investigations are being done to assess long-term survival in patients undergoing RFAs. Other investigations include assessing the feasibility and efficacy of concurrent laparoscopic colon resections for colorectal cancer along with laparoscopic RFA of liver metastases. Long-term results are needed to determine if redo laparoscopic RFAs are justified in patients with recurrent disease. One promising aspect of this new technique is for cirrhotic patients with hepatocellular carcinoma, as laparoscopic RFA can serve as a "bridge" to liver transplantation.

SURGICAL TIPS

1. Ports should be vented during laparoscopic argon beam coagulation to increased intra-abdominal pressures from the infusion of argon gas.
2. Fibrin glue applied laparoscopically to the transected liver can provide additional hemostasis and can seal small bile leaks.
3. When a surgeon is unsure of the extra- or intrahepatic biliary anatomy, laparoscopic cholangiography should be utilized.
4. Laparoscopic ultrasound is an important and essential tool to assess the liver lesions and to assess the intrahepatic vascular and biliary anatomy to plan resections or ablations.
5. Laparoscopic cholecystectomy is often performed first to assist in treating liver lesions close to the gallbladder bed.
6. Most small postoperative bile leaks will resolve spontaneously, whereas major bile leaks must be intervened endoscopically, percutaneously, or surgically.
7. Track ablation is useful in establishing hemostasis during the withdrawal of the ablation catheter from the liver.
8. Temperature monitoring of the patient is an important function of the anesthesiologist during radiofrequency ablations.
9. 10 mm trocars are used to allow laparoscopic ultrasound probes and CUSA to be used interchangeably.
10. Laparoscopic liver resections can be converted to laparoscopic-assisted procedure by using a 6 cm midline minilaparotomy.

SELECTED READINGS

Berber E, Foroutani A, Garland AM, Rogers SJ, Engle KL, Ryan TL, Siperstein AE. Use of CT Hounsfield unit density to identify ablated tumor after laparoscopic radiofrequency ablation of hepatic tumors. *Surg Endosc* 2000;14:799–804.

Bilchik AJ, Wood TF, Allegra DP. Radiofrequency ablation of unresectable hepatic malignancies. *Oncologist* 2001; 6:24–33.

Cherqui D, Husson E, Hammoud R, Malassagne B, Stephan F, Bensaid S, Rotman N, Fagniez PL. Laparoscopic liver resections: a feasibility study in 30 patients. *Ann Surg* 2000; 232(6):753–762.

Descottes B, Lachachi F, Sodji M, Valleix D, Durand-Fontanier S, de Laclause B, Grousseau D. Early experience with laparoscopic approach for solid liver tumors: initial 16 cases. *Ann Surg* 2000; 232(5):641–645.

Foroutani A, Garland AM, Berber E, String A, Engle K, Ryan TL, Pearl JM, Siperstein AE. Laparoscopic ultrasound vs triphasic computed tomography for detecting liver tumors. *Arch Surg* 2000; 135:933–938.

Franklin ME, Jr., Norem RF, Stubbs R. Laparoscopic approach for regional hepatic chemotherapy in the treatment of primary or metastatic malignancy. In: Green FL, Rosen RD, eds. Minimal Access Surgical Oncology. New York: Radcliffe Medical Press, Inc., 1995:153–157.

Hashizume M, Shimada M, Sugimachi K. Laparoscopic hepatectomy: new approach for hepatocellular carcinoma. *J Hepatobiliary Pancreat Surg* 2000; 7:270–275.

Kathouda N, Mavor E, Gugenheim J, Mouiel J. Laparoscopic management of benign cystic lesions of the liver. *J Hepatobiliary Pancreat Surg* 2000; 7:212–217.

Siperstein A, Garlan A, Engle K, Rogers S, Berber E, Foroutani A, String A, Ryan T, Ituarte P. Local recurrence after laparoscopic radiofrequency thermal ablation of hepatic tumors. *Ann Surg Oncol* 2000; 7(2):106–113.

Siperstein A, Garlan A, Engle K, Rogers S, Berber E, String A, Foroutani A, Ryan T. Laparoscopic radiofrequency ablation of primary and metastatic liver tumors. *Surg Endosc* 2000; 14:400–405.

Urbach DR, Herron DM, Khajanchee YS, Swanstrom LL, Hansen PD. Laparoscopic hepatic artery infusion pump placement. *Arch Surg* 2001; 136(6):700–704.

Wu JS, Strasberg SM, Luttmann DR, Meininger TA, Talcott MR, Soper NJ. Laparoscopic hepatic lobectomy in the porcine model. *Surg Endosc* 1998; 12:232–235.

17

Ventral Hernia Repair

THOMAS K. VARGHESE, ANDREW WU, and KENRIC M. MURAYAMA

Northwestern University, Feinberg School of Medicine
Chicago, Illinois, U.S.A.

I. BACKGROUND

Approximately 90,000 ventral hernia repairs are performed each year in the United States, making it the second most common type of abdominal hernia operation. In patients who undergo laparotomy, incisional hernias develop in about 2–11%, with incidence rates greater than 40% in those who develop postoperative wound infections. Unfortunately, open repairs of these defects often are unsatisfactory, with recurrence rates ranging from 25% to 52%.

In an attempt to improve results with ventral hernia repairs, the technique described initially by Rives and popularized by Stoppa and Wantz came into favor. This approach involved placement of a large piece of prosthetic material on top of the peritoneum but behind the rectus muscles with a large overlap in all directions. Recurrence rates of less than 3% with this technique have been reported; however, the major drawback to the procedure is the associated morbidity. The repair requires a long incision, wide fascial dissection, flap creation, and usually drain placement. Wound complications occur in 18–20% of patients undergoing this type of repair.

Using the Rives-Stoppa-Wantz method as the underlying principle, the laparoscopic method was developed. First described by Leblanc and Booth in 1993, the laparoscopic repair of ventral hernias uses a minimally invasive approach to obtain the benefits of an open mesh herniorraphy while attempting to minimize the postoperative morbidity. The laparoscopic repair allows for the application of mesh one layer deeper than the Rives-Stoppa-Wantz method and eliminates the need for extensive soft tissue dissection. Theoretical advantages are similar to other laparoscopic procedures in that patients have shorter hospital stays, decreased narcotic requirements, and quicker return of bowel function. In addition, the repair entails an approach of the hernia from a lateral direction to place the mesh, thus lowering wound complication rates and hence recurrence rates.

Ventral hernia refers to any fascial defect and protrusion through the anterior abdominal wall. They may be primary, originating in the umbilicus, epigastrium, or linea semilunaris (Spigelian hernia), or the more common secondary type, developing at the site of a previous abdominal incision. They are associated with potential incarceration; thus, such hernias need to be repaired to prevent strangulation. The goal in repairing ventral hernias laparoscopically is to reduce the contents of the hernia sac and obliterate the defect by placement of a prosthetic mesh that is used to buttress the fascial defect. This mesh is placed intraperitoneally with the prosthesis extending far beyond the borders of the fascia defect and held in place by sutures/staples, intra-abdominal pressure, and later by fibrinous growth. Patients with incisional hernias often have dense adhesions from prior abdominal operations that can impair visualization or prevent safe access. Multiple episodes of previous repair under tension, with or without insertion of prosthesis, followed by failure of the repair leads to a "Swiss cheese" abdomen, harboring multiple hernias through the old incisions and holes at previous suture sites. Careful and meticulous laparoscopic adhesiolysis is therefore required.

II. CLINICAL PRESENTATION

A. Symptoms

A typical ventral hernia appears as a diffuse bulge in the anterior abdominal wall, the bulge appearing in a portion of a healed incision in the case of an incisional hernia. The defect may be in the incision itself or may be created when one of the sutures used for the prior closure tears through tissue.

The signs and symptoms of a ventral hernia are due to congestion and stretching of the viscera in the hernia sac, intermittent bowel obstruction, ischemia of the skin overlying the hernia, and eventual loss of domain of the contents of the hernia. Stretching the attachments of the bowel mesentery occurs because abdominal contents rush into the hernia sac during any effort or straining that increases intra-abdominal pressure. This results in dull, gnawing discomfort, sometimes associated with mild nausea. Bowel obstruction due to the hernia may be related to incarceration of bowel within the hernia sac but more often is due to adhesions around the hernia orifice that kink or otherwise partially or totally occlude the lumen of a segment of small bowel.

Steady enlargement of a ventral hernia brings about atrophy and displacement of the subcutaneous fat and then stretching of the skin over the hernia. The skin can become quite thin and progressively more ischemic. Loss of domain occurs when unreduced viscera are present in an external hernia sac over a relatively long period. The abdominal cavity proper accommodates to the smaller volume of its residual contents. Sudden reduction of abdominal contents in these cases can lead to respiratory as well as cardiovascular compromise due to pressure on the diaphragm and inferior vena cava, respectively. Historically pneumoperitoneum was used to treat these cases, and hence intuitively laparoscopic surgery would be expected to be beneficial.

B. Physical Examination

Ventral hernias are often best initially evaluated with the patient in the supine position. Valsalva or straight leg raises nearly always demonstrate the presence of an abdominal wall defect and a bulge. Difficulties in evaluation may arise in patients with significant adipose tissue in the subcutaneous layer of the abdominal wall. Particular discomfort with pressure over the area of suspected hernia with Valsalva maneuver should increase suspicion of hernia in these cases but is not diagnostic. The reducibility of the hernia, the size of the defect, and the proportion of abdominal contents chronically outside the confines of the abdominal cavity are important factors. Previous scars and any changes in the overlying skin are also meaningful.

C. Differential Diagnosis

Ventral hernias are at times difficult to discern from other abdominal wall masses in the obese. These include lipomas, leiomyomas, and soft tissue sarcomas. The majority of ventral hernias are incisional, and hence the presence of a previous incision often lends itself to the diagnosis.

III. DIAGNOSTIC TESTS

Rarely are any imaging studies required to diagnose ventral hernias. A good physical examination in most cases makes the diagnosis. However, in the case of large, irreducible hernias and small, poorly defined hernias in an obese abdomen, computed tomography (CT) can help differentiate ventral hernias from abdominal wall masses. CT scan, as compared to other imaging studies, can delineate abdominal wall and pelvic wall structures and often identifies wall defects, as well as the presence of any previously placed prosthetic material. Gas, fluid collections, and contrast within bowel outside the confines of the abdominal or pelvic walls are frequently demonstrable with CT. It thus also aids in the planning of acceptable laparoscopic trocar placement.

IV. NONOPERATIVE TREATMENT

Unfortunately, no medical treatment can by itself sufficiently treat patients with ventral hernias. Abdominal binders may help the ventral hernia from increasing in size and reduce the discomfort associated with ventral hernias. However, abdominal binders may compromise bowel that gets incarcerated during times of increased intra-abdominal pressure. Surgical therapy remains the main therapy for ventral hernias.

Before hernia repair, the factors that have contributed to the development of the hernia must be investigated, particularly in the case of primary ventral hernias. Contributing elements must first be nullified or alleviated as much as possible. Increased intra-abdominal pressure due to obstructive uropathy or ascites should be reversed before repairing the hernia. Partially obstructing rectal cancer as a cause of increased intra-abdominal pressure should be evaluated by history, occult blood testing and screening sigmoidoscopy where necessary. Chronic cough should be treated to the extent possible.

In some cases of massive hernias, the skin stretched over the hernia thins and even ulcerates. Moreover, dependency of a large sac leads to lymphedema, dermatoses, and occasionally cellulitis of the overlying skin. Open sound in the region of the hernia should be allowed to heal if at all possible before the repair and must be healed before the use of a nonabsorbable prosthesis as part of the repair. Skin ulceration, dermatoses, and cellulitis must be treated before the hernia repair. Split-thickness grafting is the best method to close large, chronic granulating wounds. Chronic corticosteroid administration should be at as low a level as possible, and antimetabolites should be discontinued.

V. OPERATIVE TREATMENT

All ventral hernias should be repaired surgically to prevent incarceration and subsequent strangulation. The presence of the hernia is the indication for its repair. Repair is done upon diagnosis in order to avoid the technical and physiological consequences and complications that occur with delay, such as loss of domain, incarceration, bowel obstruction, and similar events. Factors to take into account when a decision for surgery is to be made include the patient's general status, associated symptoms, and the size of the hernia. Hernia size is generally the most important factor in determining the need for a prosthetic repair. In general, fascial defects smaller than 3 cm^2 can be repaired with a standard open approach. However, the difficulty in repairing Spigelian hernias, no matter the size, favors repair by the laparoscopic approach, as these small, difficult-to-localize hernias can be easily visualized through laparoscopy.

Larger ventral hernias can be repaired with prosthetic material. Contraindications to repair include end-stage cardiac, liver, and pulmonary diseases. In addition, several physical conditions may make the laparoscopic approach less than ideal. These include extremely large ventral hernias occupied by much of the abdominal viscera, as there may be significant loss of abdominal domain, precluding safe laparoscopic surgery. Additionally, patients with end-stage renal disease with previous peritoneal dialysis should be approached with caution, as there may be obliteration of the peritoneal space by extremely dense adhesions. Performance of laparoscopic surgery in those with cirrhosis and portal hypertension can lead to an increased risk of peritonitis and bleeding. Potential migration of mesh can occur in the pediatric population, and hence laparoscopic repair should be avoided in these individuals.

A. Equipment

Necessary equipment includes:

> General laparoscopy instrument set
> Ioban—skin barrier
> 5 mm 30-degree angled laparoscope
> 10 or 12 mm port
> Two 5 mm ports
> 5 mm circular surgical tack applicator
> Endoclose (U.S. Surgical, Norwalk, CT)
> No. 11 knife blade
> 2-0 polypropylene sutures
> Expanded polytetrafluoroethylene (ePTFE) mesh (Gore-Tex DualMesh Biomaterial,
>   WL Gore, Flagstaff, AZ)
> Surgical marking pen

B. Preoperative Preparation

Poor cutaneous hygiene in skinfolds below the hernia is quite common on patients with ventral hernias. The presence of prosthesis within a wound disrupts normal host defense mechanisms that protect against the low level of bacterial contamination that occurs in every surgical wound. Thus, administration of perioperative antibiotics is warranted. A full dose of a parenteral antibiotic with activity against staphylococci and common aerobic gram-negative coliforms, such as *Escherichia coli*, should be administered with induction of anesthesia. The infusion of antibiotic should be completed just before the skin incision is made. A second dose of antibiotic should be given if the operation lasts more than 3 hours.

All patients at our center undergo preoperative bowel prep in the event that any type of bowel injury should occur. The most challenging aspect of a laparoscopic ventral hernia repair is the lysis of adhesions and reduction of chronically incarcerated viscera. The incidence of enterotomies in laparoscopic ventral hernia repairs has ranged from 0 to 2%. In our initial experience, although no enterotomies were seen, one patient did have an additional bowel resection performed. In this patient, after lysis of adhesions and the remainder of the laparoscopic ventral hernia repair were completed, a second inspection of the previously incarcerated bowel was undertaken. On further inspection the bowel segment appeared dusky and nonviable, and a laparoscope-assisted small bowel resection was performed. Though not initially planned, the bowel resection was possible as the bowel was prepped, and there was no spillage of contents with contamination of mesh.

Other factors to account for in these patients with large incisional hernias include increased risk for postoperative septic complications, respiratory dysfunction, and pulmonary emboli. Preoperative and postoperative prophylaxis for these problems is essential.

C. Operating Room and Patient Setup

The patient is placed on the operating table in supine position. The procedure is performed under general anesthesia. An orogastric tube is inserted to decompress the stomach, and a urinary catheter is inserted to decompress the bladder after induction of general anesthesia. The abdomen is prepped and draped in sterile fashion. Ioban placement prevents ePTFE contact with the skin as well as facilitating mesh positioning. The surgeon usually stands to the right of the patient, with the assistant and scrub nurse on the opposite side. Video monitors may be placed either at the foot end of the table or at the head, depending on surgeon preference (Fig. 1).

D. Surgical Technique

1. Port Placement

Port placement is extremely important and is a major determinant of operative success (Fig. 2). Because the location of a ventral hernia is never in the same area, there is no specific pattern for port placement. General principles that are followed with regard to port placement enable access to all ventral hernias and facilitate repairs.

The 5 mm camera port needs to be placed at least 10 cm from the closest margin of the fascial defect so as to allow for a complete view in addition to providing for enough space to manipulate the mesh. This is the site used to achieve pneumoperitoneum with either a closed or open technique. An angled 5 mm laparoscope is then inserted after the abdominal cavity is insufflated with CO_2 to a pressure of 15 mmHg.

At least two additional ports (5 and 12 mm) will be needed as well. The ports are placed under direct vision. These ports need to be lateral enough from the fascial defect so as to allow room for movement and dissection. Most operating ports should be inserted and placed at the level of the anterior axillary line for midline hernias to allow free movement of instruments. This location also avoids complications of vascular injuries to the epigastric vessels that typically are displaced laterally due to the hernia. A 12 mm port

Anesthesiologist

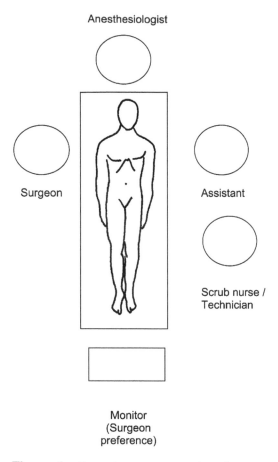

Surgeon

Assistant

Scrub nurse /
Technician

Monitor
(Surgeon
preference)

Figure 1   Operating room setup for a laparoscopic ventral hernia repair.

is used for the surgical tack applicator and introduction of mesh into the abdominal cavity. A roticulating and angled stapler may alternatively be used in lieu of the surgical tack applicator.

2.   Hernia Identification and Mesh Placement

The most difficult part of ventral hernia repairs is the adhesiolysis and reduction of the hernia contents (Fig. 3). The pneumoperitoneum stretches the abdominal wall and suspends intra-abdominal contents, facilitating adhesiolysis as well as helping to return the viscera to the abdomen. Countertraction applied to adherent pieces of bowel and omentum is necessary. The majority of the adhesions are filmy and avascular, and sharp dissection with scissors is initiated in the area. At least 3–5 cm circumferential margin of clean healthy aponeurotic tissue is cleared for placement of the mesh. Often more than one defect can be found in the anterior abdominal wall. It is important to clearly delineate all defects so that adequate mesh size can be determined for successful repair. The peritoneal sac itself is left in situ.

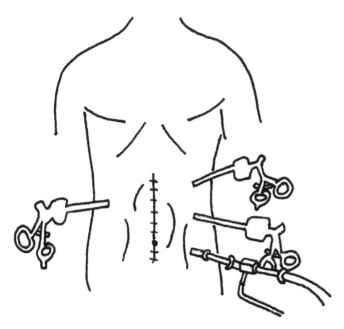

Figure 2 Port placement for laparoscopic ventral hernia repair.

The edges of the hernia defect are delineated by direct vision and palpation, and their location is drawn on the abdomen. Use of prosthesis in the repair of ventral hernias prevents peritoneal eventration in two ways: by rendering the visceral sac indistensible and by solidly uniting and consolidating the abdominal wall. ePTFE Dual-mesh is ideal for use in the repair of ventral hernias. This Gore-tex mesh is a dual synthetic composite of prosthetic mesh, with a smooth side facing the viscera and the rough side pinned towards the body wall, encouraging fibroblast and collagen ingrowth and attachment to the mesh. The mesh is cut to an appropriate size so as to overlap all defects by a margin of at least 3 cm in all directions (Fig. 4). 2-0 polypropylene sutures are then placed at the edge of the mesh at four to six equidistant points. After being oriented and marked with figures to corresponding points on the anterior abdominal wall, the mesh with the sutures are then rolled and inserted through the 12 mm port into the peritoneal cavity and subsequently flattened out. Positioning of the mesh intracorporeally is facilitated with the aid of the

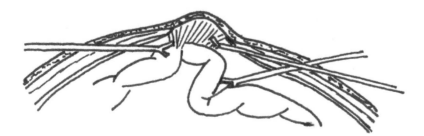

Figure 3 Adhesiolysis and reduction of hernia contents.

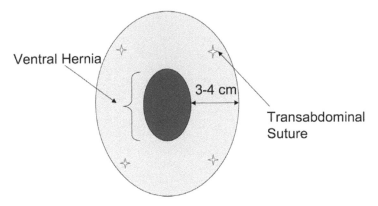

Figure 4 Patch position with respect to ventral hernia defect.

corresponding marked figures. Skin incisions of 1–2 mm are made on the previously marked sites. A suture grasper such as the Endoclose is then inserted, advanced through the abdominal wall and into the abdomen (Fig. 5). The corresponding sutures along the mesh are grasped and drawn through the incision with separate passes. The sutures are then tied extracorporeally, thus incorporating the full thickness of the abdominal wall

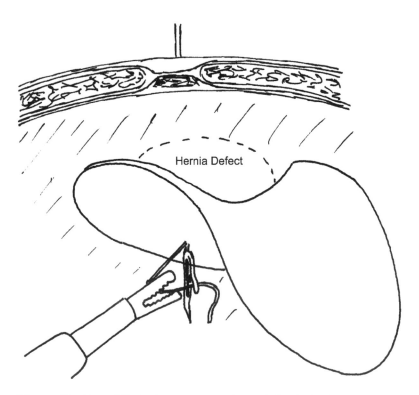

Figure 5 Use of Endoclose to secure transabdominal suture.

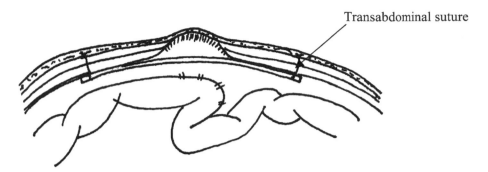

Figure 6   Mesh position on securement of transabdominal sutures.

musculature so that the knots lie in the subcutaneous tissue (Fig. 6). Once the sutures are tied, the mesh is additionally secured with the aid of 5 mm tacks placed circumferentially at intervals of <1 cm. Fascial defects in ports greater than 5 mm are closed with nonabsorbable sutures, which can also be done with the aid of the Endoclose. The skin is closed with absorbable subcuticular sutures and steri-strips.

VI.   POSTOPERATIVE CARE

The majority of patients can drink clear liquids within a few hours of surgery, and diet is then advanced accordingly. Patients should be admitted for overnight observation as often the laparoscopic ventral hernia repair can be associated with considerable pain during the first 24 hours. This also allows for monitoring of any signs of bowel compromise. Ambulation is encouraged on the day of surgery. Longer hospital stays may be needed if significant intestinal manipulation during surgery results in an ileus. This usually resolves by the second or third postoperative day in these cases. It is recommended that physical activity should be restricted for 2–4 weeks following the operation in order to allow the mesh to be properly and firmly secured. Though not routinely used, abdominal binders can be applied in order to minimize seroma formation.

The first postdischarge outpatient visit usually takes place approximately 2 weeks after surgery. The most common sequela of laparoscopic ventral hernia repair is the formation of a seroma, which presents as a firm, round mass, mimicking the appearance and feel of the original hernia. The rate of seroma formation has been reported between 1 and 16% after laparoscopic ventral hernia repair. This compares to 5–16% incidence after open procedures. Initially conservative management is utilized for seromas, as they have been observed to resolve spontaneously over 4–6 weeks. Intervention is usually reserved for those with persistent discomfort, in which case careful percutaneous aspiration can be performed. Ultrasonography can be used to exclude recurrence of hernias in these cases.

VII.   OUTCOMES AND COSTS

Although the ideal randomized, prospective controlled comparison has yet to be done, multiple retrospective and nonrandomized, prospective studies have shown good short-term results (Table 1). Perhaps the greatest benefit of performing ventral hernia repairs laparoscopically is the significant decrease in complications. The reported incidence of

Table 1

Series	No. of patients	Complication rate (%)	Hospital stay (days)	Follow-up (months)	Recurrence rate (%)
Kyzer et al.	53	11	Median 3	Median 17	0
Park et al.	56	18	Mean 3	Mean 24	11
Ramshaw et al.	79	19	Mean 2	Mean 21	3
LeBlanc et al.	96	14	Mean 1	Mean 51	9
Heniford and Ramshaw	100	13	Mean 2	Mean 23	3
Carbajo et al.	100	15	Mean 1	Mean 30	2
Franklin et al.	112	5	Range 1–12	Mean 30	1
Toy et al.	144	24	Mean 2	Mean 7	4
Heniford et al.	407	13	Mean 2	Mean 23	3
Mean	Total = 1147	15			4

major wound infections is around 3% of patients undergoing laparoscopic repair as compared with 22% of patients undergoing open herniorraphy. The apparent lower rate of infection in laparoscopic repair may be due to the avoidance of long incisions, wide dissection or flap creation, opening of the hernia sac, and placement of drains, all of which can increase the risk of perioperative bacterial contamination and infection. The total facility costs for the laparoscopic repair group has been reported by Heniford et al. to be $8,273 compared to an average of $12,461 for open repair. The majority of the cost savings was reflective of shorter hospital stays as well as decreased incidence of wound complications.

VIII. COMPLICATIONS AND MANAGEMENT

In various series of laparoscopic ventral hernia repairs, the short-term recurrence rate ranged from 3 to 11%. Although none of these are randomized prospective studies, these recurrence rates are comparable to the historical control of 3% for open repairs by the Stoppa method and 23% for traditional open repair with mesh. Mean OR times ranging from 86 to 120 minutes have been reported, while the mean length of stay has ranged from 1 to 3.4 days.

Stoppa first described the importance of peripheral sutures transfixing the abdominal wall in the repair of incisional hernias. Many authors have found a higher recurrence rate in those laparoscopic repairs where only a single fixation method of the mesh to the abdominal wall was used. In our initial institutional experience, although two fixation techniques were used routinely, we had two recurrences. Both patients had ventral hernias extending to the inguinal region. Neither patient had transabdominal fixation sutures placed in the inferior portion of the mesh. A recurrent hernia was noted at this region in each patient within 2 months of surgery. It is possible that the recurrences could have been prevented by further dissection in the inguinal region for placement of the inferior transabdominal suture, either laparoscopically or by a separate inguinal incision. Whether suturing the pubis, iliopubic tract, or other substantial pelvic tissue can alleviate recurrence in hernias extending to the inguinal ligament remains to be seen.

Other complications besides wound infections also exist. In nine large series, the overall complication rate was 15% (range 5–24%) (Table 1). Complication rates related to trocar insertions and with regard to bleeding and infection are similar to other minimally invasive procedures. These include cellulitis of a trocar site, intestinal injury, hematoma or postoperative bleeding, prolonged ileus, urinary retention, respiratory distress, fever, intra-abdominal abscess, and trocar site herniation.

IX. CURRENT STATUS AND FUTURE INVESTIGATION

Although there has been significant success with laparoscopic ventral hernia repairs, further evaluation in long-term clinical trials has yet to be determined. Laparoscopic ventral hernia repairs have proved to be highly effective in several series with short-term follow-up. Avoidance of large incisions and creation of large dissection flaps have resulted in lower wound complication rates and shorter hospitalization stays as compared to the traditional open techniques. Multiple reports in the literature from various centers reiterate the feasibility of laparoscopic repair and successful outcome in the treatment of these difficult clinical entities.

SURGICAL TIPS

1. Attention to skin hygiene: failure to control skin inflammation and infection preoperatively increases the risk of subcutaneous wound infection, contamination of the prosthesis, and eventual recurrence of the hernia.
2. All patients should ideally undergo preoperative bowel prep.
3. A full dose of a parenteral antibiotic with activity against staphylococci and common aerobic gram-negative coliforms such as *Escherichia coli* should be administered with induction of anesthesia.
4. Both of the patient's arms should be tucked at the side.
5. Stomach and bladder decompression is done with an orogastric tube and Foley catheter, respectively.
6. Meticulous adhesiolysis and reduction of incarcerated bowel should be performed.
7. Convert to open procedure if gross contamination as a result of enterotomy should occur.
8. Use ePTFE Dual-Mesh, fashioned so as to overlap all defects by at least 3 cm in all directions.
9. Two methods of fixation should be used for securing mesh.
10. Transabdominal fixation sutures should be present in all four quadrants.

SELECTED READINGS

Carbajo MA, del Olmo JC, Blanco JI, de la Cuesta C, Martin F, Toledano M, Perna C, Vaquero C. Laparoscopic treatment of ventral abdominal wall hernias: preliminary results in 100 patients. JSLS 2000; 4(2):141–145.

Carlson MA, Ludwig KA, Condon RE. Ventral hernia and other complications of 1,000 midline incisions.

Franklin ME, Dorman JP, Glass JL, Balli JE, Gonzalez JJ. Laparoscopic ventral and incisional hernia repair. Surg Laparosc Endosc. 1998; 8:294–299.

Heniford BT, Park A, Ramshaw BJ, Voeller G. Laparoscopic ventral and incisional hernia repair in 407 patients. J Am Coll Surg. 2000; 190:645–650.

Heniford BT, Ramshaw BJ. Laparoscopic ventral hernia repair. A report of 100 consecutive cases. Surg Endosc. 2000; 14:419–423.

Kyzer S, Alis M, Aloni Y, Charuzi I. Laparoscopic repair of postoperation ventral hernia. Early postoperation results. Surg Endosc. 1999; 13:928–931.

LeBlanc KA, Booth WV, Whitaker JM, Bellanger DE. Laparoscopic incisional and ventral herniorraphy in 100 patients. Am J Surg. 2000; 180:193–197.

Mudge M, Hughes LE. Incisional hernia: a 10-year prospective study of incidence and attitudes. Br J Surg. 1985; 72:70–71.

Park A, Birch DW, Lovrics P. Laparoscopic and open incisional hernia repair: a comparison study. Surgery. 1998; 124:816–822.

Ramshaw BJ, Esartia P, Schwab J, Mason EM, Wilson RA, Duncan TD, Miller J, Lucas GW, Promes J. Comparison of laparoscopic and open ventral herniorraphy. Am Surg. 1999; 65:827–831.

Stoppa RE. The treatment of complicated groin and incisional hernias. World J Surg. 1989; 13:545–554.

Toy FK, Bailey RW, Carey S, Chappius CW, Gagner M, Josephs LG, Mangiante EC, Park AE, Pomp A, Smoot RT, Uddo JF Jr, Voeller GR. Prospective multicenter study of laparoscopic ventral hernioplasty: preliminary results. Surg Endosc. 1998; 12:955–959.

Varghese T, Denham D, Dawes L, Murayama K, Prystowsky J, and Joehl R. Laparoscopic ventral hernia repair: an initial institutional experience. J Surg Res 2002. In press.

18

Triaging for Trauma

WILLIAM M. BOWLING

University of Texas Southwestern Medical Center
Dallas, Texas, U.S.A.

Historically, abdominal trauma in hemodynamically stable patients was evaluated by serial examination or paracentesis; any abnormal findings prompted laparotomy. The introduction of diagnostic peritoneal lavage (DPL) in 1965 provided a sensitive test for the presence of intraperitoneal blood, which was deemed an indicator of serious intra-abdominal injury sufficient to determine the need for surgery. The drawback of DPL is its relative lack of specificity, which is associated with nontherapeutic laparotomy rates of 20%. Computed tomography (CT) and ultrasonography (US) have also been used to evaluate abdominal trauma but are similarly limited: CT has associated rates of nontherapeutic laparotomy of up to 30%; it requires transport of the patient to the CT suite and that experienced technicians and radiologists be available. Ultrasound appears to be as sensitive as DPL for the presence of intra-abdominal fluid, but neither can determine the rate of bleeding or whether the injury is continuing to bleed or whether the injuries causing the bleeding require surgical intervention unless serial studies are performed. Furthermore, neither test reliably detects injuries to a hollow viscus, the diaphragm, or retroperitoneum.

Laparoscopy may be able to overcome these limitations. Diagnostic laparoscopy should allow the trauma surgeon to directly observe the injuries and more accurately determine whether they require surgical intervention. Diaphragmatic injuries, which can rarely be detected by other methods, can be identified and even repaired laparoscopically. However, before diagnostic laparoscopy becomes a routine part of a trauma surgeon's armamentarium, several questions must be addressed.

First, are currently available laparoscopic instruments and techniques suitable for the accurate evaluation of abdominal injuries? Second, which patients will benefit from the use of laparoscopy? Finally, will the use of laparoscopy improve the care of the trauma patient by assisting the surgeon to accurately identify patients who need surgery and avoid laparotomy in those who do not? Two secondary issues, which are related to the last question and must be evaluated, are the effects of laparoscopy on length of stay and costs of care.

The first modern report on laparoscopy in a trauma patient was published by Heselson in 1970. In this study the criterion for laparotomy was the presence of any blood in the peritoneum. Only a primitive direct-vision scope was used, which allows only the operator to view the abdomen, compared with a modern video camera/monitor system, which allows the entire surgical team to see the abdomen and thus assist. Furthermore, no additional instruments were used to manipulate the abdominal contents to allow evaluation of areas not immediately visible upon entering the abdomen. Nevertheless, the author was able to avoid laparotomy in 9 of 21 blunt trauma patients and 6 of 10 penetrating trauma patients.

In 1976, Gazzaniga et al. reported their experience with 132 consecutive patients. As in Heselson's study, this series was limited by the use of a direct-vision laparoscope, but a blunt needle was added to move the omentum. These patients had already been selected for laparotomy based on their condition and the results of DPL. Of these patients, 37 underwent laparoscopy first. Laparotomy was safely avoided in 14 of these patients. Of the 23 who subsequently underwent laparotomy, there were six nontherapeutic laparotomies, for a false-positive rate of 25%. Overall, through the use of laparoscopy in this group, 21%; of the laparotomies performed could have been avoided. An added benefit noted in this study was that the length of stay was reduced to 2 days in the laparoscopy-only group.

Carnevale et al. reported a similar study in 1977: 20 patients previously selected for laparotomy based on clinical examination and laboratory studies, including the analysis of peritoneal fluid, underwent laparoscopy before formal laparotomy. In this study a direct-vision laparoscope was also used, with a blunt-tipped probe inserted if needed. Laparotomy was avoided in 12 of the 20 patients (60%) based on the laparoscopic findings. It was also noted that the average length of hospital stay in the laparoscopy-only group was 4.5 days compared with a minimum of 7 days in the laparotomy group.

A group from Los Angeles headed by Morgenstern reported their initial experience with laparoscopy in 1980 and followed this with a more extensive update 3 years later. In their first brief report, they performed laparoscopy on 15 patients with one or more of the following: altered sensorium, multiple system trauma, unexplained hypotension, or an equivocal finding on abdominal examination. As with the previously described studies, they used a direct-vision laparoscope with a blunt-tipped probe inserted if necessary to manipulate the abdominal contents. They were the first to report using a 30-degree laparoscope. Laparoscopic findings were normal in six patients. In an additional seven patients, injuries were either seen directly or presumed to be present because of blood in the peritoneum. These injuries were felt to be self-limited and did not require laparotomy. The remaining two patients had ileal injuries and required laparotomy. Overall, laparotomy was avoided in 86% of these patients. In the updated report, they described 96 additional patients using the same criteria and techniques for laparoscopy. In the updated report, they described 96 additional patients using the same criteria and techniques for laparoscopy. In 47 patients no blood or succus entericus was seen, and these patients were observed without complications or need for laparotomy. In 27 patients with hemoperitoneum, either no injury or only self-limiting injuries were found, and none of these patients required laparotomy. Of the remaining 22 patients, all had severe hemoperitoneum and identifiable injuries, and all but one individual, in whom no injury could be found, underwent therapeutic laparotomy. Thus, surgery was avoided in more than 80% of patients who would otherwise have undergone laparotomy.

Two series from Europe have been reported. The first, from Italy in 1987, included 106 patients who had suffered blunt abdominal trauma, unexplained shock, or other injuries known to be associated with intra-abdominal pathology. Forty patients were safely observed without complications, as demonstrated by supplemental studies and their subsequent clinical course. There were two false-positive and two false-negative findings among the 66 patients who underwent laparotomy. The two false-negative findings involved extraperitoneal bladder injuries that were discovered after a nontherapeutic laparotomy. The two false-positive findings were determined to result from omental bleeding.

The second study, from England in 1988, was a randomized study of 55 patients. Patients with blunt abdominal trauma, stable vital signs, and a positive abdominal examination were randomized to either DPL or laparoscopy. Fifteen patients in the DPL group and 12 patients in the laparoscopy group had negative results (i.e., no hemoperitoneum or succus entericus). These patients were managed nonoperatively, and none required surgical intervention. Among patients with positive results, 3 of 11 in the DPL group (27%) and 1 of 13 (8%) in the laparoscopy group had negative laparotomies. No complications were reported in this series.

Berci et al. reported in 1991 on 150 blunt abdominal trauma patients in whom laparoscopy was used for evaluation. Patients were selected based on obscure or equivocal physical findings, unexplained hypotension, or history of abdominal trauma. No exploration was performed in the 84 patients who had a negative laparoscopic finding, and none subsequently required exploration. Of the 38 patients who had minimal hemoperitoneum but who did not undergo an exploratory procedure, one subsequently required exploration. In this patient there was blood in the left paracolic gutter and a perforated sigmoid colon that was not recognized at laparoscopy, but was identified and repaired after the patient's clinical condition deteriorated. Among those with positive laparoscopic findings who underwent exploration, all had significant injuries requiring surgical intervention except one patient. In this patient 700 mL of peritoneal blood was noted, but no source was found. This group also reported one complication—a patient with a minimal hemoperitoneum from an omental injury during trocar insertion. The overall sensitivity and specificity in this series were 97% and 99%, respectively.

In a small 1992 series, Sosa et al. were able to avoid laparotomy in six patients by ruling out peritoneal perforation by laparoscopy. A slightly larger series reported by Livingston et al. in 1992 included 15 gunshot wounds and 16 stab wounds as well as eight victims of blunt trauma. These patients were clinically stable but had already been selected to undergo laparotomy based on standard clinical criteria. These investigators were the first to report the use of a camera and monitor with a 0-degree laparoscope. This equipment leaves the surgeon's hands free to examine the abdomen and, since the entire surgical team can view the procedure, allows the surgeon to operate in concert with an assistant. Four patients with minimal hemoperitoneum underwent laparotomy at which no injuries or active bleeding was found; laparotomy was avoided without complication in another seven patients. Livingston et al. also reported one death in a patient with severe preexisting liver disease and a retroperitoneal hematoma who succumbed to progressive liver failure. The authors cited the ability to rule out peritoneal perforation as a major benefit of laparoscopy, but that the search for intra-abdominal injuries was limited by their inability to visualize the spleen, evacuate clot, and fully examine the small bowel. They recommended rotating the patient to improve visualization as well as the use of a 30-degree laparoscope in conjunction with intra-abdominal retractors.

The utility of laparoscopy in the evaluation of the intrathoracid abdomen was demonstrated in a series reported by Ivatury et al. in 1992. Hemodynamically stable patients with injuries to the intrathoracic or upper abdomen were eligible for laparoscopy. Among the 40 patients with potential injuries who underwent laparoscopy, the absence of peritoneal perforation was documented in 20 patients. Among the patients with positive laparoscopic findings, laparotomy was avoided in one, who recovered uneventfully. Among the remaining patients, laparotomy was therapeutic in only 50%. However, there were two injuries found at laparotomy that were not seen at laparoscopy. Two complications were also reported: one was insufflation of the preperitoneal space in an obese patient, and the second was a tension pneumothorax that developed during insufflation in a patient with an unrecognized diaphragmatic laceration. One death occurred as a result of acute respiratory distress syndrome (ARDS), which was unrelated to laparoscopy.

A brief report in 1993 by Sosa et al. described 20 additional patients with gunshot wound (GSW) of the abdomen along with the 8 previously reported. These patients were clinically stable and without overt evidence of peritoneal perforation. Laparotomy was avoided in 22 patients who had no evidence of peritoneal penetration. Among the 6 patients with peritoneal penetration, 4 underwent therapeutic laparotomy. The remaining 2 had isolated nonbleeding liver lacerations. One underwent a nontherapeutic laparotomy, and the second was observed without the need for a delayed laparotomy. No complications or missed injuries were reported.

Fabian et al. reported a larger series of 182 patients in 1993. These patients had either a penetrating or blunt trauma injury. The penetrating trauma patients were selected on the basis of equivocal evidence of peritoneal penetration or intra-abdominal injury. Blunt trauma patients were those with a positive finding either on DPL or abdominal CT. Fifty-three percent of these patients had a negative laparoscopic result and were treated successfully by observation. Of the remaining patients, 32% underwent therapeutic laparotomy and the remaining 15% had nontherapeutic laparotomies. Sosa et al. also reported a notable decrease in length of stay in patients with a negative laparoscopic result compared with the length of stay for patients who underwent either a therapeutic or nontherapeutic laparotomy, but they did not report on the significance of this difference. In a cost comparison (based on intention to treat) off negative laparotomy with laparoscopy performed in the operating room with the patient under general anesthesia, no cost savings were demonstrated for laparoscopy. They suggested that minilaparoscopy using local anesthesia might result in significant cost savings. Another important issue raised in the discussion was the difficulty they encountered in completely examining the abdomen with only a 0-degree laparoscope and cholecystectomy instruments.

In 1993, Salvino et al. compared DPL with laparoscopy in 75 trauma patients who were judged to require a DPL based on standard advanced trauma life support (ATLS) criteria. Forty-two patients (56%) had both negative DPL and negative laparoscopic findings and were managed nonoperatively without sequelae. Twenty patients (27%) had negative DPL results and insignificant findings on laparoscopy. These patients were also managed nonoperatively without complications. Three patients (4%) with negative DPL findings had diaphragmatic lacerations that were found by laparoscopy. Of the remaining 10 patients (13%), 3 had negative DPL results, but all had significant injuries on laparoscopy. Notably, 60% of the patients in this series underwent laparoscopy under local anesthesia. The authors felt that laparoscopy was useful in reducing the number of unnecessary laparotomies among patients with positive DPL results but did not recommend that the "occasional" laparoscopist employ this procedure. There was no cost comparison among the study groups in this series, but based on the usual charges at Loyola

University Medical Center, ED laparoscopy would have saved $2600 or more per patient when compared with laparoscopy or laparotomy performed in the operating room.

In 1993, Ivatury et al. evaluated 100 stable patients with penetrating abdominal trauma with laparoscopy. Forty-two percent of these patients had no evidence of peritoneal penetration by laparoscopy and were managed nonoperatively. Of the remaining patients, all but 3 required laparotomy for injuries identified on laparoscopy. Of the 3 patients who did not undergo laparotomy, one had omental herniation and 2 had nonbleeding liver lacerations. There were 7 patients who had bowel injuries that were missed on laparoscopy but were identified at laparotomy, which was undertaken for other injuries identified at laparoscopy. There was a significant 50% reduction in length of stay when the negative laparoscopy group was compared with case-controls from the same time period. The author cautioned that limitations in their ability to "run the bowel" resulted in seven missed injuries; however, these patients all had other indications for laparotomy.

A study published by Townsend et al. in 1993 compared CT with laparoscopy in 15 patients with blunt abdominal trauma. These patients, with CT evidence indicating nine splenic and eight hepatic injuries, underwent laparoscopy before laparotomy. Laparoscopy confirmed 15 of the 17 injuries, and in addition demonstrated two unsuspected hollow viscus injuries. Four additional patients had ongoing bleeding seen on laparoscopy and also underwent laparotomy, along with one patient in whom visualization was poor. The remaining 8 patients were managed nonoperatively without complication; however, there was no reduction in length of stay in this group.

Rossi et al. in 1993 studied 32 patients with blunt and penetrating abdominal trauma who had already been selected to undergo laparotomy based on clinical examination and DPL and/or CT results. Eleven of the 26 patients with penetrating trauma had no evidence of peritoneal penetration and no injuries seen at laparotomy. Among the remaining 15 patients, 36 injuries were found at laparotomy compared with only 29 seen at laparoscopy, resulting in a missed injury rate of 19%. However, all but one of the patients with missed injuries had other indications for laparotomy seen at laparoscopy. In the case of blunt trauma, nine injuries were seen at laparotomy, whereas only seven were found at laparoscopy, resulting in a missed injury rate of 22%. One of these injuries was a grade II liver injury that did not require repair; however, the other was a transection of the pancreas that required a distal pancreatectomy. These injuries were missed despite the use of two additional trocars to examine the stomach, elevate the omentum and run the small bowel.

A second study with significant missed injury rates was reported in 1994 by Brandt et al. They performed laparoscopy on 21 hemodynamically stable trauma patients, 10 with blunt injuries and 11 with penetrating injuries, who had already been selected for laparotomy based on clinical examination and results of DPL and/or CT. Nine patients showed no evidence of injury at laparoscopy or only injuries that were deemed not to require laparotomy. These findings were confirmed at laparotomy. Twelve patients were thought to require laparotomy based on the laparoscopic findings, and this was confirmed at laparotomy. However, when the injuries found at laparotomy were compared with the laparoscopic findings, laparoscopy had missed 53% of the injuries despite the use of accessory trocars to completely examine the abdomen. Despite this apparent poor performance of laparoscopy, the authors were able to accurately predict the need for laparotomy based on the laparoscopic findings. The injuries that were missed were either of no clinical significance or occurred in patients who already had other indications for laparotomy.

Finally, Carey et al. reported in 1995 on the use of laparoscopy in 35 patients with blunt and penetrating trauma. Laparoscopy identified 14 patients with significant findings and this was confirmed at laparotomy in 12 cases. Of the three false-positive findings, two resulted from bleeding from the abdominal wall and a third from an expanding hematoma over the iliac vessels. The authors also noted a minor but insignificant reduction in length of stay in the negative laparoscopy group, but no cost savings was identified in the laparoscopy group.

Eight additional studies were published in the 2 years following the first edition of this review. In 1996, Ditmars and Bongard reported on their experience with laparoscopy in 106 patients with penetrating abdominal trauma. Based on the results of laparoscopy, 38 of these patients underwent laparotomy, of which 19 (50%) were therapeutic. Lengths of stay and hospital charges were compared for those who underwent laparotomy and those who did not. After excluding patients who also had tube thoracostomy, there was an average reduction in length of stay of 2.1 days ($p < 0.01$). The average nonsurgical charges for patients who underwent laparotomy were \$4,513 more than those who underwent laparoscopy only. This comparison did not include surgical charges.

Three retrospective studies published in 1997 and 1998 by Zantut et al., Block et al., and Hallfeldt et al. reviewed their experiences with 510, 20, and 43 patients, respectively, with penetrating abdominal trauma. Their results were similar to those of Rossi et al. in that laparoscopy did not identify all of the injuries found at laparotomy but was very accurate in predicting the need for laparotomy. Zantut and Block also demonstrated reductions in length of stay. A fourth prospective study from MIEMSS by Elliott et al. confirmed laparoscopy's poor sensitivity at identifying injuries to hollow viscera, but also confirmed its accuracy in determining the need for laparotomy.

Three studies have focused on laparoscopy's ability to assess thoracoabdominal injuries, injuries frequently missed by other modalities. In 1996, Ortega et al. reported on 24 patients with penetrating thoracoabdominal trauma who were hemodynamically stable and for whom there was a high index of suspicion for peritoneal or diaphragmatic injury. No peritoneal penetration was demonstrated by laparoscopy in three patients and no injuries were found at laparotomy. In the remaining patients, laparoscopy had very good sensitivity and specificity for solid organ injury and diaphragmatic injury but performed poorly in evaluating hollow organ injury. The authors concluded that laparoscopy is of greatest value in evaluating the diaphragm and upper abdominal solid organs.

A second study, also from the University of Southern California by Murray et al., evaluated 119 patients with left thoracoabdominal penetrating trauma. Fifty patients had indications for laparotomy, and of these 60% had diaphragmatic injuries. Fifty-seven patients without indications for laparotomy underwent laparoscopy, and 26% of these patients had occult diaphragmatic injuries. The authors concluded that the incidence of diaphragmatic injuries associated with penetrating left thoracoabdominal trauma was high, that clinical and roentgenographic sign were unreliable, and that laparoscopy has an important role in ruling out these injuries. In 1998, this same group reported on 110 patients with penetrating left thoracoabdominal injuries and no indications for laparotomy. They prospectively evaluated these patients with laparoscopy and found a 24% incidence of occult diaphragmatic injury. They concluded that patients with penetrating left thoracoabdominal trauma who have no other indication for laparotomy should undergo laparoscopy to rule out occult diaphragmatic injury.

A final study from Poland by Majewski prospectively compared 120 patients with acute abdomen, including 24 with trauma, with 310 patients managed without laparoscopy. The patients managed with laparoscopy had lower morbidity and mortality, and shorter hospital stays. In subgroup analysis of the 24 trauma patients, laparoscopy was 100% sensitive and specific in predicting the need for laparotomy.

The most important consideration is whether laparoscopy improves diagnosis and treatment of trauma patients. Despite the differences in patient selection criteria in these studies, the majority show that laparotomy can be avoided in a significant number of patients who would otherwise have undergone laparotomy based on current criteria. The sensitivities and specificities are high, probably as a result of the use of conservative criteria in a population with a high prevalence and a high *a priori* probability of needing a laparotomy. Furthermore, none of the studies were blinded or measured interrater reliability, and the studies may have allowed retrospective patient reclassification. The value of avoiding laparotomy seems to be especially significant in patients with penetrating trauma, where laparoscopy can exclude peritoneal penetration in equivocal cases. Furthermore, in cases of peritoneal penetration, laparoscopy can distinguish whether the injuries require operative intervention. This advantage is somewhat less clear in patients with blunt abdominal trauma, because the entire abdomen must be examined to identify all injuries. Finally, the literature to date yields no clear consensus on the correct place of laparoscopy in the assessment algorithm. Further work will be required to decide which test or sequence of tests is most appropriate.

The second consideration is whether laparoscopy is technically advanced enough to perform all of the maneuvers necessary to completely examine the abdomen. Many of the early studies used only the direct-viewing 0-degree laparoscopes, occasionally with the assistance of a single probe. In these cases the surgeons were limited to evaluating whatever was readily visible to the scope or could be made visible with a single blunt probe. With the use of a suction-irrigator as a probe, it became possible to evacuate any hemoperitoneum and note any reaccumulation of blood, giving a better assessment of the rate of ongoing bleeding. As more procedures began to be performed laparoscopically, more and better became available, such as atraumatic graspers, endo-Babcock clamps, video laparoscopes, and angled laparoscopes. The angled laparoscope, especially the 30-degree scope used in many of the more recent studies, allows better visualization of structures such as the diaphragm, lateral gutters, and the lesser sac. The newer instruments allow the surgeon to manipulate and run the bowel, to enter the lesser sac, and mobilize the ascending and descending colon. These capabilities have also improved the evaluation of the evaluation of the retroperitoneum. With the instruments currently available, it is often possible to repair injuries through the laparoscope.

A third concern is whether the surgeon is able to fully use the available technology and perform a laparoscopic examination. In the last few years laparoscopic procedures have shifted from being ones that are performed by subspecialists and investigators at tertiary institutions to ones that can be performed by most general surgeons at community hospitals. However, the ability to do one or two procedures on elective patients does not compare with the skills required to perform a complete examination of the abdomen. Thus, the surgeon who only occasionally performs elective laparoscopy does not necessarily have the skills to be using this technique on trauma patients. For the same reason, this is not a procedure to be performed by emergency room physicians or other nonsurgical professionals. The surgeon who wishes to incorporate diagnostic laparoscopy into the assessment algorithm is thus obligated to acquire and maintain the necessary skills to safely use laparoscopy.

Although none of the more recent studies (since 1996) have compared laparoscopy with CT or ultrasound, advances in these two modalities have almost certainly diminished the role of laparoscopy as a primary evaluation tool. The advent of rapid, helical CT scanners permits the completion of technically better studies in much less time. Furthermore, the introduction and widespread use of ultrasound at the bedside, especially the FAST exam, with the convenience of frequent repeat examinations, seems to be the most efficient initial assessment modality. The exception is in the evaluation of penetrating thoracoabdominal trauma, where laparoscopy seems the preferred method of assessment.

Finally, the cost savings of using laparoscopy must be considered. Only a few studies look carefully at the charge for laparoscopy compared with that for laparotomy. However, when laparoscopy is used in the resuscitation area there could be as much as an 80% reduction in charges. The data on length of stay are somewhat stronger. When the length of stay is corrected for associated injuries, there is a significant reduction, with patients often going home the day after laparoscopy.

In summary, advancements in CT and ultrasound have limited the role of laparoscopy in the evaluation of abdominal trauma with the notable exception of thoracoabdominal trauma. Laparoscopy remains a procedure for skilled laparoscopic surgeons with the necessary awareness of the limitations of the laparoscopic exam and a willingness to convert to laparotomy when the conclusions of laparoscopy are in doubt. There are moderately strong data to support a decreased length of stay in patients who are spared laparotomy by the use of laparoscopy. The question of economic savings from laparoscopy remains unanswered, for these studies are compromised by evaluation of charges rather than cost and failure to take into account reimbursement.

SELECTED READINGS

Berci G, Dunkelman D, Michel SL, Sanders G, Wahlstrom E, Morgenstern L. Emergency minilaparoscopy in abdominal trauma: An update. Am J Surg. 1983; 146:261–265.

Berci G, Sackier JM, Paz-Partlow M. Emergency laparoscopy. Am J Surg. 1991; 161:332–335.

Brandt CP, Priebe PP, Jacobs DG. Potential of laparoscopy to reduce non-therapeutic trauma laparotomies. Am Surg. 1994; 6:416–420.

Carey JE, Koo R, Miller R, Stein M. Laparoscopy and thoracoscopy in evalution of abdominal trauma. Am Surg. 1995; 61:92–95.

Carnevale N, Baron N, Delany HM. Peritoneoscopy as aid in the diagnosis of abdominal trauma: A preliminary report. J Trauma 1977; 17:634–641.

Cortesi N, Manenti A, Gibertini G, Rossi A. Emergency laparoscopy in multiple trauma patients: Experience with 106 cases. Arch Chir Belg. 1987; 87:239–241.

Cuschieri A, Hennessy TPJ, Stephens RB, Berci G. Diagnosis of significant abdominal trauma after road accidents: Preliminary results of a multicentre clinical trial comparing minilaparoscopy with peritoneal lavage. Ann R Coll Surg Engl. 1988; 70:153–155.

Fabian TC, Croce MA, Stewart RM, Pritchard FE, Minard G, Kudsk KA. A prospective analysis of diagnostic laparoscopy in trauma. Ann Surg. 1993; 217:557–565.

Gazzaniga AB, Stanton WW, Bartlett RH. Laparoscopy in the diagnosis of blunt and penetrating injuries to the abdomen. Am J Surg. 1976; 131:315–318.

Heselson J. Peritoneoscopy in abdominal trauma. S Afr J Surg. 1970; 8:53–61.

Ivatury RR, Simon RJ, Stahl WM. A critical evaluation of laparoscopy in penetrating abdominal trauma. J Trauma. 1993; 34:822–828.

Ivatury RR, Simon RJ, Weksler B, Bayard V, Stahl WM. Laparoscopy in the evaluation of the intrathoracic abdomen after penetrating injury. J Trauma. 1992; 33:101–109.

Liu M, Lee C-H, P'eng F-K. Prospective comparison of diagnostic peritoneal lavage, computed tomographic scanning, and ultrasonography for the diagnosis of blunt abdominal trauma. J Trauma. 1993; 35:267–270.

Livingston DH, Tortella BJ, Blackwood J, Machiedo GW, Rush BF. The role of laparoscopy in abdominal trauma. J Trauma. 1992; 33:417–425.

McKenney M, Lentz K, Nunez D, Sosa JL, Sleeman D, Axelrad A, Martin L, Kirton O, Oldham C. Can ultrasound replace diagnostic peritoneal lavage in the assessment of blunt trauma? J Trauma. 1994; 37:439–441.

Pevec WC, Peitzman AB, Udekwu AO, McCoy B, Straub W. Computed tomography in the evaluation of blunt abdominal trauma. Surg Gynecol Obstet. 1991; 173:262–267.

Root HO, Hauser CW, McKinley CR, Lafave JW, Mendiola RP. Diagnostic peritoneal lavage. Surgery. 1965; 57:633–637.

Rossi P, Mullins D, Thal E. Role of laparoscopy in the evaluation of abdominal trauma. Am J Surg. 1993; 166:707–711.

Salvino CK, Esposito TJ, Marshall WJ, Dries DJ, Morris RC, Gamelli RL. The role of diagnostic laparoscopy in the management of trauma patients: A preliminary assessment. J Trauma. 1993; 34:506–515.

Sherwood R, Berci G, Austin E, Morgenstern L. Minilaparoscopy for blunt abdominal trauma. Arch Surg. 1980; 115:672–673.

Smith RS, Fry WR, Morabito DJ, Koehler RH, Organ CH. Therapeutic laparoscopy in trauma. AM J Surg. 1995; 170:632–637.

Soderstrom CA, DuPriest RW, Cowley RA. Pitfalls of peritoneal lavage in blunt abdominal trauma. Surg Gynecol Obstet. 1980; 151:513.

Sosa JL, Markley M, Sleeman D, Puente I, Carrillo E. Laparoscopy in abdominal gunshot wounds. Surgical Laparosc Endosc. 1993; 3:417–419.

Sosa JL, Sims D, Martin L, Zeppa R. Laparoscopic evaluation of tangential abdominal gunshot wounds. Arch Surg. 1992; 127:109–110.

Townsend MC, Flancbaum L, Choban PS, Cloutier CT. Diagnostic laparoscopy as an adjunct to selective conservative management of solid organ injuries after blunt abdominal trauma. J Trauma. 1993; 35:647–653.

19

Cholecystectomy

ELIZABETH C. HAMILTON

University of Texas Southwestern Medical Center
Dallas, Texas, U.S.A.

DANIEL B. JONES

Beth Israel Deaconess Medical Center
Harvard Medical School
Boston, Massachusetts, U.S.A.

I. INTRODUCTION

Gallstone disease is a common human ailment—over 1 million new cases are diagnosed per year. Approximately 10% of the American population have gallstones, with the incidence as high as 75% in some female ethnic populations. The first cholecystectomy, utilizing minimally invasive techniques, was performed in 1985 by E. Mühe of Germany. The French gynecologist Phillipe Mouret further developed the technique, and it is he who is credited with popularizing the technique in Europe. Following acceptance of the procedure in Europe, private practice physicians and then academicians in the United States embraced the new approach to gall bladder removal and started performing the operation at rates unprecedented in American surgery. Laparoscopic cholecystectomy is now considered the gold standard therapy for symptomatic cholelithiasis.

II. SYMPTOMS

Approximately 20% of patients with cholelithiasis experience symptoms attributable to gallstones. Nevertheless, cholecystectomy is usually only recommended for patients with symptomatic disease. Once symptomatic, the likelihood of subsequent attacks increases substantially. Fortunately, most patients with gallstones present with benign biliary colic before developing serious complications. When complications do occur, they may include abdominal pain, acute or chronic cholecystitis, cholangitis, biliary pancreatitis, common bile duct obstruction, biliary enteric fistulization, and gallbladder perforation.

Cholelithiasis and cholecystitis are the two most common causes of abdominal pain of biliary etiology. Pain from cholelithiasis, or biliary colic, results from contraction of the gallbladder behind an obstruction caused by a stone lodged in the infundibulum or cystic duct. The pain of biliary colic is commonly described as being constant (colic being a misnomer) and localized to the midepigastrium or right upper quadrant. It often radiates around to the right scapula. The pain may begin suddenly and increase in severity before subsiding abruptly. Discomfort may be triggered by eating certain foods (high in fat) or it may begin spontaneously. Constitutional symptoms do not usually accompany simple biliary colic.

Pain from cholecystitis, on the other hand, is more unremitting in nature. Due to the somatic nature of the pain, it may be exacerbated by palpation of the right upper quadrant. Murphy's sign, the abrupt cessation of inspiration on deep palpation of the right upper quadrant, is strongly suggestive of acute cholecystitis. Unlike symptomatic cholelithiasis, the pain of acute cholecystitis may be accompanied by constitutional symptoms including fever, nausea, and loss of appetite.

Although removal of the gallbladder is usually only recommended for patients who are symptomatic from gallstones, a few patient groups may also be candidates for cholecystectomy in the absence of symptoms. This population includes patients with porcelain gallbladder, and those who are immunosuppressed. Asymptomatic cholelithiasis in a diabetic is no longer considered a hard indication for cholecystectomy. Occasionally, typical biliary symptoms may also exist in patients without documented gallstones and may be caused by biliary dyskinesia, sludge, and microcalcifications.

III. DIAGNOSIS

A. Laboratory

Simple cholelithiasis resulting from obstruction of the infundibulum of the gallbladder or the cystic duct typically does not result in any laboratory abnormalities. As stated earlier, acute cholecystitis may result in leukocytosis and mild elevation of alkaline phosphatase and serum liver transaminases. Serum bilirubin is usually normal unless there is concomitant obstruction of the common bile duct.

B. Radiology

Plain radiographs of the abdomen are rarely useful in diagnosing cholelithiasis. Only gallstones with a high calcium concentration are radiolucent enough to be well visualized on a plain radiograph. Transcutaneous ultrasound of the right upper quadrant is very useful, however, and should be the diagnostic tool of choice in patients with suspected biliary pathology. Ultrasound is 95% sensitive and 98% specific in detecting gallstones and may also demonstrate thickness of the gallbladder wall, pericholecystic fluid collections, choledocolithiasis, sludge, polyps, microcalcifications, and the diameter of the common bile duct. The pancreas, liver, and right kidney may also be evaluated on ultrasound examination.

When the ultrasound is normal and typical biliary symptoms persist, cholecystokinin (CCK)–stimulated biliary scintigraphy demonstrating a low gallbladder ejection fraction (< 30%) and/or reproducing pain after CCK administration suggests the presence of acalculous cholecystitis or biliary dyskinesia. If atypical symptoms are present, a more extensive workup, including upper GI contrast radiographs or endoscopy, computed tomography (CT), or cardiac evaluation, should be considered before cholecystectomy is performed.

Although abdominal computed tomography (CT) scanning is a very useful assessment tool for evaluating intra-abdominal pathology, it is not as useful as ultrasound in evaluating biliary tract disease. CT scan has only a 60% sensitivity for detecting gallstones due to the fact that bile and gallstones are of equivalent density on CT. CT is useful, however, for detecting other pathology including pancreatic masses, hepatic abscess, cirrhosis, or free air.

IV. MEDICAL THERAPY

A. Oral Dissolution

Oral dissolution of gallstones is based on the concept that gallstones form from supersaturation of cholesterol and that reversal of the ratio of cholesterol to bile salts with administration of the primary bile salt chenodeoxycholic acid may cause dissolution of gallstones. In general, treatment with oral dissolution agents is unrewarding and is only successful in patients with small, noncalcified stones, and a functioning gallbladder. Fifty to sixty percent of cholesterol stones less than 1 cm in size will respond. However, complete treatment can require over 6 months of therapy with serial monitoring. Gallstones recur in half the people within 5 years.

B. Lithotripsy

Extracorporeal shock wave lithotripsy (ESWL) utilizes high-energy sound waves to fragment stones into small enough pieces to pass through the cystic duct, common bile duct, and enteric canal. Selection criteria for ESWL usually include three or fewer noncalcified stones that are less than 2–3 cm in diameter, with a functioning gallbladder. Bile acids are often used in conjunction with ESWL to dissolve stone fragments. Most biliary calculi can be fragmented when strict inclusion criteria are met, but complications include biliary colic, hemobilia, and pancreatitis. Approximately one third of patients have recurrent stones within 5 years.

Patients who are not candidates for operation may be managed medically, as described above, or by percutaneous cholecystostomy.

V. SURGICAL THERAPY

Laparoscopic cholecystectomy is recommended for symptomatic gallbladder disease (see below). Most laparoscopic cholecystectomies are performed for symptomatic cholelithiasis. Once a patient has documented attack of biliary colic and gallstones have been confirmed, an elective laparoscopic cholecystectomy should be scheduled. Any history of jaundice, acholic stools, pruritis, pancreatitis, elevated liver enzymes, or evidence of enlarged cystic duct or choledocolithiasis on ultrasound examination should prompt evaluation of the common bile duct radiographically either pre-, intra-, or postoperatively. Acute cholecystitis may be more difficult to treat operatively because of inflammation and edema of the gallbladder wall. Despite the historical recommendations that patients with acute cholecystitis be allowed to "cool off" before performing a laparoscopic cholecystectomy, several prospective, randomized controlled trials have confirmed an advantage of early versus delayed surgical management of the disease. Higher conversion rates to open cholecystectomy are anticipated for these patients.

Acalculous cholecystitis, most commonly seen only in postoperative and critically ill patients, can be treated effectively by laparoscopic cholecystectomy.

VI. INDICATIONS AND CONTRAINDICATIONS FOR LAPAROSCOPIC CHOLECYSTECTOMY

Indications:

Symptomatic cholelithiasis
Acute cholecystitis
Chronic cholecystitis
Biliary dyskinesia

Contraindications:

Inability to tolerate general anesthesia
Uncorrected coagulopathy
Peritonitis/cholangitis
Late pregnancy
Biliary fistula
Suspected carcinoma
Generalized peritonitis
Other conditions requiring laparotomy

Preoperative evaluation should be the same as that performed for an open operation and should include, when possible, knowledge of any preexisting medical or surgical conditions that may affect the patient's ability to tolerate general anesthesia and the operation. Absolute contraindications include inability to tolerate general anesthesia, uncorrectable coagulopathy, diffuse adhesions preventing safe entry into the peritoneal cavity, cholecystoenteric fistula, and suspected gallbladder cancer. Numerous relative contraindications (previous abdominal surgery, obesity, pregnancy) exist but pose little problem for the experienced laparoscopic surgeon.

Symptomatic gallstone disease is sometimes detected during pregnancy. Symptoms of suspected biliary tract origin should be assessed using ultrasound as this modality is safe for the mother or fetus. In the past, cholecystectomy of any type was considered unsafe because of the risk of fetal loss, preterm delivery, or injury to the uterus. With advances in anesthesia and surgical care, however, laparoscopic cholecystectomy during all stages of pregnancy is considered relatively safe.

VII. PREOPERATIVE PREPARATION

The setup of the operating room and its personnel requires consideration. The surgeon stands to the left of the patient for cross-table access to the patient's right upper quadrant (Fig. 1). The first assistant stands to the patient's right to manipulate the gallbladder and provide exposure. A laparoscopic video camera operator, who stands below the surgeon, assumes the important responsibility of serving as "the surgeon's eyes" in the abdomen.

The operation is performed under general anesthesia and should only be attempted in a fully equipped operating room. Patients are fasted for approximately 8 hours before elective operations and admitted to the hospital the morning of surgery. Routine administration of intravenous antibiotics for prophylaxis against wound infections is not mandatory in uncomplicated cases of cholelithiasis. When administered, a single

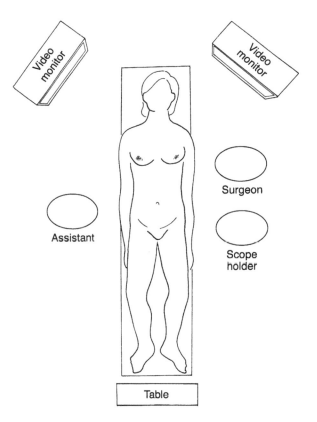

Figure 1 Operating room setup for laparoscopic cholecystectomy. The surgeon stands at the patient's left, and the first assistant is to the patient's right. The electronic laparoscopic equipment is placed on protective carts and the monitors are positioned to allow clear visualization by the entire surgical team. Irrigation, suction, and electrocautery come off the head of the table on the left side.

preoperative dose of intravenous cephalosporin should be given so that peak drug levels are present at the time of skin incision. Prior to induction of anesthesia, some form of deep venous thrombosis prophylaxis should be utilized and may include sequential compression stockings, TED hose, or low-dose subcutaneous heparin. After induction of anesthesia, a urinary bladder catheter and a naso/orogastric tube are generally placed to decompress these hollow organs. The abdomen is prepared in standard fashion.

Equipment used is as follows:

Two 5 mm ports
Two 10 mm ports
Three 5 mm ratcheted graspers
One 5 mm scissors
One 5 mm hook cautery
One 5 mm curved dissectors
One 10 mm claw grasper
One entrapment sack
One loop ligature (optional)

VIII.   SURGICAL TECHNIQUE

A.   Port Placement

A pneumoperitoneum (CO_2) is created to facilitate safe placement of trocars into the abdomen and in general, should be limited to 15 mmHg. Careful attention should be paid to the patient's hemodynamics during this time. If hemodynamic compromise develops, the pneumoperitoneum (CO_2) should be promptly evacuated until vital signs normalize. The pneumoperitoneum can be established using either a closed or an open technique. A 1.5 cm skin incision (vertical or horizontal) is made in the infraumbilical skinfold. After the pneumoperitoneum has been established, the initial large (10/11 mm) port is placed at the infraumbilical incision. Open insertion of the initial port may take longer than the closed technique, but extraction of the gallbladder at the conclusion of the operation is easier. The open technique is particularly helpful in patients with previous periumbilical incisions, patients in whom insertion of the Veress needle is not performed satisfactorily, and those with large (>2.5 cm) gallstones or acute cholecystitis.

With a 10 mm laparoscope, the retroperitoneum immediately posterior to the umbilicus and the pelvis are viewed to ensure that there is no injury as a result of insertion of the trocar or sheath. The pelvic viscera, anterior surface of the intestines, omentum, and stomach are examined for abnormalities. The secured patient is then placed in a reverse Trendelenburg position of 30–40 degrees while the table is rotated to the patient's left by 15–20 degrees. This maneuver generally allows the colon and duodenum to fall away from the liver edge. The falciform ligament and both lobes of the liver are closely examined for pathology. The inferior margin of the liver is then visualized to determine the location of the gallbladder. Usually the gallbladder can be seen protruding beyond the edge of the liver; however, sometimes the gallbladder is not visible without carefully elevating the liver and/or taking down adhesions.

Two 5 mm subcostal ports are then placed in the right upper quadrant. The first port is placed in the anterior to middle axillary line between the twelfth rib and the iliac crest inferior to the gallbladder fundus and liver edge. A second 5 mm port is inserted midway between the axillary sheath and the xiphoid process. Through these ports two grasping forceps secure the gallbladder. The assistant (standing on the right side of the table) manipulates the lateral grasping forceps, which are used to elevate the liver edge to expose the fundus of the gallbladder. The surgeon (standing to the left of the patient) uses a dissecting forceps to raise a serosal "fold" of the most dependent portion of the fundus. The assistant's heavy grasping forceps are then locked onto this fold using either a spring or ratchet device to push in a lateral and cephalad direction, so that the entire right lobe of the liver rolls cephalad. The successful performance of the maneuver is important to expose the porta hepatis and gallbladder.

In patients with few adhesions to the gallbladder, pushing the fundus cephalad exposes the entire gallbladder, cystic duct, and porta hepatis. However, most patients have adhesions between the gallbladder and the omentum, hepatic flexure, or duodenum. These adhesions are generally avascular and may be lysed bluntly by grasping them with a dissecting forceps at their site of attachment to the gallbladder wall and gently "stripping" them down toward the infundibulum. Vascular adhesions may be divided with a hook cautery. After exposing the infundibulum, blunt grasping forceps are placed through the midclavicular trocar for traction on the neck of the gallbladder. The operative field is thereby established, and the final working port is then inserted.

The last 10/11 mm trocar is placed through a transverse or longitudinal skin incision in the midline of the epigastrium. In general, this is placed 5 cm below the xiphoid process, but the position depends on the location of the gallbladder and the size of the medial segment of the left liver lobe. The trocar is angled just to the right of the falciform ligament while aiming toward the gallbladder. The basic positions for placement of the various ports are shown in Figure 2.

B. Exposure

Having established the positions of all trocars, the first assistant retracts the fundus superiorly and the infundibulum of the gallbladder under tension away from the common bile duct (CBD) in the inferolateral direction. Then, either a one-handed or two-handed dissection technique may be used, depending on whether the surgeon or the assistant manipulates the gallbladder infundibulum. With the fundus and neck of the gallbladder under tension, a fine tipped dissecting forceps is used to tease away the overlying fibroareolar structures from the gallbladder infundibulum and Hartmann's pouch. This is done with a blunt stripping action, always starting on the gallbladder and pulling the tissue toward the porta hepatis.

C. Dissection

During this initial dissection around the gallbladder neck, the peritoneum is lysed with the blunt dissector similar to the technique by which the peritoneum is incised and pushed bluntly with a Kittner dissector during a traditional open cholecystectomy. With the

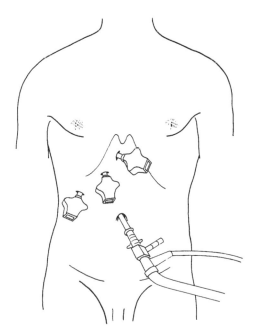

Figure 2 Port placement for laparoscopic cholecystectomy.

laparoscopic dissection performed under two-dimensional optics, it is vital to clearly identify the structures contained within two triangles: the hepatocystic triangle and its reverse side. The hepatocystic triangle (Calot's triangles) is the ventral aspect of the area bounded by the cystic duct, hepatic duct, and liver edge. The reverse side of the hepatocystic triangle is the dorsal aspect of this space. The triangle is placed on tension and maximally exposed by retracting the gallbladder infundibulum inferiorly and laterally while pushing the fundus superiorly and medially (Fig. 3A). A lymph node usually overlies the cystic artery, and occasionally a brief application of electrical current is required to obtain hemostasis as the lymph node is swept away. The assistant then places the infundibulum of the gallbladder on stretch in a superior and medial direction while pushing the fundus superiorly and laterally, thereby exposing the reverse of the hepatocystic triangle, an area defined by the cystic duct, the inferior lateral border of the gallbladder, and right lobe of the liver (Fig. 3B). Further blunt dissection is used to identify precisely the junction between the infundibulum and the origin of the cystic duct. Identification of this junction is the critical maneuver in the operation; certainly, no structure should be sharply divided until the cystic duct is clearly identified. Curved dissecting forceps are helpful in creating a "window" around the posterior aspect of the cystic duct to skeletonize the duct (Fig. 4). Alternatively, the tip of a hook-shaped cautery probe can be used to encircle and expose the duct. The cystic artery may be separated from the surrounding tissue by similar blunt dissection either at this time or later, depending upon its anatomical location. In the usual position, the cystic duct is dissected and divided first, as it is the structure presenting more anteriorly in the field.

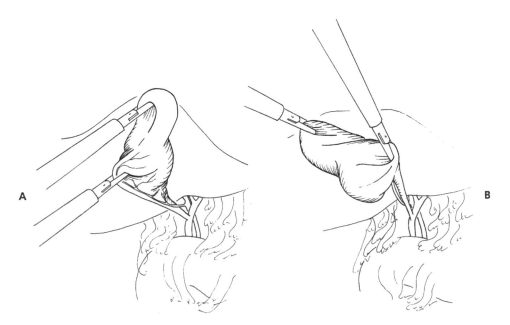

Figure 3   The hepatocystic triangle is exposed by manipulating the gallbladder with traction applied by the assistant's grasping forceps. B. The reverse (dorsal aspect) of the hepatocystic triangle is shown.

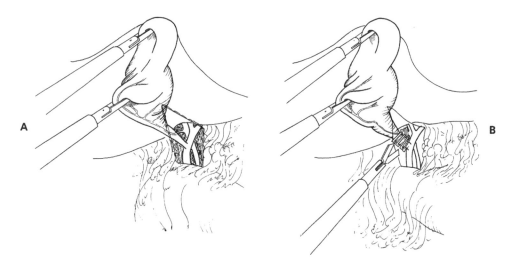

Figure 4 The "critical view" of the cystic duct and cystic artery is identified before any structure is divided (A) and after clipping the duct and artery (B).

D. Intraoperative Evaluation for CBD Stones

After initial dissection of the cystic duct, static or fluoroscopic cholangiography may be performed on a routine or selective basis. First, the dissecting forceps is used to squeeze the cystic duct gently in the direction of the gallbladder, thereby "milking" cystic duct stones back into the gallbladder. A clip applier placed through the epigastric sheath is used to apply a single clip at the junction of the cystic duct with the gallbladder. A scissors inserted through the axillary or midclavicular trocar is used to incise the anterolateral wall of the cystic duct. Then, a 4 to 5 Fr catheter that has been thoroughly flushed to eliminate all air bubbles (that could be confused with ductal stones) is gently inserted into the ductotomy and secured lightly with a clip. The cholangiocatheter should be attached to a three-way stopcock that connects two syringes—one containing radio-opaque contrast and the other saline. The cholangiogram should be scrutinized for the following: (1) the size of the CBD, (2) the location of the junction between the cystic duct and CBD, (3) the presence of intraluminal filling defects, (4) free flow of contrast medium into the duodenum, (5) the anatomy of the proximal biliary tree including identification of the "rabbit ears" (common hepatic duct branching into left and right branches), and (6) aberrant biliary radicles entering the gallbladder directly.

After removing the cholangiocatheter, the cystic duct is doubly clipped near its junction with the CBD and divided. As is the case every time a clip is placed, the posterior jaw of the clip applier must be visualized before applying each clip to avoid injury to surrounding structures. Great care should be taken so that the CBD is not tented up into the clip. If the cystic duct is particularly large or friable, it may be preferable to replace one of the clips with a preformed loop ligature or suture.

E. Completion of the Cholecystectomy

Attention is then directed to the cystic artery. The assistant places the infundibulum of the gallbladder on tension, and the surgeon dissects the cystic artery bluntly from the surrounding tissue. The surgeon must ascertain that the structure is the cystic artery and not the right hepatic artery looping up onto the neck of the gallbladder, as may be seen. After an appropriate length of cystic artery has been separated from the surrounding tissue, it is clipped proximally and distally and divided by sharp dissection.

The ligated stumps of the duct and cystic artery are then examined to ensure that neither bile nor blood has leaked, that the clips are securely placed, and that the clips compress the entire lumen of the structures without impinging on adjacent tissue. To avoid injury to structures in the porta hepatis, no dissection is undertaken medial to the stumps. A suction-irrigation catheter is used to remove any debris or blood that has accumulated during the dissection of the duct and artery, but care is taken not to dislodge the clips by overzealous suctioning. The heavy grasping forceps traversing the midclavicular trocar are repositioned on the proximal end of the gallbladder at Hartmann's pouch. The infundibulum is retracted superiorly and laterally, as well as distracted anteriorly away from its hepatic bed. The surgeon uses the dissecting forceps to thin out the tissue that tethers the neck of the gallbladder and to ensure that no other sizable tubular structures are traversing the space. Dissection of the hepatic fossa is then initiated using a thermal source to divide and coagulate small vessels and lymphatics. Occasionally a larger blood vessel or aberrant small bile duct will require placement of a clip for control.

Separation of the gallbladder from its bed is performed with sharp dissection, monopolar electrocautery, or laser-based instruments (Fig. 5). With the tissue connecting the gallbladder to its fossa placed under tension, the surgeon uses an electrocautery spatula

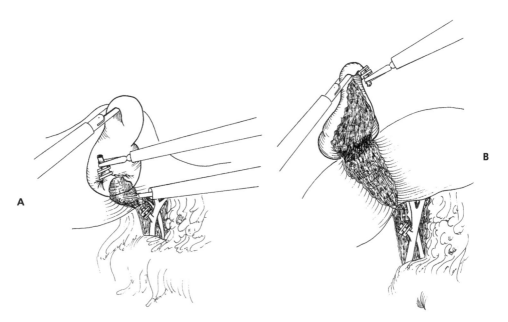

Figure 5   Separation of the gallbladder from its bed by dissecting with a blunt-tipped thermal energy probe. A. The neck of the gallbladder is placed on traction in a superior direction and then twisted to the left and right to place tension on the junction between the gallbladder and hepatic fossa. B. Before completely removing the gallbladder, the cystic duct and artery are carefully inspected to confirm hemostasis and clip placement.

or hook in a gentle sweeping motion with low-power wattage (25–30 W) to coagulate and divide this tissue. Using the cautery probe, the surgeon can also perform blunt dissection, pushing the tissue to facilitate exposure of the proper plane. Occasionally, hemorrhage from the liver bed or gallbladder obscures precise identification of the anatomy. Small liver lacerations frequently stop with direct pressure, further electrocauterization, or application of a topical hemostatic agent. One should avoid blind placement of clips to stop hemorrhage as important structures may be damaged. Frequent irrigation through the port of the electrocautery instrument during this dissection clarifies visualization of the plane.

Dissection of the gallbladder fossa continues from the infundibulum to the fundus, intermittently moving the midclavicular grasping forceps to a position closer to the plane of dissection to allow maximal countertraction. The dissection proceeds until the gallbladder is attached by only a thin bridge of tissue. At this point, before losing visualization of the operative field afforded by cephalad traction applied to the gallbladder, the hepatic fossa and porta hepatis are once again inspected for hemostasis and bile leakage. The clips are reinspected to ensure that they did not inadvertently dislodge during dissection of the gallbladder fossa. Small bleeding points are coagulated with the electrocautery. The right upper quadrant is then liberally irrigated and aspirated dry. The final attachments of the gallbladder are lysed, and the liver edge is once again examined for hemostasis.

After performing the cholecystectomy, the gallbladder is removed from the abdominal cavity. Although the process is costly and usually unnecessary, the gallbladder may be placed in an entrapment sack to assist in extraction. We recommend bagging if the gallbladder is purulent, fragmented, or perforated with multiple small stones or the presence of carcinoma is suspected. The gallbladder is usually removed through the umbilicus under direct visualization from the laparoscope that has been transferred to the midepigastric port. Removal through the umbilical port is attractive because there are no muscle layers and only one fascial plane to traverse. Also, if the fascial opening needs to be enlarged because of large or numerous stones, extending the umbilical incision causes less postoperative pain than would enlarging the subxiphoid entry site. Removal of the gallbladder from the abdominal cavity is facilitated by using a large "claw" grasping forceps. The assistant presents the gallbladder neck into the jaws of the grasper so that it is lined up parallel to the axis of the forceps. The assistant then releases the gallbladder, and its infundibulum is pulled up into the umbilical sheath. The forceps, sheath, and gallbladder neck are then retracted as a unit through the umbilical incision taking care not to tear the gallbladder or the entrapment bag (if used). The neck of the gallbladder is thus exposed on the anterior abdominal wall, with the distended fundus remaining within the abdominal cavity (Fig. 6).

If the gallbladder is not distended with bile or stones, it can be simply withdrawn with gentle traction. In other cases, a suction catheter is introduced into the gallbladder to aspirate bile and small stones. A stone forceps can be placed into the gallbladder to extract or crush calculi if necessary. Occasionally, the fascial incision must be dilated or extended to deliver larger stones.

Each incision may be infiltrated with local anesthetic and irrigated with saline solution. The fascia of the umbilical incision is closed with one or two large absorbable sutures. Failure to adequately approximate fascial edges has resulted in incisional hernia. The skin of the subxiphoid and umbilical incisions is closed with subcuticular absorbable sutures, and Steri-Strips (3M Health Care, St. Paul, MN) are applied to each incision.

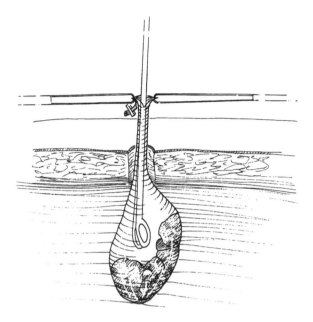

Figure 6 Gallstones contained within the fundus may be crushed or removed after delivering the neck of the gallbladder through the umbilical incision.

IX. POSTOPERATIVE CARE

To monitor for immediate complications, patients may be observed overnight in the hospital or discharged later the same day following laparoscopic cholecystectomy. Although major complications are rare, major hemorrhage or cardiopulmonary complications may occur as in any patient having undergone a major abdominal operation. Clear liquids are resumed postoperatively and advanced to a regular diet as tolerated. Nausea and mild shoulder discomfort from diaphragmatic irritation may occur in the early postoperative period. No activity restrictions are placed on the patient, because functional status depends entirely on the degree of abdominal tenderness. The patient may return to work as soon as the abdominal discomfort is tolerable but is encouraged to do so within 1 week. We routinely evaluate patients in the office 2 weeks after the operation.

X. MANAGEMENT OF COMPLICATIONS

Complications of laparoscopic cholecystectomy include the following: bile duct injury, bile leaks, biliary stricture, hemorrhage, perforated gallbladder, retained stones, pancreatitis, wound infections, incisional hernia, and duodenal injury.

A. Bile Duct Injury

Injuries to the bile ducts occur in approximately 0.5% of laparoscopic cholecystectomies, several times the rate of injury seen with open cholecystectomy. The most common cause of bile duct injury during laparoscopic cholecystectomy is misidentification of a major bile duct for the cystic duct. Causes for misidentification are usually technical and result from superior traction (not enough lateral traction) on the gallbladder aligning the cystic and common ducts. The CBD may be "tented up" because of the vigorous superior traction placed on the gallbladder, making it susceptible to injury during placement of clips. Meticulous dissection of the hepatocystic triangle should expose the "critical view" of the structures surrounding the neck of the gallbladder and decrease these types of injuries. If the anatomy remains unclear, a cholangiogram should be performed before clipping or dividing tissue.

Management of bile duct injuries depends on the level of injury and whether the injury is detected intraoperatively or postoperatively. When detected intraoperatively, immediate repair with interrupted absorbable sutures should be performed. High ductal injuries are more ominous, and delay in their diagnosis may cause an already difficult repair to be even more challenging. Referral to a surgeon experienced in hepatobiliary surgery may be appropriate so that the initial repair is as optimal as possible. Because of the morbidity and mortality associated with ductal injuries, extreme care must be taken to avoid this complication.

The gastroenterologist and radiologist play an important role in the diagnosis and management of bile duct injuries discovered postoperatively. When a ductal injury is suspected because of anorexia, abdominal distention, jaundice, or biliary pain, ultrasound or computed tomography (CT) scan is performed to exclude a fluid collection or ductal dilatation resulting from obstruction. Percutaneous drainage may confirm the diagnosis of a biloma and should control the bile fistula. Endoscopic retrograde cholangiopancreatography (ERCP) or percutaneous transhepatic cholangiography (PTC) is generally performed to define the level of injury and direct treatment. In general, repair of ductal injuries in which the diagnosis has been delayed should be postponed until fluid collections (blood or bile) have been adequately drained, antibiotics have been administered, and the patient's nutritional status optimized.

Bile leaks in the absence of major ductal injury occur either because a duct is not ligated or a clip has slipped. Most leaks (most commonly from the cystic duct stump) will resolve spontaneously and not require reoperation. Superficial aberrant ducts in the gallbladder bed (ducts of Luschka) may be divided and not recognized at the time of surgery until formation of a biloma is noted postoperatively. Therefore, during dissection, superficial ducts in the gallbladder bed should be sought and ligated. Large edematous or short cystic ducts may not be suitable for closure by clips alone, and these cystic stumps should also be loop ligated or sutured for added security. Accumulation of sterile bile may be asymptomatic or may cause nonspecific vague abdominal discomfort and should be evaluated by ultrasound or CT scan in a patient who is slow to recuperate after laparoscopic cholecystectomy. Endoscopic placement of a temporary stent across the sphincter will decrease biliary pressure and allow the fistula to close within a few weeks. Fluid collections may also require percutaneous drainage. However, if bile peritonitis ensues, laparoscopy or a laparotomy may be required to irrigate the abdominal cavity and repair the fistula.

B. Hemorrhage

Anatomical variations of the cystic artery and right hepatic artery may be confusing. Dissection in the region of the lateral wall of the common bile duct may cause bleeding from its nutrient vessels; monopolar electrocautery should not be used near the porta hepatis to prevent devascularization injuries. After careful dissection, clips should be applied at right angles to the cystic artery and clearly include the whole structure to avoid later slippage. Electrocautery should not be used for this division, because the current may be transmitted to the proximal clips, leading to subsequent necrosis and hemorrhage. A common error is to dissect and divide the anterior branch of the cystic artery, mistaking it for the main cystic artery. This may result in hemorrhage from the posterior branch during dissection of the gallbladder fossa. Before exsufflation at the end of the procedure, the hepatic fossa and porta hepatis are once again inspected for hemostasis and to ensure that clips were not inadvertently dislodged during dissection of the gallbladder fossa.

C. Gallstone Spillage

During laparoscopic cholecystectomy, gallbladder perforation with leakage of bile and/or gallstones into the abdominal cavity occurs frequently. Perforation may occur secondary to traction applied by the grasping forceps or because of thermal injury during removal of the gallbladder from its bed. Escaped stones composed primarily of cholesterol probably pose little threat of infection; however, pigment stones frequently harbor viable bacteria and may potentially lead to subsequent infectious complications if allowed to remain in the peritoneal cavity. When spill occurs, bile is aspirated completely, the abdominal cavity is irrigated liberally, and all retrievable stones are removed. A second dose of intravenous antibiotics may also be administered. Gallbladder spillage, when treated in this manner, results in no adverse short- or long-term complications.

D. Conversion to an Open Operation

The decision to convert to an open operation is a matter of judgment. Experienced surgeons do not hesitate to convert to a traditional open cholecystectomy if the anatomy is unclear or if complications arise. Conversion to an open operation should not be considered a complication in and of itself. Some complications requiring laparotomy are obvious, such as massive hemorrhage, bowel perforation, or major injury to the bile duct. Laparotomy is also indicated when inflammation, adhesions, or anomalies obscure delineation of anatomy. Finally, the demonstration of potentially resectable carcinoma dictates open exploration.

E. Gallbladder Cancer

Carcinoma of the gallbladder is rare and occurs at a rate of 1–3 per 100,000 individuals. It is associated with the presence of gallstones, particularly single large stones or a porcelain gallbladder. Because of this, all pathology reports should be reviewed by the surgeon. If carcinoma is identified after the gallbladder has been removed, open operation with resection of liver parenchyma from the gallbladder fossa and lymph node dissection are indicated. Survival from gallbladder carcinoma is poor with only 5% 5-year survival.

XI. SURGICAL TIPS

Higher insufflation pressures may be required to obtain an adequate working space in morbidly obese patients.

Insufflation pressures, kept below 15 mmHg, reduce the risk of cardiorespiratory problems.

A motorized surgical table facilitates repositioning the patient intraoperatively.

When one is uncertain about the appropriate trocar position, a Veress needle may first be placed at the proposed site to determine whether its location and angle of insertion are optimal.

Countertension to the plane of dissection facilitates dissection.

Electrocautery should not be used to divide the cystic artery, because the current may be transmitted to the proximal clips, leading to subsequent necrosis and hemorrhage.

Clips should be fastened at right angles and clearly include the whole structure to avoid later slippage.

Gentle irrigation while pushing away the periductal structures aids precise visualization.

Tears in the gallbladder wall may be clipped or loop ligated to prevent stone spillage and further bile leak.

All port sites larger than 5 mm must be closed or risk herniation.

Identification of the "critical view" should be obtained before clipping the cystic duct.

All necessary laparoscopic equipment should be available in or near the operating room including instruments to perform an intraoperative cholangiogram and common bile duct exploration.

The cholangiogram catheter should be well flushed to avoid air bubbles.

XII. OUTCOMES

The major benefits of gallbladder removal using the minimally invasive technique include decreased patient morbidity from avoiding the large subcostal incision. Most series of laparoscopic cholecystectomies report an uneventful postoperative course in the vast majority of patients, with 90% of patients being discharged from the hospital within 24 hours of surgery and only 10% requiring parenteral administration of narcotics after leaving the recovery room.

Similarly, the duration of disability is minimal: the average postoperative interval to return to full activity is 9 days. These results compare favorably with those of traditional open cholecystectomy, after which duration of hospitalization is 3–5 days, with return to work at 1 month postoperatively. Mortality, which is rare after this procedure, usually is attributable to unrelated events, and the rate of conversion from laparoscopy to an open operation is usually less than 10%. Major complications, such as bile duct injury, are also relatively rare in the hands of an experienced surgeon, but the incidence is generally greater early in a surgeon's experience with the procedure.

XIII. CURRENT STATUS AND FUTURE INVESTIGATION

Laparoscopic management of gallstones has rapidly become the standard therapy for removal of the gallbladder in the United States and throughout much of the world. Most cases of symptomatic gallstones can be treated laparoscopically without complications. Careful dissection of the "critical view" is essential to avoiding technical errors, and intraoperative cholangiography may further clarify anatomical relationships. Occasionally, anatomical or physiological considerations will preclude use of the laparoscopic approach. Elective conversion to an open operation reflects sound surgical judgment and should not be considered a complication.

Advances in robotics, three-dimensional video systems, articulating instrumentation, and laparoscopic ultrasonography may facilitate completion of laparoscopic cholecystectomy in the near future. Teleproctoring will allow expert surgeons to train and credential surgeons from distant locations. Today laparoscopic cholecystectomy may be performed safely, and most patients benefit from less postoperative pain, early hospital discharge, and rapid recuperation.

SELECTED READINGS

Barkun JS, Barkun AN, Sampalis JS, Fried G, Taylor B, Wexler MJ, Goresky CA, Meakins JL. Randomized controlled trial of laparoscopic vs. mini-cholecystectomy. Lancet. 1992; 340:1116–1119.

Bass EB, Pitt HA, Lillemoe KD. Cost-effectiveness of laparoscopic cholecystectomy versus open cholecystectomy. Am J Surg. 1993; 165:466–471.

Jones DB, Dunnegan DL, Brewer JD, Soper NJ. The influence of intraoperative gallbladder perforation or long-term outcome after laparoscopic cholecystectomy. Surg Endosc. 1995; 9:977–980.

Jones DB, Dunnegan DL, Soper NJ. Results of a change to routine fluorocholangiography during laparoscopic cholecystectomy. Surgery. 1995; 118:693–702.

Jones DB, Soper NJ, Brewer JD, Quasebarth M, Swanson PE, Strasberg SM, Brunt CM. Chronic acalculous cholecystitis: laparoscopic treatment. Surg Laparosc Endosc. 1996; 6:114–122.

McMahon AJ, Russell IT, Baxter JN, Ross JR, Morran CG, Sunderland G, Galloway D, Ramsay G, O'Dwyer PJ. Laparoscopic versus minilaparotomy cholecystectomy: a randomized trial. Lancet. 1994; 343:135–138.

National Institutes of Health Consensus Development Conference Statement on Gallstones and Laparoscopic Cholecystectomy. Am J Surg. 1993; 165:390–398.

Soper NJ. Laparoscopic cholecystectomy. Curr Probl Surg. 1991; 28:585–655.

20

Common Bile Duct Stones

ELIZABETH C. HAMILTON

University of Texas Southwestern Medical Center
Dallas, Texas, U.S.A.

DANIEL B. JONES

Beth Israel Deaconess Medical Center
Harvard Medical School
Boston, Massachusetts, U.S.A.

Choledocholithiasis is a common clinical condition. Approximately 10% of patients with symptomatic cholelithiasis have common bile duct stones. While the optimal method for treatment of common bile duct (CBD) stones is controversial, surgeons with advanced laparoscopic skill have numerous options, which include the following: (1) observation, (2) postoperative endoscopic retrograde cholangiopancreatography (ERCP) ± sphincterotomy (S), (3) open common bile duct exploration (CBDE), (4) transcystic laparoscopic CBDE, and (5) transductal laparoscopic CBDE.

Many therapeutic modalities exist, and the ultimate choice of therapy for choledocholithiasis depends on a variety of factors including the patient's condition and the relative local expertise in laparoscopy, endoscopy, and interventional radiology. Whether common duct stones are detected before, during, or after cholecystectomy also plays an important role. Rather than performing a laparotomy and managing CBD stones with a choledochotomy and T tube in all cases, stones may now be retrieved transcystically without incising the common duct or placing a T tube. Alternatively, therapeutic endoscopists may use endoscopic retrograde cholangiography with endoscopic sphincterotomy (ERC/ES) to extract stones, and interventional radiologists may dislodge or disintegrate stones by percutaneous transhepatic cholangiography (PTC).

In this chapter we will review the following subjects as they relate to common bile duct stones: presenting symptoms, modes of diagnosis, operative technique, anticipated results, and complications. An algorithm is proposed for quick reference but assumes the surgeon has advanced laparoscopic biliary experience and has excellent endoscopic and radiological support available at his or her institution (see Fig. 1). The obvious goal of

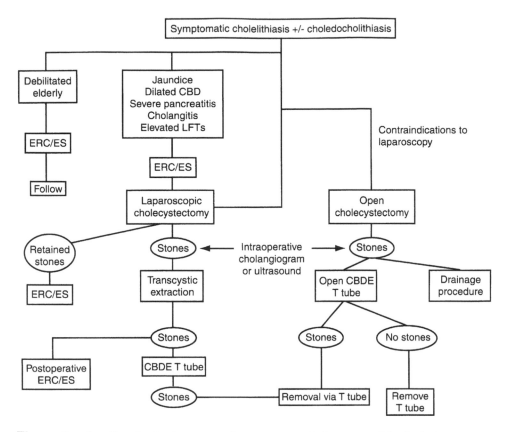

Figure 1 Algorithm for the laparoscopic management of common bile duct stones.

therapy is to achieve ductal clearance with the fewest interventions, the least morbidity, and the lowest cost.

I. SYMPTOMS

Approximately 25–50% of patients with choledocholithiasis develop symptoms attributable to common bile duct obstruction. Commonly, right upper quadrant pain, jaundice, dark urine, or acholic stools are the presenting symptoms. A thorough history may elucidate a pattern of jaundice that may give clues as to the pathology at hand. For example, progressive, persistent jaundice may indicate an impacted common bile duct stone or an obstructing tumor. Prolonged obstruction in the common bile duct may lead to infection and systemic illness. Cholangitis classically presents with the triad of right upper quadrant abdominal pain, fever, and jaundice (Charcot's triad). A subset of patients with cholangitis deteriorate further, developing mental status changes and shock (Reynold's pentad). Cholangitis is considered a medical emergency and requires prompt fluid resuscitative measures, antibiotics, and biliary drainage.

II. DIAGNOSIS

Preoperative predictors of common bile duct stones are insensitive. In patients with known gallstones, approximately 20% of patients with one abnormal serum laboratory value (bilirubin, alkaline phosphatase, ALT, AST, or GGT) harbor common bile duct stones. With two elevated values, the incidence of choledocholithiasis increases to 40%, and CBD stones are present in more than half of patients with three elevated enzymes. The presence of a dilated CBD or choledocholithiasis on ultrasound examination offers little more sensitivity. Nevertheless, surgeons often use this information to direct further treatment. Due to the cost, morbidity (5–10%), and low therapeutic rates (11% for all cases, 33% when ERCP done on selected patients) of ERCP, its routine use is not justified. ERCP is very useful however, when concomitant pancreatitis, malignancy, stricture, or cholangitis are suspected. In addition to liver function tests, serum coagulation markers and serum amylase may be useful. After prolonged common duct obstruction, patients may have a prolonged prothrombin time due to impaired intestinal bile–dependent vitamin K absorption. This abnormality can be corrected with vitamin K replacement.

III. RADIOLOGICAL EVALUATION

Preoperative evaluation of patients with suspected uncomplicated common bile duct stones should include ultrasound examination of the gall bladder, common bile duct, liver, and pancreas. Transabdominal ultrasonography has an accuracy of 55–80% with the two primary indications of choledocholithiasis being duct dilatation (> 7 mm) and echogenic foci within the duct. Ultrasound is now also being used to evaluate the biliary tree intraoperatively. Advantages of this technique include no exposure to radiation, lack of dependence on radiological ancillary support or cumbersome fluoroscopy equipment, speed, as well as the ability to gain anatomical information about surrounding structures. Results, however, are operator dependent, and obstacles such as fatty liver or pancreas or small ducts can prevent thorough imaging. Results reported in the literature for laparoscopic ultrasound range from 70% to 100%, and a learning curve probably exists. Today, magnetic resonance cholangiopancreatography (MRCP) is emerging as yet another alternative for preoperative biliary tract imaging. This radiological procedure offers excellent anatomical detail and has a negligible morbidity rate. MRCP is costly, however, requires radiological support, and is not available in all institutions. Therefore, at this time, intraoperative fluoroscopic cholangiography remains the gold standard to which all other procedures are compared.

Advocates of routine cholangiography cite several reasons why cholangiogram should be performed on every person undergoing elective laparoscopic cholecystectomy. These reasons include the following: (1) some retained stones cause problems in the postoperative period, (2) preoperative predictors of choledocholithiasis are insensitive, (3) ERCP is not available or appropriate in all cases, (4) management of choledocholithiasis at the time of operation saves money and avoids another invasive procedure, and, finally, (5) laparoscopic common bile duct exploration can be performed by the surgeon quickly, safely, and effectively. For those surgeons choosing not to perform routine cholangiography, indications for intraoperative cholangiogram and/or CBDE are listed in (Table 1).

IV. OPERATIVE TECHNIQUE

Trocar placement for laparoscopic common bile duct exploration is similar to that used for routine laparoscopic cholecystectomy. A 30-degree laparoscope is introduced through the 10 mm subumbilical trocar. Next, two 5 mm trocars are placed in the right upper quadrant—halfway between the inferior costal margin and the superior anterior iliac crest

Table 1   Indications for Common Bile Duct Evaluation

Preoperative indications
  Elevated serum liver enzymes: bilirubin, alkaline phosphatase, transaminases
  History of jaundice, pancreatitis, or acholic stools
  Ultrasonographic findings
    Dilated common bile duct (>6 mm)
    Choledocholithiasis
  ERC ± sphincterotomy
  Biliary dyskinesia

Intraoperative indications
  Cystic duct stones
  Unclear anatomy
  Dilated cystic duct (>4 mm)

in the midaxillary line and the other midclavicular inferior to the costal margin. Placement of the latter trocar as lateral and close to the costal margin as possible facilitates use of this port for the cystic ductotomy and later for the choledochoscope. An additional 10 mm trocar is placed in the epigastric region midline and serves as the main working port for the surgeon's right hand.

After the cystic duct is dissected, a cholangiogram is performed. To begin, the cystic duct is clipped where it enters the gallbladder. Next, a small, full-thickness transverse cystic ductotomy is created with scissors. Bile is milked retrograde. A catheter over a 14-gauge introducer needle is inserted percutaneously through the abdominal wall at a point halfway between the midclavicular and midepigastric ports. (*Note:* On the back table, the catheter should be thoroughly flushed of all air bubbles before insertion into the duct to minimize false positives from air bubbles.) Once inside the abdominal cavity, the needle is withdrawn and the cholangiogram catheter is guided into the cystic ductomy using graspers. Alternatively, a cholangiogram may be performed directly through the fundus of the gallbladder. With the catheter properly positioned in the cystic duct, a second clip is used to secure the catheter in place. At this time, a cholangiogram is performed.

Accurate interpretation of intraoperative cholangiography is necessary for successful laparoscopic common bile duct exploration. The entire common bile duct should be visualized including identification of the cystic duct–common bile duct junction, right and left hepatic ducts, intrahepatic biliary radicals, and free flow of contrast into the duodenum. Once all pertinent anatomy has been identified, the common bile duct should be examined for stricture, stones, mass effect, or other abnormalities, including deviant anatomy. Although static images can be used, digital fluoroscopy is much faster and adds minimal time to the overall operative time. If the cholangiogram is negative, the surgeon removes the catheter and proceeds by clipping the distal side of the cystic duct as well as the cystic artery, transecting both structures and completing the laparoscopic cholecystectomy.

If common duct stones are detected, the surgeon may attempt to clear the duct under fluoroscopic guidance alone initially until the choledochoscope is ready. All operating room personnel should be appropriately protected with lead aprons or protective shields to minimize exposure to radiation. The surgeon may begin by flushing the duct with sterile saline. Prior to flushing, the anesthesiologist administers 1 mg of glucagon intravenously to decrease tone in the sphincter of Oddi. Frequently very small stones and debris are cleared using this technique, but larger stones remain intact. In this case, a basket or balloon catheter may be utilized.

Use of a flexible choledochoscope provides direct visualization of the common bile duct and facilitates more precise stone removal. When selecting a scope, choosing one with a minimum 2.4 mm outer diameter and 1.2 mm working channel is useful. Before insertion, a 5 Fr introducer sheath should be positioned so that it traverses the abdominal wall and facilitates safe passage of the choledochoscope into and out of the abdominal cavity. Once inside the peritoneal cavity, the scope is directed into the cystic duct directly using padded graspers, or it may be introduced over a wire. Manipulation of the scope should always take place away from tip where delicate fiberoptic filaments are most vulnerable. Placement of a wire, although not mandatory, facilitates the atraumatic placement of subsequent instruments into the duct system. With the introducer catheter and a 0.35-in. guidewire in place, the choledochoscope (or ureteroscope) is inserted over the wire using a push-pull technique to keep the wire inside the common bile duct. Under direct visualization, the surgeon can then use a variety of graspers, baskets, and balloons to extract stones from the bile duct. Instruments are placed through the working channel of the scope, requiring the instruments to be smaller than 1.2 mm or 3.6 Fr in size. When a basket is used, it is introduced through the working port of the choledochoscope in the closed position. Once past the stone, the basket is opened and the stone is snared inside the wires of the basket. For stones in difficult positions, it is helpful to remember that the direction of the basket is manipulated by directing the tip of the choledochoscope to point directly at the stone. Some baskets require two-handed coordination at the time the basket is closed to prevent loss of the stone while the basket is being closed. A small pushing maneuver should be performed to compensate for the slight withdrawal from the duct that occurs when the basket is closed. When removing a stone from the duct, the scope, basket, and stone should be withdrawn as a unit. While doing so, gentle traction should be kept on the basket to keep the stone taut against the end of the choledochoscope. When basket techniques do not work, it is helpful for the surgeon to be familiar with other instruments and techniques that might be useful depending on different case scenarios. For example, a balloon catheter (Fogarty) may also be used in either a push or pull fashion. When using this instrument, the balloon tip is advanced past the stone into the duodenum and then inflated and withdrawn slowly. Care should be taken when traversing the sphincter (balloon should be deflated) to prevent ampullary trauma that could result in postoperative edema and jaundice or pancreatitis. In addition, caution should be taken to avoid pulling the stone into the proximal biliary tree.

Sometimes the cystic duct is too small in diameter to accommodate the choledochoscope or a common bile duct stone identified on cholangiography. In that case, a balloon angioplasty catheter is introduced into the cystic duct over a guide wire. The balloon angioplasty (5 Fr) catheter is positioned so that the deflated balloon rests with one third of the balloon visible from the cystic ductotomy and the remaining two thirds hidden within the cystic duct. Once properly positioned, the balloon is slowly inflated to the insufflation pressure recommended by the manufacturer. The balloon is left in position for 4–5 minutes to achieve adequate dilatation. With experience, most cystic ducts can be dilated to upwards of 7 mm without complication. The goal for dilation is to accommodate the largest stone identified on cholangiography. Cystic ducts should not be dilated larger than the internal diameter of the CBD, however. Due to the dilatation and attenuation of the cystic duct during these manipulations, the surgeon may choose to ligate the cystic duct with an endoloop instead of clips at the conclusion of the exploration.

If attempts to clear the common duct by the transcystic approach are unsuccessful or the stones are larger than 6 mm, a direct ductal (choledochotomy) approach may be taken. This is performed before the gallbladder is removed so that the gallbladder may be used to provide traction on the common duct. To begin, the anterior wall of the common bile duct is dissected. Next, two stay sutures are placed at either end of the proposed ductotomy. Next, a longitudinal incision (the length of the largest stone) is made on the common duct near the insertion of the cystic duct. If bleeding occurs during this maneuver, a suture should be placed using an absorbable 4.0 suture. To perform the ductotomy, two techniques may be used. First, scissors may be used to make a very small initial transverse incision before extending the incisional longitudinally. Alternatively, an 11 blade placed over a needle-driver can be used to make the entire incision. Disadvantages of the first option include a greater possibility of leak and the possibility of a more difficult closure if a cruciate type of incision is accidentally created. Once the ductotomy has been made, stones can often be milked out of the common duct using the graspers. When the choledochoscope is necessary, it is introduced in the direction of the stones targeted for removal. Through the working port of the scope, irrigation, graspers, baskets, balloons, and lithotripsy devices may be used to facilitate stone removal. As with the transcystic approach, cholangiography is often performed after completion to document a clear duct.

If the duct is cleared of stones (documented with cholangiography and with a choledochoscope), one must decide whether a drainage procedure is necessary. A common bile duct of ample size may be closed primarily with interrupted nonabsorbable sutures. Advocates of primary closure suggest the risk of bile leak after T tube removal is increased after laparoscopic procedures because of an apparent smaller amount of adhesion formation. If the surgeon is unsure if the duct is completely clear or if a stone is intentionally left behind, a drainage tube should be placed. A T tube can be positioned in the common bile duct with the long end pointed distally and the short end proximally. The remainder of the ductotomy is then closed using intracorporeal suturing techniques. Proficiency at intracorporeal suturing is a necessity for this portion of the operation. Nonabsorbable 4.0 suture is used so that the suture does not serve as a nidus for later stone formation. If a T tube is used, it is brought out through a lateral port site and may then be used as access for later cholangiography or endoscopic manipulation of the common bile duct.

V. ANTICIPATED RESULTS

With experience, laparoscopic common bile duct exploration is successful at clearing the bile duct approximately 85–95% of the time (see Table 2).

VI. TROUBLESHOOTING

Sometimes, certain clinical challenges arise that may necessitate alternative action by the surgeon. Below (see Table 3) is a list of scenarios commonly encountered during LCBDE. Therapeutic alternatives are included.

Table 2 Success Rates of Experienced Laparoscopic Surgeons Performing LCBDE

Total LCBDE cases	No. transcystic (%)	No. transductal (%)	Success clearing duct (%)
20	20(100)	0(0)	17(85)
120	111(93)	9(8)	112(93)
197	173(88)	24(12)	189(96)
148	3(2)	145(98)	140(95)
181	147(81)	34(19)	170(94)

Source: SAGES 2001.

Table 3 Clinical Scenarios and Therapeutic Options

Scenario	Management options (in recommended order)
Small diameter (< 6 mm) CBD	Transcystic approach, basket, balloon, choledochoscope, try to avoid choledochotomy and stricture
Obstructed cystic duct	Milk stones back toward gallbladder, repeat cystic ductotomy closer to CBD junction, pass guide wire through cholangiocatheter, make cystic ductotomy over obstructing stone
Impacted stone in CBD	Irrigation (distend the wall allowing a basket to be used), Fogarty catheter, graspers or lithotripsy, conversion to open CBD exploration
Stone in proximal biliary tree	Postural positioning, suction-irrigation, IV glucagon, complete cystic duct dissection (to minimize the angle limitation of the scope), direct transductal approach
Big (> 6 mm) CBD stone	Choledochotomy with scope instrumentation, balloon or basket, placement of T tube or primary closure
Multiple stones in CBD	Biliary bypass with choledocoduodenostomy or hepaticojejunostomy
Bleeding from CBD	Irrigation with cold saline or tamponade with balloon angioplasty catheter
Retained CBD stone	Perform biliary drainage (transcystic tube or T tube) and access for postoperative ERCP
Biliary stenosis	T tube, laparoscopic CBD stent placement, laparoscopic anterograde sphincterotomy if malignancy is ruled out
Cystic duct injury	Ligation of cystic duct with endoloop or intracorporeal suturing
Visual impairment	Flush with saline through working port on scope

VII. COMPLICATIONS

The minor and major morbidity rates quoted in the literature for transcystic laparoscopic common bile duct exploration are 8% and 6%, respectively. In addition, a 1% mortality rate is quoted. Complications related specifically to laparoscopic common bile duct exploration can be divided into five broad categories: (1) failure to clear the common bile duct of stones, (2) injury to the common bile duct, (3) bile leaks, (4) pancreatitis, and, finally, (5) other complications. Patients undergoing transcystic LCBDE usually recover

Table 4   Results of Therapy for Choledocholithiasis

Method	Success rate (%)	Postoperative hospitalization (days)	Return to work (days)
Transcystic duct extraction	80–95	1–2	7–10
Laparoscopic CBDE	85–100	4–7	14–30
Open CBDE	90–100	5–10	20–42
ERC/ES	85–95	2–3	7–14

CBDE = common bile duct exploration; ERC = endoscopic retrograde cholangiography; ES = endoscopic sphincterotomy.

quickly, and the surgeon should suspect morbidity when a patient fails to thrive within 24–48 hours at home. Patients who have undergone transductal LCBDE may take slightly longer to recover, but the recovery time is usually substantially less than with open CBDE because the large subcostal incision is avoided.

After laparoscopic common bile duct exploration, retained stones may occur in up to 10–20% of patients. Not all retained stones cause problems in the postoperative period, however. Single small (< 3 mm) stones will usually pass by themselves and probably do not need to be aggressively pursued unless the patient has a history of gallstone pancreatitis. Stones in the common hepatic duct may be easily missed because the proximal biliary tree is usually not visible by choledochoscope via the transcystic approach. In addition, retained stones may be present after preoperative ERCP. Because of this, completion cholangiography should be performed after LCBDE and routine cholangiography considered in those who have undergone preoperative ERCP. If the surgeon is not sure he has cleared the duct based on completion cholangiography, biliary drainage with a transcystic tube or T tube is prudent and can greatly facilitate postoperative access to the biliary tree for imaging and therapeutic procedures.

Abdominal pain, jaundice, and anorexia after a laparoscopic cholecystectomy or CBD exploration should raise the question of bile leak. Injury to the common hepatic duct, common bile duct, right or left hepatic ducts or an accessory duct are all possible. Damage to these structures can occur from electrocautery or instrumentation and occasionally T tubes become dislodged. In this situation, prompt imaging with CT scan or ultrasound to identify a fluid collection and to guide percutaneous drainage is warranted. Drainage should be followed by contrast imaging with ERCP or percutaneous transhepatic cholangiography (PTC) to define the anatomy. Placement of a covered stent and sphincterotomy at the time of ERCP or PTC may also be considered. Injury to the duodenum or bowel must also be suspected when patients deteriorate in the postoperative period. Failure to make a progressive, complete recovery should prompt a timely, thorough investigation and may require reexploration.

Injury to the common bile duct from ischemia (with subsequent stricture) can occur with overzealous dissection of the duct, especially with electrocautery, and indiscriminant clipping of unidentified structures. Bleeding, if encountered, may often be controlled with direct pressure and the liberal use of suction/irrigation. If more is needed, intracorporeal suturing is recommended. Injury to the common bile duct may also occur from instrumentation if the common duct is too small. Stones within common bile ducts of ≤ 6 mm may best be managed with postoperative ERCP. Avulsion of the cystic duct from the common bile duct may also occur. In this case, intracorporeal suturing skills are necessary for repair, or a T tube may be placed through the site of avulsion.

Pancreatitis after a laparoscopic CBDE can be caused by retained stones, cholangiography, ampullary edema/stenosis, or excessive manipulation/fragmentation of stones in the duct. Avoiding trauma and manipulation of the ampulla can help diminish the risk of pancreatitis in the postoperative period. When using a balloon catheter to clear the common duct, care should be taken to deflate the balloon while traversing the ampulla. If pancreatitis is suspected clinically by exam and serum laboratory values, a retained common bile duct should be excluded by contrast imaging.

Other postoperative complications occur besides those mentioned above and include intra-abdominal abscess from infected stones left in the peritoneal cavity. Numerous studies have examined this issue and it is generally accepted that the rate of intra-abdominal abscess from free stones is minimal if all recoverable stones are removed from the abdominal cavity at the completion of the operation and the right upper quadrant is copiously irrigated and aspirated. Occasionally, circumstances are encountered that necessitate conversion of the laparoscopic procedure to the open approach.

VIII. TRADITIONAL MANAGEMENT

Laparotomy with choledochotomy remains a viable option for managing CBD stones and has a low morbidity rate ($<1\%$) in young patients. We reserve open choledochotomy for patients in whom laparoscopic CBD exploration fails and intraoperative management is indicated and/or when endoscopy is not feasible.

Most impacted stones may be removed through the choledochotomy. Occasionally, however, duodenostomy with sphincterotomy or sphincteroplasty may be necessary to remove the stone.

CBD stones may be left behind for postoperative endoscopic clearance when the stones are small and unlikely to obstruct, the CBD is small and prone to injury, there is no evidence of complete biliary obstruction, or the patient is considered a high operative risk.

IX. CONCLUSION

In conclusion, laparoscopic choledocholithotomy represents an exciting option in the armamentarium of experienced laparoscopic surgeons for the management of common bile duct stones. The literature suggests that this technique is not only feasible, but also safe and effective. A learning curve does exist, however, and multicenter randomized trials comparing laparoscopic, endoscopic, and combined techniques for ductal clearance will be necessary to establish the optimal therapy of choledocholithiasis.

There are two ways to approach laparoscopic common bile duct exploration: via the cystic duct or the direct ductal approach. Both approaches are highly effective, with the transcystic approach representing the less invasive technique. Biliary tract surgeons should consider the laparoscopic management of common bile duct stones as a cost-effective, minimally invasive, safe alternative to ERCP and open common bile duct exploration.

SURGICAL TIPS

A 4 Fr embolectomy catheter may be advanced past the stone, the balloon inflated, and the impacted stone gently pulled back into a more dilated common duct.

If the CBD stone is larger than the lumen of the cystic duct, the cystic duct may be balloon dilated to a maximum of 8 mm in diameter.

Transcystic techniques should be attempted before choledochotomy is considered.

If a choledochoscope is not available, a ureteroscope works well.

Because of tissue edema secondary to ductal dilation and manipulation, the cystic duct stump is ligated (rather than clipped) for added security after choledochoscopy.

Every effort should be made to avoid a choledochotomy in small-diameter (< 6 mm) bile ducts because of the risk of subsequent stenosis.

The choledochotomy should be closed with absorbable 4-0 sutures, because nonabsorbable suture may serve as a nidus for subsequent stone formation.

If stone extraction is not successful, a cholangiocatheter may be left in the bile duct to aid in postoperative ERC/ES.

Proficiency in intracorporeal suturing requires dedicated practice.

SELECTED READINGS

Crawford DL. Laparoscopic common bile duct exploration. World J Surg 1999; 23(4):343–349.

Franklin ME Jr., Pharand D, Rosenthal D. Laparoscopic common bile duct exploration. Surg Laparosc Endosc 1994; 4(2):119–124.

Giurgiu DI. Laparoscopic common bile duct exploration: long term outcome. Arch Surg 1999; 134(8):839–843.

Jones DB, Dunnegan DL, Brewer JD, Soper NJ. The influence of intraoperative gallbladder perforation on long-term outcome after laparoscopic cholecystectomy. Surg Endosc 1995; 9:977–980.

Jones DB, Dunnegan DL, Soper NJ. Results of a change to routine fluorocholangiography during laparoscopic cholecystectomy. Surgery 1995; 118:693–702.

Lakos S, Tompkins R, Turnispeed W, et al. Operative cholangiography during routine cholecystectomy. Arch Surg 1972; 104:484–488.

Lauth DM. Laparoscopic common bile duct exploration in the management of choledocholithiasis. Am J Surg 2000; 179(5):372–374.

SAGES 2001 Hands-On Course II, St. Louis, MO.

Urbach DR. Cost effective management of common bile duct stones, a decision analysis of the use of endoscopic retrograde cholangiopancreatography (ERCP), intraoperative cholangiography, and laparoscopic common bile duct exploration. Surg Endosc 2001; 15(1):4–13.

21

Biliary Bypass

JUSTIN S. WU

*Kaiser Permanente Medical Center
and University of California, San Diego
San Diego, California, U.S.A.*

W. STEPHEN EUBANKS

*Duke University Medical Center
Durham, North Carolina, U.S.A.*

I. BRIEF HISTORY

The incidence of periampullary carcinoma has increased significantly during the past five decades. Approximately 30,000 new cases of pancreatic cancer will be diagnosed this year in the United States, accounting for 85% of all periampullary malignancies. Carcinoma of the pancreas is the second most frequent cause of death from gastrointestinal malignancies and fourth from all types of cancer. The most common type of pancreatic cancer is ductal adenocarcinoma of the head of the pancreas; other types include cystadenocarcinoma and various APUDomas. The remaining 15% of the periampullary malignancies consist of duodenal carcinoma, ampullary carcinoma, carcinomas of the lower common bile duct, lymphomas, sarcomas, and metastatic cancer.

Because periampullary tumors are insidious and often invade surrounding structures early in their growth, surgical resection with curative intent is feasible in less than 10% of patients. For the 90% of patients who have unresectable disease, the principal goal of surgical therapy is to maximize the quality of life by relieving jaundice, pruritis, and gastric outlet obstruction. These palliative procedures include cholecystojejunostomy (CCJ), choledochojejunostomy (CDJ), and gastrojejunostomy (GJ). The implementation of laparoscopic surgery can further optimize the outcome of palliative procedures by reducing postoperative pain, shortening the length of hospital stay, and allowing the patient to return to baseline functioning more rapidly.

Laparoscopic CCJ was first reported in 1992, and most reports subsequently have involved only small numbers of patients. Early data have been promising, with patients discharged between postoperative days 2–12 compared retrospectively to open procedures in which patients had been discharged between 11 and 17 days postoperatively. A recent study at Duke University Medical Center revealed similar lengths of operative time and postoperative hospital stay, comparable rates of perioperative morbidity and mortality, and good long-term palliative results following both open and laparoscopic CCJ.

II. CLINICAL PRESENTATION

The mean age of patients with periampullary carcinoma is 60 years. The *sine qua non* presentation of malignant biliary obstruction is painless jaundice: 65–75% of patients with pancreatic cancer present with jaundice. Thirty percent of patients present with nausea, vomiting, and malnutrition, and of these, 20% ultimately will have duodenal obstruction. Other symptoms include weight loss, coagulopathy, pruritis, and liver failure. Although most patients do not report abdominal pain, patients with advanced malignancy may complain of mild to moderate abdominal or mid-back pain. Abdominal pain associated with jaundice in a patient with malignant biliary obstruction is an ominous finding since it often indicates extension of the tumor into tissue surrounding the pancreas.

III. DIAGNOSTIC TESTS

Abdominal ultrasonography (US) and computed tomography (CT) are established methods to evaluate patients with biliary obstruction. Dilation of the extrahepatic biliary tree, with or without intrahepatic bile duct dilation, or gallbladder distention, can be reliably demonstrated by both imaging studies. A dilated main pancreatic duct may also be demonstrated in these patients. CT is generally considered more useful, however, for detecting pancreatic or hepatic masses as small as 1 cm in size and for demonstrating local vascular invasion.

Cholangiography is often next performed, either by endoscopic retrograde cholangiography (ERCP) or percutaneous transhepatic cholangiography (PTC). The choice between the two largely depends on local expertise, but ERCP is usually selected for the workup of suspected tumors of the distal biliary tree or ampulla. Tissue diagnosis can be confirmed by histological or cytological analysis using either CT-guided needle biopsy or endoscopic brushings and biopsy, although both techniques have high false-negative rates.

Cholangiography is also useful to map the cystic duct and its site of entry to the common hepatic duct. This will allow a decision on whether the patient is suitable for CCJ. If the tumor involves the duodenum causing a potential gastric outlet obstruction, then GJ may also be required.

In the absence of a histological diagnosis by biopsy, laparoscopic exploration can allow assessment of the lesion and the peritoneal surfaces throughout the entire abdomen. Diagnostic laparoscopy can proceed to definitive laparoscopic bypass if unresectable disease is established or can be deferred until biopsies confirm the diagnosis. In most cases, the presence of any metastatic disease confirms the diagnosis and renders biopsy of the primary tumor unnecessary.

Magnetic resonance imaging (MRI) and endoscopic ultrasonography (EUS) have been sporadically applied and are not well established in the diagnosis and staging of malignant obstructive jaundice. Of note, it is essential that benign diseases such as gallstones or chronic pancreatitis, which occasionally mimic tumor, be excluded.

IV. NONOPERATIVE THERAPY

The role and type of palliative procedures for unresectable periampullary carcinoma are controversial. Surgical biliary bypass has been the traditional therapeutic intervention. However, with the advent of percutaneous transhepatic biliary drainage (PTBD) and endoscopic stenting, there are reasonable but often debatable alternatives to operative decompression for treating unresectable periampullary carcinoma. Many reports have concluded that these nonoperative palliative procedures are just as effective for the short-term treatment of biliary obstruction but have lower complication rates, procedure-related mortality rates, and shorter initial periods of hospitalization compared to the surgical biliary bypass procedures. Nevertheless, recent reports indicate that nonoperative palliation is more frequently associated with subsequent complications of recurrent jaundice, stent obstruction, cholangitis, and gastric outlet obstruction.

V. SURGICAL THERAPY

The most appropriate palliative procedure to relieve malignant obstructive jaundice caused by unresectable periampullary tumors is surgical biliary bypass, e.g., CDJ or CCJ. Unresectability of the tumor for cure is defined by nodal involvement, extensive involvement of local structures such as the portal vein or celiac artery, peritoneal or hepatic metastases, or the patient's poor general condition precluding a major resective procedure.

Because of recent advances in laparoscopic techniques, laparoscopic biliary bypass has been added to the armamentarium of the various palliative procedures for malignant biliary obstruction. The best method for palliative biliary bypass is controversial. Both Roux-en-Y jejunal limb and jejunal loop reconstruction is acceptable for the creation of a biliary-jejuno anastomosis. Several authors advocate CDJ as the biliary bypass of choice due to lower morbidity rates or a more effective reduction of bilirubin. Others, however, support CJ as the preferred biliary bypass citing similar morbidity rates. Rappaport and Villalba also support CJ over CDJ because of the simplicity of the procedure and shorter operative times, in conjunction with a comparable relief of symptoms. De Rooij et al. also favor CJ and reported a reduction of morbidity rate from 31% to 21% when comparing CDJ and CJ, respectively.

Absolute contraindications to laparoscopic biliary bypass include patients who cannot tolerate general anesthesia or laparotomy, uncorrectable coagulopathy, prior biliary tract operations such as cholecystectomy or biliary bypass, or certain anatomical locations of the tumor. The latter category includes hilar obstruction (including common hepatic duct stricture) or tumor involving or encroaching on (< 1 cm) the hepatocystic junction. Relative contraindications include prior abdominal surgery causing scarring and adhesions.

In a recent study from Duke University, the majority of patients with malignant obstructive jaundice were shown to be ineligible for laparoscopic CCJ because of the contraindications just discussed; only 22 of 218 or 10% of patients presenting with malignant obstructive jaundice during a 2-year period were candidates for the laparoscopic procedure. Nevertheless, for these few acceptable candidates, the laparoscopic approach remains a desirable option due to its potential benefits.

VI. PREOPERATIVE PREPARATION

The patient must be informed of the benefits and risks of the procedure, including the possibility that the operation will be converted to an open procedure.

Healthy patients can be admitted the day of operation after an overnight fast. In the operating room, the patient is placed in a supine position with the arms tucked to the sides. After induction of general anesthesia, the stomach is decompressed with a nasogastric tube and the bladder is emptied with a urinary catheter. The abdomen is prepped and draped sterilely. Antibiotic prophylaxis is administered (cephalosporin and metronidazole).

VII. OPERATING ROOM AND PATIENT SETUP

The surgeon stands to the patient's right side, and the assistant and the scrub nurse stand opposite the surgeon on the patient's left side (Fig. 1A). Video monitors placed at either side of the head of the table are viewed easily by all members of the operating team. Irrigation, suction, and electrocautery connections come off the head of the table on the patient's left side. Special instruments include an angled (30° or 45°) telescope, atraumatic grasping forceps, atraumatic liver retracter, needle holder, 3-0 absorbable sutures, external anchoring suture, rubber-shod suture holder, linear cutter/stapler, and a suction/aspirator device.

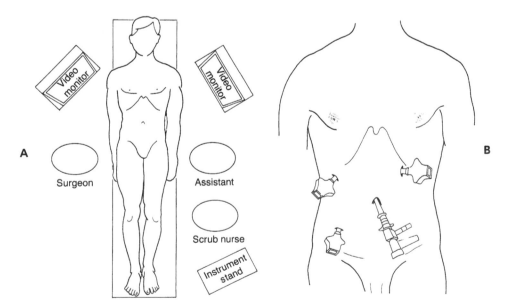

Figure 1   (A) Operating room setup. (B) Port placement for cholecystojejunostomy.

VIII. SURGICAL TECHNIQUE

A. Port Placement

Adequate pneumoperitoneum is achieved either with a closed or open technique in the peri-umbilical location using CO_2 at 15 mmHg pressure. A 10 mm trocar is inserted in this location (Fig. 1B). A 5 mm trocar is placed in the right hypochondrium close to the costal margin. Below this, a 12 mm trocar is placed in the right iliac fossa to introduce the endoscopic cutting/stapling device. A 5 mm port is placed in the left mid-clavicular line for manipulation and suturing.

B. Exposure and Dissection

Examination of the abdomen is initially performed to assess the tumor and the presence or absence of metastases. The inferior surface of the liver is first inspected with a fan-shaped liver retracter which lifts the liver in a cephalad direction. The transverse colon and omentum are then reflected anterior and cephalad to the stomach. This is made easier by placing the patient in the Trendelenburg position and tilting the table to the left. The assistant can then maintain the transverse colon in this position with one grasper through the left trocar. Meanwhile, the surgeon, using two atraumatic graspers, can follow the small bowel proximally by "walking" in a "hand-over-hand" technique until the distal duodenum is reached. Examination of the root of the mesentery is performed with exposure of the ligament of Treitz. The small bowel is then followed down, and a suitable point, approximately 40–50 cm from the ligament of Treitz, is chosen for the anastomosis. The transverse colon is allowed to fall back into position and the small bowel is brought up to the gallbladder in an antecolic fashion (in case a GJ will also be performed).

C. Cholecystojejunostomy: Stapled and Sutured Anastomosis

The loop of proximal jejunum is brought close to the dilated gallbladder. An external 3-0 silk or polypropylene suture on a straight needle is passed through the right lateral abdominal wall. A laparoscopic needle holder grasps the needle, passes it through the fundus of the gallbladder and the jejunum, and then back out the abdominal wall (Fig. 2). Another option is to place two stay sutures at the ends of the selected anastomotic site between the gallbladder and the jejunum. Both techniques can provide appropriate countertraction for the insertion of the linear stapler. The gallbladder is decompressed by aspirating its contents using a long needle. A 1 cm cholecystotomy and enterotomy are made using an endo-scissors with electrocautery (Fig. 3). An endoscopic linear cutter/stapling device is then introduced through the right subcostal trocar; it should be in line with the long axis of the gallbladder and jejunum to easily slip its jaws into the newly created openings (Fig. 4). The device is fired to create two staple lines in a V pattern, thus forming the anterior and posterior walls of the anastomosis (Fig. 5).

The anastomosis is completed by using an intracorporeal 3-0 running suture to close the common openings in the gallbladder and the jejunum (Fig. 6). Sutures are placed by taking bites of tissue 5 mm apart, incorporating full thickness of the gallbladder wall and seromuscular layer of the jejunum (Fig. 7). Another method of closure is by firing a stapler across the base of the openings; if this technique is used, great care must be exercised to avoid narrowing the anastomosis.

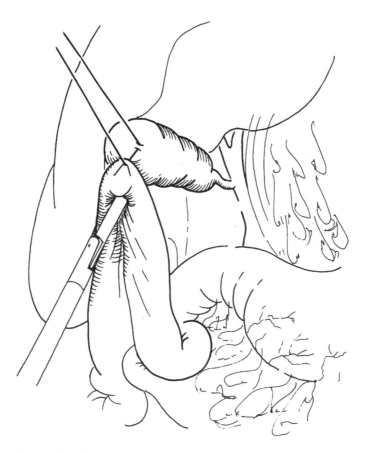

Figure 2   An external anchoring suture is inserted through the abdominal wall, fundus of the gallbladder, and the jejunum.

D.   Cholecystojejunostomy: Sutured Anastomosis

Another method to create a cholecystojejunostomy is by performing a complete single-layer suture technique. Two sutures are used, one for the posterior and the other for the anterior sections of the anastomosis. After selection of the proposed anastomotic sites on the jejunum and the fundus of the gallbladder (as described above), a 25 mm mark is made with the electrocautery on the antimesenteric border and the serosa of the gallbladder fundus. These marks not only identify the incision site, but also maintain the surgeon's orientation during suturing.

A 3-0 absorbable suture is prepared extracorporeally by forming a jamming loop knot at the tail of the suture. The suture is introduced into the peritoneal cavity slowly to prevent inadvertent closure of the loop. The needle is passed through the tissue and the loop, which is then closed by pulling on the body of the suture with the needle holder. Bites of tissue 5 mm apart incorporate the full thickness of the gallbladder wall and the seromuscular layer of the jejunum, thus creating a continuous posterior approximation (Fig. 8). After each suture bite, tension is maintained by the assistant grasping the suture with a rubber-shod or atraumatic grasping forceps.

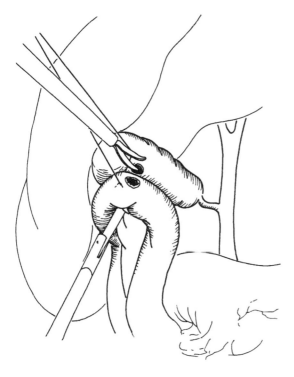

Figure 3 A cholecystotomy and an enterotomy are performed using scissors with electrocautery.

Upon completion of the posterior layer, a reef knot is tied. Both the gallbladder and the jejunum are opened along the 25 mm cautery line and aspirated dry to minimize spillage of their contents (Fig. 9). A second suture with a pretied jamming loop knot is introduced at the apex, and the anterior layer of the anastomosis is sutured in a similar fashion (Fig. 10).

IX. POSTOPERATIVE CARE

Routine prophylactic measures are taken to prevent deep venous thrombosis and stress ulceration. The nasogastric tube may be removed as early as 6 hours postop if drainage is minimal and bowel peristalsis is present. With no complications, the patient should be ready for discharge on postoperative day 2–4.

X. OUTCOMES AND COSTS

In a recent study, open and laparoscopic CCJ had comparable length of surgical time (mean of 1.5 hr with a range of 1–4 hr), similar perioperative mortality and postoperative morbidity rates, and good long-term palliation. However, the laparoscopic group had a shorter postoperative hospital stay. Other series also reported laparoscopic patients being discharged 2–12 days postoperatively compared to open procedures in which patients

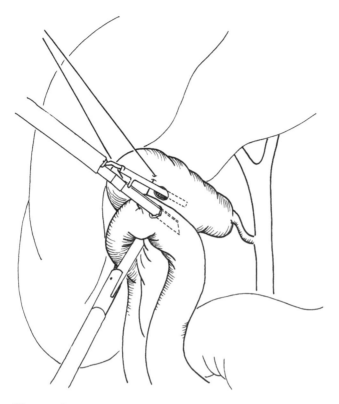

Figure 4 An endoscopic cutter/stapler is introduced into the newly created openings of the gallbladder and jejunum.

were discharged between postoperative days 11–17. The 6-month survival rates were similar with open and closed approaches—58% and 62%, respectively. In the same series, the average hospital cost for the conventional procedure was approximately $15,600 compared to $14,400 in the laparoscopic group.

XI. COMPLICATIONS AND MANAGEMENT

Postoperative complications include ileus, anastomostic edema, anastomotic hemorrhage, bile leak, wound infection, intra-abdominal abscess, and pancreatitis. Ileus and anastomostic edema are managed conservatively with a nasogastric tube and bowel rest for several days until spontaneous resolution.

XII. CURRENT STATUS AND FUTURE INVESTIGATION

Laparoscopic CCJ has recently joined the open surgical bypass and nonoperative stenting as options for palliating patients with malignant obstructive jaundice. It has the advantages of the open surgery, in terms of long-term patency and decompression of the biliary tree with its large diameter stoma, but causes less postoperative disability. Future outcome studies and assessment of pain, satisfaction, and return to work are necessary to confirm

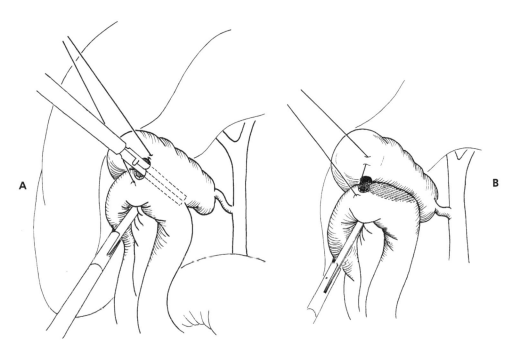

Figure 5 (A) The anastomosis is formed after firing the endoscopic cutter/stapler. (B) The stapled cholecystojejunostomy.

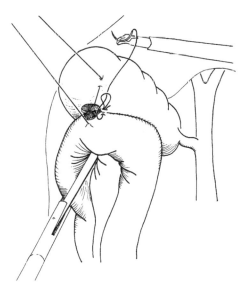

Figure 6 Intracorporeal 3-0 running suture sewing the anastomosis between the gallbladder and the jejunum.

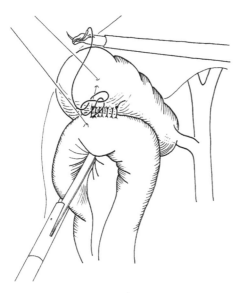

Figure 7   Suture bites 5 mm apart incorporate full thickness of the gallbladder wall and seromuscular layer of the jejunum.

the use of the laparoscopic technique as the modality of choice for palliation of unresectable periampullary tumors in carefully selected patients.

Currently, our group is investigating laparoscopic CDJ as another means for biliary bypass using a porcine model. So far we have successfully performed seven CDJ using entirely laparoscopic intracorporeal sutures.

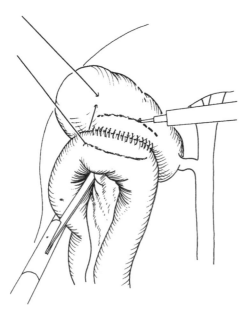

Figure 8   Creation of the posterior layer of the anastomosis.

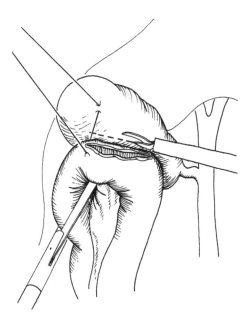

Figure 9   Opening of the gallbladder and the jejunum with scissors.

SURGICAL TIPS

1. Countertraction should be applied prior to the insertion of a linear stapler into the gallbladder and the jejunum.
2. Adequate aspiration of the gallbladder contents is suggested prior to the cholecystotomy.

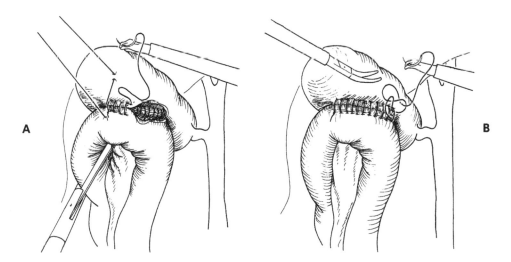

Figure 10   (A) Creation of the anterior layer of the anastomosis. (B) Securing the anterior layer of the anastomosis with intracorporeal knots.

3. The endoscopic linear cutter/stapler can be introduced through either the right subcostal or the right iliac fossa trocar, whichever provides a direct line of fire into the gallbladder and the jejunum.
4. Remember, suture full thickness of the gallbladder wall and the seromuscular layer of the jejunum.
5. The stapling closure of the openings is faster but can easily narrow the anastomosis.
6. Jamming loop knots require practice (see Chapter 7).
7. The above is also true for reef knots.
8. Initially, the Trendelenburg position can help mobilization of the small bowel; reverse Trendelenburg is preferred while performing the anastomosis.
9. The assistant should help provide tension on the suture after each bite.
10. Periodic aspiration of the jejunal contents may be required to avoid spillage into the abdominal cavity.

SELECTED READINGS

Chekan EG, Clark L, Wu J, Pappas TN, Eubanks S. Laparoscopic biliary and enteric bypass. Semin Surg Oncol 1999; 16:313–320.

Cuschieri A, Berci G. Laparoscopic management of pancreatic cancer. In: Laparoscopic Biliary Surgery. Oxford: Blackwell Scientific Publications, 1992: 170–182.

Nordback IH, Cameron JL. Periampullary cancer. In: Cameron JL, ed. Current Surgical Therapy, 4th ed. St. Louis: Mosby-Year Book, Inc., 992:441–448.

O'Rourke N, Nathanson L. Laparoscopic biliary-enteric bypass. In: Paterson-Brown S and Garden J., eds. Principles and Practice of Surgical Laparoscopy. London: WB Saunders Co Ltd, 1994: 179–189.

Tarnasky PR, England RE, Lail LM, et al. Cystic duct patency in malignant obstructive jaundice. Ann Surg 1995; 221(3):265–271.

Wu JS, Centers DS, Eubanks WS. Open versus laparoscopic palliative procedures for unresectable periampullary tumors. South Med J 1994; 87(9):S129.

22

Gastrostomy and Jejunostomy

JUSTIN S. WU

*Kaiser Permanente Medical Center
and University of California, San Diego
San Diego, California, U.S.A.*

NATHANIEL J. SOPER

*Northwestern University, Feinberg School of Medicine
Chicago, Illinois, U.S.A.*

I. BRIEF HISTORY

Enteral feeding has clearly been demonstrated to be the preferred choice of nutritional supplementation for patients with a functioning gastrointestinal tract. This can best be provided through a gastric or jejunal tube, which has traditionally been surgically placed via a laparotomy. The gastrostomy tube was first described by Egeberg in 1837 and first successfully performed in a human by Sedillot in 1849. However, there were numerous complications of intra-abdominal leakage until Verneuil in 1876 devised a method to appose the stomach to the abdominal wall using a silver wire. Verneuil's patient was the first to survive following gastrostomy. Subsequently, there were many modifications, including those by Witzel (1891), Senn (1896), Stamm (1894), and Janeway (1906). The most common technique for open gastrostomy currently is still the century-old Stamm gastrostomy. This procedure uses concentric purse string sutures to hold the catheter in the stomach. The first jejunostomy tube was placed by a French surgeon in 1879. Again, several modifications have occurred over the next century. The most common technique for open jejunostomy currently is the Witzel jejunostomy, which uses a serosal tunnel to prevent intra-abdominal leakage from the catheter entrance site.

Since its introduction in 1980 by Gauderer and Ponsky, percutaneous endoscopic gastrostomy (PEG) has replaced the Stamm gastrostomy in most patients because it is less invasive and less expensive. The endoscopy-assisted technique, however, has not been as successful for jejunostomy, so most are currently performed via a laparotomy. Fluoroscopy-assisted and ultrasonography-assisted gastrostomy and jejunostomy techniques have recently been developed by interventional radiologists; the former technique is just beginning to become popularized, while the latter method has not been widely accepted. In 1984, Russell et al. described a new endoscopically assisted insertion of a percutaneous tube gastrostomy adapting Seldinger's vascular technique. The authors emphasized only a single passage of the endoscope to observe intraluminally the insertion of a needle, guidewire, dilator, sheath, and gastrostomy (Foley) tube. In 1991, the laparoscopic method of gastrostomy tube insertion, using the Russell percutaneous technique, was first published by Edelman et al. Subsequently, the use of Brown/Mueller T-fasteners to anchor the stomach or jejunum to the abdominal wall during laparoscopic gastrostomy or jejunostomy has been a further advancement of the technique.

II. CLINICAL PRESENTATION

Gastrostomy and jejunostomy are common procedures used to provide long-term nutritional support for patients who are malnourished and still have a functioning gut with the ability to absorb and digest nutrients but who are unable to consume sufficient calories to meet their metabolic demands. Gastrostomy is also used to vent the stomach to prevent vomiting or aspiration in patients with mechanical or functional gastric outlet obstruction. These patients can have a variety of underlying diseases including neurological disorders associated with an abnormality in swallowing, oropharyngeal trauma, diabetes mellitus with gastroparesis, gastroesophageal reflux disease (GERD), and tumors of the head and neck, esophagus, stomach, duodenum, or pancreas. These diseases cause various symptoms including anorexia, weakness, vomiting, and weight loss.

III. DIAGNOSTIC TESTS

The tests required are those for the patient's underlying symptoms and disease.

IV. NONOPERATIVE THERAPY

Both gastrostomy and jejunostomy are long-term methods to treat or to prevent malnutrition by feeding enterally. The advantages of enteral over parenteral feeding are its lower cost (5- to 25-fold less than total parental nutrition) and fewer septic complications (especially pneumonia, abdominal infections, and wound infections). Other issues that influence the choice of enteral nutrition or total parenteral nutrition are intraluminal bacterial overgrowth, intestinal mucosal barrier, bacterial and endotoxin translocation, host humoral responses, and cellular immune function. In patients who require short-term enteral feeding, a nasogastric or nasojejunal feeding tube is usually adequate. For those who require longer periods of enteral feeding, gastrostomy or jejunostomy tubes are advised because they are more comfortable and reliable. For enteral feeding, gastrostomy is preferred over jejunostomy because the gastrostomy catheter is larger bore and easier to care for. In addition, bolus feeding through the gastrostomy is more physiological, better tolerated, has less chance of producing osmotic diarrhea, and is less expensive than jejunostomy feeding. When gastrostomy is indicated, PEG is preferred over standard operative gastrostomy because it is technically simpler, less expensive, and can be performed in a minor procedure room. Complications of PEG include intraperitoneal gastric leakage due to the lack of fixation between the stomach and the abdominal wall and injury to hollow or solid viscera since the intra-abdominal contents are not directly visualized.

Jejunostomy is usually performed if gastrostomy is contraindicated, difficult, or has failed. In addition, patients who have had partial or complete gastrectomy, gastric outlet obstruction, severe gastroparesis, or GERD with potential aspiration are ideal candidates for jejunostomies. Currently, percutaneous endoscopic jejunostomies (PEJ) have not been widely used. At our institution, interventional radiology commonly places gastrojejunostomy (GJ) catheters, specially designed so that the proximal port in the stomach is used for decompression while the distal port in the jejunum is used for feeding. However, the technique is somewhat cumbersome and associated with a relatively high rate of tube migration back into the stomach.

V. SURGICAL THERAPY

A surgical gastrostomy is required in patients who are candidates for long-term gastric feeding or decompression but in whom PEG is difficult or has failed, and in those patients with anatomical barriers to placement of a tube by the percutaneous endoscopic method. These barriers include obstructing tumors or strictures of the head and neck, esophagus, stomach, or duodenum, oropharyngeal trauma, liver or colon overlying the stomach, intra-abdominal adhesions secondary to prior abdominal surgery, or a morbidly obese abdominal wall precluding endoscopic transillumination.

Surgical jejunostomies are currently indicated for all patients with indications for jejunostomies in general, i.e., those patients who do not have a functioning stomach with a need for enteral nutrition. The advantage of the laparoscopic approach over the open approaches to gastrostomy and jejunostomy include minimal invasiveness, lower incidence of wound infection, less pain, decreased incidence and length of ileus, earlier postoperative recovery, and better cosmesis. Open techniques are generally indicated only if the laparoscopic technique fails.

The indications and contraindications for laparoscopic gastrostomy and jejunostomy are listed in Tables 1 and 2, respectively. Various techniques for performing laparoscopic gastrostomies and jejunostomies have recently been developed including adaptation of the Janeway, Witzel, and Stamm gastrostomies as well as the Witzel jejunostomy. In this chapter we describe the T-fastener technique that is commonly used by the authors. We also mention the laparoscopic Janeway (permanent) gastrostomy and the laparoscopic knot-tying jejunostomy as alternatives. All methods are safe, effective, and relatively simple.

VI. PREOPERATIVE PREPARATION

The benefits and risks of a laparoscopic gastrostomy or jejunostomy are discussed with the patient. As with other laparoscopic procedures, it is made clear that if at any point a laparoscopic operation cannot be continued safely, the operation will be converted to an open approach. Prophylactic antibiotics are administered, and either general or local anesthesia is used. The stomach is decompressed with a nasogastric tube (NGT) or an orogastric tube (OGT) during trocar insertion to avoid inadvertent injury. The bladder is emptied either by voiding immediately preoperatively or by placing a urinary catheter. The patient is placed in the reverse Trendelenburg position to allow the bowel to fall away from the upper abdomen by gravity. The abdomen is prepped and draped sterilely.

Table 1 Indications

General indications for gastrostomy (endoscopic, laparoscopic, or open)
  To prevent or treat malnutrition
    Inability to swallow due to neurological deficits
      (stroke, Guillain-Barré syndrome, head injury, etc.)
    Obstruction due to stricture or cancer (head and neck, esophageal)
  To vent the stomach to prevent aspiration
    Gastric outlet obstruction, severe gastric ileus

Specific indications for laparoscopic gastrostomy
  Difficult or dangerous percutaneous endoscopic gastrostomy
    Poor transillumination of light through the abdomen (obesity)
    Endoscopy difficult or impossible because of esophageal obstruction
    Severe intra-abdominal adhesions from prior operations
  Failed percutaneous endoscopic gastrostomy
    Early catheter dislodgement with a free gastric perforation
  Concomitant laparoscopy or general anesthesia for other procedures

General indications for jejunostomy (laparoscopic, open, or endoscopic)
  To prevent or treat malnutrition in patients who do not have a functioning stomach
    Gastric outlet obstruction
    Gastroparesis
    Gastroesophageal reflux with aspiration of gastric contents
  Difficult or failed gastrostomy

Specific indications for laparoscopic jejunostomy
  All patients with indications for jejunostomy
  Concomitant laparoscopy or general anesthesia for other procedures
  Difficult laparoscopic gastrostomy

VII. OPERATING ROOM AND PATIENT SETUP

The surgeon stands either at the patient's right or left side, depending on which technique
is used (described below). The assistant and the scrub nurse stand opposite the surgeon.
Video monitors placed at either side of the head of the table are viewed easily by all

Table 2 Contraindications

General contraindications for gastrostomy (endoscopic, laparoscopic, or open)
  No functioning bowel (total parenteral nutrition indicated)
  No functioning stomach (jejunostomy indicated)

Specific contraindications for laparoscopic gastrostomy
  Laparoscopy contraindicated: severe ascites, peritonitis, pregnancy

General contraindications for jejunostomy (laparoscopic, open, or endoscopic)
  No functioning bowel (total parenteral nutrition indicated)

Specific contraindications for laparoscopic jejunostomy
  Laparoscopy contraindicated: severe ascites, peritonitis, pregnancy
  Proximal jejunum cannot be identified due to severe adhesions

members of the operating team. Special instruments include an angled (30° or 45°) laparoscope, atraumatic grasping instruments, Flexiflo Lap G™ Kit (Ross Product Division, Abbott Laboratories, Columbus, OH) for the T-fastener gastrostomy technique, Flexiflo Lap J™ Kit (Ross Product Division, Abbott Laboratories, Columbus, OH) for the T-fastener jejunostomy technique (Table 3).

VIII. SURGICAL TECHNIQUE

A. Port Placement and Exposure

Adequate pneumoperitoneum is achieved either with a closed or open technique in the peri-umbilical location using CO_2 at 12–15 mmHg pressure. A 5 or 10 mm trocar is inserted in this location, and the laparoscope is placed to perform diagnostic laparoscopy.

B. Laparoscopic Gastrostomy

1. Technique #1: Laparoscopic Gastrostomy Using T-Fasteners

This technique utilizes the prepackaged Flexiflo Lap G™ Kit (Ross Product Division, Abbott Laboratories, Columbus, OH), which includes a Brown/Mueller T-Fastener™ Set. The T-fastener is a 1 cm T-bar attached to a nylon suture that is loaded onto a slotted needle (Fig. 1). The surgeon stands on the patient's left side. The stomach is insufflated fully with room air using the previously placed NGT or OGT (Fig. 2). This maneuver separates the anterior and posterior gastric walls. The greater curvature of the stomach is used as the gastrostomy site. If the omentum or transverse colon obscures this site, a 5 mm port can be inserted in the right upper or left lower quadrant through which an atraumatic grasper can be introduced for manipulation. The grasper can also be used to retract and to provide tension on the stomach while placing the T-fasteners.

The T-fastener is introduced into the stomach lumen percutaneously after the pneumoperitoneum pressure is lowered to 5–10 mmHg (Fig. 3). The site of skin puncture is determined by indenting the abdominal wall to appose the gastric wall from the external side and viewing it laparoscopically. This site is usually several cm below the costal margin, ideally through the rectus abdominis muscle. The T-fasteners allow the anterior stomach to be drawn up against the anterior abdominal wall without tension. No endoscopy, laparoscopic suturing, or transabdominal percutaneous suturing of the stomach is required. The first T-fastener is placed farthest from the laparoscope (more proximal on the stomach, closer to the lesser curvature). Once the T-fastener pierces the gastric wall, the T-bar is dislodged by a stylet (Fig. 4). The needle and stylet are then withdrawn simultaneously, leaving the T-bar in the lumen of the stomach. Three additional T-fasteners are placed at 1 or 2 cm distances to form a 4 cm square or diamond pattern around the selected gastrostomy site. The fourth T-fastener should be the closest to the greater curvature of the stomach.

The stomach is gently retracted to the abdominal wall with the T-fasteners, which are temporarily anchored with Kelly clamps or manual retraction (Fig. 5). A J-guidewire is inserted through the center of the T-fastener square via an 18-gauge needle (Fig. 6). At this point, confirmation of the guidewire placement is performed by visualization after loosening the T-fasteners. A 0.5 cm skin incision is made at the guidewire entrance site and carried down through the subcutaneous layer and the abdominal wall fascia. The stoma tract is then serially dilated with lubricated dilators over the J-guidewire, ranging

Table 3 Specific Equipment

0° or angled (30° or 45°) laparoscope
Atraumatic graspers

Gastrostomy
  1. T-fastener technique
    Flexiflo Lap G™ kit:
      Brown/Mueller T-Fastener™ set
        18 ga slotted, beveled needle with stylet
        5 stainless steel/suture T-fastener assemblies
      Flexiflo gastrostomy tube (18 Fr)
      J-guidewire (80 cm)
      #11 scalpel
      Needle, 18 ga × 2 3/4″
      Syringes, 5 cc and 20 cc
      12, 14, 16, 18, 20, 22 Fr dilators
      Gastrostomy-tube stylet
      Nasogastric tube
    Kelly clamps
    Hemostat
  2. Janeway technique
    Two 5 mm trocars
    30 mm endoscopic stapler/cutter
    24 Fr gastrostomy tube

Jejunostomy
  1. T-fastener technique
    Flexiflo Lap J™ kit:
      Brown/Mueller T-Fastener™ set
        18 ga slotted, beveled needle with stylet
        5 stainless steel/suture T-fastener assemblies
      Flexiflo jejunostomy tube (10 Fr), with skin anchor
      Peel away sheath/dilator
      J-guidewire (80 cm)
      #11 scalpel
      Needle, 18 ga × 2 3/4″
      Nasogastric tube
      Syringe, 5 cc
    Kelly clamps
    Hemostat

  2. Knot-tying technique
    5 mm and 10 mm trocars
    Needle holder
    Straight needle with suture
    12 Fr venous introducer kit
      needle
      guidewire
      peel-away introducer/dilator
    10 Fr red rubber catheter

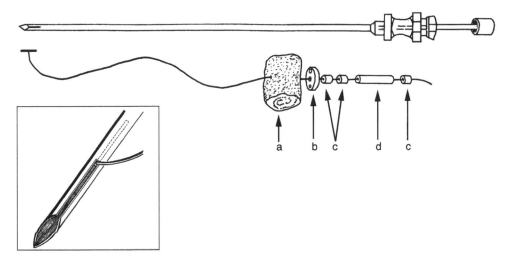

Figure 1 Ancillary components that facilitate securing of the suture line are preloaded on the proximal end of the nylon suture. They are (a) a cotton pledget, (b) a nylon washer, (c) aluminum crimps, and (d) a 4 Fr sleeve. (Inset) A 23 cm, 18 gauge needle with beveled tip is fashioned with a 7 mm longitudinal side slot. A 1 cm T-shaped single piece of stainless steel is carried in the needle so that the T-bar is positioned in the lumen at the tip of the needle. The T-fastener suture protrudes from the slot and trails alongside the needle.

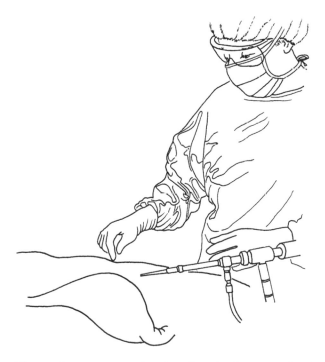

Figure 2 The stomach is insufflated using a previously placed nasogastric or orogastric tube. A gastrostomy site is selected on greater curvature of stomach.

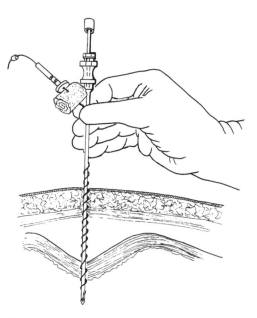

Figure 3   The abdominal cavity is partially decompressed to 5–10 mmHg while gastric insufflation is maintained. The first T-fastener is placed farthest from the laparoscope, into the peritoneum and the stomach.

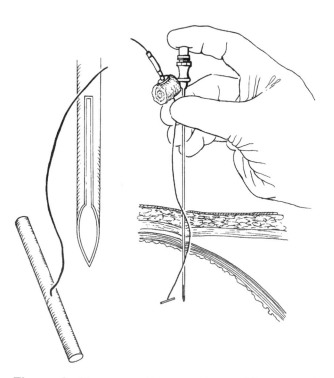

Figure 4   The cm markings are observed for penetration depth. The T-bar is dislodged using a stylet.

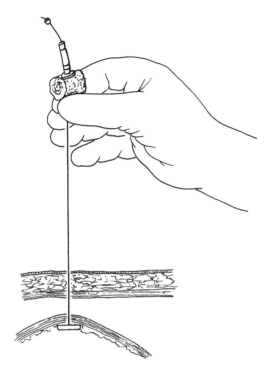

Figure 5 The needle and stylet are withdrawn; this is repeated until four T-fasteners are placed to form a square pattern around the gastrostomy site. The stomach is retracted gently to abdominal wall using T-fasteners. The T-fasteners can be temporarily secured with Kelly clamps or manual retraction.

from 12 to 22 Fr. The 18 Fr balloon-tipped G-tube catheter is placed over the stylet and inserted over the J-wire into the stomach (Fig. 7). This catheter is held in place by inflating the balloon with sterile water and by an external skin disk, which may or may not be sutured to the skin. Again, the T-fasteners can be loosened to confirm tube placement laparoscopically. Further confirmation of the placement can be performed under fluoroscopy by injecting contrast media through the tube.

The stomach is then affixed to the abdominal wall by retightening the T-fasteners, sliding the nylon washers down against the cotton pledgets, and crimping the two aluminum T-fastener crimps with a hemostat (Fig. 8). This strong apposition of the serosal surface of the stomach to the abdominal wall creates a watertight seal, which should prevent leakage of intestinal contents into the abdominal cavity. The stylet and the J-guidewire are removed. Finally, the abdomen is thoroughly examined with the laparoscope for hemostasis and for leakage around the gastrostomy.

2. Technique #2: Laparoscopic Janeway Gastrostomy

Janeway gastrostomy is a permanent stoma with a mucosal-lined gastric tract from the abdominal skin to the stomach. After diagnostic laparoscopy is performed, two 5-mm ports are placed in the left and right midclavicular lines at the level of the umbilicus. The gastrostomy skin site is selected by indenting the left upper quadrant of the abdomen with

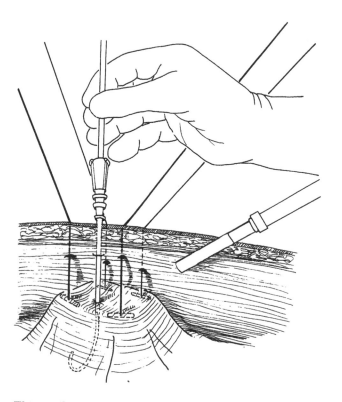

Figure 6   After insertion of an 18 gauge needle through center of T-fastener square, a J-guidewire is inserted through the needle. The needle is removed, leaving the J-guidewire in place. The surgeon observes and confirms the guidewire placement by loosening T-fasteners and viewing them laparoscopically; then the tract is dilated with a series of dilators over the J-guidewire.

a finger and lifting the stomach with grasping forceps to determine the location which will not require excessive tension. A 12 mm port is then placed at this location (Fig. 9) through which a 30 mm endoscopic linear stapler is inserted. The stomach is then held by the two grasping forceps so that the stapler can be applied across the anterior gastric wall close to the greater curvature (Fig. 10). After careful positioning and inspection, the stapler is fired, creating a 3 cm gastric tube or diverticulum (Fig. 11). The diverticulum may be lengthened, if desired, by reapplying and refiring the stapler or using a 60 mm stapler. A 5 mm grasper is then passed down the 12 mm port, and the gastric tube is withdrawn into the port. The port and tube are then pulled out to the skin (Fig. 12). The pneumoperitoneum is released to 5–10 mmHg, allowing the anterior gastric wall to contact the interior abdominal wall. The gastric tube is opened using a scalpel or electrocautery and sutured circumferentially to the skin using 3-0 absorbable sutures (Fig. 13). A 24 Fr gastrostomy tube is inserted, the bulb inflated, and the tube pulled up until the bulb is felt to be snugged against the abdominal wall. Finally, the abdomen is examined laparoscopically for hemostasis and for leakage around the gastrostomy. Further confirmation of the placement can be performed fluoroscopically while injecting contrast through the tube.

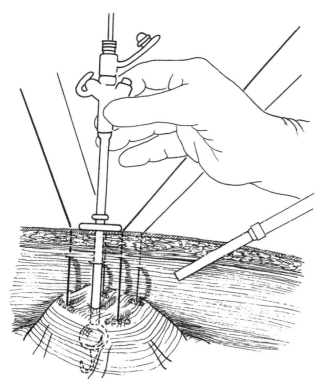

Figure 7 The gastric tube is placed over the stylet and the assembly is inserted over the J-guidewire into stomach. The balloon is filled with sterile water. The T-fasteners are loosened to confirm tube placement laparoscopically.

C. Laparoscopic Jejunostomy

1. Technique #1: Laparoscopic Jejunostomy Using T-Fasteners

This technique utilizes the prepackaged Flexiflo Lap J™ Kit (Ross Product Division, Abbott Laboratories, Columbus, OH), which includes the Brown/Mueller T-Fastener™ Set. The surgeon stands on the patient's left side. Two 5 mm trocars are placed in the left lower quadrant and the right upper quadrant of the abdomen. Atraumatic grasping forceps introduced through these ports can manipulate the omentum and the transverse colon to provide access to the jejunum. The proximal jejunum is insufflated using the previously placed NGT or OGT. Using the grasper, the bowel is "walked" down using a "hand-over-hand" maneuver to the ligament of Treitz and then selecting a point 30 cm distally. This jejunostomy site should provide enough length to reach the abdominal wall without tension. After partially decompressing the abdominal cavity, the proximal jejunum is lifted up to the abdominal wall and a T-fastener is inserted percutaneously into the lumen on the antimesenteric border (Fig. 14). The surgeon should feel the resistance drop as the needle is advanced into the lumen and observe the cm markings for penetration depth before dislodging the T-bar with the stylet (Fig. 15). The needle and the stylet are then withdrawn simultaneously. The first T-fastener is the most difficult to place. It should be located farthest from the laparoscope (closest to the ligament of Treitz); this facilitates

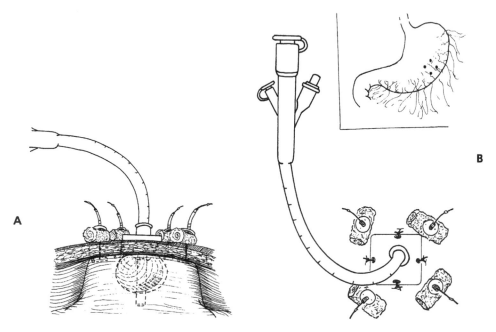

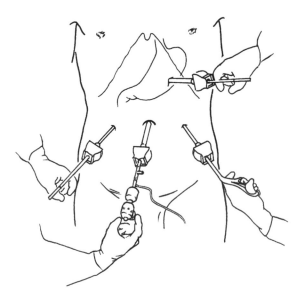

Figure 8   (A) The stomach is affixed to abdominal wall by retightening T-fastener crimps. The stylet and J guidewire are removed. In 10–14 days, the T-fastener sutures are cut, allowing T-bars to pass. (B) The completed gastrostomy.

Figure 9   Port placement and the positions for laparoscopic Janeway gastrostomy.

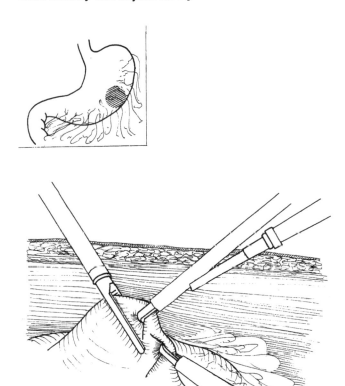

Figure 10 The anterior gastric wall, close to the greater curvature, is grasped by atraumatic forceps and positioned into the jaws of the stapler.

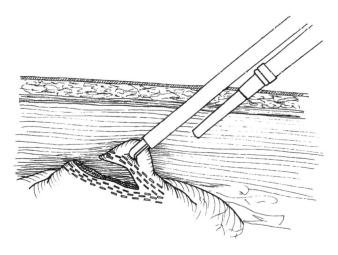

Figure 11 A gastric diverticulum is created after firing the endoscopic stapler.

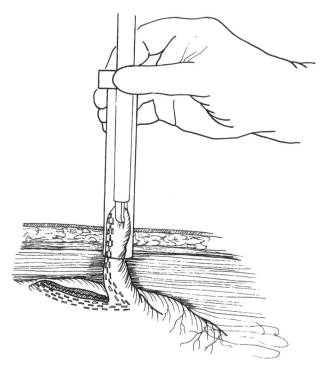

Figure 12   The diverticulum is pulled out through the 12 mm port and opened using a scalpel or electrocautery.

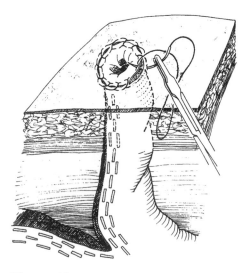

Figure 13   The ostomy is created by suturing the opened diverticulum circumferentially to the skin. A gastric tube can then be placed through the stoma and into the stomach.

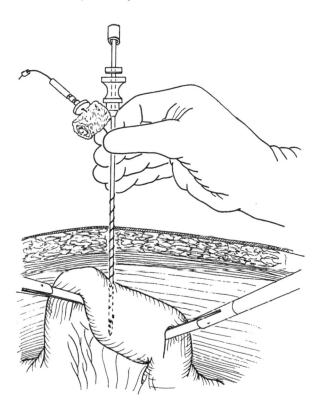

Figure 14 The abdominal cavity is partially decompressed while jejunal insufflation is maintained. The T-fastener is placed farthest from the laparoscope and closest to the ligament of Treitz into the peritoneum and the jejunal lumen.

placement of subsequent T-fasteners. Three additional T-fasteners are repeated to form a 3 cm diamond-shaped area on the antimesenteric border of the proximal jejunum. If the bowel was difficult to insufflate, one can now use the T-fastener needle without the stylet to insufflate; a quick injection of air with resulting intraluminal insufflation confirms that the needle is in the lumen. The small bowel is then gently pulled up to the abdominal wall using all four T-fasteners, which are then temporarily secured with Kelly clamps or manual retraction.

A J-guidewire is inserted through the center of the T-fastener diamond into the lumen of the jejunum via an 18-gauge needle (Fig. 16). Confirmation of the J-guidewire placement is performed by loosening the T-fasteners and viewing it laparoscopically. The distal T-fasteners can be lowered so that the small bowel angles away from the abdominal wall to minimize the possibility of posterior bowel wall penetration. A 0.5 cm skin incision is made at the J-wire site and carried down through the abdominal wall fascia. The tract is dilated with an 11 Fr peel-away sheath/introducer by inserting it over the J-guidewire into the jejunum. The 10 Fr J-tube is inserted through the introducer 10 cm beyond the internal jejunostomy site (Fig. 17). The sheath is then peeled away and removed. The jejunum is again lowered by loosening the T-fasteners, and the tube's placement is confirmed laparoscopically. Further evidence of correct placement can be made by fluoroscopy after injecting contrast.

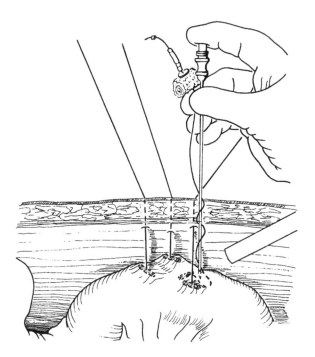

Figure 15   The cm markings are observed for penetration depth. The T-bar is dislodged using the stylet.

The jejunum is affixed to the abdominal wall by retightening the T-fasteners, sliding the nylon washer down against the cotton pledget, and crimping the two aluminum T-fastener crimps with a hemostat. This strong apposition of the serosal surface of the jejunum to the abdominal wall creates a watertight seal, which should prevent dislodgement of the bowel and leakage of intestinal contents into the abdominal cavity. The stylet and the J-guidewire are removed. The abdomen is thoroughly examined with a laparoscope for hemostasis and for leakage around the gastrostomy. Finally, the J-tube is further secured by the external skin disk to the skin (Fig. 18).

2.   Technique #2: Laparoscopic Jejunostomy Using Knot-Tying

After a diagnostic laparoscopy is performed, two additional ports are placed, a 5 mm port in the epigastrium and a 10 mm port in the right lower quadrant. The laparoscope is then transferred to the right lower quadrant position, and the umbilical port becomes the primary operating site. The surgeon stands on the patient's right side. Using grasping forceps the jejunum is followed down to the ligament of Treitz, and a suitable jejunostomy site 30 cm distal to the ligament is brought up to the abdominal wall in the left upper quadrant. An external 3-0 silk or polypropylene suture on a straight needle is introduced through the left lateral abdominal wall, passing through the jejunum, and then inserted back out of the abdominal wall. This suture can be either tied or temporarily secured with a Kelly clamp. Another option is to suture the jejunum to the abdominal wall, using a tapered semicircular needle and tied either intracorporeally or extracorporeally and pushed into place (Fig. 19).

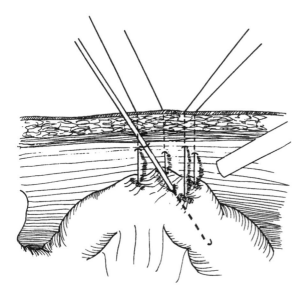

Figure 16 The process shown in Figures 4–15 is repeated until four T-fasteners are placed in a diamond pattern around the jejunostomy site. The small bowel is gently retracted to the abdominal wall using T-fasteners; these are temporarily secured with Kelly clamps or by manual retraction. An 18-gauge needle is inserted through the center of the T-fastener diamond and into jejunal lumen. Then a J-guidewire is inserted through the needle. The needle is removed, leaving the J-guidewire in place. J-guidewire placement is confirmed by loosening the T-fasteners and viewing them laparoscopically.

After the jejunum is securely anchored to the posterior peritoneum with three sutures, thus creating a triangular pattern, a standard 12-Fr venous introducer kit is used to gain access to the jejununal lumen. Adapting the Seldinger technique, a needle is passed through the abdominal wall to the jejunum in the middle of the triangle (Fig. 20). A guidewire is placed through the needle into the lumen of the bowel, and the needle is removed. The dilator and introducer are subsequently placed over the guidewire (Fig. 21). After the dilater is withdrawn, a 10 Fr red rubber catheter can now be placed through the introducer and guided 10 cm distally in the jejunum by an atraumatic grasper. The introducer is peeled apart and removed, leaving the catheter in place (Fig. 22). If an external anchoring suture was used, the surgeon sutures the jejunum to the abdominal wall with three 3-0 stitches that can be tied either intra- or extracorporeally; the anchoring suture can then be removed. After the abdomen is thoroughly examined with a laparoscope for hemostasis and for leakage around the gastrostomy, the J-tube is additionally secured by suturing to the skin. Further confirmation of the placement can be performed fluoroscopically.

IX. POSTOPERATIVE CARE

Both gastrostomy and jejunostomy catheters can be used for feeding immediately after the procedure, but is generally recommended to wait until the following morning. The catheters should be irrigated with 30–60 mL of saline every 4–6 hours or before and after

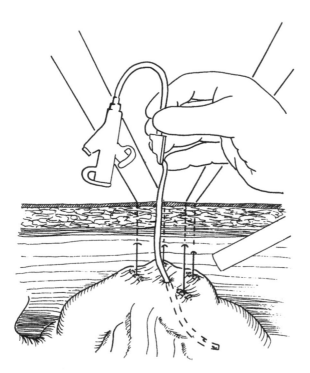

Figure 17 After dilation of the tract by inserting a peel-away sheath/dilator over the J-guidewire into the jejunum, the dilator and J-guidewire are removed. Then the J-tube is threaded through the peel-away sheath to 10 cm beyond the internal jejunostomy site. The peel-away sheath is removed; the jejunum is lowered by loosening the T-fasteners, and tube placement is confirmed laparoscopically. Placement is further confirmed radiologically including a check for extravasation by injecting contrast media through the tube.

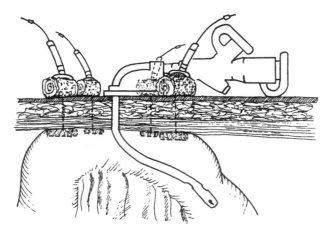

Figure 18 The jejunum is affixed to the abdominal wall by retightening the T-fasteners and crimping the aluminum T-fastener crimps. The J tube is sutured to the skin anchor to prevent slippage, and the skin anchor is sutured to the skin. In 10–14 days, the T-fastener sutures are cut, allowing T-bars to pass.

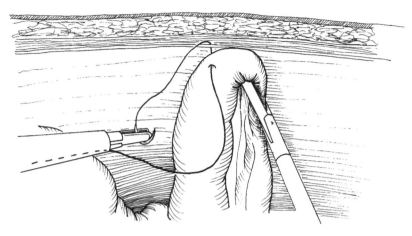

Figure 19 The jejunum is sutured to the abdominal wall from the inside and secured with a knot tied either intra- or extracorporeally and pushed into place.

each feeding. In 10–14 days, after maturation of the stoma tract, the T-fasteners are removed by cutting the nylon sutures at the skin level. The 1 cm stainless steel T-bars are allowed to pass in the stool.

Any medications administered through both tubes should be crushed thoroughly to keep the catheter patent. Diarrhea is not uncommon, especially with jejunostomy tube feedings. This can usually be controlled by slowing the rate of the tube feeds temporarily, by changing to an isotonic formula, or by adding Kaopectate or paregoric to the formula.

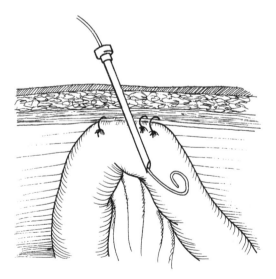

Figure 20 A needle is inserted percutaneously into the jejunum. The guidewire is then placed through the needle.

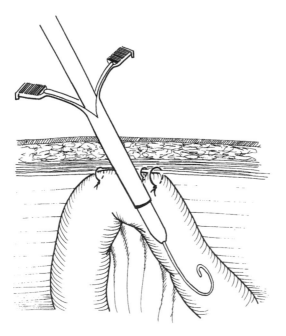

Figure 21   After removing the needle, a 12 Fr peel-away sheath and dilator are passed over the wire into the jejunum.

X.   OUTCOMES AND COSTS

Since laparoscopic gastrostomies and jejunostomies are relatively new procedures, there are few published data regarding the outcomes and costs. Sangster and Swanstrom in 1993 described laparoscopic jejunostomies in 23 patients using the knot-tying technique. The average operative time was 45 minutes. All patients were receiving full nutritional support within 48° of the tube placement. The only complications were a superficial abscess in one patient and minor skin breakdown in two patients. The authors also reported the operating room and GI lab charges for various procedures: $873.85 for PEJ, $1,676.87 for open jejunostomy, and $2,398.07 for laparoscopic jejunostomy.

In 1994, Edelman et al. looked at 20 consecutive patients with laparoscopic gastrostomies and reported an average operating time of 20 minutes (range 10–25 min) and blood loss of < 10 mL with no morbidity or mortality. Duh and Way in 1995 described 25 consecutive laparoscopic T-fastener gastrostomies with no morbidity or mortality. They also performed 31 consecutive laparoscopic T-fastener jejunostomies with 6% morbidity (one patient with a cutaneous fistula and another with wound infection) and no mortality. Murayama et al. in 1995 compared 32 patients who had laparoscopic T-fastener gastrostomies with 37 patients who had open gastrostomies. The operative time was significantly shorter in the laparoscopic gastrostomy group (38 min vs. 62 min). The rate of major complications for the laparoscopic gastrostomy was 6% compared to 11% for the open gastrostomy. There were no procedure-related deaths in the former group, whereas three patients in the latter group died in the immediate postoperative period.

Duh et al. in 1999 prospectively randomized patients undergoing laparoscopic gastrostomy and jejunostomy to general versus local anesthesia. Of the 48 patients studied,

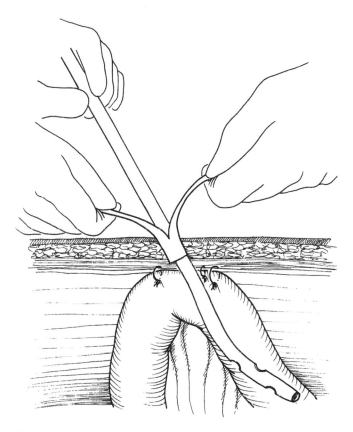

Figure 22 After the dilator is removed, a 10 Fr red rubber J-tube is passed through the peel-away catheter, and the sheath is then removed.

there were no differences in success rates, complications, total mean cost, and procedure time in the two groups. Some patients in the local anesthesia group complain of abdominal discomfort, which seemed to be the diaphragmatic irritation due to carbon dioxide pneumoperitoneum. This problem was alleviated by providing deeper (level 2) sedation or by lowering pneumoperitoneum pressure (4–6 mmHg). Using nitrous oxide pneumoperitoneum or the gasless technique may decrease the amount of intravenous sedation required. Nevertheless, the authors remarked that potential savings are possible from the operating room or anesthesiologist costs if the procedures are performed in an endoscopy suite without monitored anesthesia care.

XI.   COMPLICATIONS AND THEIR MANAGEMENT

Some of the potential complications include the usual risks of laparoscopy: local wound infection; injury to the abdominal organs, which can be repaired by laparoscopic or open suturing; and penetration of the posterior gastric or jejunal wall. The best way to confirm proper placement of the catheter and to prevent the latter complication is by temporarily dropping the stomach or jejunum away from the abdominal wall and identifying the catheter entrance. In the jejunostomy placement technique, 5 mL of air can be injected into the bowel in order to document the intraluminal position of the needle. Other complications include dislodgement of the catheters and leaks around the catheter at the skin site. Both situations can be managed by replacement with a larger gastrostomy or jejunostomy tube at bedside.

XII. CURRENT STATUS AND FUTURE INVESTIGATION

Recent developments and improvements in laparoscopy have allowed new methods of feeding tube placement. Although PEG is still considered the preferred method for enteric access, surgical gastrostomies and jejunostomies are commonly employed in patients who are not candidates for the percutaneous endoscopic techniques. A large prospective study is needed to compare open and laparoscopic approaches and to evaluate issues such as operative time, postoperative pain, complication rates, recovery time, length of hospitalization, and costs. In addition, further studies should compare the PEG, laparoscopic technique, and fluoroscopy-guided placement of gastrostomy tubes.

SURGICAL TIPS

1. Maintaining gastric or jejunal insufflation via an NGT/OGT helps prevent inappropriate T-fastener placement.
2. If the stomach or bowel is too difficult to insufflate, use the T-fastener needle without the stylet to insufflate.
3. The gastrostomy site should be selected on the greater curvature of the stomach or the antimesenteric side of the jejunum to ensure good laparoscopic visualization.
4. Sequence of multiple T-fastener or suture placement is important to allow maximal laparoscopic visualization. Work toward the laparoscope.
5. Retract the stomach or the jejunum *gently* to help prevent tearing by the T-fasteners or sutures.
6. For definitive G-tube or J-tube placement, location can be confirmed radiologically.
7. Proficiency in intracorporeal suturing requires dedicated practice.
8. The pneumoperitoneum can be released temporarily to 5–10 mmHg to allow the gastric or jejunal wall to contact the anterior abdominal wall.
9. The jejunum can be followed to the ligament of Treitz with graspers in a "hand-over-hand" technique.
10. Peel the peel-away sheath/dilator in a smooth and slow fashion while the assistant holds the J-tube with forceps.

SELECTED READINGS

Brown AS, Mueller PR, Ferruci JT Jr. Controlled percutaneous gastrostomy: nylon T-fastener for fixation of the anterior gastric wall. Radiology 1986; 158:543–545.

Duh QY. Laparoscopic gastrostomy and jejunostomy. Surg Rounds 1995 (April):143–151.

Duh QY, Senokozlieff AL, Choe YS, Siperstein AE, Rowland K, Way LW. Laparoscopic gastrostomy and jejunostomy. Arch Surg 1999; 134:151–156.

Edelman DS and Unger SW. Laparoscopic gastrostomy and jejunostomy. Surg Lap Endosc 1994; 4(4):297–300.

Murayama KM, Schneider PD, Thompson JS. Laparoscopic gastrostomy: a safe method for obtaining enteral access. J Surg Res 1995; 58:1–5.

Russell TR, Brotman M, Norris F. Percutaneous gastrostomy—a new simplified and cost-effective technique. Am J Surg 1984; 148:132–137.

Watson TJ and Peters JH. Laparoscopic feeding gastrostomy and jejunostomy. In: Peters JH and DeMeeste TR, eds. Minimally Invasive Surgery of the Foregut. St. Louis: Quality Medical Publishing, Inc., 1994; 309–324.

23

Paraesophageal Hiatal Hernias

EDWARD LIN and C. DANIEL SMITH

Emory University School of Medicine
Atlanta, Georgia, U.S.A.

I. TERMINOLOGY

Degeneration of the stabilizing attachments at the esophageal hiatus ultimately manifests as paraesophageal hernias. Although the etiology for this acquired defect is not fully understood, its association with advanced age implicates chronic stress to the ligamentous phrenoesophageal membrane of the crura as a causative factor (Fig. 1).

Paraesophageal hernias are classified into three types, but a fourth type has been increasingly used in nomenclature (Fig. 2). Approximately 90% of paraesophageal hernias are the type I sliding hiatal hernia, which more commonly affect women after the fifth decade of life. Indeed, hiatal hernias are the most commonly described abnormalities found on barium studies of the foregut. The hiatal hernia is characterized by the upward migration of the gastroesophageal junction into the posterior mediastinum. While surgeons disagree on the existence of a true hernia sac in hiatal hernias, there is little debate that the phrenoesophageal membrane is attenuated and elongated in a type I defect.

Accounting for 5–10% of all hiatal hernias, type II and III defects are true paraesophageal hernias because the gastric fundus herniates through the hiatal defect and is juxtaposed with the esophagus. Furthermore, type II and III hernias have true hernia sacs that accompany the herniated stomach. This hernia sac is comprised of the visceral peritoneum on the undersurface, the phrenoesophageal membrane, and the pleural lining on the superior aspect. The type II paraesophageal hernia is characterized by herniation of the gastric fundus through the hiatus anterior to the esophagus while the gastroesophageal junction remains fixed to its normal position. The type III paraesophageal hernia, or *mixed* type, is characterized by displacement of both the gastric fundus and the gastroesophageal junction into the mediastinum. Typically, type I hernias are simply referred to as hiatal hernias, while type II and III are paraesophageal hernias. Of the paraesophageal hernias, the type III variant makes up 90% of the cases encountered. Moreover, large variants of

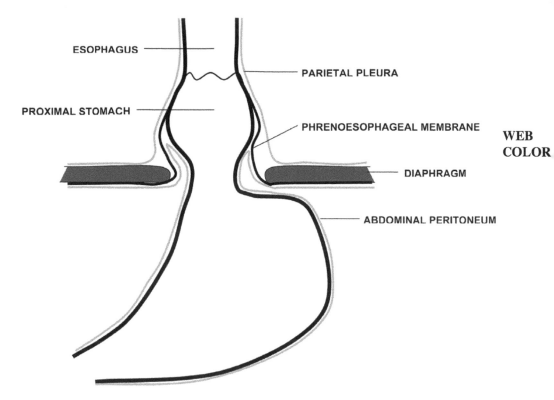

WEB COLOR

Figure 1 Depiction of a sliding (type I) hiatal hernia with the gastroesophageal junction protruding above the diaphragm. The phrenoesophageal membrane normally anchors the gastroesophageal junction at the level of the hiatus, but is stretched into the mediastinum in a hiatal hernia. The abdominal peritoneum is similarly drawn into the mediastinum, forming a potential hernia sac.

type II and III hernias have been alternatively called *giant* paraesophageal hernias, but this designation is often arbitrary. Most paraesophageal hernias occur in adults greater than 50 years of age, while the type I hiatal hernia is not uncommon in younger adults.

Difficulties in the management of paraesophageal hernias can be compounded by the presence of a gastric volvulus. Most reports of gastric volvulus associated with large paraesophageal hernias describe an approximate incidence of 5%, but tertiary thoracic surgical centers have reported incidences up to 50%! As the hernias enlarge, lax ligamentous anchors of the stomach permit 180-degree gastric rotation around its longitudinal axis, known as an *organoaxial* volvulus (Fig. 3). Consequently, the posterior aspect of the gastric wall sits anteriorly and a closed-loop obstruction of the stomach is formed. A much less common form of gastric volvulus is the *mesenteroaxial* rotation, where the antrum rotates around a transverse axis in the mid-stomach, frequently causing partial upper gastrointestinal obstructions (Fig. 3). A combination of the two rotations within the hernia sac is possible, but this is extremely rare.

When encountered in the literature, type IV hernias refer to gastric herniation into the chest along with intra-abdominal organs such as the colon, omentum, and spleen.

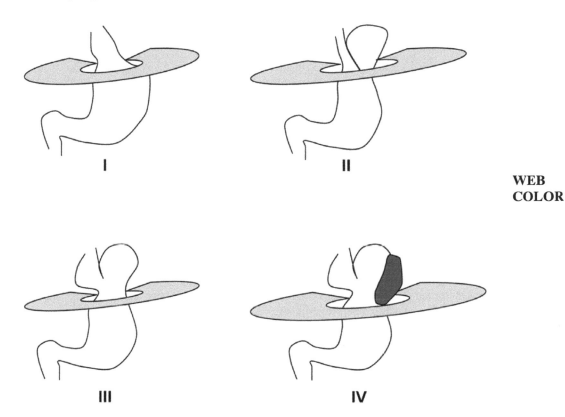

Figure 2 Types of paraesophageal hiatal hernias. Type I is a sliding hiatal hernia with the gastroesophageal junction and the proximal stomach protruding above the diaphragm. Type II paraesophageal hernias have a fixed intra-abdominal gastroesophageal junction, but a portion of the stomach herniates through the hiatus alongside the esophagus. Type III is a mixed paraesophageal hernia with herniation of both the stomach and gastroesophageal junction into the mediastinum. The Type IV paraesophageal hernia is not a universally accepted classification but refers to herniation of the stomach along with other intra-abdominal organs such as the spleen, omentum and colon.

II. PRESENTATION

Many hiatal hernias are asymptomatic and do not warrant intervention. Symptomatic type I hiatal hernias typically present in association with gastroesophageal reflux symptoms that include chest pain, cough, dysphagia, regurgitation, heartburn, vocal hoarseness, and respiratory complaints. Occult upper gastrointestinal bleeding should also be considered in patients with chronic hiatal hernias due to traumatic fluctuation of the proximal stomach through the hiatus. It should be noted that while 50% of patients with gastroesophageal reflux disease have hiatal hernias, the hernia is more likely a factor that augments ongoing reflux esophageal injury and not a primary cause of the disease.

Symptoms related to paraesophageal hernias (types II and III) are distinct from hiatal hernias, and if they are not surgically corrected, traditional dogma suggests a

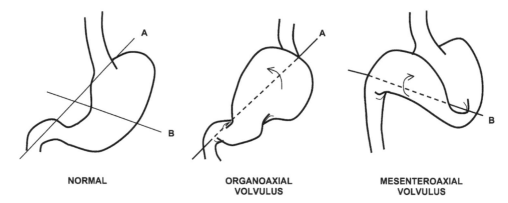

NORMAL   ORGANOAXIAL   MESENTEROAXIAL
                VOLVULUS   VOLVULUS

Figure 3 Gastric volvulus along a rotational axis can be a potential complication of longstanding paraesophageal hernias. (A) Rotation along a longitudinal axis is an organoaxial volvulus, with the posterior stomach now oriented anteriorly. This results in a closed-loop obstruction of the stomach. (B) Folding of the stomach along a transverse axis is a mesenteroaxial volvulus, which divides the distal stomach from the proximal. This can result in a partial gastric outlet obstruction.

morbidity and mortality rate that approaches 30–50%. However, while the need for emergent surgery is considerably lower in most current series (Table 1), there is no debate that grave complications are associated with emergent surgery for incarcerated or strangulated hernia contents. Not all patients diagnosed with paraesophageal hernias are symptomatic. However, more discriminating patient questioning often will confirm a history of vague abdominal symptoms with variable duration (Table 1). The most significant symptoms are related to upper gastrointestinal obstruction such as early satiety, postprandial distress or pain, vomiting, and dysphagia. Anemia is present in 25% of patients with paraesophageal hernias, some requiring repeated blood transfusions. Other serious complications of paraesophageal hernias include restrictive pulmonary disease, strangulation, ulceration, and perforation. Type III paraesophageal hernias commonly present with gastroesophageal reflux symptoms due to the sliding gastroesophageal junction. The notion that type II paraesophageal hernias do not have reflux symptoms due to a normally positioned gastroesophageal junction is a fallacy. In fact, whenever complete studies are feasible, 70% of patients with type II paraesophageal hernias have pathological acid reflux or incompetent lower esophageal sphincters documented by 24-hour pH studies and manometry, respectively.

When symptoms are present, those associated with paraesophageal hernias (dysphagia, chest pain, bloating, and respiratory distress) tend to be more severe than those associated with sliding hiatal hernias.

III. DIAGNOSIS

The diagnosis of type I hiatal hernias is most commonly achieved by endoscopy and barium studies. In many cases, characteristic lower esophageal sphincter manometry profiles ("double hump") lend support to the diagnosis (Fig. 4).

Table 1 Clinical Presentation for Paraesophageal Hernias (Excluding Type I) from Centers Reporting Consecutive Experience with More Than 90 Patients

Group (Ref.)	Year	N	Age	Female: Male	Postprandial discomfort/ substernal pain (%)	Regurgitation/ emesis (%)	Heartburn (%)	Dysphagia (%)	Anemia/UGI bleed (%)	Volvulus (%)	Respiratory dysfunction (%)	Emergent surgery (%)
Lahey Clinic (31)	1993	119	64	75:44	74	50	33	50	26	7	—	6
Mayo Clinic–Rochester (1)	1993	147	69	93:54	59	31	16	30	23	5	13	3
Toronto General (14)	1998	94	64	60:34	56	15	31	48	38	50	19	2
University of Illinois–Chicago (5)	2000	100	73	61:39	90	89	74	20	18	16	—	20
University of Pittsburgh (11)	2000	100	64	62:38	31	37	55	—	26	29[a]	11	4
Emory University (13)	2002	125	64	85:40	30	17	23	25	17	4[b]	—	3
Summary (Averages)		681 Total	66	1.8:1 Ratio	56	40	39	35	25	19	14	6

[a]From Ref. 21.
[b]From Ref. 27.

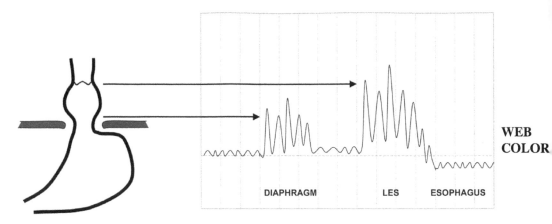

WEB
COLOR

Figure 4 Manometric tracing of a sliding hiatal hernia demonstrating a "double-hump" configuration. The first set of pressure tracings are generated from the diaphragm. The second set of pressure tracings are from the lower esophageal sphincter, which has an intrathoracic position. The esophageal pressure tracings deflect below the baseline because of the negative intrathoracid pressure.

A. Endoscopy

Many hiatal and paraesophageal hernias are diagnosed incidentally by endoscopy performed for other reasons. Diagnosis of these hernias can be made by retroflex view with the endoscope. The gastroesophageal junction can often be found within or at the orifice of the herniated stomach (Fig. 5). The most telling indication of a paraesophageal hernia is the presence of gastric rugal folds above the diaphragm. Endoscopy is limited by its inability to differentiate large sliding hiatal hernias with paraesophageal hernias. Large hernia sacs that compress the esophagus may render false estimates of esophageal length or impede passage of the endoscope below the area of obstruction. Nevertheless, whenever feasible, endoscopy should be performed to determine the presence of esophagitis, gastritis, ulcers, or tumors. On occasion, endoscopy may offer temporary decompression of incarcerated portions of the stomach.

The inability to pass a nasogastric tube into the stomach or termination of the distal tip in the intrathoracic stomach is often the initial indicator of a large paraesophageal hernia. Furthermore, Borchardt's triad of epigastric pain, inability to vomit, and the inability to pass a nasogastric tube into the stomach can be suggestive of impending gangrene.

B. Radiological Studies

Paraesophageal hernias are often discovered incidentally by plain upright chest radiographs. Retrocardiac air-fluid levels can be demonstrated by these studies, particularly in the lateral view (Fig. 6). The barium esophagram remains the most utilized and informative for diagnosing paraesophageal hernias (Fig. 7). Although not always feasible, the position of the gastroesophageal junction should be noted in these studies. The position of the gastroesophageal junction can sometimes be identified by a double contrast (air and barium) technique (Fig. 8). Barium enema studies for the colon

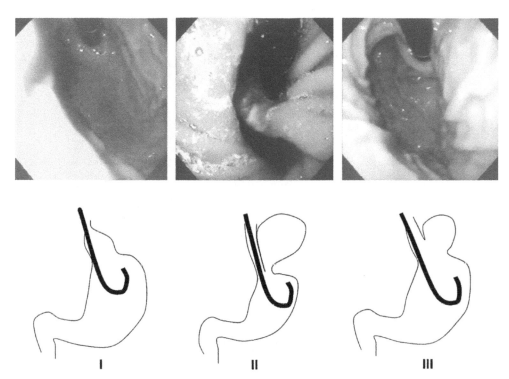

Figure 5 Endoscopic retroflex ("J") view of the three types of paraesophageal hernias. (I) A large sliding (Type I) hiatal hernia. (II) A Type II paraesophageal hernia with a fixed gastroesophageal junction and a narrow orifice through which the gastric fundus herniates into the mediastinum. Note the gastric rugal folds ascending into the hernia sac. (III) A Type III paraesophageal hernia with the gastroesophageal junction emerging midway along the side of the hernia. Again, gastric rugal folds are ascending past the hernia orifice into the mediastinum. It is often difficult to differentiate a Type III paraesophageal hernia from a large Type I hiatal hernia.

can also demonstrate intrathoracic stomach and bowel, confirming a paraesophageal hernia.

Computed tomography (CT) scans are often performed early in the patient's work-up, not necessarily to find paraesophageal hernias but to investigate the cause for symptoms such as weight loss and early satiety. In addition, three-dimensional reconstruction of the paraesophageal hernia in relation to adjacent structures can be readily obtained. However, these studies do not contribute much to the treatment algorithm for paraesophageal hernias, particularly in the symptomatic patient.

C. Esophageal Motility and pH Studies

Many patients presenting for elective management of paraesophageal hernias will have had manometry and 24-hour pH studies. Of these studies, many will be inconclusive or incomplete because of difficulties in passing the catheters and unusual pressure tracings that render uninterpretable results. There is, however, the potential to glean information about cricopharyngeal function and esophageal body motility from these studies.

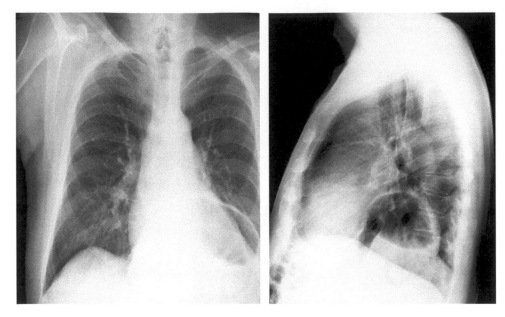

Figure 6 Chest radiograph of a patient with complaints of early satiety and upper abdominal pain. A retrocardiac gastric bubble can be seen in the anterior-posterior view, and if unclear, the lateral view demonstrates the gastric bubble above the diaphragm.

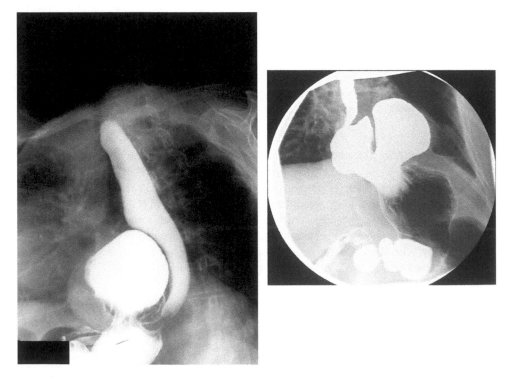

Figure 7 Barium esophagrams for a Type II paraesophageal hernia (left) with the gastroesophageal junction located at the hiatus, and a Type III paraesophageal hernia (right) with mediastinal herniation of both the gastroesophageal junction and the stomach.

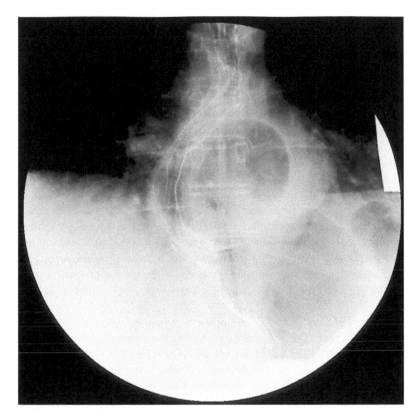

Figure 8   Double contrast (air and barium) studies can often ascertain the position of the gastroesophageal junction, which is situated below the diaphragm in this esophagram. This is a Type II paraesophageal hernia.

IV. SURGICAL TREATMENT

Hiatal hernias that are asymptomatic generally do not require therapy. Problematic hiatal hernias usually present in conjunction with gastroesophageal reflux symptoms. These patients are likely to undergo an unspecified period of acid reduction medication and postpone surgical management until the disease is recalcitrant to medication or when compliance becomes an issue. Given that both incompetent lower esophageal sphincter function and hiatal hernias are mechanical derangements, surgical correction should be considered early.

With the potential morbid complications for untreated type II or type III paraesophageal hernias, patients with known paraesophageal hernias should undergo surgery when their physical status is optimal. The principles of surgical repair are the same for open cases and for laparoscopic cases. These are to return the herniated contents to their anatomically correct positions below the diaphragm, to repair the defect, and to prevent recurrence.

There are several pivotal issues that surround the operative management of paraesophageal hernias.

A. Role of Antireflux Procedures in Paraesophageal Hernia Repairs

Few studies have objectively evaluated this issue. With the anatomical and functional derangements of the lower esophageal sphincter in type I and type III hernias, it is intuitive that antireflux procedures should be part of the repair. Despite the fact that most data to date have average follow-ups of less than 30 months after surgery, the overall favorable outcome following combined paraesophageal hernia repairs and antireflux procedures leaves few who are willing to prospectively compare the dual procedure with the hernia repair alone.

As much as half of the patients who present for management of paraesophageal hernias will give a remote history consistent with gastroesophageal reflux. In addition, the vast majority of patients with type II paraesophageal hernias who were amenable to 24-hour pH and motility studies have documented diminution in lower esophageal sphincter function, even though the gastroesophageal junction is intra-abdominal. Furthermore, circumferential mobilization of the gastroesophageal junction during surgery effectively disrupts any intrinsic contribution of the hiatus to lower esophageal sphincter function. Taken together, an antireflux procedure in paraesophageal hernia surgery will very likely avert the unmasking of gastroesophageal reflux disorders following hernia repair.

Lastly, a fundoplication also serves as an anchor to tether the stomach below the diaphragm after the hernia repair. The practice of anchoring the stomach stems from the beginning of open repairs, but there are no studies to support or refute this procedure. Tube gastrostomies have been advocated by some to anchor the anterior stomach to the abdominal wall in place of a fundoplication, but there have been reports of recurrent herniations of the free posterior stomach—particularly if a hernia sac posterior to the esophagus was missed.

B. Hernia Sac Removal

The primary rationale for completely resecting any hernia sac is to prevent recurrence. Early experience from the Mount Sinai Medical Center had a 20% hernia recurrence 6 months after surgery when the hernia sac was not excised. Initial experience with laparoscopic paraesophageal hernia repairs without excising the hernia sac resulted in fluid collections in the posterior mediastinum postoperatively. Moreover, larger sacs compressed the esophagus causing dysphagia and perpetuated pulmonary restriction. Laparoscopic resection of the hernia sac can be a tedious task particularly in complex and recurrent hernias because of potential injury to the esophagus, the vagus nerves and structures within the mediastinum. Advocates for leaving the hernia sac in place argue that risks such as a tension pneumothorax outweigh any benefits, and that proper crura closure and anchoring of the fundoplication below the diaphragm are more effective in preventing hernia recurrence than sac excision. Most centers with demonstrated expertise in laparoscopic paraesophageal hernia repairs presently favor hernia sac excision whenever feasible (Table 2). Anesthesiologists familiar with these procedures have heightened awareness for potential cardiopulmonary complications during hiatus dissection. Lighted esophageal bougies and endoscopy are invariably employed when structural identification is difficult. In most complications encountered during hiatal and hernia sac dissection, early recognition and remedy averts any long-term sequelae.

Table 2 Overview of Laparoscopic Paraesophageal Hernia (Excluding Type I) Repairs Reported in a 6-Year Period

Group (Ref.)	Year	N	Age (yr)	Hernia sac excision	Preferred fundoplication type	Esophageal lengthening (%)	Open conversion (%)	Early complication rate—Major and Minor (%)	30-day mortality (%)	Preferred crura closure	Late hernia recurrence (%)	Post-op GERD symptoms (%)	Months follow-up (% patients)
Boise, ID VAMC (8)	1997	58	67	Yes	Posterior	0	2	7	2	Primary posterior	0	0	12 (78%)
Morristown Hospital, NJ (30)	1997	30	68	Yes	7 None 23 Posterior	0	0	27	0	Mesh	0	10	N/A (N/A)
Mayo Clinic–Jacksonville (18)	1997	65	64	Yes	Posterior	0	3	13	0	Primary posterior	5	3	18 (81%)
Mt. Sinai, NY (3)	1998	55	68	25 No 30 Yes	42 Posterior 13 None	0	5	5	0	Mixed mesh/primary	9	20	29 (89%)
UCSF (4)	1998	55	67	Yes	Posterior	0	9	7	2	Primary posterior	4	2	11 (N/A)
Washington University (32)	1999	38	67	12 No 26 Yes	10 None 28 Posterior	0	3	11	5	6 Mesh 32 Posterior	28	21	12 (74%)
Legacy Health, OR (25)	1999	52	63	Yes	Posterior	13	0	6	0	Primary posterior	8	10	18 (96%)
University of Washington (7)	1999	41	67	Yes	Posterior	0	5	17	2	Primary posterior	2	0	36 (100%)
University of Southern California (6)	2000	27	68	Yes (freed from hernia only)	Posterior	3	7	26	0	Primary posterior	42	23	17 (77%)
University of Pittsburgh (11)	2000	100	68	Yes	Posterior	27	3	28	0	Primary posterior	1	10	12 (90%)
Allegheny General, PA (29)	2001	60	57	Yes	Posterior	0	10	3	2	Primary posterior	5	5	19 (100%)
Swedish Medical Center, Washington (9)	2002	52	70	Yes	Hill repair	0	7	13	0	Primary posterior	32	19	39 (71%)
Emory University (13)	2002	125	64	Yes	Posterior	5	2	10	2	Primary posterior	33	7	40 (66%)
Summary 758 Patients			66 Mean	Most	Posterior fundoplication	Selected centers	< 10%	3–30%	≤ 2%	Primary posterior/ selective mesh use	0–42%	11–40%	11–40 mos. (66–100%)

C. Options for Crura Closure

Most crura closures are performed with interrupted, nonabsorbable sutures. Pledgets are recommended to buttress these sutures. Most crura closures are performed posterior to the esophagus to capitalize on a low tension area of the diaphragmatic crura. Occasionally, one or two sutures may be required anteriorly for large hernia orifices. A complete anterior crura closure can also be performed for smaller hernias, but this precludes a posterior fundoplication wrap.

The various prosthetic materials available to reinforce the crura repair have had some appeal. Polypropylene has been proposed because it permits tissue incorporation into the mesh surrounding the hiatus. There are also ongoing investigations in the use of biomaterials to close the hernia orifice. The inflammatory reaction and potential to contract for both these materials have been known to cause esophageal strictures and erosions. Polytetrafluoroethylene may be an alternative material that does not contract or allow for fibrous ingrowth, but infections have been reported with this mesh. Furthermore, the lack of tissue incorporation with polytetrafluoroethylene makes the repair prone to reherniation. Most surgeons are disinclined to place a prosthetic material around the esophagus because complications to the esophagus are often unforgiving.

Some groups have reported primary crura closure for large tension-prone hernia defects and to create relaxing incisions remote to the hiatus that are closed with prosthetic material. The prospects of this approach and its outcome remain to be validated.

In addition to determining the most appropriate prosthetic materials, the hernia size at which primary closure should be abandoned in favor of prosthetic closure remain active areas of investigation.

D. The Short Esophagus

While the incidence of shortened esophagus encountered with paraesophageal hernias are unknown, approximately 15–20% of the patients presenting for antireflux surgery have preoperatively determined short esophagus (i.e., lower esophageal sphincter above the diaphragm). Of this group, significantly fewer will require esophageal lengthening procedures after maximum intraoperative mobilization of the esophagus (Table 2). The indications for esophageal lengthening stems from the desire to return the gastroesophageal junction below the diaphragm and to enable tension-free crura closure around the esophagus. A fundoplication performed around a short esophagus is likely to disrupt or slip down around the stomach under tension. Alternatively, an intact fundoplication around a short esophagus can also retract into the mediastinum, making any hiatal repairs futile. Preliminary reports from centers performing more esophageal lengthening procedures seem to infer fewer hernia recurrences in the first 12 months after surgery. However, there does not appear to be any advantage in reducing reflux symptoms postoperatively.

The surgeon repairing paraesophageal hernias laparoscopically or thorascopically should be aware of the potential need for an esophageal lengthening procedure, particularly for patients with esophageal strictures or large hiatal hernias (> 5 cm diameter). As alluded to previously, complete mobilization of the esophagus may obviate the need for a lengthening procedure. While some advocate thoracic mobilization, it is possible to laparoscopically mobilize the esophagus to the level of the aortic arch. To accomplish this, surgeons are mindful that the left side of the esophagus is intimately associated with the left parietal pleura. Finally, the formation of a neoesophagus is not a physiological norm, and data remain sparse regarding the long-term sequelae.

V. LAPAROSCOPIC REPAIR

The techniques for laparoscopic paraesophageal hernia repairs do not differ from laparoscopic antireflux surgeries, with similar operating room settings and port placements (Fig. 9). However, many patients with paraesophageal hernias are elderly with comorbid

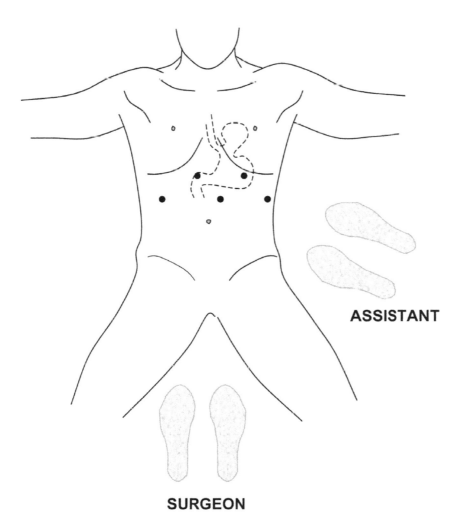

ASSISTANT

SURGEON

Figure 9 Patient positioning is similar to that for laparoscopic antireflux procedures. 10 mm trocars are used for the laparoscope and the righthand port. All other ports use a 5 mm trocar. If procedures such as endostapling for esophageal lengthening are required, one of the ports will be extended to accommodate a larger port. A mechanical liver retractor usually enables the procedure to be performed by one surgeon.

conditions and frail from malnutrition. The procedure can generally be performed between 90 to 240 minutes, depending on hernia size and amount of adhesions.

The initial step is to reduce the hernia contents, which occurs spontaneously in most cases with pneumoperitoneum. Hernias that do not reduce easily may first require excision of the hernia sac. The sac is incised along the hernia orifice and detached from the hiatal arch (Fig. 10). Following this, blunt dissection is used to deliver the sac out of the mediastinum. The vagus nerves are preserved, and in difficult cases a lighted bougie can help identify the cord-like structure. Most perforations can be repaired laparoscopically when encountered. Routine use of endoscopy or methylene blue intraoperatively can minimize missed perforations.

The crura is approximated posterior to the esophagus with nonabsorbable sutures. Pledgets are often used to bolster the suture closure and prevent tearing. Most surgeons favor a fundoplication and gastropexy, primarily to buttress the stomach to the diaphragm. When indicated, tube gastrostomies are used not to anchor the stomach within the abdomen, but for patients in whom delayed gastric emptying is significant.

Small pneumothoraces from breaches in the parietal pleura are more frequently encountered after paraesophageal hernia repairs than for antireflux surgery alone.

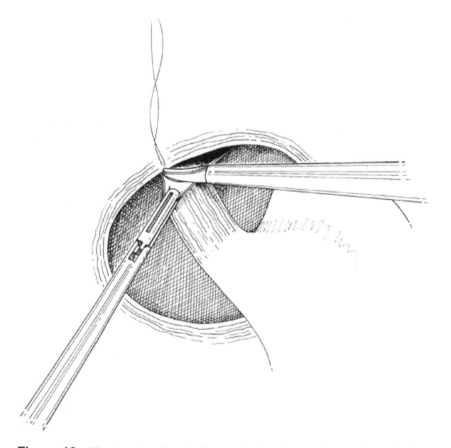

Figure 10 The hernia orifice is dissected circumferentially free from the hiatal arch using cautery and endoshears. Subsequent blunt dissection can be used to free the sac from the mediastinum.

Table 3 Total Reported Types of Early Postoperative
Complications Following 758 Laparoscopic Paraesophageal Hernia
Repairs

Complication type	Total numbers reported out of 758 cases
Respiratory (atelactasis, ARDS, pneumonia, etc.)	26
Cardiac (arrhythmia, CHF, MI, etc.)	19
Dysphagia early	15
Pulmonary embolus	8
Surgical bleeding	8
Leak/perforation	7
Wrap disruption (immediate repair)	6
Urinary retention/UTI	6
Prolonged ileus/small bowel obstruction	5
Wound infection	2
Esophageal obstruction	2
Gastric necrosis/dead gut	2
Gastric volvulus	1
Cerebrovascular accident	1
Intra-abdominal abscess	1
Deep vein thrombosis	1
Dehydration	1
Renal failure (transient)	1
Infectious colitis	1
Alcohol withdrawal	1

However, this frequently only requires watchful observation because the diffusion coefficient of carbon dioxide ensures rapid absorption.

A water-soluble esophagram is performed on the first postoperative day prior to beginning fluids. Patients go home 2 days after surgery on a soft mechanical diet.

Results to date for elective laparoscopic paraesophageal hernia repairs show early recovery and acceptable major complication rates. Most postoperative complications, albeit infrequent, are related to nonfatal pulmonary or cardiac issues (Table 3).

Early reports of laparoscopic paraesophageal hernia repairs estimated hernia recurrence rates of less than 15%. However, recent reports of large paraesophageal hernia repairs have found overall recurrence rates of 30–40% with the laparoscopic approach—a rate higher than in open surgeries (Table 2). Interestingly, less than half of these recurrences are symptomatic, which further attest to the importance of a properly performed antireflux procedure with hernia repairs. Even with the lower recurrence rates reported by some centers, the recent results cast the spotlight again on the controversies surrounding crura closure methods, and management of the short esophagus.

SELECTED READINGS

Allen MS, Trastek VF, Deschamps C, Pairolero PC. Intrathoracic stomach. J Thorac Cardiovasc Surg 1993; 105:253–259.

Geha AS, Massad MG, Snow NJ, Baue AE. A 32-year experience in 100 patients with giant paraesophageal hernia: the case for abdominal approach and selective antireflux repair. Surgery 2000; 128:623–630.

Hashemi M, Peters JH, DeMeester TR, Huprich JE, Quek M, Hagen JA, Crookes PF, Theisen J, DeMeester SR, Sillin LF, Bremner CG. Laparoscopic repair of large type III hiatal hernia: objective followup reveals high recurrence rate. J Am Coll Surg 2000; 190:539–547.

Jobe BA, Aye RW, Deveney CW, Domreis JS, Hill LD. Laparoscopic management of giant type III hiatal hernia and short esophagus: objective follow-up at three years. J Gastrointest Surg 2002; 6:181–188.

Kercher KW, Matthews BD, Ponsky JL, Goldstein SL, Yavorski RT, Sing RF, Heniford BT. Minimally invasive management of paraesophageal herniation in the high-risk surgical patient. Am J Surg 2001; 182:510–514.

Luketich JD, Raja S, Fernando HC, Campbell W, Christie NA, Buenaventura PO, Weigel TL, Keenan RJ, Schauer PR. Laparoscopic repair of giant paraesophageal hernia: 100 consecutive cases. Ann Surg 2000; 232:608–618.

Mattar SG, Bowers SP, Galloway KD, Hunter JG, Smith CD. Long-term outcome of laparoscopic repair of paraesophageal hernia. Surg Endosc 2002; 16:745–749.

Ruhl CE, Everhart JE. Relationship of iron-deficiency anemia with esophagitis and hiatal hernia: hospital findings from a prospective, population-based study. Am J Gastroenterol 2001; 96:322–326.

Schauer PR, Ikramuddin S, McLaughlin RH, Graham TO, Slivka A, Lee KKW, Schraut WH, Luketich JD. Comparison of laparoscopic versus open repair of paraesophageal hernia. Am J Surg 1998; 176:659–665.

Seelig MH, Hinder RA, Klingler PJ, Floch NR, Branton SA, Smith SL. Paraesophageal herniation as a complication following laparoscopic antireflux surgery. J Gastrointest Surg 1999; 3:95–99.

Skandalakis JE, Ellis H. Embryologic and anatomic basis of esophageal surgery. Surg Clin North Am 2000; 80:85–155.

Smith CD. Esophagus. In: Norton JA, et al., eds. Surgery: Scientific Basis and Clinical Evidence. Springer-Verlag, New York, 2001;455–488.

Swanstrom LL, Jobe BA, Kinzie LR, Horvath KD. Esophageal motility and outcomes following laparoscopic paraesophageal hernia repair and fundoplication. Am J Surg 1999; 177:359–363.

Terry M, Smith CD, Branum GD, Galloway K, Waring JP, Hunter JG. Outcomes of laparoscopic fundoplication for gastroesophageal reflux disease and paraesophageal hernia. Surg Endosc 2001; 15:691–699.

Urbach DR, Khajanchee YS, Glasgow RE, Hansen PD, Swanstrom LL. Preoperative determinants of an esophageal lengthening procedure in laparoscopic antireflux surgery. Surg Endosc 2001; 15:1408–1412.

Wiechmann RJ, Ferguson MK, Naunheim KS, McKesey P, Hazelrigg SJ, Santucci TS, Macherey RS, Landreneau RJ. Laparoscopic management of giant paraesophageal herniation. Ann Thorac Surg 2001; 71:1080–1087.

Wu JS, Dunnegan DL, Soper NJ. Clinical and radiologic assessment of laparoscopic paraesophageal hernia repair. Surg Endosc 1999; 13:497–502.

24

Nissen Fundoplication

KETAN M. DESAI

Washington University School of Medicine
St. Louis, Missouri, U.S.A.

NATHANIEL J. SOPER

Northwestern University, Feinberg School of Medicine
Chicago, Illinois, U.S.A.

DANIEL B. JONES

Beth Israel Deaconess Medical Center
Harvard Medical School
Boston, Massachusetts, U.S.A.

Laparoscopic antireflux surgery (LARS) has assumed a major role in the treatment of gastroesophageal reflux disease (GERD). The advancement in laparoscopic techniques and instrumentation over the past decade has led to an increase in the number of antireflux operations. Although the operation is fundamentally similar to open antireflux procedures, clear benefits to the laparoscopic approach have been described.

In 1955, Rudolf Nissen reported the efficacy of a 360° gastric wrap through an upper abdominal incision to control reflux symptoms. A prospective randomized trial in the 1980s through a Veterans Administration cooperative trial compared the results of transabdominal open Nissen fundoplication with those of medical therapy in patients with complicated gastroesophageal reflux disease (GERD). Those patients who were treated surgically had better control of symptoms and had more complete healing of endoscopically documented esophagitis. Despite these findings, many patients and physicians still opted for lifelong medication and significant lifestyle limitations. It was not until 1991 that the first laparoscopic Nissen fundoplication was reported. From that point, acceptance on the part of patients and physicians to proceed with surgical treatment began to grow. Although the minimally invasive approach follows the same surgical principles as the open operation, LARS reduces postoperative pain, shortens the hospital stay and recovery period, and achieves a short-term functional outcome that is similar to that of the open operation.

I. CLINICAL PRESENTATION

GERD is the most common upper gastrointestinal disorder in western society. Patients with GERD can present with typical or atypical symptoms. Typical symptoms include heartburn, regurgitation, and dysphagia. Atypical symptoms include chest pain, postprandial fullness, belching odynophagia, nocturnal aspiration, chronic cough, wheezing, and hoarseness.

An incompetent or dysfunctional lower esophageal sphincter usually causes gastroesophageal reflux. However, other diseases that impair esophageal clearance and/or gastric emptying such as achalasia, esophageal spasm, esophageal carcinoma, and pyloric stenosis may initially present with symptoms similar to those of GERD. Reflux symptoms may be confused with symptomatic cholelithiasis, peptic ulcer disease, or coronary artery disease. Therefore, before operative therapy is undertaken a thorough evaluation is essential, since antireflux operations are designed solely to correct a mechanically defective gastroesophageal sphincter.

II. DIAGNOSTIC TESTS

The majority of patients with GERD experience relatively mild symptoms and can be managed medically without diagnostic studies. With refractory symptoms of GERD and in those patients being considered for surgical therapy, a host of diagnostic tests are considered. Radiographic, endoscopic, and physiological evaluation is performed as part of the complete workup. Prior to pursuing a surgical approach, the diagnosis of GERD must be secure. Patients with typical symptoms (heartburn or regurgitation) require at least one other piece of objective evidence of reflux such as an abnormal 24-hour pH test or esophagitis on endoscopic evaluation. For patients with atypical symptoms two other objective measures of GERD are required. Esophagogastroduodenoscopy (EGD) and contrast radiographs of the esophagus and stomach help to define anatomical complications such as ulceration, stricture, hiatal hernia, or foreshortened esophagus. Endoscopic evaluation also determines the extent and severity of esophagitis and excludes Barrett's metaplasia or malignancy. However, the most sensitive and specific test to document GERD is the 24-hour pH test. Esophageal pH monitoring objectively records the frequency and duration of gastroesophageal reflux, and event recording correlates symptoms with reflux episodes. Esophageal manometry characterizes the location and tone of the lower esophageal sphincter and rules out primary esophageal motility disorders by measuring amplitude of esophageal peristalsis and the adequacy of propagation of each swallow.

III. NONOPERATIVE TREATMENT

The majority of GERD patients are managed medically. Lifestyle modification and/or acid reduction medication are initial treatment options for patients with uncomplicated GERD. Eating within 2 hours of bedtime is discouraged, since reflux is often aggravated while asleep. The head of the bed is elevated to promote nocturnal gravity-dependent clearance of the esophagus. Patients are directed to lose weight if they are obese and are advised to avoid foods and other substances known to diminish lower esophageal sphincter tone, especially fats, chocolate, onions, peppermint, alcohol, and tobacco. Commonly prescribed medications such as theophylline, calcium channel blockers, nitrates, and tricyclic antidepressants also promote reflux and should be substituted if possible.

Medical therapy decreases the patient's gastric acidity and reduces esophageal exposure to gastric contents. Antacids neutralize corrosive gastric juices, and H_2 blockers inhibit gastric acid secretions. Metoclopramide may enhance gastric emptying and augment lower esophageal sphincter tone, thereby decreasing intragastric pressure and improving esophageal clearance. Proton pump inhibitors (PPI) have become the primary treatment for patients with GERD in the United States. Patients usually undergo a short-term (2-month) trial of intensive medical therapy before an antireflux operation is considered. However, many patients require escalating doses over time, relapse quickly when medication is stopped, or desire to be free of medications. It is this group of patients who may benefit greatly from LARS.

Complications of GERD may develop if reflux is not adequately controlled. Ulceration, stricture, and bleeding are commonplace, whereas malignancy occurs rarely. Such findings are also indications for surgical treatment in select patients.

IV. OPERATIVE TREATMENT

LARS augments the lower esophageal sphincter barrier and is generally recommended for patients with documented GERD whose symptoms are unresponsive to a trial of medical therapy, whose symptoms interfere with desired lifestyle, or who develop complications. The most common indications for operation in patients with documented GERD include symptoms refractory to medical therapy, high-grade esophagitis (ulceration, stricture, Barrett's esophagus) and children with severe esophagitis, recurrent pneumonia, or failure to thrive. Ideal patients for the Nissen fundoplication have an incompetent lower esophageal sphincter with normal proximal esophageal peristaltic contraction amplitude, esophagitis documented by endoscopic biopsy, symptoms responsive to proton pump inhibitors, and 24-hour esophageal pH monitoring that demonstrates frequent reflux events.

The few absolute contraindications to LARS include a patient's inability to tolerate general anesthesia or the presence of an uncorrectable coagulopathy. A number of conditions make LARS more difficult and should be considered relative contraindications. Severe, longstanding reflux, resulting in stricturing and shortening of the esophagus, may prevent the creation of a tension-free intra-abdominal fundoplication and may result in an anatomical failure (wrap disruption or intrathoracic migration). The propulsive force of the esophagus must also be sufficient to propel food across a reconstructed valve. If peristalsis is markedly diminished, a partial wrap may be preferable. Prior upper abdominal surgery (especially fundoplication, vagotomy, or gastrectomy) with secondary scarring and adhesion formation may also distort anatomy and render the dissection more difficult.

A. Preoperative Preparation

The expected results and risks of a laparoscopic Nissen fundoplication are discussed with the patient. Patients are counseled that if at any point a laparoscopic operation cannot be continued safely, the operation will be converted to an open approach. A healthy patient is admitted the day of surgery after an overnight fast. In the operating room, the patient is placed in a modified lithotomy position on a beanbag cushion (Fig. 1). After induction of

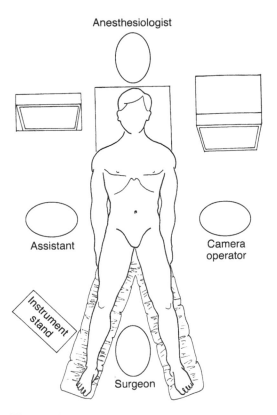

Figure 1 Operating room layout. The patient is supine with legs abducted.

general anesthesia, the stomach is decompressed with an orogastric tube and the bladder emptied by voiding immediately preoperatively. The arms are tucked and protected at the sides. Inflatable compression stockings are worn on the lower extremities for deep venous thrombosis prophylaxis. The legs are abducted and supported on cushioned spreader bars. The beanbag is aspirated while "cupping" the patient's body wall and perineum, thereby preventing subsequent slippage during extremes of tilt of the operating room table. The abdomen is prepared and draped sterilely.

B. Operation Room and Patient Setup

The operating room personnel and equipment are arranged with the surgeon between the patient's legs, the assistant surgeon on the patient's right, and the camera holder to the left. Other surgeons prefer to work from the patient's side for the entire procedure or position the assistant to the patient's left. Video monitors placed at either side of the head of the table can be viewed easily by all members of the operating team. Irrigation, suction, and electrocautery connections come off the head of the table on the patient's left side. Special instruments include endoscopic Babcock graspers, cautery scissors, curved dissectors, clip applier, atraumatic liver retractor, 5 mm needle holders, and ultrasonic coagulating shears.

C. Surgical Technique

1. Port Placement

Access to the abdominal cavity is achieved by either a closed or an open technique superior to the umbilicus. A port is placed in the left mid-rectus muscle approximately 12–15 cm below the xiphoid process. The entire abdomen is explored with an angled laparoscope (usually 30-degree oblique) beginning at the area deep to the insertion site. Adhesiolysis may be necessary if the patient has had previous surgery. After thorough inspection of the pelvis, and upper abdomen, four additional ports are placed under direct vision of the laparoscope. Ports are typically placed in the following locations to optimize visualization, tissue manipulation, and facilitate suturing (Fig. 2): right subcostal, 15 cm from the xiphoid process; a point midway between the first two ports in the right mid-rectus region; in the left subcostal region 8–10 cm from the xiphoid; and in the right paramedian location at the same horizontal level as the left subcostal trocar (usually 5 cm inferior to the xiphoid process). This port arrangement allows access to the hiatus and permits comfortable suturing by placing the optics between the surgeon's hands. The gastroesophageal junction is usually deep to the xiphoid, and from a point 15 cm distant, only half of the laparoscopic instrument must be introduced to reach the hiatus. This distance establishes the fulcrum at the midpoint of the instrument and maximizes its range of motion during tissue manipulation. With excellent 5 mm equipment and optics, we generally use only one 10–12 port, for the surgeon's right hand, to allow insertion of a SH needle.

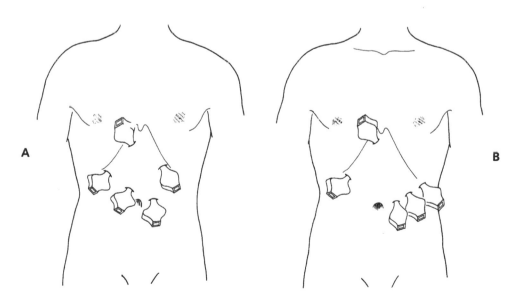

Figure 2   Port placement. (A) Standard placement if the surgeon stands between the patient's legs. (B) Alternate port placement if the surgeon prefers to work from the patient's side.

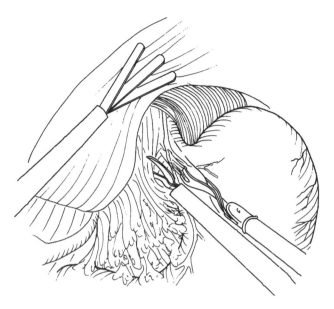

Figure 3 Retraction of the liver exposes the esophageal hiatus while the phrenoesophageal ligament is divided.

2. Exposure

Once access is safely achieved, exposure of the esophageal hiatus is facilitated by gravity and maintained by an assistant. Positioning the patient in reverse Trendelenburg (Fowler's) position uses gravity to displace the bowel and stomach from the diaphragm. A skilled camera holder and the use of an angled laparoscope are important. The assistant introduces a self-retaining liver retractor through the right subcostal port, and a Babcock grasper is introduced through the right mid-rectus port to pull the stomach and epiphrenic fat pad inferiorly and to the left (Fig. 3). The left triangular ligament is not divided but is left to aid in retraction of the liver anteriorly. Next, both crura and the anterior vagus nerve are identified after opening the phrenoesophageal ligament.

3. Dissection

If a hiatal hernia is present, it is reduced into the abdominal cavity with gentle traction after cutting all adhesions to the hernia sac. The right crus is retracted laterally, and the right side of the esophagus is carefully dissected to visualize the aortoesophageal groove and posterior vagus nerve (Fig. 4). On the other side of the esophagus, the left crus is similarly dissected from the esophagus and fundus to its point or origin from the right crural leaflet. A "window" is created between the crura and posterior esophageal wall under direct vision using the angled laparoscope.

The fundus is then fully mobilized by dividing the proximal gastrosplenic ligament. Beginning at a point on the greater curve 8–10 cm distal to the esophageal junction, the short gastric vessels are placed on traction and a window is created into the lesser sac. The short gastric vessels are then divided by serial application of the LaparoSonic Coagulating Shears (LCS) (Ethicon Endo-Surgery, Inc., Cincinnati, OH) or by clipping and dividing

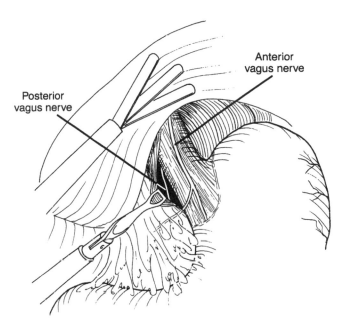

Posterior
vagus nerve

Anterior
vagus nerve

Figure 4 With the right crus retracted laterally, the anterior and posterior vagus nerves are clearly visible.

them (Fig. 5). To fully mobilize the proximal stomach, all posterior retroperitoneal adhesions to the fundus are divided.

4. Fundoplication

After mobilizing the fundus, a Babcock clamp is passed right to left in front of both crura and behind the esophagus (Fig. 6). The Babcock clamp grasps the fundus near the insertion of the short gastric vessels and pulls the fundus left to right around the esophagus (Fig. 7). When the surgeon releases the fundus it should lie in place. If the fundus springs back around the esophagus, the wrap is too tight. The hiatal defect is closed with several interrupted 0-Ethibond sutures. Retroesophageal exposure of the crura is gained either by using the mobilized fundus to retract the esophagus anteriorly and to the left or by placing a Penrose drain around the distal esophagus for retraction. Approximation of the right and left crura is usually performed posterior to the esophagus (Fig. 8), although anterior closure may be appropriate in select cases.

Next, the esophagus is serially dilated with a 50–60 Fr Maloney dilator. The dilator calibrates the wrap and prevents excessive narrowing of the esophagus during the actual fundoplication. Dilation must be performed cautiously if the patient has esophageal stricture or severe inflammation. The surgeon should watch the bougie pass smoothly through the gastroesophageal junction as a bulge on the video monitor. If the bougie appears to be hung up at the gastroesophageal junction, the surgeon can sometimes improve the angulation by retracting the stomach anteriorly or caudally. With the dilator in the esophagus, a "short, floppy" Nissen fundoplication is performed using three interrupted, braided 0- or 2-0 polyester sutures. Seromuscular bites of fundus to the left of the esophagus, the anterior esophageal wall away from the anterior vagus nerve, and the

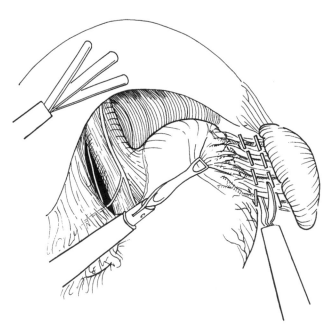

Figure 5 The short gastric vessels are divided from an inferior to a superior direction until the fundus is completely mobilized.

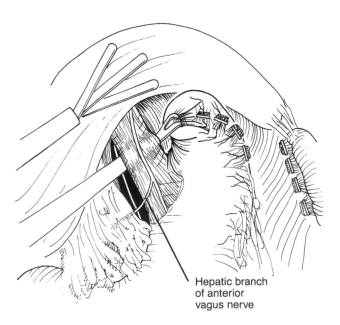

Hepatic branch
of anterior
vagus nerve

Figure 6 A Babcock clamp is passed through the "window" posterior to the esophagus to grasp the lateral wall of the gastric fundus.

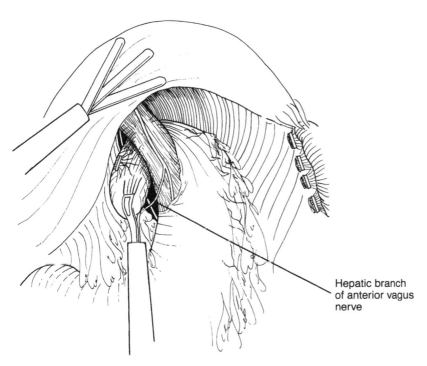

Hepatic branch
of anterior vagus
nerve

Figure 7   The fundus is wrapped posterior to the esophagus and anterior to the crura and posterior branch of the vagus nerve. The 360° fundoplication is constructed over a 50–60 Fr esophageal dilator. A tension-free wrap will not recoil back around the esophagus when the Babcock clamp releases the fundus.

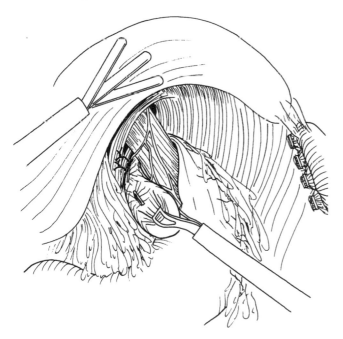

Figure 8   The crura are approximated beginning posteriorly and inferiorly. Closure is usually performed posterior to the esophagus.

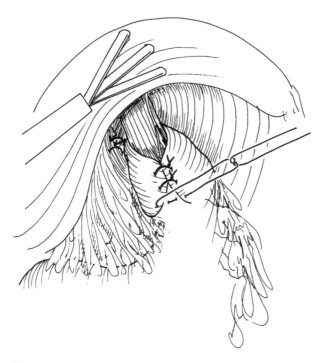

Figure 9   The fundoplication is secured with three braided 0-polyester sutures. Sutures should include bites of the seromuscular left fundus, superficial anterior esophageal wall, and seromuscular right fundus.

fundus to the right are all incorporated in the 360-degree fundoplication (Fig. 9). The esophageal wall should be incorporated in at least one of the sutures to prevent slippage of the wrap around the body of the stomach or into the thoracic cavity. Our practice has been to use extracorporeal knotting techniques, tying square knots and pushing them into position (Fig. 10), whereas other surgeons prefer intracorporeal suturing. Regardless, the surgeon should take generous tissue bites and oppose the gastric wall without strangulating tissue. Ideally, the wrap should be ≥ 2 cm in length. After three sutures secure the fundoplication; additional sutures may be placed from the wrap to the crura for stabilization, although we currently do not perform this step. The esophageal dilator is withdrawn by the anesthesiologist. At this point the laparoscopic Nissen fundoplication is complete.

At the end of the operation, the abdominal cavity is thoroughly irrigated with saline and aspirated dry. The suture line is inspected to assure that there is no leak or hemorrhage. A 10-mm instrument should slide easily under a loose wrap. The pneumoperitoneum is evacuated, and the ports are removed under direct vision as a last check to assure no bleeding from the trocar sites. Incision sites are irrigated with saline and infiltrated with the remaining 0.5% bupivacaine (maximal dose 2.5 mg/kg). The fascia of each incision > 5 mm is closed using an absorbable 1-Vicryl suture, and the skin is closed using running subcuticular 4-0 absorbable sutures.

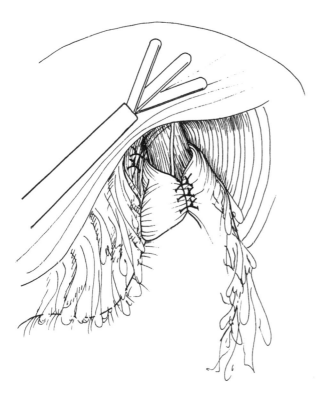

Figure 10 View of the completed laparoscopic Nissen fundoplication.

V. POSTOPERATIVE CARE

Pneumatic compression stockings are left in place until the patient is awake and ambulating. For the first 24 hours after surgery, patients are given intermittent intravenous ondansetron and ketorolac. Nasogastric tubes are not used. Injectable and/or oral narcotics are administered as needed for pain control. Postoperatively, all antireflux and antacid medications (antacids, H_2 blockers, proton pump inhibitors, and metoclopramide) may be discontinued. Clear liquids are permitted on the evening after surgery. The patient is advanced to an esophageal diet, mechanical soft foods, as tolerated and maintained for 2–3 weeks while esophageal edema resolves. Most patients are discharged the day after operation and may return to work at one week. We generally prohibit lifting of objects heavy enough to require Valsalva (e.g., weight lifting) for 4–6 weeks postoperatively.

VI. COMPLICATIONS

LARS is a safe operation when performed by an experienced surgeon. Although rare, intraoperative complications include gastric or esophageal perforation, liver or splenic injury, short gastric vessel bleeding, and pneumothorax or pneumomediastinum. Directly grasping the esophagus with any instrument should be avoided, due to the risk of esophageal perforation. Instead, for retracting the esophagus, the side of the instrument should be used to nudge the esophagus to the right or left. Since perforation of the esophagus is potentially life threatening, this complication should be suspected in any postoperative patient who manifests severe chest pain or signs of infection (fever, pain, tenderness, leukocytosis). Bleeding from the liver or spleen usually results from retractor or instrument trauma. These injuries are usually recognized at the time of surgery and can be managed with simple pressure or electrocautery. Pleural injuries can also occur during a difficult dissection; however, intervention (tube thoracostomy) is rarely necessary secondary to the rapid reabsorption of CO_2. If a pleural tear occurs and leads to hypotension or increased airway pressure, desufflating the abdomen and then reinsufflating with a lower pressure limit (e.g., 10 mm) usually resolves the problem.

Postoperative sequelae are usually minor and self-limiting. They include nausea, ileus, urinary retention, dysphagia, and abdominal bloating. Complications ($>$ grade 2) such as deep venous thrombosis, COPD exacerbation, and myocardial infarction are extremely rare in the postoperative period.

Problems most commonly associated with the Nissen fundoplication are technical. Anatomical failures occur after LARS and may be more common in the hands of a less experienced surgeon. Anatomical fundoplication failures can be classified as those secondary to displacement (intrathoracic migration or slippage aborally onto the proximal stomach) or disruption of the fundoplication.

VII. OUTCOMES AND COSTS

LARS provides marked reduction in GERD symptoms and antisecretory medication use at long-term follow-up. Improvement in esophageal symptoms and overall satisfaction is excellent by outcomes analysis. Gas bloat and mild dysphagia are reported in the early postoperative period, but are usually self-limiting. Following LARS, patients have less postoperative pain, shorter hospitalization, and faster recovery when compared to an open approach. Operative time ranges from 1 to 3 hours, with a mean of 2 hours. After an open Nissen fundoplication, patients are discharged on average 5–10 days postoperatively, whereas after a laparoscopic Nissen fundoplication, patients are usually discharged within 24–48 hours and return to work and/or full activity within 2 weeks of surgery. Early hospital discharge and discontinuation of expensive medication represent substantial savings in health care dollars, while rapid return to employment should markedly decrease indirect costs.

VIII. CURRENT STATUS

The laparoscopic Nissen fundoplication has proved to be a highly effective treatment for gastroesophageal reflux disease in several large series. Since the laparoscopic fundoplication follows well-established principles of antireflux surgery, patients should enjoy the same effective long-term control of GERD as with open Nissen fundoplication. Moreover, by avoiding a major laparotomy incision, patients experience less pain, shorter hospitalization, faster recovery to full activity, and improved cosmesis with the laparoscopic operation compared with its open counterpart. For these reasons, patients who previously endured significant lifestyle restrictions and chronic medication are now experiencing the benefits of operative therapy of GERD.

SURGICAL TIPS

1. The laparoscopic Nissen fundoplication is deceptively simple; for the best results the surgeon must be knowledgeable in esophageal physiology and skilled in advanced laparoscopic techniques.
2. Proper selection of patients is necessary to achieve excellent postoperative results.
3. Securing the patient to the table using a beanbag will allow steep reverse Trendelenburg positioning for gravity displacement of the bowel and maximum exposure of the gastroesophageal junction.
4. Port placement is critical, because the uppermost ports must reach the gastroesophageal junction for dissection and suturing.
5. Dividing the short gastric vessels will freely mobilize the fundus.
6. Adequacy of fundic mobilization is checked by releasing the fundus and watching whether the fundus rests in place or recoils under tension.
7. A short, floppy wrap ≤ 2 cm in length is ideal.
8. A 360-degree wrap is too tight if a 10 Babcock clamp does not easily pass under the wrap.
9. Never grasp the esophagus with an instrument, as it may perforate.
10. Diet should be advanced first with a mechanical soft feeding; otherwise, edema may cause transient dysphagia.

SELECTED READINGS

Bowery DJ, Peters JH. Laparoscopic esophageal surgery. Surg Clin North Am 2000; 80(4):1213–1242.

Clavien PA, Sanabria JR, Strasberg SM. Proposed classification of complications of surgery with examples of utility in cholecystectomy. Surgery 1992; 111:518–526.

Hunter JG, Trus TL, Branum GD, et al. A physiologic approach to laparoscopic fundoplication for gastroesophageal reflux disease. Ann Surg 1996; 223:673–685.

Jones DB, Soper NJ. Laparoscopic Nissen fundoplication. Surg Rounds 1994; 17:573–581.

Peters JH, DeMeester TR, Crookes P, et al. The treatment of gastroesophageal reflux disease with laparoscopic Nissen fundoplication: prospective evaluation of 100 patients with "typical" symptoms. Ann Surg 1998; 228:40–50.

Soper NJ. Laparoscopic management of hiatal hernia and gastroesophageal reflux. Curr Probl Surg 1999; 36:765–840.

Soper NJ, Dunnegan D. Anatomic fundoplication failure after laparoscopic antireflux surgery. Ann Surg 1999; 229:669–677.

Spechler SJ. Comparison of medical and surgical therapy for complicated gastroesophageal reflux disease in veterans. N Engl J Med 1992; 326:786–792.

Stein HJ, DeMeester TR, Hinder RA. Outpatient and physiologic testing and surgical management of foregut motility disorders. Curr Probl Surg 1992; 31:415–555.

25

Heller Myotomy

LEONARDO VILLEGAS

Beth Israel Deaconess Medical Center
Harvard Medical School
Boston, Massachusetts, U.S.A.

ROBERT V. REGE

University of Texas Southwestern Medical Center
Dallas, Texas, U.S.A.

The advent of laparoscopic techniques for esophageal surgery provides a minimally invasive approach with known advantages for patients with esophageal motility disorders. This new modality has resulted in a resurgence of the surgeon's role in management of esophageal disorders and has dramatically changed the operative approach to the distal esophagus.

In 1914 Heller described a surgical procedure for cardiospasm of the esophagus, known today as achalasia. Before that time the only effective treatment was esophageal dilatation. Originally, he performed an extramucosal myotomy on the anterior and posterior walls of the distal esophagus. The patient noted great relief of the dysphagia initially after surgery, but marked reflux resulted and was associated with significant morbidity. Late recurrence of dysphagia was common due to a peptic stricture.

Many surgeons described modifications of Heller's procedure. However, the morbidity of the open operation led the majority of physicians to continue to recommend, and patients to choose, dilatation, especially with the introduction of pneumodilatation using a balloon system. This situation did not change until the late 1980s, when Cuschieri performed the first laparoscopic modified Heller myotomy. The advantages of this minimally invasive procedure include decreased pain, lower operative morbidity, shorter hospital stay, and quicker return to full unrestricted activity. Although the procedure is technically demanding and requires advanced laparoscopic skills, the magnification afforded by the video laparoscopic system allows the surgeon to visualize all muscle layers and to more accurately perform the myotomy. When combined with intraoperative intraluminal endoscopy and/or manometry, the laparoscopic approach leads to optimum outcomes.

I. CLINICAL PRESENTATION

Achalasia is an idiopathic primary motor disorder of the esophagus, involving the body and the lower esophageal sphincter (LES). Microscopically, the disease is manifest by an absence of the myenteric neural plexus, a monocellular infiltrate and with marked hypertrophy of esophageal muscle. Although the exact cause of the problem has not been found, it has been associated with the class II antigen DQW1, and it has been suggested to be an autoimmune disease. Others have associated achalasia with herpes zoster and measles virus infections. As a consequence, the therapeutic approach remains palliative, aimed at symptomatic relief of LES obstruction. Achalasia occurs equally in both sexes and has a typical onset in the third or fourth decade.

Early symptoms include heartburn, mild dysphagia, and chest pain. Patients are often misdiagnosed as having gastroesophageal reflux disease, but the dysphagia and chest pain are not typical for that disease. Late symptoms reflect more severe disease and consist of increasing dysphagia and chest pain, weight loss, and regurgitation of undigested food, especially at night. Symptoms tend to be of gradual onset and insidious, distinguishing them from the dysphagia with esophageal cancer, which progresses much more rapidly. Patients may report that dysphagia is overcome by drinking liquids or by assuming unusual postures that facilitate passage of the food bolus, including straightening their back and raising their hands over their heads or by jumping up and down. Over time, the esophagus dilates and retains undigested food. It becomes tortuous, and dysphagia may subside and even disappear. Nighttime regurgitation becomes common and leads to aspiration, manifested as cough or pneumonia.

II. DIAGNOSTIC TESTS

Diagnosis of achalasia is suggested by the clinical presentation and the time course. A barium upper gastrointestinal study reveals moderate dilatation of the esophagus with tapering at the gastroesophageal junction, producing a typical "bird's beak" deformity. This feature is distinctly different from the "apple core" lesion classically observed with esophageal cancer. End-stage achalasia presents with a large, tortuous esophagus, which assumes a sigmoid configuration, and substantial amounts of retained food.

Upper gastrointestinal endoscopy and esophageal manometry are the two tests that confirm the diagnoses. Endoscopy excludes other causes of dysphagia, such as cancer, esophageal webs, and benign strictures. Distal esophagitis may be encountered, but this is more likely to be due to retention of food and oral bacteria than to gastroesophageal reflux. Usually the LES is closed. The endoscope, however, passes if continuous, gentle pressure is applied. Esophageal motility studies reveal a typical pattern for achalasia—absence of peristalsis of the body of the esophagus and a nonrelaxing or incompletely relaxing LES. If swallowing initiates esophageal contractions, they are simultaneous rather than peristaltic, demonstrating that the esophagus has lost its normal propulsive action. LES pressure is usually much higher than normal, but patients can present with normal LES pressure, although the LES fails to relax normally.

A proper diagnosis of the underlying disease is crucial. It is extremely important to be sure that patients do not have malignancy at or near to the esophageal junction. Submucosal spread of carcinoma in the cardia of the stomach may lead to signs and symptoms clinically indistinguishable from achalasia. This syndrome has been termed pseudoachalasia. Patients with gastroesophageal reflux mistakenly diagnosed with achalasia experience increasing reflux after the myotomy. On the other hand, many patients with achalasia have gastrointestinal reflux, or will develop it postoperatively after myotomy. Controversy exists about performance of a fundoplication with myotomy, and to date no preoperative feature of the disease or test can predict which patients will benefit from myotomy.

At the time of evaluating the initial treatment for achalasia, patient preferences and local expertise should be taken into consideration. Recent publications have shown that after 10 years, there is a small difference in quality-adjusted survival between laparoscopic Heller myotomy with partial fundoplication and pneumatic dilatation or botulinum injection. Pneumatic dilation is less expensive than the two other treatments.

Speiss et al. in 1989 performed a meta-analysis and reported that in a single controlled trial (prospective and randomized) comparing pneumatic dilation (39 patient) with Heller myotomy (42 patient by thoracotomy), surgery was found superior to dilation (95% vs. 51% nearly complete symptom resolution; $p < 0.01$) after 5 years. In uncontrolled trials pneumatic dilation is 72% effective versus 84% for Heller myotomy. The limitation of perforation is the 3% incidence of esophageal perforation.

III. NONOPERATIVE TREATMENT

Medical management includes the use of drugs for smooth muscle relaxants, such as amyl nitrate, sublingual nitroglycerin, and theophylline and calcium channel blockers, to reduce LES pressure. Patients experience some improvement, but benefit is soon lost since patients develop tachyphalaxis to the medications. Medications are rarely used for definitive treatment of patients but may be used as a bridge to surgery or esophageal dilatation.

Botulinum toxin may be directly injected into the LES by endoscopy and has been shown to decrease LES pressure by about 33% in humans. About 30% of patients obtain relief from botulinum toxin, but regrowth of synapses and of terminal axons overcomes the effects of the toxin, usually within a year from treatment. Only about half of the patients respond to retreatment. Although results do not compare pneumatic dilatation or operative myotomy, botulinum injection may be helpful in patients with severe comorbidities who are not good risks for dilatation or operation and who have limited life expectancy. Its effects last for only about one year.

Endoscopic pneumatic balloon dilation is an effective treatment for achalasia. A specially designed balloon catheter is fluoroscopically guided across the esophagus to the region of the LES. The low-pressure balloon is then insufflated to between 3 and 4 cm in diameter, disrupting the esophageal muscle of the LES. Patients need to be sedated since they will experience chest or epigastric pain. The success rate increases as the balloon size increases from 3 to 4 cm, but so does the perforation rate. Dilatation to 3.5 cm seems to be the optimum balance between success and complication in most patients. The range of symptomatic improvement has been reported in 48–78% of patients, but in experienced hands initial rates of success should be over 70%. Retreatment will increase success rates to about 80%. These success rates are comparable to those obtained with open thoracotomy or laparotomy. There may be a small amount of bleeding, but this is self-limiting. The major complication of this procedure is esophageal perforation, which occurs in about 0.2% of patients. Perforation rates increase with repeat dilatations, and dilation is performed with large balloons. Repeat dilatation is reasonable if the first treatment is not completely successful, but two sessions should be considered a reasonable trial of this method and referral for surgery should be considered if the patient is at good operative risk. Recent studies also report an incidence of 0.07% for major bleeding requiring transfusion or surgery. Endoscopic dilatation is much more difficult in patients with a markedly dilated esophagus, and such patients are not considered good patients for pneumatic dilation.

A controlled trial reported in 1997 comparing botulinum toxin to pneumatic dilation found a substantial symptomatic response in 32% of botulinum toxin patients compared with 70% of the pneumatic dilation group at 12 months ($p < 0.01$).

It is important to recognize and treat perforations promptly. If there is any question about the integrity of the esophagus, a barium or gastrografin study should be performed immediately. Perforations most often require operative therapy and, when recognized promptly, should be managed by closing the perforation and performing a myotomy on the opposite side of the esophagus.

IV. OPERATIVE TREATMENT

The surgical treatment for achalasia is the esophagomyotomy, which divides the muscle fibers of the LES. The current approach differs from the double myotomy introduced by Heller, although the procedure continues to be called a Heller or modified-Heller myotomy. A single myotomy suffices, but the length of the myotomy is still controversial. It is imperative that the myotomy encompasses the entire zone of high pressure and that it is carried onto the stomach, but a myotomy that is too long may result in severe gastroesophageal reflux. The second controversy is concerned with the need for an antireflux procedure. If done, the antireflux procedure should prevent reflux, but should not result in a distal barrier to swallowing causing dysphagia. The decision to perform operative treatment rather than pneumatic dilatation is a complex one, which must weigh the outcomes of both procedures and the operative risk of the patient. However, after two sessions of unsuccessful pneumatic dilation, the treatment of choice is clearly surgery in patients who have reasonable operative risk. The operation is now most often performed with the laparoscope.

V. PREOPERATIVE PREPARATIONS

Prior to surgery, the surgeon should advise patients to remain on a liquid diet during the 2–3 days preceding the operation; this diet decreases the risk of aspiration during intubation. Antibiotics are given prior to surgery to reduce the risk of infection in the event of mucosal perforation. Although a normal esophagus harbors very low amounts of bacteria, the esophagus in achalasia is essentially obstructed and contains debris with high bacterial counts.

The expected results and risks are discussed with the patient, and the patient is counseled that if at any time the operation cannot be continued safely, the operation will be converted to an open approach. Although small perforations of the mucosa may be repaired using laparoscopic techniques, it may be necessary in some cases to convert to an open operation to obtain an optimal repair.

VI. OPERATION ROOM AND PATIENT SETUP

The patient is placed in a modified lithotomy position on a beanbag cushion, which is used to hold the patient on the table when the patient is placed in reverse Trendelenburg position. After induction of general anesthesia, the esophagus and stomach are decompressed with an orogastric tube and the bladder emptied with a urinary catheter. The arms are tucked and protected at the sides. Inflatable compression devices on the lower extremities, or other appropriate deep venous thrombosis prophylaxis, are used to prevent deep venous thrombosis.

The operating room personnel and equipment are arranged as follows: the surgeon stands between the patient's legs, the assistant surgeon on the patient's right and the camera holder on the left. All members of the team can view video monitors placed at either side of the head of the table. The patient is prepped and the abdomen draped in a sterile manner.

VII. SURGICAL TECHNIQUE

A. Port Placement

Pneumoperitoneum is created through an open or closed technique at the umbilicus. A 12 mm port is placed in the midline above the umbilicus, and a 30-degree oblique laparoscope is used to explore the entire abdomen. The exact placements of this point various with body habitus. Four additional 10 mm ports are placed under direct vision with the video laparoscope as follows: two are placed in the midclavicular line below the costal margin, and the other two are placed laterally in the anterior axilar line below the costal margin (Fig. 1). The placement of ports is similar to that used for Nissen fundoplication since the distal esophagus and proximal stomach are the focus of the operation. Some surgeons routinely perform an antireflux operation; others use a wrap when a mucosa perforation occurs to protect the area.

B. Exposure

The patient is placed in the reverse Trendelenburg position. This facilitates the exposure of the esophageal hiatus. The assistant elevates the left lobe of the liver with a retractor introduced through the right midrectus port. The use of a self-retaining retractor system to hold the liver frees the assistants to help with other aspects of the operation. Both crura and the anterior vagus are identified after opening the phrenoesophageal ligament. A Babcock is then used to grasp the stomach caudally.

C. Dissection

The hepatogastric ligament is divided using the harmonic scalpel, and the right crus is retracted laterally. The right side of the esophagus is carefully dissected to visualize the posterior vagus nerve. The left crus is similarly dissected to its point of origin from the right crural leaflet. The extent of division of the short gastric vessels varies depending on whether an antireflux procedure is anticipated. A "window" is created behind the esophagus wall, and a Penrose is placed behind the esophagus and traction is placed caudally for mobilizing it so at least 6–8 cm of the esophagus is below the hiatus. The hiatus is later closed using sutures.

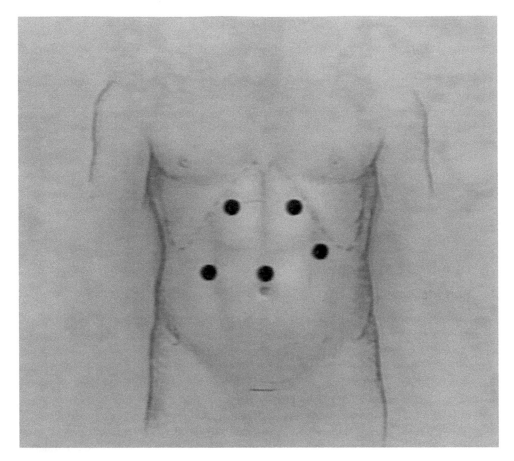

Figure 1   Port placement.

D.   Myotomy

An endoscope is placed through the mouth of the patient toward the hiatus while a Babcock clamp retracts down the cardioesophageal junction. The endoscopist identifies the zone of high pressure, and the surgeon marks the zone using the light from the scope. A 7–10 cm esophagomyotomy is performed (Fig. 2), its length depending on the length of the zone of high pressure. The circular fibers of the LES are then divided initially by lifting individual fibers away from the mucosa with the electrocautery hook, and then by dividing them with a short burst of current. Alternately, the harmonic scalpel or bipolar scissors may be used to perform the myotomy. Once the submucosal plane is exposed, the remainder of the myotomy is more easily performed. It is important to bluntly separate the muscle fibers from the mucosa lateral to the myotomy, allowing the mucosa to bulge through the myotomy incision. When this is done correctly, the mucosa will be exposed for at least 40% of its circumference preventing closure of the myotomy. Transillumination, provided by the endoscope, plays a key role by helping identify muscle fibers and ensures complete division of the muscle fibers. Although the rule of thumb is that the myotomy should be extended onto the stomach about 1–1.5 cm, the endoscopist is also helpful in determining if the myotomy is complete by documenting complete opening through the area of high pressure. This is particularly important when

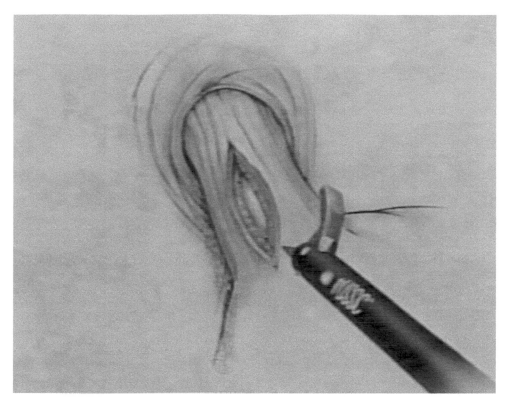

Figure 2   Laparoscopic Heller myotomy.

the myotomy is carried onto the stomach by verifying that the entire LES has been divided before the myotomy is carried onto the stomach too far. When completed, the myotomy is tested by examining it with the endoscope and insufflating air, while the esophagus is submerged under saline. Then the endoscope is removed.

E.   Fundoplication

A fundoplication may be performed, and many antireflux procedures have been described in conjunction with myotomy. Whether to perform a fundoplication and the ideal antireflux procedure following laparoscopic Heller myotomy is controversial.

Shiino and coworkers reviewed the literature and found that the quality of life was not improved by an antireflux operation if the myotomy was performed through a thoracotomy, but results were markedly improved after the abdominal approach. It was felt that mobilization of the esophagus through the abdomen disrupts anatomical relationships that are important in preventing reflux. Since the laparoscopic approach is similar to the open abdominal approach, results may be extrapolated to this operation, but not enough experience exists to definitively answer the question. Some surgeons do not perform an antireflux procedure and report excellent results or advocate myotomy with minimal mobilization of the esophagus. Most surgeons perform a partial wrap because of their concern about causing dysphagia. The Dor fundoplication, or partial anterior wrap, is the most common antireflux procedure used.

We reported a small series of patients performing a laparoscopic Heller myotomy with bolstering partial posterior fundoplication (Fig. 3). The anterior wall of the gastric

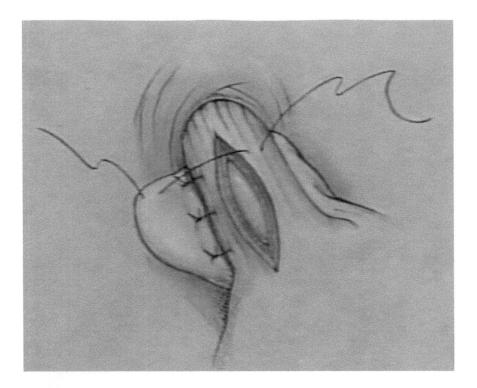

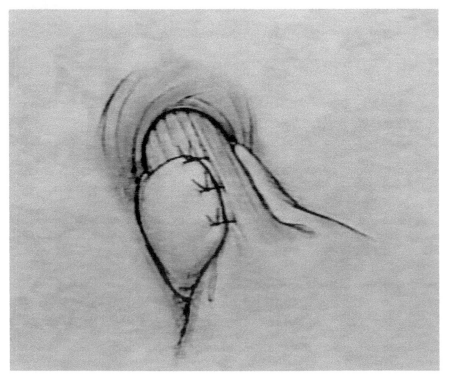

Figure 3   (A) Partial fundoplication; (B) bolstering myotomy.

fundus is sutured to the edges of the myotomy and to the crura. This helps to keep the edges of the myotomy open and provides protection and support for the exposed mucosa. We did not find symptom of gastroesophageal reflux after the procedure; we believe it is an effective antireflux procedure. Furthermore, bolstering the myotomy may help heal small esophageal perforations and keep the myotomy opened.

At the end of the procedure, all of the operative accesses are examined and bleeding control is performed. The port site is then closed, and the skin is closed with subcuticular 4-0 sutures.

VIII. POSTOPERATIVE CARE

Patients are left fasting for 12–24 hours postoperatively. If liquids are tolerated, a soft diet is started. In case of a repaired esophageal perforation, patients usually are kept fasting for an additional 36–48 hours, and often a barium swallow is performed to ensure that the perforation is well closed. Patients may progress to normal diet as tolerated, but most patients require soft diet for 2–4 weeks. Patients are discharged when they tolerate diet and have good pain control, usually between 2 and 3 days. Postoperative testing is not required if the patient is markedly improved, but 24-hour pH monitoring and manometry may be required to diagnose reflux or causes of persistent symptoms.

IX. MANAGEMENT OF COMPLICATIONS

Operative complications of laparoscopic esophagomyotomy include those related to administration of a general anesthetic, complications common to all laparoscopic operations such as injury to other organs during trocar placement or dissection or bleeding, and problems related directly to performance of the myotomy. The two most common myotomy-related complications are bleeding and mucosal injury, specifically perforation. Bleeding usually is controlled by laparoscopic approach, but, if not controlled, conversion to open procedure should be performed.

Mucosal injuries can be early or late. Early injuries are usually due to placement of instrumentation (nasogastric tubes, bougies, or endoscopes) in the esophageal lumen or entry into the lumen while the myotomy is being performed. The latter complication may occur in as many as 5–10% of cases and, if recognized, can be repaired laparoscopically in most cases. The perforation is repaired using a 4-0 or 5-0 suture, and the stomach can be used to cover the hole after suturing. A gastric wrap is indicated to buttress the repair when perforation occurs, and a barium swallow should be done prior to discharge to verify healing. Failure to obtain an adequate repair laparoscopically may necessitate conversion to open operation. The injury most often occurs as the myotomy is carried onto the stomach since the mucosa and muscle layers are more difficult to separate in this area and the mucosal layer is thinner in this region. Late perforation may be related to ischemia from the electrocautery, which results in late necrosis.

Late problems that occur after myotomy include failure to improve swallowing, progression of disease, gastroesophageal reflux, failure or slippage of fundoplication if used, and stricture of the distal esophagus. Problems with failed myotomy and stricture at the myotomy site can be minimized by meticulous detail at the initial operation. The inappropriate use of an antireflux procedure at the time of myotomy may lead to a functional postoperative obstruction requiring a reoperative procedure. Most surgeons feel this problem can be avoided by using a partial fundoplication at a time of myotomy.

Patients with achalasia are at higher risk to develop esophageal carcinoma, which must be excluded when patients present with late worsening or new-onset symptoms.

SURGICAL TIPS

1. Laparoscopic Heller myotomy is an excellent treatment option for achalasia. Success rates in experienced hands exceed 90%. Results are worst in patients who present with markedly dilated esophagus.
2. Upper gastrointestinal endoscopy, esophageal manometry, and a 24-hour pH are useful diagnostic studies in achalasia. Endoscopy excludes malignancy, manometry identifies the underlining esophageal motility disorder, and pH studies may be helpful with decisions concerning antireflux procedures.
3. Success of esophagomyotomy depends on an accurate diagnosis and careful selection of patients who are operative candidates.
4. Experience with advanced laparoscopic techniques is critical for effective performance of the operation.
5. Outcome requires a myotomy sufficient to disrupt the entire zone of high LES pressure; a myotomy that is too long predisposes to gastroesophageal reflux.
6. Intraoperative esophogoscopy is useful in determining myotomy length and may ensure safety of the procedure by excluding perforation.
7. Early recognition and prompt repair of perforation is essential. Postoperative barium swallow should be used liberally if there is any question about esophageal integrity.
8. Postoperative dysphagia may be due to an inadequate myotomy, progression of disease, or an antireflux procedure that results in either functional or anatomical obstruction.
9. The need for an antireflux procedure is not fully established and needs further study.
10. When recognized promptly, perforation from pneumatic dilatation should be managed by closing the perforation and performing a myotomy on the opposite side of the esophagus.

XI. CURRENT STATUS AND FUTURE INVESTIGATIONS

Laparoscopic esophagomyotomy is a safe and effective treatment for achalasia. Symptoms of dysphagia and regurgitation resolve in 80–90% of the patients. Length of hospital stay, amount of pain medication required, and time to full recovery are much less than with the open approach. Approximately 5–25% of patients suffer from symptomatic gastro-esophageal reflux after myotomy, and many surgeons perform an antireflux operation in conjunction with the myotomy, usually a partial wrap. The need for an antireflux operation is, however, still controversial. Although video-assisted thoracic surgical (VATS) approaches have also been used, this method is technically more demanding and relief of dysphagia is obtained in only about 80% of the patients. Most surgeons using this approach have adopted the abdominal approach.

Since precise myotomy is the key to obtaining optimum results and avoiding significant myotomy-related complications, new modalities like robotically assisted laparoscopy have been proposed for Heller myotomy. The prediction is that robotic assistance will increase the precision and accuracy of the procedure since it should eliminate tremor and fatigue of the human hand. Likewise, the operator's hand movements can be modulated to produce smaller, more precise movement of the instruments improving accuracy. The benefits of extra magnification and three-dimensional imaging can help prevent esophageal perforation and identify residual circular fibers. The current status of robotics in surgery, and especially in esophagomyotomy, is investigational, and few data exist to determine if robotics will result in a significantly better clinical outcome for this procedure.

SELECTED READINGS

Ancona E, Anselmino M, Zaninotto G, et al. Esophageal achalasia: laparoscopic versus conventional open Heller-Dor operation. Am J Surg 1995; 170:265–270.

Bruley des Varannes S, Scarpignato C. Current trends in the management of achalasia. Dig Liver Dis 2001; 33(3):266–277.

Ellis H. Reoperation for failed myotomy. In G Pearson, ed. Esophageal Surgery. New York: Churchill Livingstone, 1995.

Eubanks TR, Pellegrini C. Laparoscopic esophageal surgery. In G Zuidema, C Yeo, eds. Survey of the Alimentary Tract. 5th ed. 2002, pp 301–312.

Little, AG. Functional disorders of the esophagus. In G Zuidema, C Yeo, eds. Surgery of the Alimentary Tract, 5th ed. 2002, pp 271–287.

Pellegrini C. Esophageal disease. In Larry R Kaiser. Thoracic Surgery. Boston: Little Brown and Company, 1993.

Pellegrini C. Surgical endoscopy for achalasia and esophageal motility disorder. In SW Eubanks. Mastery of Endoscopic and Laparoscopic Surgery. 2000, pp 174–182.

Raiser F, Perdikis G, Hinder R, et al. Heller myotomy via minimal-access surgery: an evaluation of antireflux procedures. Arch Surg 1996; 131:593–598.

Richter JE. Comparation and cost analysis of different treatment strategies in achalasia. Gastrointest Endosc Clin North Am 2001; 11(2):359–370.

Shiino Y, Filipi C, Awad ZT, et al. Surgery for achalasia. J Gastrointest Surg 1999; 3(5):447–455.

Speiss AS, Kahrilas P. Treating achalasia from whalebone to laparoscopy. JAMA 1998; 280(7):638–642.

Urbach DR, Hansen PD, Khajanchee YS, Swanstrom LL. A decision analysis of the optimal initial approach to achalasia: laparoscopic Heller myotomy with partial fundoplication, thoracoscopic Heller myotomy, pneumatic dilatation, or botulinum toxin injection. J Gastrointest Surg 2001; 5(2):192–205.

Villegas L, Rege RV, Jones DB. Laparoscopic Heller myotomy with bolstering partial posterior fundoplication for achlasia. J Laparoendosc Adv Surg Techniques 13(1):1–4.

26

Peptic Ulcer Disease

TIMOTHY T. HAMILTON and ROBERT V. REGE

Center for Minimally Invasive Surgery
University of Texas Southwestern Medical Center
Dallas, Texas

I. BACKGROUND

A. Duodenal Ulcer

Duodenal ulceration is fundamentally a disease of excess acid load in the duodenum, although alterations in protective factors also play a role. Gastric acid secretion is under the regulatory control of three important influences: parasympathetic stimulation via the vagus nerve, histaminergic receptor agonism, and gastrin produced by the antrum. The role of the vagus nerve in regulating gastric acid secretion, as delineated by Prout, Beaumont, Pavlov, Dragsted and others, coupled with the anatomical descriptions of the vagus nerve, beginning with those attributed to Galen, led to the development of a number of highly effective operations designed to minimize acid production in keeping with Schwarz's dictum of "no acid, no ulcer." Consequently, peptic ulcer disease (PUD) of the duodenum was one of the most common indications for elective gastric surgery as recently as the 1960s and early 1970s.

However, better understanding of the pathophysiology of PUD and the cellular events responsible for gastric acid secretion led to the development of effective medications for the treatment of PUD. This so-called antisecretory therapy, first achieved with histamine receptor antagonists (H_2 blockers, e.g., cimetidine) and more recently with proton pump inhibitors (PPIs, e.g., omeprazole), has revolutionized the treatment of PUD by controlling pain, healing ulcers, and preventing recurrence and complications in a majority of patients. PPIs essentially eliminate acid secretion so that most ulcers encountered today by surgeons have mitigating circumstances.

Chronic infection with *Helicobacter pylori* is felt to be important in promoting peptic ulceration as well. Fully 95% of patients with duodenal ulcer and 50–85% of patients with gastric ulcer harbor the organism. In contrast, as many as 50% of normal adults also harbor the organism but will never develop symptoms of peptic ulceration, leading to the confusion regarding the significance of *H. pylori* infestation. A number of combination drug therapies, often combining bismuth subsalicylate and metronidazole or amoxicillin or tetracycline with a PPI such as omeprazole, have been shown to be effective in eradicating the organism in 85–95% of patients depending on the combination of drugs used. These regimens essentially eliminate ulcer recurrence if the organism is successfully eradicated. Treatment failure due to recurrent *H. pylori* infection is on the increase due to the development of organisms resistant to conventional antibiotic therapy.

B.   Gastric Ulcer

Gastric ulcers are considered separate entities and have been categorized with respect to both location and pathophysiology. Type I ulcers are found on the lesser curve, and type IV ulcers are found high on the lesser curve near the esophagogastric junction. Gastric ulcers generally result from a breakdown in the mucosal defense mechanism rather than excess acid production. In fact, many gastric ulcers occur in achlorhydric patients. The mucosal defense breakdown theory is reinforced by the typically poor healing rates of gastric ulcers associated with antisecretory therapy. Gastric ulcers are also associated with use of anti-inflammatory agents, medications that effect the protective system by inhibiting prostaglandin production.

Type II and III gastric ulcers differ in that they seem to arise as a consequence of excess acid production, similar to duodenal ulcers. Type II ulcers are located in the mid-body of the stomach and exist in conjunction with duodenal ulcers. Type III ulcers are pyloric or prepyloric ulcers that occur without associated duodenal ulcers.

Gastric malignancies commonly present as ulcerations. Consequently, all gastric ulcers are assumed to represent malignancy until proven otherwise and should therefore be biopsied endoscopically upon their diagnosis. Documented benign gastric ulcers are typically treated with agents, such as sucralfate, that help to restore the mucosal defense mechanism and promote ulcer healing. Consideration should also be given to a trial of proton pump inhibitor therapy in the setting of type II and III gastric ulcers. *H. pylori* is felt to be much less important in the pathogenesis of gastric ulceration than in duodenal ulcer disease, but the standard currently is to treat *H. pylori* when infestation accompanies gastric ulceration.

Chronic nonsteroidal anti-inflammatory drug (NSAID) administration has clearly been linked to the development of both gastric and duodenal ulceration, as prostaglandins are of great importance in maintaining adequate mucosal blood flow. Indeed, given sufficient time, virtually 100% of long-term NSAID users will develop gastric ulceration of one degree of another. Other agents that predispose to gastric ulceration include alcohol and tobacco use and abuse, corticosteroids, and aspirin. Withdrawal of such ulcerogenic agents is, of course, a first step in the treatment of gastric ulceration.

II.   COMPLICATIONS OF PUD

A.   Bleeding

Chronic peptic ulcer disease may result in a slow insidious loss of blood resulting in a microcytic anemia related to iron deficiency. This presentation, however, is more characteristic of a gastrointestinal malignancy. Duodenal ulcers may erode posteriorly into the gastroduodenal artery producing brisk, life-threatening upper gastrointestinal hemorrhage (UGIB). Gastric ulcers may likewise erode into the rich submucosal vasculature resulting in similarly impressive acute blood loss. Although only 10–20% of all UGIB patients will be found to have PUD, as many as 50% of patients with severe UGIB suffer from peptic ulceration. Patients with acute, severe UGIB from peptic ulceration may present in extremis and mandate aggressive volume resuscitation, blood transfusion, and early upper endoscopy. If bleeding does not resolve spontaneously, or if patient factors predispose to recurrent bleeding (e.g., a visible vessel in the ulcer base), endoscopic treatments such as heater probe coagulation, epinephrine injection, and/or laser therapy may be useful. Surgery is indicated if bleeding cannot be adequately controlled endoscopically.

B. Perforation

Ulcers located on the anterior wall of the duodenal bulb may erode through the serosa, resulting in free intraperitoneal perforation. A patient with an acute duodenal perforation will typically present with acute severe pain, a rigid abdomen, and, depending upon the duration of the perforation, may show signs of septic shock. Posteriorly located duodenal ulcers may penetrate into the substance of the pancreas producing a more chronic course of abdominal pain and chronic pancreatitis. Gastric ulcers >5 cm in diameter (giant gastric ulcers) put patients at high risk for both free perforation and bleeding. Perforation is the complication most frequently requiring operative intervention today.

C. Obstruction

Chronic duodenal bulb ulcers as well as type II and type III (pyloric and prepyloric) gastric ulcers may result in gastric outlet obstruction (GOO). Patients with GOO typically present with progressive weight loss, intractable nausea and vomiting, inability to tolerate oral nutrition, and frequently suffer from severe fluid and electrolyte imbalances. The classic example is a hypochloremic, hypokalemic metabolic alkalosis and severe volume deficit. Patients are also typically malnourished due to the chronicity of the condition. Total parenteral nutrition (TPN), aggressive fluid resuscitation with saline supplemented by potassium, and gastric decompression are mainstays of initial therapy. Although surgery is almost universally indicated, it is best postponed for approximately 7 days to ensure adequate preparation of the patient, unless urgent exploration is otherwise indicated.

III. THE ROLE OF SURGERY

As recently as the 1960s, procedures designed to reduce acid secretion by interrupting the vagal innervation of the parietal cell mass of the stomach were routinely performed on an elective basis and surgery was the primary treatment option for PUD. The advances in pharmacotherapy, coupled with the natural steady decline in prevalence of the disease from the 1940s through the 1970s, have resulted in a significant reduction in the performance of elective acid-reducing procedures. Consequently, in today's world, surgery is now rarely performed strictly to eliminate gastric acid secretion, and elective surgery for PUD is reserved for the minority of patients refractory to medical therapy or felt to be unable to fully comply with the medication regimen prescribed.

More commonly, patients come to operation for the treatment of complications of PUD, frequently emergently, and very often at the limits of physiological reserve. Despite the medical advances outlined above, the incidence of surgical exploration for the emergent treatment of acute exsanguinating hemorrhage, duodenal perforation, or gastric outlet obstruction is actually on the rise. Controversy exists concerning the performance of an acid-reducing procedure in addition to control of the complication for which the operation is performed.

IV. SURGICAL OPTIONS

A. Acid Reduction

Primary acid-reducing procedures are predicated on interruption of the vagal fibers innervating the parietal cell mass. This may be accomplished by sectioning the right and left vagus nerves (anterior and posterior trunks) as they enter the abdomen (total abdominal or truncal vagotomy), by dividing the vagi on the proximal stomach after they have given off the hepatic and celiac branches (selective gastric vagotomy), or by selectively dividing only those branches innervating the parietal cells (parietal cell vagotomy, proximal gastric vagotomy, highly selective gastric vagotomy). The extent of vagotomy largely influences the effectiveness of the procedure as well as the incidence of subsequent untoward side effects. The vagus nerve, in addition to stimulating acid secretion from the parietal cells, innervates the antrum and pylorus helping to regulate the reservoir function of the distal stomach and relaxation of the pylorus. Both truncal vagotomy and selective gastric vagotomy result in significant loss of the reservoir function of the antrum, as well as persistent, tonic contraction of the pylorus. The antral pumping mechanism may also be lost, resulting in gastroparesis. Consequently, each procedure must be accompanied by some form of gastric drainage procedure to overcome the functional gastric outlet obstruction produced by denervation of the pylorus. Highly selective gastric vagotomy (parietal cell vagotomy, proximal gastric vagotomy) divides only the vagal branches innervating the parietal cell mass, limiting side effects, but also reducing efficacy somewhat.

The most effective acid-reduction operation has historically been truncal vagotomy with antrectomy (V&A). The inclusion of antrectomy, when combined with total abdominal vagotomy, further reduces stimuli for acid secretion by removing the G-cells (gastrin-producing cells) of the antrum. Antrectomy involves resection of the pylorus, and gastrointestinal continuity may be reestablished by either a Billroth I (gastroduodenostomy) or Billroth II (loop gastrojejunostomy) reconstruction. However, as gastric reservoir function is impaired and the pylorus no longer slows the entry of chyme into the proximal small bowel, osmotic diarrhea and dumping symptoms are likely to occur. Recurrence of PUD after V&A is infrequent ($<2\%$), but the procedure carries with it significant operative morbidity, and long-term side effects such as diarrhea and dumping are common, thus limiting the clinical utility of the operation. V&A remains the operation of choice for type III gastric ulcers as well as most forms of benign GOO. V&A can be safely performed laparoscopically, and several series have reported results comparable to those achieved with open techniques.

A less morbid alternative is to perform a truncal vagotomy, leaving the antrum intact. As with V&A, division of the vagal trunks denervates the pylorus, leading to tonic contraction and an inability for the stomach to empty. Thus, truncal vagotomy must be combined with some sort of gastric drainage procedure. The most commonly performed vagotomy and drainage procedure in the United States is the truncal vagotomy and pyloroplasty (V&P), typically employing the Heineke-Mikulicz (two layer) or Weinberg (single layer) pyloroplasty. The V&P avoids resection of stomach and duodenum, thereby reducing the technical demands and operative morbidity considerably. V&P is an effective procedure for the elective treatment of PUD with an approximate 10% recurrence rate at 10 years. Unfortunately, however, dumping and diarrhea may still complicate long-term postoperative management up to 20% of the time. Other vagotomy and drainage options include vagotomy with either loop or Roux-en-Y gastrojejunostomy. These are far less attractive options and are not routinely recommended. V&P is the operation of choice in the emergent surgical treatment of bleeding duodenal ulceration. Since the proximal duodenum must be opened to control bleeding from the gastroduodenal artery, the same longitudinal incision can be extended onto the distal stomach and closed transversely, creating the standard Heineke-Mikulicz pyloroplasty. Vagotomy and pyloroplasty, like the VA, is a procedure that also lends itself to laparoscopic techniques with good result.

An attractive option for the surgical treatment of PUD is selective interruption of the vagal fibers innervating the parietal cell mass while preserving innervation of the pylorus (parietal cell vagotomy, PCV). The PCV, when performed by skilled operators, can effectively reduce acid secretion while preserving pyloric physiology. Thus, the recurrence rate of PUD is acceptably low (5–20%), and the incidence of postvagotomy syndrome should be near zero. Although the recurrence rates after PCV are significantly higher than those of V&A or V&P, the PCV is considered by many to be the best first option for the elective surgical treatment of PUD, due to the significantly reduced risk of operative complications and long-term side effects. In suitable candidates, laparoscopic PCV may be a more attractive first-line treatment option than standard medical therapy. Those patients who do develop recurrent PUD after PCV can usually be managed successfully with medical antisecretory therapy.

B. Perforated Duodenal Ulcer

Perforation of a duodenal ulcer is a frequent presentation of chronic PUD requiring emergent surgical management. The operative approach for the management of perforated duodenal ulcer is frequently a matter of some controversy. In addition to addressing the perforation, should a primary acid-reducing procedure be performed at the same operation, and, if so, which one, or should the perforation be closed and the patient's PUD be managed medically postoperatively? The most appropriate course of action is dependent upon the clinical situation at the time of surgery. Three fundamental concepts must be foremost in the surgeon's mind: (1) close the perforation; (2) irrigate the abdomen thoroughly; (3) perform no more surgery than the patient will safely tolerate. Whether or not to proceed with a primary acid-reducing procedure is an individual decision. In selected young patients who present early after perforation, are otherwise relatively healthy, have not demonstrated physiological decompensation, and have failed initial medical therapy or have risk factors predisposing to failure of medical therapy, an acid-reducing procedure may appropriately be added after closure of the perforation. Patients who present with perforation as the first sign of peptic ulcer disease are likely to respond to medical therapy and do not need an acid-reducing procedure. Similarly, the majority of patients operated upon for complications of known peptic ulcer disease represent failure of medical therapy. As such, the addition of an acid-reducing procedure should be considered in any patient felt to be able to tolerate the additional procedure. Our practice is to perform a PCV in such a setting. Laparoscopic Graham patch closure of duodenal ulcer perforation both with and without simultaneous PCV can safely be performed. Among the few series describing the approach, good short- and intermediate-term results have been reported.

C. Bleeding Duodenal Ulcer

Patients typically come to operation for bleeding duodenal ulceration only after unsuccessful endoscopic management. Such patients have likely bled considerably, been resuscitated for hemorrhagic shock, and are frequently physiologically compromised. It makes sense, then, to perform the most expedient operation in one's armamentarium and return the patient to the intensive care unit for further resuscitation. The operation of choice in this setting is usually the V&P. The usual culprit in bleeding duodenal ulceration is the gastro-duodenal artery deep to the posterior wall of the duodenal bulb. Access to the artery is via a longitudinal duodenotomy extending 2–3 cm distal to the pylorus. The vessel is usually visible in the ulcer base. The vessel must be ligated with a three-stitch approach: two single interrupted sutures above and below the ulcer to control the vessel proximally and distally, and the so-called U-stitch in the ulcer base to control the feeding dorsal pancreatic branch of the gastroduodenal artery. Once the bleeding is controlled, the duodenotomy is extended proximally across the pylorus approximately 4–5 cm onto the distal stomach. The resultant gastro-pyloroduodenotomy is then closed transversely in Heineke-Mikulicz fashion. If the pylorus is heavily scarred, a Finney or Jaboulay pyloroplasty may also be opted for. Truncal vagotomy is then performed, adding little extra time to the procedure. Although this procedure may be performed laparoscopically as well, the friability of the duodenum and the limited tactile feedback of current laparoscopic instruments make suture placement within the ulcer base difficult. In the setting of massive upper GI hemorrhage and associated hemorrhagic shock described above, is not recommended that V&P be performed using laparoscopic techniques.

D.   Obstruction

Benign duodenal obstruction and GOO secondary to PUD are best managed with truncal vagotomy and antrectomy. That said, special circumstances may preclude safe dissection of the proximal duodenum, making the operation hazardous. The oft-mentioned "difficult duodenum" dictates an alternate approach. The Finney stricturoplasty or the Jaboulay pyloroplasty (actually a gastroduodenostomy) are both acceptable solutions. Occasionally, the inflammatory process is so intense that duodenal mobilization is impossible and even these techniques cannot safely be performed. In such a case, simple loop gastro-jejunostomy with truncal vagotomy may be the most appropriate operation. Each has been performed laparoscopically with good result.

E.   Gastric Ulcer

Patients who present with gastric ulcer, especially type I ulcers, are best treated by gastric resection. The ulcer is removed allowing definitive diagnosis, excluding malignancy and the portion of the stomach at risk for subsequent ulcers is removed. Antrectomy has been discussed previously. Proximal ulcers may be removed by wedge resection, but type IV ulcers are difficult to resection without compromising the esophagus. They are best handled by open operation.

V. TECHNIQUES

A. Laparoscopic Parietal Cell Vagotomy

After appropriate preoperative evaluation has been completed, the patient is counseled regarding surgical options and patient expectations as well as the potential complications of the procedure including conversion to an open technique, recurrence, and so forth. Perioperative antibiotic prophylaxis (usually a first-generation cephalosporin or equivalent) is given to reduce the risk of wound infection. Pneumatic compression boots are placed before induction of general endotracheal anesthesia to minimize DVT formation. Once successfully anesthetized, the patient is positioned (see Fig. 1). We prefer the open technique to place the initial 10 mm Hasson cannula in the infraumbilical position. The 10 mm 30° laparoscope is placed through this port, and four additional ports (one 5 mm and three 10 mm) are placed under direct vision (see Fig. 2). The operating table is then positioned in a gentle head-up position.

Thorough exploration of the abdomen is then undertaken. If the operation is performed in the setting of duodenal perforation, thorough peritoneal lavage is likewise carried out. If not already placed, a nasogastric tube is inserted by the anesthesiologist and visualized through the laparoscope as it passes along the greater curve of the stomach. A liver retractor is inserted through the right upper quadrant port to retract the left lobe of the liver cranially. It is sometimes necessary to divide the left triangular ligament to facilitate exposure. We prefer to use the harmonic scalpel for this. A Babcock retractor is used to

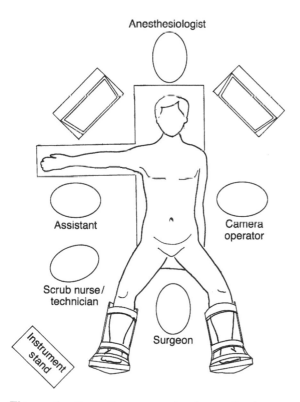

Figure 1   Operating room setup for peptic ulcer operations.

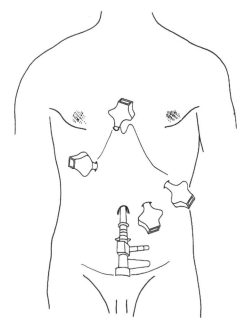

Figure 2 Port placement for peptic ulcer operations.

grasp the nasogastric tube through the greater curve of the stomach and apply gentle traction caudad and to the left. Care must be taken not to tear the stomach or avulse the vasa breva to the spleen with undue tension. Complete visualization and identification of both vagal trunks, both nerves of Laterjet, and the hepatic and celiac branches of the vagi is next performed. Complete familiarity with the vagal anatomy before undertaking any dissection is imperative and cannot be overemphasized.

The surgeon then begins the vagotomy at a point 6 cm proximal to the pylorus along the lesser curve. Division of the vagal branches to the stomach proximal to this point ensures that the crow's foot will be preserved and postoperative pyloric function will be maintained. Countertraction of the anterior leaf of the lesser omentum in a craniad direction allows division of the vagal branches close to the anterior gastric wall with the harmonic scalpel. The dissection is continued proximally parallel to the lesser curve to the cardia. The middle and posterior leaves of the lesser omentum are dissected in a similar fashion from 6 cm proximal to the pylorus to the cardia using the harmonic scalpel, again taking care to preserve the nerves of Laterjet. The dissection is then continued anteriorly at least 6 cm up the right side of distal esophagus. The laparoscope provides excellent visualization of the vagi facilitating division of all vagal branches to the fundus taking care to preserve the anterior and posterior vagal trunks and hepatic and celiac branches of the vagus. The phreno-esophageal membrane is then opened from the right and a Penrose drain passed behind the esophagus. The assistant then provides constant downward and leftward traction of the esophagogastric junction which will "banjo string" the vagal trunks. The lesser sac is then entered and posterior adhesions are divided. The left side of the esophagus is then cleared of vagal fibers for at least 6 cm proximally. The first two to three sets of short gastric vessels are next divided close to the greater curve (approximately 10 cm of greater curve from the fundus inferiorly should be so mobilized to ensure vagal division). The lesser sac is then entered through a window conveniently placed in the gastrocolic ligament and the stomach retracted anteriorly. Visual inspection confirms complete division of posterior vagal branches to the fundus. Remaining fibers are divided at this time completing the dissection. To minimize the risk of lesser curve necrosis, the anterior and posterior surfaces of the lesser curve are then oversewn with running 3-0 silk.

The abdomen is again irrigated and meticulously examined for hemostasis. All ports are withdrawn under direct vision. All 10 mm fascial defects are closed with the fascial closure device. The skin is closed with absorbable 4-0 monofilament subcuticular sutures. Sterile dressings are applied.

B. Postoperative Care

The gastric tube and urinary catheter are removed in the operating room. The patient may resume oral intake of fluids immediately, and the diet is advanced as tolerated. Pain control is usually achievable with opiates administered via a PCA for 24 hours and then discontinued in favor of oral analgesics as the diet is advanced. The patient may be discharged from the hospital as early as postoperative day 2 or 3, depending upon the individual.

VI. OTHER PROCEDURES

A. Laparoscopic Management of Duodenal Perforation

In the case of known or suspected duodenal perforation, the principles outlined above hold true for the laparoscopic approach as well. The perforation must be closed, the abdomen must be thoroughly irrigated and drained, and the decision as to whether or not to perform definitive ulcer surgery at the same setting must be made in the context of the individual patient and the clinical scenario. In general, the approach most often used to close duodenal perforation involves suture plication of the perforation incorporating an omental overlay patch (Graham patch). This procedure may be carried out using the same port placement as for PCV, facilitating subsequent performance of the PCV in appropriate patients. Interrupted 3-0 or 2-0 silk sutures are placed 5–10 mm to either side of the perforation and sequentially tied either intra- or extracorporeally, leaving the tails long. A tongue of omentum is then mobilized from a convenient location and placed over the repair. The tails are then tied over the omental patch, securing it in place. As with the open approach, a PCV may next be carried out as described above.

B. Laparoscopic Truncal Vagotomy and Pyloroplasty

The same port sites as described for PCV are used. Once the abdomen has been thoroughly inspected, attention is turned to the phrenoesophageal membrane, where a 1 cm window is made to the right of the esophagus and carried around circumferentially. A Penrose drain is then placed around the esophagus and secured with clips. Traction is then provided to the left and downward, resulting in banjo-stringing of the vagal trunks. Once the vagal trunks are identified, they are divided between clips and excised performing an approximately 1 cm vagectomy. The specimens are sent to pathology for frozen section confirmation of neural tissue.

With the stomach still on traction to the patient's left, a full-thickness longitudinal pyloromyotomy is next performed using either cautery or the ultrasonic shears extending

3–4 cm onto the stomach and 2–3 cm onto the duodenum. Traction sutures of 3-0 silk are placed at the midpoint of the opening both above and below. A single-layer running intracorporeal 2-0 silk suture is then used to close the pyloromyotomy transversely incorporating full-thickness bites. Two sutures may be used, one starting superiorly and one inferiorly, tied at the midpoint of the suture line.

C. Laparoscopic Posterior Truncal Vagotomy and Anterior Seromyotomy

This (so-called Taylor) procedure incorporates division and excision of a segment of the posterior vagal trunk at the distal esophagus (as with truncal vagotomy) and a seromyotomy parallel to and 1.5 cm inferior to the lesser curve of the stomach extending from the crow's foot (5–7 cm proximal to the pylorus) to the posterior aspect of the angle of His. The posterior truncal vagotomy is performed first, as described above. Again, the specimen is sent for pathological confirmation. The seromyotomy may be performed with the ultrasonic shears or the hook cautery. The muscular layers of the gastric wall are opened sequentially until the bluish-hued mucosa bulges into the wound. Air insufflation of the stomach combined with careful visual inspection will identify inadvertent gastric perforation. The serosa is then closed over the myotomy in an overlapping fashion with running intracorporeal 2-0 silk to prevent reinnervation of the lesser curve.

VII. CONCLUSIONS

Laparoscopic approaches to the surgical treatment of peptic ulcer disease and the attendant complications of PUD are becoming an important part of the surgical armamentarium. Among the majority of patients presenting with complications of peptic ulcer disease, surgery in general continues to be reserved for the treatment of the complication only without performing an antiulcer procedure at the same setting (see Table 1). However, with widespread application of minimally invasive techniques, an antiulcer procedure

Table 1 Surgery Reserved for Management of Complications Only

Initial presentation is with a complication, i.e., no previous PUD history.
No history of NSAID therapy, or patient can stop NSAID therapy without ill effects.
Patient able to maintain a high degree of medication compliance.
Patient hemodynamically unstable at presentation, or presentation late after perforation.

Table 2 Antiulcer Procedure as an Adjunct During Operation for Complication

Previous history of peptic ulcers.
Medical treatment failure.
Requires NSAIDs long-term.
Patient unable to maintain compliance with medical regimen.
Hemodynamically stable patient.
Highly experienced surgeon.
Other risk factors for treatment failure, i.e., tobacco abuse.

surgery may become a viable alternative to long-term antisecretory therapy in the absence of complications in selected higher-risk patients or as an adjunct to operative management of a PUD complication performed at the same setting (see Table 2). Above all, the operative treatment should be tailored to the individual needs of each patient.

SELECTED READINGS

Casas AT, Gadacz TR. Laparoscopic management of peptic ulcer disease. Surg Clin North Am 1996; 76:515–522.

Dubois F. New surgical strategy for gastroduodenal ulcer: laparoscopic approach. World J Surg 2000; 24:270–276.

Jones DB, Rege RV. Operations for peptic ulcer and their complications. In: Feldman M, Friedman LS, Sleisenger MH, editors. Sleisenger and Fordtan's Gastrointestinal and Liver Disease, 7th edition, New York: W. B. Saunders 2002, p. 797–809.

Khoursheed M, Fuad M, Safar H, Dashti H, Behbehani A. Laparoscopic closure of perforated duodenal ulcer. Surg Endosc 2000; 14:56–58.

Taylor TV, Lythgo JP, McFarland JB, et al. Anterior lesser curve seromyotomy and posterior truncal vagotomy versus truncal vagotomy and pyloroplasty in the treatment of chronic duodenal ulcer. Br J Surg 1990; 77:1007–1009.

27

Gastrectomy

TIMOTHY T. HAMILTON and ROBERT V. REGE

Center for Minimally Invasive Surgery
University of Texas Southwestern Medical Center
Dallas, Texas, U.S.A.

I. BACKGROUND

A. History

Theodur Billroth performed the first successful partial gastrectomy in Vienna in 1881. The indication for surgery was an apple-sized mass palpable in the mid-epigastrium. He performed an antrectomy and reestablished gastrointestinal continuity by anastomosing the duodenal stump to the lesser curve of the stomach. He later modified this reconstructive approach to anastomose the duodenum to the greater curve in what is now classically referred to as the Billroth I (or BI) operation. Pathological examination of the specimen revealed adenocarcinoma of the antrum.

Since surgical resection offers the only realistic chance for cure of gastric cancer and virtually all carcinomas of the stomach eventually obstruct or bleed, necessitating palliative surgery in the absence of curative resection, a less invasive approach to gastric cancer surgery is an attractive option. A number of reports describing series of laparoscopic distal, subtotal, and total gastrectomy published within the past 5 years demonstrate excellent short- and long-term results that are at least equivalent to the open approach. The laparoscopic approach may be superior in terms of patient satisfaction, postoperative pain, and time to return of normal activities. However, these procedures demand significant advanced laparoscopic skill and experience on the part of the surgeon.

Standard indications for partial, subtotal, or total gastrectomy can be broadly divided into malignant and benign conditions. The most common malignant disease leading to gastrectomy is adenocarcinoma (95%) with fewer cases of lymphoma and sarcoma (< 5%). Benign conditions include submucosal tumors of uncertain biological behavior (gastrointestinal stromal tumors) and, more commonly, complications of peptic ulcer disease (PUD) such as perforation, bleeding, and gastric outlet obstruction. Vagotomy and antrectomy remain the most effective elective procedures for the surgical treatment of PUD, with a recurrence rate of < 2%, but have significant operative morbidity and long-term sequelae. Highly selective vagotomy (and vagotomy with pyloraplasty) has a high recurrence rate (8–12%), but fewer complications. However, with the great success of pharmacological therapy for PUD, operations are now performed infrequently.

B. Anatomy

The stomach is an elongated bag-shaped organ occupying the mid upper abdomen and left upper quadrant. The stomach represents an incomplete diverticularization of the foregut with differentiation of the mucosa into acid-secreting (parietal or oxyntic) cells and proteolytic enzyme–secreting (peptic or chief) cells. The distal stomach or antrum produces the hormone gastrin, which controls the gastric phase of gastric secretion.

The stomach possess a rich, redundant blood supply, with both the lesser and greater curves receiving nourishment from two major arteries. This provides an explanation for the exsanguinating hemorrhage occasionally observed in cases of gastric ulceration. The right and left gastric arteries, which supply the lesser curve, arise ultimately from the celiac axis, with the left coming directly from the celiac and the right arising as a branch of the common hepatic artery. The arteries supplying the greater curve, the right and left gastroepiploic arteries, arise from the gastroduodenal and splenic arteries, respectively. Generally, any three of the four primary arteries may be sacrificed in order to allow mobilization of the stomach without compromising tissue viability. This may be particularly important when length is at a premium, for example, when performing an esophagectomy and reconstructing the GI tract by creating a gastric tube pulled into the chest or neck for esophagogastrectomy. The proximal-most portion of the greater curvature and the gastric fundus are also supplied by the short gastric arteries arising from the splenic artery.

The stomach is intimately related to the pancreas posteriorly, the spleen superior-laterally, the transverse colon inferiorly, and the liver anteriorly and superiorly. These anatomical relationships must be recognized during mobilization of the stomach. Undue traction inferiorly and medially may injure the spleen, resulting in bothersome hemorrhage. In addition, mobilization of the posterior surface of the stomach must be done with care to avoid injuring the pancreas. Not infrequently, the left lobe of the liver must be mobilized and retracted cephalad in order to expose the esophagogastric junction adequately. Finally, the transverse mesocolon and greater omentum are separated by only a single cell layer, and care must be taken not to injure the middle colic artery within the mesocolon when mobilizing the greater curvature of the stomach from the omentum.

II. OPERATIVE TECHNIQUES

As with most laparoscopic procedures, the techniques described are essentially analogous to those used for open operations. These laparoscopic approaches, therefore, require advanced laparoscopic skills including excellent technique for dissection, suturing, and intra- and extracorporeal knot tying.

A. Laparoscopic Distal Gastrectomy and Billroth I Reconstruction

After appropriate preoperative evaluation has been completed, the patient is counseled regarding surgical options and patient expectations as well as the potential complications of the procedure including conversion to an open technique, recurrence, and so forth. Perioperative antibiotic prophylaxis (usually a first-generation cephalosporin or equivalent) is given to reduce the risk of wound infection. Pneumatic compression boots are placed before induction of general endotracheal anesthesia to minimize DVT formation. Once successfully anesthetized, the patient is positioned (Fig. 1). We prefer the open technique to place the initial 10 mm Hasson cannula in the infraumbilical position. A 0° 10 mm camera is inserted and a thorough evaluation of the abdomen is conducted. If conditions are considered appropriate, the 10 mm 30° laparoscope is placed through this port, and five additional ports (one 12 or 18 mm port and four 10 mm ports) are placed under direct vision (Fig. 2). The operating table is then positioned in a gentle head-up position.

The anterior surface of the stomach is examined and the angularis incisura is identified just proximal to the crow's foot on the lesser curve. The ramification of the left and right gastroepiploic arteries is then identified on the greater curve. A line connecting these two points (roughly perpendicular to the long axis of the stomach) denotes the margin of proximal resection. Cautery is used to score the serosa along this line. The left gastric artery is identified near the angularis incisura and is divided with the harmonic scalpel or between clips. The greater curve of the stomach is mobilized by dividing the branches of the right gastroepiploic artery and vein close to the stomach wall using the harmonic scalpel. This dissection is continued as far to the right as possible. The lesser curve of the stomach is similarly mobilized by dividing the branches of the right gastric artery and vein close to the stomach. The nerves of laterjet and the hepatic braches of the vagus nerve are left intact.

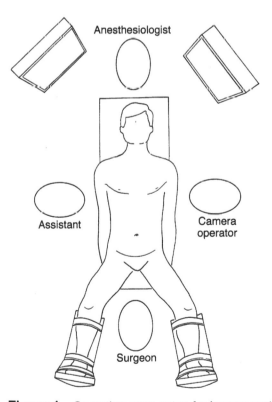

Figure 1   Operating room setup for laparoscopic gastrectomy.

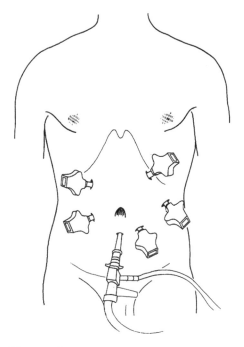

Figure 2 Port placement for laparoscopic gastrectomy.

Having completely devascularized the portion of the stomach to be resected, a generous Kocher maneuver is performed with cautery and blunt dissection, and the duodenum is divided distal to the pylorus, taking care to identify and avoid the common bile duct posteriorly. Superior and inferior traction sutures may be placed and cautery used to divide the anterior and posterior duodenal walls. Alternatively, the duodenum may be divided using a GIA stapler. We prefer to divide the duodenum with cautery and leave the lumen open as the length lost by stapling may preclude a BI reconstruction in some cases. The stomach is next divided with a GIA stapler from the lesser curve towards the greater curve, leaving an opening similar in size to the duodenum. The stapler is left engaged after the last firing to act as a retractor to bring the stomach and duodenum together. If there appears to be any tension, the Kocher maneuver is enlarged to allow greater duodenal mobility. The stapler is then fired and the gastric remnant removed in an endo-pouch via a convenient port. A hand-sewn single-layer anastomosis is fashioned between the stomach and duodenum. Stay sutures are placed on the corners but not tied, and the posterior suture line is completed from inside the anastomosis using interrupted 3-0 Vicryl stitches tied intra- or extracorporeally. The stay sutures are then tied and the anterior suture line is completed in a similar fashion. Additional Lembert sutures are placed at any sites of concern. A three-corner reinforcement stitch is placed at the "angle of sorrows," where the staple line and suture line meet. A drain may be placed via a port site if desired. All port sites are closed in the standard fashion.

B. Laparoscopic Distal Gastrectomy and Billroth II Reconstruction

A Billroth II reconstruction is appropriate in cases of significant duodenal inflammation making mobilization dangerous or if there is undue tension at the proposed BI anastomotic site. The initial dissection is the same as for BI gastrectomy. In the case of BII reconstruction, the duodenum is divided with a GIA stapler and the staple line reinforced with 3-0 silk Lembert sutures tied intra- or extracorporeally. The stomach is divided with an endoscopic GIA stapler. The stapler may be left engaged after the final firing to act as a retractor. The distal stomach is flipped cephalad to expose the posterior wall. A convenient loop of jejunum 15–20 cm distal to the ligament of Treitz is grasped and brought into the lesser sac through a window made in the transverse mesocolon. Care must be taken to avoid the middle colic artery and vein. An enterotomy is made on the antimesenteric border of the jejunum. A gastrotomy is made on the posterior wall of the stomach approximately 1 cm cephalad from the staple line. A hand-sewn anastomosis may be fashioned as described for BI gastrectomy, or a GIA 60 stapler may be used and the resultant enterotomy closed with a TA 30. Lembert stitches of 3-0 silk are placed wherever needed. The anastomosis is then gently caudally pulled through the mesocolic defect and the stomach sutured to the mesocolon with interrupted sutures. A drain may be placed adjacent to the anastomosis through a port site if desired. All port sites are closed in the standard fashion after removing the specimen in an endopouch.

C. Laparoscopic Wedge Resection

A wedge resection may be indicated for resection of a chronic gastric ulcer, to biopsy a lesion of uncertain malignant potential, or as definite therapy for small submucosal lesions. The set-up is similar to that for a gastrectomy, but, generally, only four trocars are required. If the lesion can be grasped with a Babcock grasper, we prefer to elevate the lesion and use multiple firings of a reticulating endo GIA stapler to resect the lesion and a suitable margin of adjacent stomach. Occasionally, the lesion is not able to be grasped satisfactorily, and seromuscular guy sutures are placed proximally and distally. Tension is applied to these sutures to elevate the lesion and the stapler fired below the lesion. Care must be taken when approaching lesions in proximity to the pylorus and cardia. In such cases, a wedge resection may result in excessive narrowing of the lumen. A distal gastrectomy may provide a better surgical option in cases involving the pylorus. Cardiac lesions may still be addressed with a wedge resection, but a bougie is often helpful in preventing luminal compromise.

D. Postoperative Management

A nasogastric tube is carefully inserted by the anesthesiologist, under laparoscopic vision, and left in place until postoperative ileus resolves. A urinary catheter is generally used until the first postoperative day. Pain control is achieved with a PCA. Oral intake may be started after the NG tube is removed and advanced as tolerated. Routine upper GI contrast examination is not necessary unless there is clinical concern for an anastomotic leak.

E. Complications

Bleeding from the suture line, anastomotic leak, and bowel obstruction are the most bothersome complications. An anastomotic leak or bowel obstruction mandates exploration. Bleeding may frequently be successfully managed endoscopically, but may require operative revision of the anastomosis if endoscopic techniques fail to achieve satisfactory hemostasis. Although follow-up data are short-term only, a number of series now published indicate that patients return to normal activity and have significantly reduced postoperative pain compared to historical controls operated upon in the open era. Long-term data are lacking regarding recurrence rates, the incidence of postoperative bowel obstruction, and the like.

F. Future Directions

There are now several published series describing laparoscopic gastrectomy for gastric malignancies including extended lymphadenectomy. At this time, however, this approach is not widely accepted as the standard surgical treatment for gastric adenocarcinoma except in a few centers. It must be emphasized that oncological principles must not be compromised in order to utilize a minimally invasive approach.

SELECTED READINGS

Fujiwara M, Kodera Y, Kasai Y, et al. Laparoscopy-assisted distal gastrectomy with systematic lymph node dissection for early gastric carcinoma: a review of 43 cases. J Am Coll Surg 2003; 196:75–81.

Mochiki E, Nakabayashi T, Kamimura H, Asao T, Kuwano H. Gastrointestinal recovery and outcome after laparoscopic-assisted versus conventional open distal gastrectomy for early gastric cancer. World J Surg 2002; 26:1145–1149.

Reyes CD, Weber KJ, Gagner M, Divino CM. Laparoscopic vs open gastrectomy. A retrospective review. Surg Endosc 2001; 15:928–931.

Shimizu S, Noshiro H, Nagai E, et al. Laparoscopic wedge resection of gastric submucosal tumors. Dig Surg 2002; 19:169–173.

28

Inguinal Hernias

DANIEL J. SCOTT

Tulane Center for Minimally Invasive Surgery
Tulane University School of Medicine
New Orleans, Louisiana, U.S.A.

DANIEL B. JONES

Beth Israel Deaconess Medical Center
Harvard Medical School
Boston, Massachusetts, USA

Each year in the United States approximately 680,000 inguinal hernia repairs are performed. Over the past two centuries hernia repairs have evolved considerably. In 1986 Lichtenstein introduced the tension-free concept and used prosthetic material to reinforce the inguinal canal floor. The tension-free repair revolutionized hernia surgery and resulted in decreased rates of recurrence and considerably less disability related to recovery from the operation.

In 1982 the first laparoscopic hernia repair was reported. However, it was not until the 1990s with the tremendous success of laparoscopic cholecystectomy that laparoscopic hernia repair gained momentum. It was also after considerable modifications in technique that the laparoscopic approach proved reliable. Early methods used laparoscopic suturing to close the hernia defect, resulting in high recurrence rates. Sutured repairs were abandoned, and tension-free repairs using mesh were adopted. Two mesh repair techniques evolved, including the transabdominal preperitoneal (TAPP) and the totally extraperitoneal (TEP) techniques. Although early experiences with TAPP and TEP repairs were fraught with high recurrence rates and nerve entrapment problems, as techniques were refined and the anatomy was more completely understood, these repairs proved safe and effective. The TAPP and TEP techniques combine a minimally invasive approach with placement of a large piece of prosthetic mesh in the preperitoneal space similar to an open Stoppa repair. Placement of the mesh in the preperitoneal space affords excellent reinforcement of emaciated tissues and prevents intrusion of the abdominal contents through any abdominal wall defect. The preperitoneal approach may be well suited for recurrent hernias since scar tissue from previous anterior repairs may be avoided. For bilateral hernias, the laparoscopic approach may also be advantageous since access to both groins may be achieved with a single set of ports and the need for two open groin incisions is obviated. For nonrecurrent, unilateral hernias, many surgeons offer a minimally invasive approach.

Despite early doubts concerning the safety and efficacy of laparoscopic repairs, a wealth of data now exists that has validated this approach. Over 30 prospective randomized trials have been performed comparing laparoscopic and open repairs. With 5-year follow-up available, these trials have shown that a recurrence rate of < 5% may be reliably achieved for both laparoscopic and open repairs and that complication rates are similar. Several differences between the two techniques have, however, been noted. First, laparoscopic repairs have been shown consistently to result in less postoperative pain. Second, recovery is shorter following laparoscopic repairs. Studies have documented improved exercise tolerance and faster resumption of full activity after TAPP and TEP repairs. Patients tend to return to work approximately one week sooner (about postop day 7) after a laparoscopic repair compared to a traditional open approach (about postop day 14).

On the other hand, laparoscopic repairs tend to cost more than open repairs by approximately $400–$800. However, if indirect cost of time away from work is considered, the laparoscopic approach may be more cost effective. Importantly, considerable expertise is needed to perform a laparoscopic repair, and the learning curve may be as high as 30 cases. While a laparoscopic repair under local and spinal anesthesia have been documented, most surgeons feel that a general anesthetic is required. Thus, for debilitated patients, an open approach under a local anesthetic may be preferable.

Because of the above-mentioned issues, significant controversy has surrounded the acceptance of laparoscopic hernia repair. Given the large body of level I evidence, it is justifiable to perform laparoscopic hernia repairs according to patient preference and surgeon qualifications. Very large scrotal hernias and incarcerated or strangulated hernias, however, may be very difficult to repair using a laparoscopic approach and may be better treated with an open approach. In appropriately selected patients, the laparoscopic approach may offer significant advantages in terms of decreased pain and faster recovery.

I. ANATOMY

Safe performance of a laparoscopic hernia repair requires knowledge of preperitoneal anatomy (Fig. 1). For beginners, the preperitoneal anatomy can be quite confusing and is considerably different than the perspective afforded by anterior groin repairs. Identifying landmarks within the preperitoneal space can be very helpful for gaining initial orientation. The pubic synthesis is directly midline, and Cooper's ligament can usually be seen just lateral to midline. The iliopubic tract runs from the pubic synthesis to the anterior superior iliac spine and is the internal equivalent of the inguinal ligament. The inferior epigastric vessels can be identified on the anterior abdominal wall and followed posteriorly to identify external iliac artery and vein. Two anatomical regions deserve mention. The *triangle of pain* refers to the area bounded inferiorly medially by the testicular vessels and superior laterally by the iliopubic tract. It is within this triangle that nerve entrapment can occur during mesh fixation. Posterior to the iliopubic tract course the lateral femoral cutaneous nerve and the femoral branch of the general femoral nerve. When mesh is fixated, care must be taken not to apply staples or tacks below the iliopubic tract in this area to avoid nerve entrapment. The *triangle of doom* is formed medially by

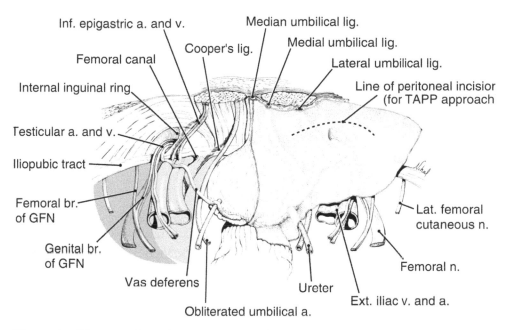

Inf. epigastric a. and v.
Median umbilical lig.
Cooper's lig.
Medial umbilical lig.
Femoral canal
Lateral umbilical lig.
Internal inguinal ring
Line of peritoneal incisior
(for TAPP approach
Testicular a. and v.
Iliopubic tract
Femoral br.
of GFN
Lat. femoral
cutaneous n.
Genital br.
of GFN
Femoral n.
Vas deferens
Ureter
Ext. iliac v. and a.
Obliterated umbilical a.

Figure 1 The preperitoneal space as viewed from within the abdomen. The dark shaded area represents the triangle of pain. The light shaded area represents the triangle of doom. *GFN*, genitofemoral nerve. (From Scott and Jones, 2000.)

the vas deferens and laterally by the testicular vessels. It is within this triangle that serious vascular injury may occur to the external iliac artery or vein if care is not taken.

From the preperitoneal space multiple hernias may be identified, reduced, and repaired. Indirect inguinal hernias course with the spermatic cord through the internal ring. Direct inguinal hernias course medial to the inferior epigastric vessels through Hesselbach's triangle, which is bounded by the inguinal ligament laterally, the rectus sheath medially, and the inferior epigastric vessels superiorly. Femoral hernias course within the femoral canal, which is bounded by Cooper's ligament medially, the external iliac vein laterally, and the iliopubic tract anteriorly. Obturator hernias course through the obturator canal along the course of the obturator neurovascular bundle.

II. CLINICAL PRESENTATION AND EVALUATION

A. Symptoms

Traditionally, both symptomatic and asymptomatic hernias are repaired to avoid the potential complications of incarceration and strangulation. Patients who are symptomatic usually present with groin pain associated with a bulge. If the hernia becomes irreducible it is referred to as incarcerated. If there is compromise to the blood supply of the herniated viscera, the hernia is termed strangulated. Incarcerated hernias must be promptly taken to the operating room, and this may best be done by an open approach.

B. Physical Examination

Physical examination is the primary method for confirming the diagnosis of hernia. During palpation of the inguinal canal during straining maneuvers, a mass or an impulse is felt pushing downward onto the examiner's fingertip. The differential diagnosis of a groin mass includes an inguinal hernia, a femoral hernia, lymphoma, lymphadenitis, lymphadenopathy, an abscess, a hematoma, a varicocele, a hydroceles, a testicular mass, testicular torsion, epididymitis, an ectopic testicle, a femoral aneurysm or pseudo aneurysm, a cyst, or a seroma. A careful history and physical can usually exclude masses other than hernias.

C. Diagnostic Tests

If the diagnosis of a hernia is in doubt on physical exam, computed tomography and ultrasound scanning may be helpful. Computed tomography may show herniated viscera into the subcutaneous fat overlying the inguinal ligament. An ultrasound scan may show bowel gas of herniated intestines.

D. Preoperative Preparation

History of urinary straining, constipation, cough, and heavy lifting should be sought as causes for increased intra-abdominal pressure. Routine workup should be pursued for patients with known or suspected comorbidities. Patients who are at prohibitive risk for undergoing a general anesthetic should be excluded. Patients should be counseled appropriately about the risk and benefits of the procedure, and consent should be obtained.

III. TRANSABDOMINAL PREPERITONEAL REPAIR

In the event of laparoscopic hernia repair, the TAPP procedure was one of the first methods to be widely adopted. This approach avoids some of the disorientation associated with preperitoneal anatomy by gaining initial access to the abdomen in an intraperitoneal fashion, similar to the approach used by surgeons for most laparoscopic operations. Once the abdomen is entered, the peritoneum is incised to gain access to the preperitoneal space and the repair is then performed.

Equipment used in this procedure includes:

General laparoscopy instrument set
5 mm laparoscopic scissors
Blunt graspers (two)
5 mm tacker
10 mm 30° laparoscope
Polypropylene mesh (12 × 15 cm)
5 mm clip applier (or suture and needle drivers)

A. TAPP Operating Room and Setup

With the patient under general anesthesia, a Foley catheter and sequential suppression devices are placed. According to surgeon preference, an antibiotic is administered prophylactically. The patient placed in a supine Trendelenburg position with both arms

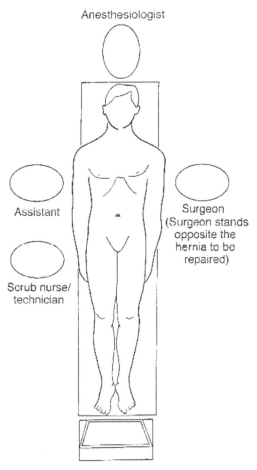

Figure 2 Operating room setup for a laparoscopic herniorrhaphy (TAPP or TEP approach). (From Molmenti E, et al. In: Jones DB, Wu J, Soper NJ, eds. Laparoscopic Surgery: Principles and Procedures. St. Louis: Quality Medical Publishing, 1997.)

tucked. The surgeon stands on the side opposite to the hernia (Fig. 2). The assistant and scrub nurse stand on the ipsilateral side. The monitor is placed at the patient's feet.

B. TAPP Surgical Technique

1. Port Placement

A pneumoperitoneum of 12–15 mmHg is achieved, and three ports are placed as shown in Figure 3. The infraumbilical port is usually a 10 mm trocar; the left and right ports may either be 5 or 10 mm ports.

2. Exposure and Dissection

The abdominal cavity is briefly explored to rule out unsuspected pathologies, and both groins are inspected. The peritoneum overlying the superior edge of the hernia defect is incised transversely from the medial umbilical ligament to the anterior superior iliac spine,

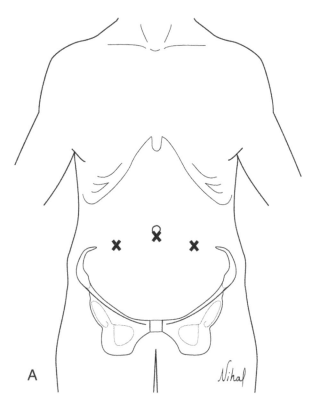

Figure 3   For the TAPP approach three ports are placed in the locations marked *X*. (From Scott and Jones, 2000.)

and peritoneal flaps are developed. The relevant anatomical landmarks are identified (Fig. 4), and blunt dissection is used to reduce the hernia. The spermatic cord is skeletonized to clearly visualize the vas deferens and the testicular artery and vein. Such skeletonization ensures that no cord lipomas or small indirect hernias are missed. If large indirect hernias are identified, the sack should be divided to limit the extent of the distal dissection. The vas deferens and gonadal vessels are separated from the peritoneum ("parietalization" of the cord) for a sufficient distance to allow placement of mesh between the peritoneum and the cord structures.

3.   Repair of the Hernia

A large piece of polypropylene mesh (at least 12×15 cm) is recommended for repair. The mesh is placed through one of the 10 mm trocars into the abdomen. The inguinal floor is covered with the mesh, and care is taken to overlap all hernia defects at least 2–3 cm. If the spermatic cord has been adequately parietalized (dissected free from the peritoneum), the mesh may be placed directly over the cord without the need for a cutting a slit and fashioning tales in the mesh. Alternatively, a slit in the mesh may be cut so that the cord may be encircled. However, encircling the cord with mesh may be associated with increased pain, a higher rate of recurrence, and scrotal seroma formation. The mesh is usually fixated to the anterior abdominal wall using helical fasteners (Fig. 5). Fasteners are

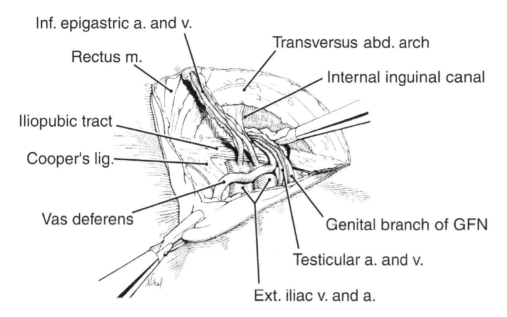

Inf. epigastric a. and v.

Rectus m.

Transversus abd. arch

Internal inguinal canal

Iliopubic tract

Cooper's lig.

Vas deferens

Genital branch of GFN

Testicular a. and v.

Ext. iliac v. and a.

Figure 4 Anatomical landmarks are identified after preperitoneal fat is dissected away. Locations for mesh fixation are marked *X*. (From Scott and Jones, 2000.)

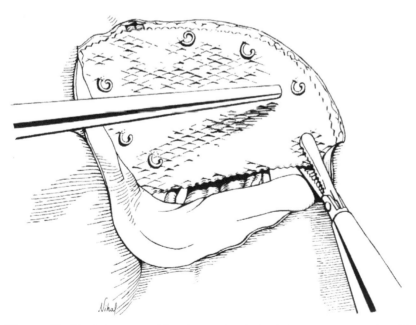

Figure 5 Mesh is secured in place using helical fasteners or staples. (From Scott and Jones, 2000.)

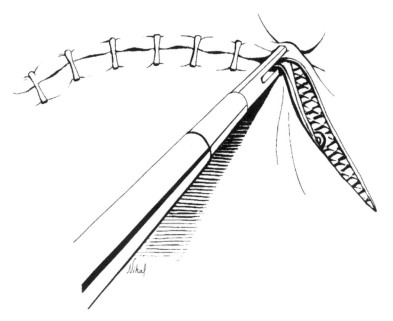

Figure 6 Clips are used to close the peritoneum. (From Scott and Jones, 2000.)

applied inferiorly to Cooper's ligament, and possibly to the rectus muscle, and superiorly and laterally to the transversus abdominis arch. No fasteners should be placed posterior to the iliopubic tract to avoid nerve entrapment. Alternatively, some authors advocate that mesh fixation is not necessary (and the risk of nerve entrapment is alleviated) if a large enough piece of mesh is used. To complete the procedure, the peritoneum is closed with clips or sutures (Fig. 6). Care must be taken to close the peritoneum without leaving gaps to prevent formation of adhesions between mesh and loops of bowel. The abdomen is reinspected to detect any inadvertent injuries. The ports are removed, and the facial openings and skin are closed.

C. Management of TAPP Complications

Potential complications include visceral injury, bleeding from the inferior epigastric or external iliac vessels, neuralgias from stapling injuries, infections, and recurrence of the hernia. Because the TAPP approach gains access to the groin via an intraperitoneal placement of ports, there is a small but real danger of injury to abdominal organs, intestinal adhesions, and bowel obstruction. The inferior epigastric vessels may be prone to injury during trocar insertion, and care must be taken to avoid these vessels. Other complications include port site hernias, and all trocars > 5 mm must be closed appropriately.

IV. TOTALLY EXTRAPERITONEAL REPAIR

The TEP repair represents the latest evolution in laparoscopic hernia repair and may be the ideal approach. The TEP technique gains access to the groins via a completely extraperitoneal approach. Thus, a peritoneal violation is avoided and the associated potential for visceral injury and adhesion formation may be diminished. However, a significant learning curve must be overcome since the preperitoneal anatomy can be disorienting and the technique is difficult.

Equipment used in the TEP procedure includes:

General laparoscopy instrument set
5 mm laparoscopic scissors
Blunt graspers (two)
5 mm tacker
10 mm 30° laparoscope
Polypropylene mesh (12 × 15 cm)
Balloon dissector

A. TEP Operating Room and Patient Setup

The operating room and patient setup are identical as for a TAPP approach.

B. TEP Surgical Technique

1. Port Placement

Ports are placed as shown in Figure 7. Initial access to the preperitoneal space is afforded through a 10 mm infraumbilical incision. The anterior rectus sheath is incised, the rectus

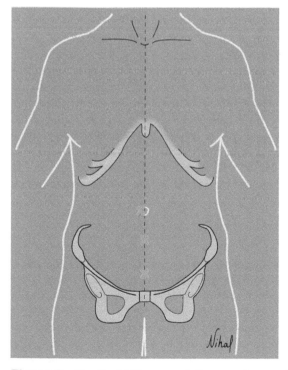

WEB
COLOUR

Figure 7 For the TEP approach three ports are placed in the locations marked X. (From Scott and Jones, 2000.)

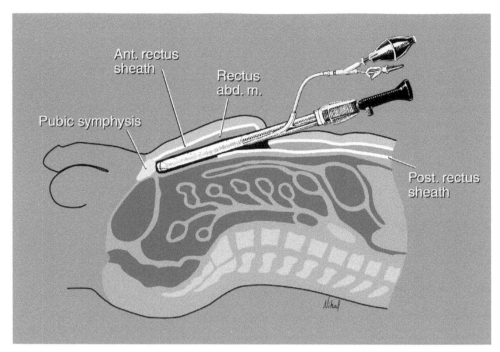

Figure 8 Access to the preperitoneal space is gained in the periumbilical area. The balloon is inserted into the preperitoneal space and is advanced to the pubic symphysis. (From Scott and Jones, 2000.)

muscle is retracted laterally, and dissection with an S-retractor along the posterior rectus sheath affords access to the preperitoneal space. Care is taken to avoid an incising midline fascia, which would result in entry through the linea alba into the peritoneal cavity. A balloon dissector is placed along the anterior surface of the posterior rectus sheath and advanced inferiorly to the pubic bone. With the patient in Trendelenburg position and the hernia maximally reduced, the balloon dissector is inflated to create a working space between the peritoneum and the abdominal wall (Figs. 8 and 9). The balloon dissector is deflated and removed (Fig. 10). A cannula is then inserted and the preperitoneal space is insufflated to 12 mmHg. Two 5 mm trocars are placed in the midline under direct visualization.

2. Exposure and Dissection

A 30° laparoscope is used, the area is inspected, and landmarks including the pubic synthesis, Cooper's ligament, the iliopubic tract, and the inferior epigastric vessels are identified. Direct hernias are frequently reduced by the balloon dissector. The cord is carefully skeletonized to reduce indirect sacks and to rule out cord lipomas. The cord is then parietalized by dissecting the peritoneum off of the vas deferens and the testicular artery and vein back to the level of the anterior superior iliac spine. This wide dissection allows for subsequent 12 × 15 cm mesh placement without the need for slitting the mesh. Care must be taken to avoid creating small tears in the peritoneum during the dissection. If this occurs a competing intra-abdominal pneumoperitoneum may compromise

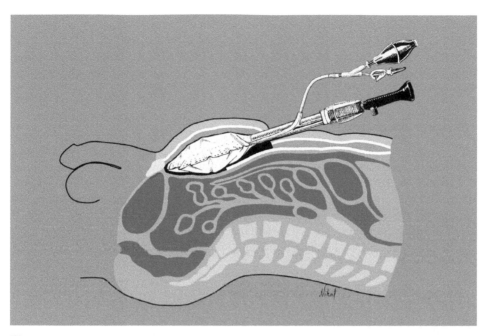

Figure 9 The balloon is inflated to create a working space. (From Scott and Jones, 2000.)

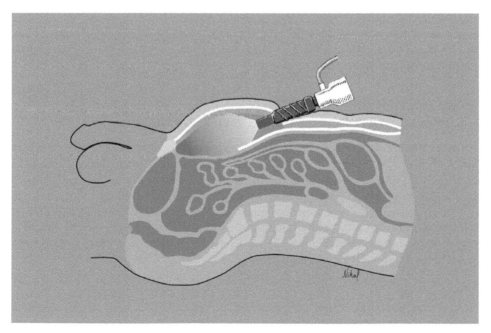

Figure 10 The balloon is deflated and removed. The preperitoneal working space is visualized with the laparoscope and other ports are placed. (From Scott and Jones, 2000.)

visualization, requiring a Veress needle to be placed into the peritoneal cavity in the upper abdomen to allow decompression. Defects must be closed with suture, endo loops, or clips so that postoperative adhesion formation or intestinal obstruction may be avoided. Alternatively, the procedure may be converted to a TAPP approach in the case of large peritoneal tears.

3. Repair of the Hernia

A 12 × 15 cm piece of polypropylene mesh is placed through the 10 mm umbilical port. The mesh is fixated to Cooper's ligament. Additional fixation to the anterior abdominal wall may not be necessary depending on the size of the hernia defect. The case is completed by the removal of the ports and evacuation of the pneumopreperitoneum. The pneumopreperitoneum is evacuated under direct visualization, while the inferior lateral edges of the mesh are held in place to ensure that the peritoneum does not slip underneath the mesh and cause an immediate recurrence.

C. Management of TEP Complications

Potential complications include visceral injury, bleeding from the inferior epigastric or external iliac vessels, neuralgias from stapling injuries, infections, and recurrence of the hernia. If peritoneal tears are not adequately repaired, there is also a risk of adhesion formation and intestinal obstruction.

V. POSTOPERATIVE CARE

The patient is discharged to home the same day of surgery once he or she is able to void spontaneously. However, there is no limitation on postoperative activity. Patients are instructed that scrotal bruising, crepitus, and seroma formation may occur and are usually self-limited. Clinical follow-up is scheduled 2–3 weeks after the procedure.

VI. CURRENT STATUS AND FUTURE INVESTIGATION

Long-term (5-year follow-up) level I data are now available that show laparoscopic hernia repair is as safe and as effective as open hernia repair while offering the advantages of quicker recovery time and less postoperative pain. Most surgeons in the United States favor the TEP approach, and it has almost entirely replaced the TAPP approach since it is felt to be safer and diminishes the potential for intra-abdominal injuries. However, a significant learning curve must be overcome to perform this procedure with good results. Data now exist that show that training on an inanimate model as part of a multimodality curriculum may result in improved operative performance during laparoscopic hernia repair (see Chapter 12). Overcoming the learning curve by using simulators may become more widespread.

Technical modifications of the procedure are ongoing. Many authors now believe that mesh fixation is unnecessary if a large enough piece of mesh is used. Avoiding mesh fixation may decrease cost and avoid nerve entrapment. Absorbable fasteners are under development, and mesh fixation using biological glues has also been anecdotally reported.

VII. TOP TEN SURGICAL TIPS

1. Place video cart and monitor at the foot of the bed.
2. Understand preperitoneal anatomy.
3. Keep the lowest port at least three finger breadths above the pubis.
4. Use a large piece of mesh with adequate overlap—the most common cause of recurrence is inadequate mesh size.
5. Most preperitoneal dissections are performed easily by gently pushing tissue—avoid sharp dissection and the use of cautery.
6. Divide large indirect sacks at the level of the internal ring—an endo loop or a ligature tied extracorporeally may be useful.
7. Excise cord lipomas to prevent postoperative pseudo-hernias.
8. Avoid placing the tacks in the triangle of pain.
9. Avoid dissection in the triangle of doom.
10. Close all peritoneal tears.

SELECTED READINGS

EU Hernia Trialists Collaboration. Laparoscopic compared with open methods of groin hernia repair: systematic review of randomized controlled trials. Br J Surg 2000; 87:860–867.

Liem MSL, Van Der Graff Y, Van Steensel CJ, et al. Comparison of conventional anterior surgery and laparoscopic surgery for inguinal-hernia repair. N Engl J Med 1997; 336:1541–1547.

Payne JH, Grininger LM, Izawa MT, Podoll EF, et al. Laparoscopic or open inguinal herniorrhaphy? A randomized prospective trial. Arch Surg 1994; 129:973–981.

Schneider BE, Castillo JM, Villegas L, Scott DJ, Jones DB. Laparoscopic totally extraperitoneal versus Lichtenstein herniorrhapy: cost comparison at teaching hospitals. Surg Laparosc Endosc Percutan Tech 2003; 13(4):261–267.

Scott DJ, Jones DB. Hernia. In: McClelland RN, ed. Selected Readings in General Surgery, Vol. 26, No. 4, Issues 1–2, 1999.

Scott DJ, Jones DB. Hernias and abdominal wall defects. In: Norton JA, Bolinger RR, Chang AE, Lowry SF, Mulvihill SJ, Pass HI, Thompson RW, eds. Surgery: Scientific Basis and Current Practice. New York: Springer-Verlag; 2000. p. 787–823.

Wright D, Paterson C, Scott N, Hair A, et al. Five-year follow-up of patients undergoing laparoscopic or open groin hernia repair: a randomized controlled trial. Ann Surg 2002; 235:333–337.

29

Appendectomy

MICHAEL ROSEN and FRED BRODY

Cleveland Clinic Foundation
Cleveland, Ohio, U.S.A.

I. INTRODUCTION

Ancient Egyptian hieroglyphics describe the appendix as the "worm of the bowel." Subsequently, it was illustrated by Leonardo da Vinci in 1492 and described by Vesalius in 1543 in his *De Humani Corporis Fabrica*. Named the "appendix vermiformis" by the Flemish anatomist Verheyen in 1710, this organ is the object of the most commonly performed emergency surgical procedures in western countries. More than 260,000 appendectomies were performed in the United States in 1997. Approximately 53% of these procedures are performed for appendicitis and 47% for incidental or prophylactic reasons. The diagnosis of acute appendicitis may be a diagnostic dilemma if the patient is at the extremes of age, is female, or has variant anatomy. Due to these diagnostic challenges, 15–45% of explorations for presumed appendicitis yield negative findings.

Claudius Amyand at St. George's Hospital in London performed the first reported appendectomy in 1735. William West Grant of Davenport, Iowa, performed the first appendectomy in the United States in 1885. The following year Reginald Fitz described the classic signs and symptoms of appendicitis and advocated appendectomy as the preferred treatment. Charles McBurney, whose name is associated with point tenderness located approximately two-thirds the distance from the umbilicus to the anterior superior iliac spine, popularized the surgical cure of this disease with his "muscle-splitting" incision. In the early 1900s the mortality rate from acute appendicitis was approximately 50%. This has declined significantly to 2–3% secondary to advances in perioperative care, surgical skills, and antibiotic therapy.

Laparoscopic appendectomy was first reported in 1977 when De Kok used a scope to remove an appendix through a minilaparotomy site. In 1983 Semm performed the first true nonacute laparoscopic appendectomy incidentally during a gynecological procedure. Schreiber reported the first laparoscopic appendectomy for acute appendicitis in 1987.

Unlike laparoscopic cholecystectomy, widespread acceptance of laparoscopic appendectomy has not occurred. Some of the typical advantages of the laparoscopic approach including small incisions, minimal postoperative discomfort, and early hospital discharge are not as readily apparent when compared to the traditional open approach. Since the traditional appendectomy is usually performed through a relatively small incision, patients usually experience minimal discomfort with short hospital stays. In addition, the open approach does not require the expensive intraoperative equipment necessary to perform a laparoscopic procedure. As these issues are addressed in prospective randomized trials, the future role of laparoscopic appendectomy will be defined.

II. CLINICAL PRESENTATION

Appendicitis presents in a number of ways depending on the location of the appendix. Appendicitis classically presents with periumbilical pain localizing to the right lower quadrant. Anorexia is a hallmark symptom, and most patients experience nausea at some point during their course. Physical examination typically reveals fever in conjunction with a tender abdomen. Pain is most severe overlying McBurney's point. Peritoneal signs are common. Examiners might induce pain in the right lower quadrant when palpating the left lower quadrant (Rovsing's sign), when rotating the hip internally (obturator sign), or when extending the hip (psoas sign). Focal tenderness may be present on rectal examination. The overall course of appendicitis is 24–36 hours from the onset of symptoms to perforation.

Despite the technological advances of the twentieth century, little diagnostic specificity has been added over the past 100 years. A deliberate and thorough history and physical examination remains the best tool to diagnose appendicitis. There has been minimal reduction of the 10–40% negative laparotomy rate. Although the added utility of the laparoscopic appendectomy may be questionable, its diagnostic capabilities may well validate its use in the treatment of appendicitis. In fact, some investigators report a decrease of approximately 75% in the number of negative laparotomies for right lower quadrant pain using laparoscopy. Also, coexisting pathological conditions are identified at virtually any location within the abdominal cavity.

III. OPERATIVE TREATMENT

A. Preoperative Preparation

Preoperative considerations are similar to an open appendectomy. The principal contraindication to laparoscopic appendectomy is multiple previous procedures of the lower abdomen. A relative contraindication is pregnancy in the first and third trimester. Performing a laparoscopic appendectomy during the second trimester is considered safe by most laparoscopists. However, the effects on the fetus of the pneumoperitoneum and hypercarbia as well as the use of intra-abdominal thermal energy sources raise separate and as yet unanswered questions.

B. Operating Room and Patient Setup

The patient is placed in the supine or occasionally the dorsal lithotomy position. The surgeon and camera operator stand on the patient's left side with the first assistant on the patient's right (Fig. 1).

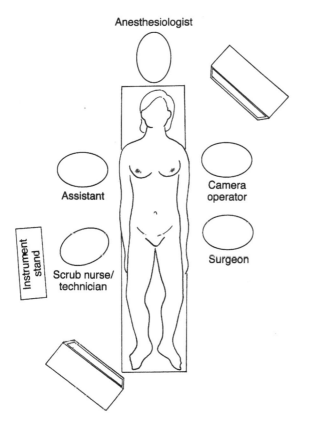

Figure 1   Operating room setup and patient positioning for a laparoscopic appendectomy.

IV.   SURGICAL TECHNIQUE

A.   Port Placement

The number and location of the laparoscopic trocars varies from only two to up to five trocars if necessary. Gotz and Pier from Grevenbroich, Germany, described a two-puncture technique in which an operative laparoscope similar to the one originally produced by Nitze is used. Typically, we use a three-trocar arrangement with a 10/12 mm port at the umbilicus, a 5 mm port in the lower midline, and a 10/12 mm port in the left lower quadrant. The placement of these ports varies somewhat depending on the patient's body habitus and location of the appendix. In order to allow adequate working space, the ports should be placed approximately 15 cm from the appendix. Additional ports can be placed in the right lower quadrant or right upper quadrant if necessary (Fig. 2).

B.   Exposure and Dissection

Following a visual abdominal exploration for concomitant pathology, the patient is placed in a slight Trendelenburg position and is rotated to the left to facilitate exposure. Locating and following the taeniae of the right colon and cecum leads directly to the appendiceal base. A retrocecal appendix may require release of the lateral peritoneal attachments and mobilization of the right colon. When releasing these attachments, the distal ileum,

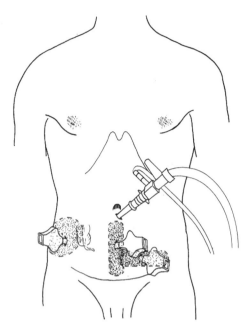

Figure 2 Port placement for a laparoscopic appendectomy.

mesenteric vessels, right ureter, and iliac vessels must be avoided. Atraumatic bowel clamps are preferred over laparoscopic Babcock clamps for grasping and manipulation of the cecum and terminal ileum. The appendix itself may be inspected and manipulated to provide mesoappendiceal traction. Alternatively, if there is significant inflammation and tissue is friable, a pretied Roeder loop may be placed around the tip of the appendix allowing gentle traction (Fig. 3).

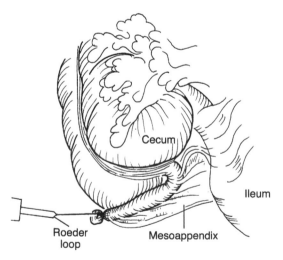

Figure 3 Retraction of the appendix with a Roeder (pretied) loop for mesoappendiceal traction.

With the mesoappendix under tension, the appendiceal artery and its branches are bluntly dissected, ligated, and divided. The remainder of the mesoappendix is likewise ligated and divided. This may be performed with endoscopic clips, bipolar cautery, ultrasonic dissection, or an endoscopic vascular stapling device (Fig. 4). With the appendix freed, two Roeder loops are placed at its base and the appendix is divided (Fig. 5A). Alternatively, the endoscopic GIA stapling device may be employed for amputation of the appendix and closure of the stump in one maneuver (Fig. 5B). The appendix can be

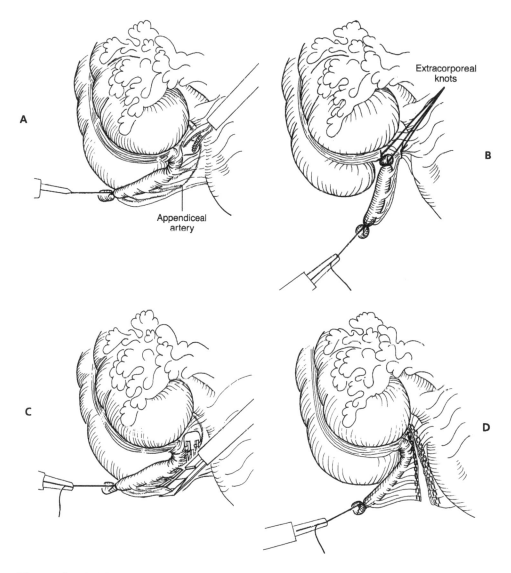

Figure 4   **A,** Dissection of the appendiceal artery. **B,** Ligation of the appendiceal artery and appendiceal base with tension/retraction using a Roeder loop on the appendiceal tip. **C,** Use of hemoclips for division of the mesoappendix and appendiceal artery branches. **D,** Ligation and division of the mesoappendix using a linear stapling device.

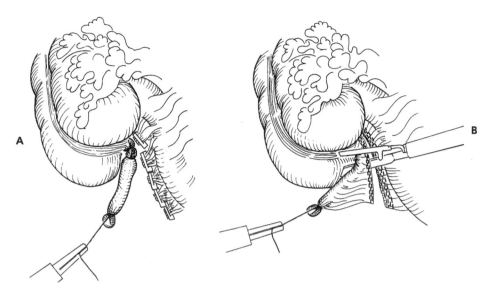

Figure 5 **A,** Placement of Roeder pretied loops for amputation of the appendix. **B,** An alternate method for appendix amputation using a linear stapler.

removed through a 10/12 mm trocar (Fig. 6A), or if it is edematous, enlarged, or friable it can be placed in a specimen retrieval bag (Fig. 6B).

After the appendix is removed, contaminated areas of the abdominal cavity are copiously irrigated and a final survey is completed. The trocars are removed under direct visualization, the pneumoperitoneum released, and the trocar sites closed in the usual

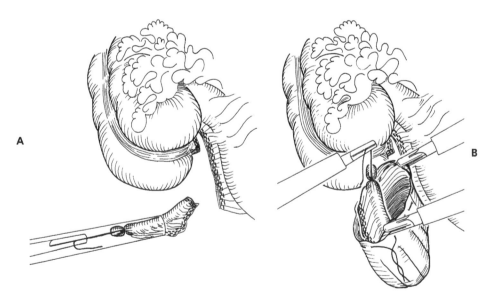

Figure 6 **A,** Removal of the appendix with a Roeder loop through a trocar. **B,** Optional removal of the appendix using a retrieval bag.

manner. Antibiotic coverage is generally employed as in open appendectomy, and as with other laparoscopic procedures, bupivacaine is often infiltrated at the trocar sites at the time of closure.

V. PROSPECTIVE RANDOMIZED TRIALS

Laparoscopic appendectomy was initially reserved for the equivocal case of right lower quadrant pain in which there is an obvious benefit of performing an abdominal exploration for other pathology. However, its indications have extended to include those cases in which the preoperative diagnosis of acute appendicitis is quite clear. Several randomized trials are presented below that specifically address some of the pertinent issues of the laparoscopic approach including complication rates, postoperative hospital stays, return to activity, and cost analysis when compared to the open approach. These studies attempt to delineate the true benefits and proper indications for laparoscopic appendectomy.

In 1994, Frazee et al. from Texas A&M University reported 75 patients randomized to open (37) or laparoscopic (38) appendectomy. In only two of the laparoscopic procedures was intraoperative conversion to an open approach necessary. Pathological confirmation of acute appendicitis was obtained in 80–85% of patients in both groups. The average duration of surgery was 87 minutes for laparoscopic procedures and 65 minutes for open procedures. There were no statistically significant differences in length of hospitalization, resumption of oral intake, or morbidity. Duration of both parenteral and oral analgesics favored laparoscopic appendectomy (2.0 days compared with 1.2 days and 8.0 days compared with 5.4 days; $p < 0.05$). Patients were able to return to full activities in an average of 25 days in the open group compared with 14 days in the laparoscopic group. The authors' conclusion was that laparoscopic appendectomy was the procedure of choice in light of the patients' lower requirements for analgesic agents and earlier return to full activities.

In 1995 Martin et al. from the University of Miami reported 169 patients with the diagnosis of acute appendicitis. Eighty-eight were randomized to traditional open and 81 to laparoscopic appendectomy. The groups were similar demographically. Thirteen (16%) of the attempted laparoscopic patients required conversion to the open procedure. The operative time was significantly longer in the laparoscopic group (102 min vs. 81.7 min; $p < 0.01$). The overall hospital stay was significantly shorter in the laparoscopic group. However, when based on pathological diagnosis there was no significant difference between the open and laparoscopic groups with the exception of perforated appendicitis having a significantly shorter hospital stay. The hospital costs were comparable for the two groups as well. In this series, patients had a similar time to return to activity or work. These authors concluded that laparoscopic appendectomy is comparable to open appendectomy with regards to complications, hospital stay, cost, return to activity, and return to work, and with the greater operative time involved with the laparoscopic technique, it does not provide any benefit over open appendectomy for the routine patient with acute appendicitis.

The role of laparoscopic appendectomy in males was addressed by a prospective randomized trial from Cox et al. from Flinders Medical Center, Australia. These authors randomized 64 men with the diagnosis of acute appendicitis into laparoscopic (33) and open appendectomy (31). Operative times were similar for both groups (51 min open vs. 59 min laparoscopic; $p = 0.13$). Complication rates were similar for both procedures as well. However, postoperative hospital stay was significantly longer for the open vs. the laparoscopic appendectomies (3.8 vs. 2.9 days; $p = 0.045$). In addition, the laparoscopic group had a quicker return to normal activities of 10.4 days as opposed to the open groups 19.7 days ($p = 0.001$). These authors concluded that the laparoscopic appendectomy in men provides significant advantages in terms of a more rapid recovery when compared to open appendectomy.

In 1998, Heikkinen et al. from the University Hospital in Oulu, Finland reported 40 patients who were randomized to open (21) and laparoscopic (19) appendectomies. These authors noted similar operative times of 91 and 82 minutes for the laparoscopic and open approaches, respectively. They reported no significant difference in postoperative pain or fatigue. However, the laparoscopic group had an earlier return to normal life (14 vs. 26.5 days; $p < 0.05$). While the median hospital costs were similar between the laparoscopic and open groups, these authors estimated a significant savings of 25% in the cost of lost work days due to the faster return to normal function in the laparoscopic group. These authors conclude that the slightly higher intraoperative costs for the laparoscopic approach are offset by the faster convalescence, and among employed patients it offers cost savings to society as a result of a faster return to work.

In 2001, Pedersen et al. from Aarhus University Hospital, Denmark, published a prospective randomized trial comparing 301 open appendectomies to 282 laparoscopic appendectomies. Sixty-five of the laparoscopic appendectomies required conversion to an open operation, and their statistical analysis was based on intention to treat. Hospital stays were equally short in both groups with a median of 2 days. However, the median time to return to normal activity (7 vs. 10 days) and work (10 vs. 16 days) was significantly shorter following laparoscopy. Laparoscopy was associated with fewer wound complications ($p < 0.03$) and improved cosmesis ($p < 0.001$). These authors concluded that the decreased wound infection rate, shorter convalescence, and improved diagnostic capability make laparoscopic appendectomy the procedure of choice.

In 2001, Long et al. from Rochester, Minnesota, and the Laparoscopic Appendectomy Interest Group published a prospective randomized trial comparing laparoscopic to open appendectomy. After a prestudy power analysis was performed, this study enrolled 200 patients with the preoperative diagnosis of acute appendicitis, of which 93 were randomized to laparoscopic appendectomy while 105 had an open appendectomy performed. These authors found statistically significant advantages favoring the laparoscopic over the open approach in analgesic requirements, days to tolerance of a general diet, postoperative hospital stay, and return to full activity. Additionally, a cost analysis revealed a significant advantage of the laparoscopic group versus the open group, secondary to earlier hospital discharge, which resulted in at least a $2,000 dollar savings in more than 60% of the cases. In a subgroup analysis comparing the complicated and noncomplicated appendectomies, similar incidences of wound infections, abscesses, technical complications, general postoperative complications, and total complications occurred between the laparoscopic and open approach. However, the small sample size for subgroup analysis prevents establishing firm conclusions for these subgroups. These authors conclude that the clinical and economic benefits favor the laparoscopic approach as the preferred method of appendectomy.

VI. CURRENT STATUS AND FUTURE INVESTIGATION

The consensus from the several prospective randomized studies reviewed here is that removal of the appendix using the laparoscope is as safe as the traditional open procedure.

While operative times are slightly longer, the patients benefit from decreased postoperative analgesic requirements, length of hospitalization, and time to resumption of normal activities. In addition, in some studies an economic benefit of decreased hospital costs as well as a benefit to society with decreased days off work favor the laparoscopic approach. However, because of the skilled laparoscopist's ability to access and view all reaches of the peritoneal space, the true utility of the laparoscope may come not just in the removal of the acutely inflamed appendix, but in excluding other concomitant intra-abdominal pathological conditions. Indeed, young women, obese patients, and those with a history and physical examination that post diagnostic dilemmas clearly seem to benefit from this approach in the management of right lower quadrant pain. The role of laparoscopy in the management of complicated appendicitis remains controversial, and larger prospective randomized trials are necessary to address these issues.

VII. TOP TEN SURGICAL TIPS

1. Diagnosis of acute appendicitis may be difficult.
2. A laparoscopic approach to a patient with right lower quadrant pain allows improved examination of the entire abdomen.
3. A retrocecal appendix requires division of the lateral attachments of the cecum.
4. The taeniae of the cecum lead directly to the base of the appendix.
5. Mesoappendix may be divided using a linear cutting (vascular) stapler, clips, harmonic scalpel, or bipolar coagulation.
6. When appendiceal tip is difficult to mobilize, the appendix can be divided at its base and removed in "retrograde" fashion.
7. If the base of the appendix is severely inflamed, a linear cutting (tissue) stapler may remove a small portion of the cecum in continuity with the appendix.
8. When conversion to an open operation is necessary, laparoscopy guides the appropriate location of the incision.
9. Laparoscopic appendectomy is particularly appropriate in patients who are obese, women of child-bearing age, and patients whose diagnosis is not clear.
10. The appendix should always be removed through an operative trocar or in a bag to avoid contact with the surgical wound. All recesses and dependent regions of the abdominal cavity should be copiously irrigated to avoid postoperative intra-abdominal infection or abscess formation.

SELECTED READINGS

Cox MR, et al. Prospective randomized comparison of open versus laparoscopic appendectomy in men. World J Surg, 1996. 20(3): p. 263–266.

Easter DW. The diagnosis and treatment of acute appendicitis with laparoscopic methods. In Hunter JG, Sackier J, eds. Minimally Invasive Surgery. New York: McGraw-Hill, 1993, pp 171–177.

Frazee RC, et al. A prospective randomized trial comparing open versus laparoscopic appendectomy. Ann Surg, 1994. 219(6): p. 725–731.

Heikkinen TJ, Haukipuro K, Hulkko A. Cost-effective appendectomy. Open or laparoscopic? A prospective randomized study. Surg Endosc, 1998. 12(10): p. 1204–1208.

Long KH, et al. A prospective randomized comparison of laparoscopic appendectomy with open appendectomy: clinical and economic analyses. Surgery, 2001. 129(4): p. 390–400.

Martin LC, et al. Open versus laparoscopic appendectomy. A prospective randomized comparison. Ann Surg, 1995. 222(3): p. 256–262.

Mori T, Bhoyrul S, Way LW. History of laparoscopic surgery. In: Mori T, Bhoyrul S, Way LW, eds. Fundamentals of Laparoscopic Surgery. New York: Churchill Livingstone, 1995, pp 6–7.

Organ BC. Laparoscopic appendectomy. In: Arregui ME, Fitzgibbons RJ Jr, Katkhouda N, McKernan JB, Teich H, eds. Principles of Laparoscopic Surgery: Basic and Advanced Techniques. New York: Springer-Verlag, 1995, pp 268–277.

Pedersen AG, Peterson OB, Wara P, Ronning H, Qvist N, Laurberg S. Randomized clinical trial of laparoscopic versus open appendectomy. Br J Surg, 2001. 88:200–205.

30

Colorectal Surgery

JAMES W. THIELE, JAMES W. FLESHMAN, and DAVID E. BECK

Institute for Minimally Invasive Surgery
Washington University School of Medicine
St. Louis, Missouri, U.S.A.

I. BACKGROUND

Despite the fact that the first laparoscopic colectomy was performed more than 10 years ago, this approach has not become the standard of care for benign or malignant colon disease in the United States. Even though a limited number of surgeons across the country have gained experience with the technique and have adopted its use into their practice, there remains resistance on the part of most general and colorectal surgeons to focus their efforts on learning the skills needed to safely and efficiently perform laparoscopic colon procedures. The technique is not readily assimilated as cholecystectomy or even Nissen fundoplication due to complexity, disease factors, operating times, anatomical variation, and limited technology. However, the ultimate role that laparoscopy will have in the treatment of diseases of the colon and rectum remains a matter of debate. The training of young surgeons and residents to perform complex laparoscopic procedures and a concerted effort by the Program Directors Association for Colorectal Surgery to emphasize laparoscopic training may overcome some of the barriers in the future.

Operations involving resection of all or part of the colon are more technically demanding than other intra-abdominal laparoscopic procedures for a variety of reasons. First, the blood supply to the colon is not an end artery, but rather a rich vascular arcade that must be largely preserved to ensure that the undiseased colon and small bowel remain viable. In addition, mobilization of the colon near vital structures such as the spleen, liver, and duodenum and the task of retrieving a large specimen intact for histological evaluation can pose further problems. Once the resected specimen is removed, the challenge of creating a functional anastomosis, either intracorporeally or extracorporeally, must also be undertaken. To successfully complete each component of the operation, the surgeon must possess advanced laparoscopic skills, including the ability to operate and recognize anatomy from multiple viewpoints.

Colon resections may be performed using exclusively intracorporeal techniques or in a laparoscopically assisted technique in which a portion of the operation is performed extracorporeally through a minilaparotomy. The recent introduction of hand-assisted laparoscopy allows the surgeon to retract or dissect with one hand inside the abdomen, often greatly reducing the time needed to complete the procedure. The limited incision used for the hand assist port can then be used for specimen removal and extracorporeal anastomosis using standard techniques.

II. PATIENT SELECTION AND PREPARATION

A. Indications

The indications for laparoscopic colectomy are essentially the same as for traditional open colectomy and include benign diseases such as polyps, inflammatory bowel disease, diverticular disease, volvulus, and ischemic colitis as well as for malignancy in some cases (Table 1). The standard therapy for colon cancer is open surgical resection, and the use of laparoscopy remains controversial. A more complete discussion of this topic will follow in the outcomes and discussion at the end of this chapter.

As with open techniques, any resection of the colon for malignant disease should include all of the lymphatic vessels, arteries, and veins supplying the segment of bowel involved with cancer. Arteries and veins should be divided at the level of the primary feeding vessel to ensure adequate resection of the cancer. In most cases this will result in a wide mesenteric resection with long proximal and distal margins, thus adding to the bulk of the specimen and possibly making it more difficult to remove through a limited incision. In benign disease processes a wide mesenteric resection is not a necessity and mobilization of the specimen can be accomplished by dividing vessels close to the bowel wall even though it is not always the best method. Laparoscopic colectomy for colonic polyps should follow the same guidelines as for colon cancer. Colotomy with polypectomy is not recommended.

The benign processes for which laparoscopic colectomy is suited encompasses the entire range of colorectal disease. Some scenarios are more easily approached laparoscopically than others, thus patients should be selected on an individual basis.

Table 1   Indications for Laparoscopic Colectomy

Benign diseases	Malignancy
Polyps; familial adenomatous polyposis	Adenocarcinoma of the colon
Localized inflammatory bowel disease	Localized for cure
Volvulus	Metastatic for palliation
Bleeding (AVM, diverticular disease)	Carcinoid tumors
Complications of diverticular disease	Malignancy within a polyp
Localized inflammation	
Stricture	
Fistula	
Bleeding	
Ischemic colitis	
Rectal prolapse	
Constipation	
Colostomy reversal	

Inflammatory disease processes such as Crohn's disease and diverticulitis may make laparoscopic resection very difficult because of adherence to adjacent structures or thickening and hardening of inflamed bowel and its mesentery. The complications of Crohn's disease and diverticulitis including abscess, fistulas, and phlegmon can usually be managed preoperatively to allow a laparoscopic approach. Care should be taken to identify the ureters intraoperatively to avoid ureteral injury during dissection of inflamed or diseased colon at or near the pelvic brim. Ureteral stents are often helpful in this regard as they can be felt through the ureter even with regular laparoscopic instruments. Other disease processes that may be amenable to laparoscopic techniques, such as colonic volvulus, may also be approached through a minilaparotomy, which has been shown to yield similar results.

B. Contraindications

In our opinion, the only absolute contraindication to laparoscopic colectomy is diffuse fecal peritonitis secondary to colonic perforation as it is impossible to adequately explore, drain, and debride the abdomen in a timely manner through laparoscopic means. All other contraindications are relative, including previous surgery, extensive neoplastic process, morbid obesity, and inflammatory bowel disease. The frequency with which it is necessary to convert to an open colectomy is dependent on surgeon skill and expertise as well as the limits established by each condition individually.

C. Diagnostic Tests and Preoperative Counseling

The limitation of laparoscopic surgery to the visual and tactical senses makes accurate preoperative identification of colonic lesions such as polyps or malignant tumors very important. In addition to standard preoperative labs, as well as medical and cardiac clearance, patients should also receive either a colonoscopic or radiographic examination to determine the site of the lesion. During colonoscopy, biopsy specimens should be obtained for microscopic evaluation and confirmation of the diagnosis. In addition, the site can be tattooed by injection into the mucosa of 0.1 cc of sterile India ink or other commercially available agents, which stain the bowel wall permanently and will be visible at the time of laparoscopy. A plain radiograph of the abdomen can also be obtained with the colonoscope pointing at the site of the lesion. Any of these maneuvers can help the surgeon locate the lesion in question during the procedure. Some surgeons, however, prefer to perform intraoperative colonoscopy to ensure precise localization.

If the lesion in question is indeed colon cancer, liver function tests and a carcinoembryonic antigen level should be obtained in addition to the standard preoperative labs. Although the liver cannot be palpated during a laparoscopic colon resection, intraoperative ultrasound can greatly enhance the surgeon's ability to evaluate the liver during the procedure. This is very operator dependent and requires cooperation of the laparoscopic surgeon and radiologist and carries a fairly steep learning curve. Alternatively, preoperative computed tomography (CT) scans of the abdomen and pelvis are routinely obtained in all colon cancer patients to evaluate the liver and provide a baseline for long-term follow-up. In patients with Crohn's disease, it is helpful to fully evaluate the small bowel preoperatively using a small bowel follow-through contrast study. This will prevent the revelation of multisegmental disease in the operative setting.

Patients who can successfully complete a mechanical bowel preparation as outpatients are generally admitted on the day of surgery. If there is any question as to the ability of the patient to comply with a complete bowel preparation or if the patient does not tolerate the preparation at home, in-hospital bowel preparation may be prudent. Prior to the procedure, the benefits and risks of a laparoscopic colon resection should be discussed with the patient and informed consent should be obtained. All patients should be counseled that if at any point a laparoscopic approach cannot be continued safely, the operation will be converted to a traditional open procedure. Conversion should not be considered a failure. The surgeon's learning curve for this technically difficult approach is between 20 and 50 cases. Even so, a 20% conversion rate to an open approach is a reasonable level for any practice. Patient selection will eventually be the major factor influencing the conversion rate as the surgeon becomes more comfortable with laparoscopic techniques.

D. Operating Room Set-Up

Proper positioning of the patient is crucial to the success of laparoscopic colon surgery. The patient will be placed at extreme angles during the procedure to allow gravity to aid in retraction of the colon. In addition, the surgeon and the assistant will need to have access to the patient from both sides as well as from between the patient's legs; thus, the patient should be placed in modified lithotomy position with the buttocks near the lower edge of the operating table, and both arms should be tucked. All bony prominences should be carefully padded to avoid nerve or pressure injuries. A beanbag mattress is helpful in securing the patient to the operating table and allows one to tilt the table laterally and in steep Trendelenburg and Fowler's position without the patient slipping. The beanbag should be attached directly to the table-top without the cushions using a Velcro strip. Compression stockings should be placed on the patient's lower extremities prior to positioning and used during the case for deep venous thrombosis prophylaxis. After the induction of anesthesia, the stomach is decompressed with an orogastric tube and the bladder is emptied by placement of an indwelling urinary catheter. Prophylactic antibiotics should be administered intravenously at some point prior to any skin incisions being made. If a transanal-stapled anastomosis is planned, the rectal lumen should be irrigated thoroughly prior to preparation and draping. The abdomen is prepared and draped for both a laparoscopic and a conventional open laparotomy.

For most cases, the surgeon and the camera holder stand on the side opposite the involved segment of colon (Fig. 1). The assistant will stand opposite the surgeon or between the patient's legs. At least two video monitors will be required: one opposite the surgeon and one opposite the assistant. The monitors will be moved between the head and the foot during the case, depending on the site of the operation. Specific necessary and optional equipment is listed in Table 2. Ureteral stents may be placed in cases of severe inflammation or mass lesions to assist in identification of the ureters intraoperatively, and while they may not prevent injury of these structures, they reduce operative time and aid in the identification and direct repair of injuries. Our indications for placement of stents apply to both open and laparoscopic cases: (1) an acute inflammatory process resulting from Crohn's disease or diverticulitis that may involve the ureter in the retroperitoneum, (2) hydroureter, (3) colovesical fistula, and (4) a large pelvic mass with the potential for involving the ureter.

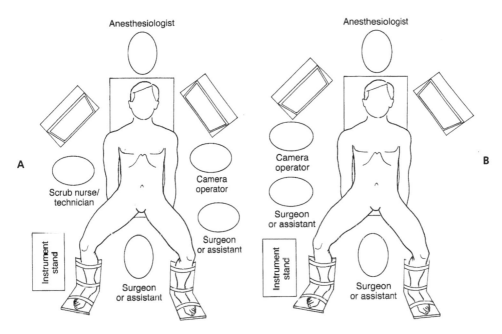

Figure 1 **A,** Operating room setup for right colectomy. **B,** Operating room setup for left colectomy, low anterior resection, and abdominal perineal resection.

III. PROCEDURES

A. Right Hemicolectomy—Surgical Technique

1. Port Placement

Access to the abdominal cavity is achieved by either a closed or an open technique at the umbilicus. After pneumoperitoneum is established, a 10/12 mm trocar is placed at the

Table 2 Equipment for Laparoscopic Colectomy

Necessary
    0 or 30-degree laparoscope (or flexible laparoscope is available)
    Atraumatic forceps for handling the bowel
    Curved dissectors
    Curved scissors (attached to monopolar cautery)
    Laparoscopic linear staplers with vascular staples
    Standard bowel stapler
    EEA stapler (for left colectomy or LAR)
    Endoscopic clip applier
    Entrapment sack or wound protector

Optional
    Hand assist port
    Endoscopic needle holder, knot pusher, and suture material
    Pretied endoscopic loop ligature devices
    Harmonic scalpel

umbilicus and a flexible or zero degree laparoscope is introduced into the peritoneal cavity. Careful inspection of the abdomen is then undertaken to ensure that there is no evidence of needle or trocar injuries, metastatic disease, or other pathology. Three additional trocars are then placed as needed under direct laparoscopic visualization in an anchor-shaped configuration: suprapubic and in the left and right lower quadrants at the level of the umbilicus in the anterior axillary line (Fig. 2). The procedure can usually be completed with only umbilical, suprapubic, and left lower quadrant trocar sites. This configuration provides the surgeon access to all quadrants of the abdomen without interference. The placement of an additional port in the right upper quadrant may be necessary if mobilization of the hepatic flexure is difficult. Position of additional ports will be dictated by the anatomy of the patient and where they will be best suited to aid in dissection. The size of the trocar is dependent on the surgeon's preference and the use of 10 mm stapling, grasping, and retrieving instruments. The suprapubic site is most useful as a 10/12 mm trocar.

2. Exposure

The small bowel is examined from the ligament of Treitz to the ileocecal valve by sequential grasping of the bowel with atraumatic bowel clamps. Placement of the patient in steep reverse Trendelenburg position will then allow the liver to drop away from the diaphragm, which allows for better inspection of both hepatic lobes for possible metastatic disease. Laparoscopic ultrasound should be used for further evaluation of any questionable lesions noted on visual inspection of the liver. A trucut needle biopsy is possible through the abdominal wall even in the presence of pneumoperitoneum and should be performed as clinically indicated. The patient is then placed in extreme Trendelenburg position and

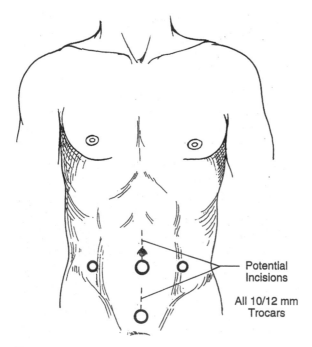

Figure 2   Anchor-shaped trocar placement with potential incision sites shown.

tilted as far to the left as possible for the initial portion of the procedure. The viscera can then be swept caudad and to the patient's left side and gravity will maintain its position.

3. Dissection

Safe dissection of the right colon requires a thorough understanding of the anatomical relationships between the right ureter, second and third portions of the duodenum, ascending colon, pancreas, and right kidney. A medial posterior approach to mobilization of the right colon is best approached by starting at the cecum, as it is mobile and easily identified in the right lower quadrant. After the patient is placed in Trendelenburg position, atraumatic grasping forceps via the suprapubic site are used to retract the terminal ileum and ascending colon in a cephalad and anteromedial direction. The junction of the visceral and parietal peritoneum is then incised using the cautery scissors through the left lower quadrant port site over the iliac vessels under the cecum (Fig. 3). After incising the peritoneum, the right colon and cecum are mobilized in this avascular plane using a sweeping motion with either the back of the endoscissors or a blunt dissecting instrument.

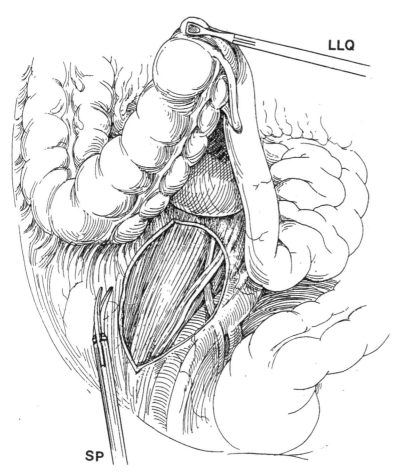

Figure 3 The cecum is retracted cephalad and the junction of the visceral and parietal peritoneum is incised.

The medial point of this triangular avascular plane leads to the third portion of the duodenum to the left of the superior mesenteric artery. Further lateral and cephalad dissection leads to the liver and avoids dissection of the ureter and vascular structures. Sharp dissection or electrocautery is not necessary in this plane. Mobilization of the colon from a posterior approach should continue until the second portion of the duodenum is identified. The duodenum should be gently swept down and dissection continued over the top of the duodenum. Attachments of the duodenum to the mesentery of the right colon may require incision or cautery at this point of the procedure.

After medial and posterior mobilization is carried over and beyond the duodenum in a cephalad direction over the right kidney, the cecum is retracted anteromedially to place the lateral peritoneal attachments (the white line of Toldt) of the ascending colon under tension. The peritoneum is divided starting over the iliac fossa with the cautery using a traction/countertraction technique (Fig. 4). When the lower pole of the kidney is reached,

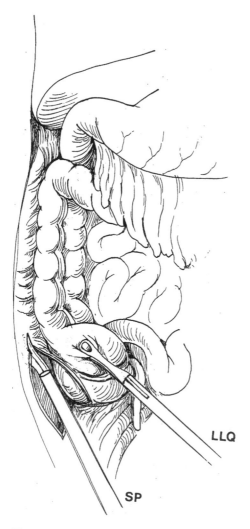

LLQ

SP

Figure 4   Division of the lateral peritoneal attachments.

the patient should be placed in extreme reverse Trendelenburg position. If the hepatic flexure ligaments are not readily visible at this point, the use of a 30° angled laparoscope positioned in an overhead, angled-down view may be helpful. The laparoscope can also be periodically moved to the right lower quadrant position to permit better visualization of the right gutter and the paraduodenal area looking toward the midline. The hepatic flexure is retracted inferiorly and medially toward the umbilicus, and the well-vascularized peritoneal attachments of the hepatic flexure are divided using cautery, harmonic scalpel, or surgical clips if cautery is ineffective in controlling bleeding (Fig. 5). This can be accomplished from a medial approach with the energy source in the left lower quadrant or a lateral approach, as shown in Figure 5. The lateral approach requires that a 5 mm trocar be placed in the right lower quadrant anterior axillary line at the level of the umbilicus.

Colonic mobilization is facilitated by detachment of the omentum from the proximal transverse colon, taking care to avoid the omental vessels by staying in the fusion plane (Fig. 6). Mobilization of the omentum off of the colon from the midtransverse colon toward the hepatic flexure is an alternative approach. The colon is pulled downward until the duodenum is exposed. It is necessary to completely free the hepatic flexure from the undersurface of the liver and the duodenum. Again, the surgeon uses blunt and sharp dissection to push the duodenum away from the adjacent colonic mesentery.

The next step is to identify and divide the blood supply to the right colon. The ileocolic artery can be identified by first returning the right colon to its normal anatomical position. The ileocolic vascular pedicle is grasped close to the right colon and the mobilized colon is suspended anteriorly toward the abdominal wall. As the mesentery is tented up, clear areas (now appear dark purple) on either side of the ridge of the ileocolic

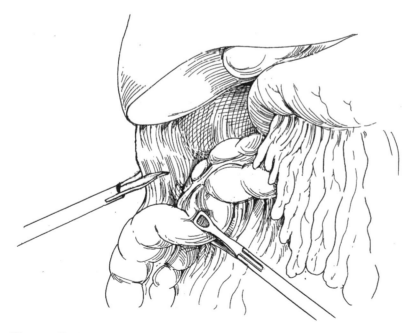

Figure 5 Division of the hepatic flexure attachments. The colon is retracted caudad through the LLQ port site while the attachments are divided via an instrument introduced through the suprapubic port.

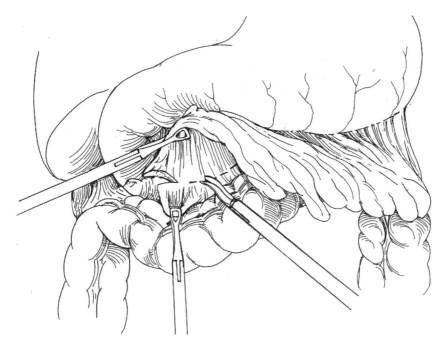

Figure 6   Detachment of the proximal transverse colon from the omentum.

vessels can be identified between the terminal ileal vessels of the superior mesenteric artery (SMA) and the ileocolic artery and between the ileocolic artery and the right colic vessels (Fig. 7). Each of these windows is opened and the vessels ligated and divided near their origin using staples that yield 0.75 mm height closure, multiple clips, ligature, or suture. The process is then repeated to divide right branch of the middle colic artery (Fig. 8). The LigaSure™ system uses low voltage and high current to liquefy and reform vascular walls resulting in fusion of the lumen and creation of a permanently welded structure, in contrast to traditional bipolar electrocautery, which desiccates tissue, causing a coagulum to form. This device can be used to seal vessels up to 7 mm without the need for clips or staples. Although more expensive than any individual endoscopic clip applier or stapling device, if multiple large vessels are going to be divided during the procedure, this device actually saves time and has been shown to be as effective as other methods of vascular control.

4.   Resection and Anastomosis

Following mobilization and division of the mesenteric vessels, the right colon should be easily mobilized to the anterior abdominal wall since it is a midline structure. The involved segment of colon can be resected either extracorporeally (laparoscopically assisted colectomy) or intracorporeally. In an extracorporeal resection, the mobilized right colon and terminal ileum are eviscerated through a small (4–6 cm) incision that is extended from the umbilical trocar port site incision. We prefer the vertical midline incision as it allows visualization of the SMA origin, including the middle colic and ileocolic arteries. This aids in completion of the dissection and allows vascular ligation, if necessary. Placement of a plastic drape or other impervious material around the wound protects the

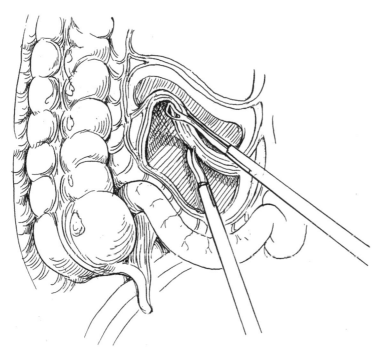

Figure 7 Dissection and isolation of the ileocolic artery.

abdominal wall and subcutaneous tissues during delivery of the specimen. The proximal and distal margins are then divided as in an open technique and a side-to-side functional end-to-end anastomosis is accomplished using conventional hand-sewn or stapled techniques (Fig. 9). After anastomosis, the resulting mesenteric defect can be approximated through the umbilical incision because the incision is positioned over the origin of the superior mesenteric artery. The bowel is then returned to the peritoneal cavity and the fascial opening is closed along with any other trocar sites.

Intracorporeal resection requires a laparoscopic 35 mm linear cutter/stapler to divide the ileum and distal margin of the bowel (Fig. 10). The specimen can then be placed in a sterile, impervious retrieval sack and removed through a small fascial incision. The mesentery is carefully inspected for bleeding after reinsufflation and preparation for the anastomosis is undertaken. Division of additional retroperitoneal attachments of the ileal mesentery may be required to ensure that a tension-free anastomosis can be constructed.

A functional end-to-end anastomosis is constructed using a 35 mm laparoscopic lineal cutter/stapler. To facilitate this, the laparoscope can be moved to the suprapubic port and the right abdominal trocar. One additional port is generally needed in the left upper quadrant to aid in alignment of the bowel, which is crucial for success of the anastomosis. First, each limb of the bowel is controlled with a grasper and a small enterotomy is created in each limb using the electrocautery scissors. Next, one limb of the stapling device is inserted into each of the enterotomies and fired (Fig. 11). If a 35 mm device is used, two or three firings will be required. The anastomosis is then inspected for bleeding and integrity, after which the stapling device and the laparoscope are switched for closure of the enterotomies (Fig. 12). Again, the staple lines

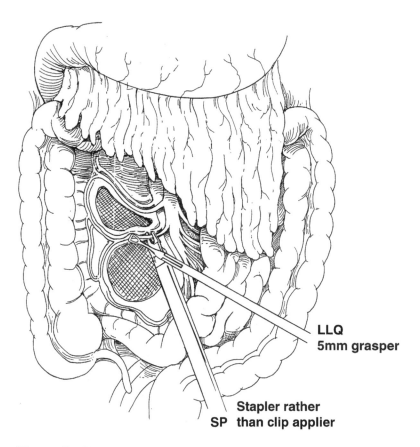

Figure 8 Division of the ileocolic artery. The right branch of the middle colic artery is divided in a similar manner.

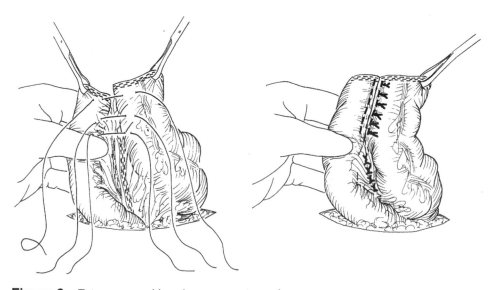

Figure 9 Extracorporeal hand-sewn anastomosis.

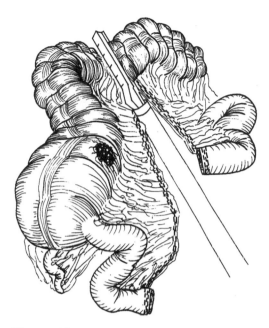

Figure 10   Endoscopic transection of the transverse colon using a linear stapler.

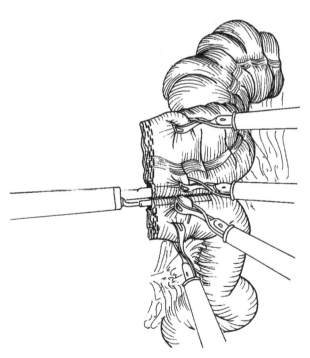

Figure 11   After alignment of bowel, endoscopic stapler is inserted into the enterotomies and then fired.

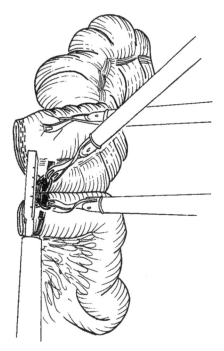

Figure 12   Closure of the enterotomies with the linear stapler.

are inspected after each firing. The mesenteric defect is generally left open after an intracorporeal resection and anastomosis but can be closed with intracorporeal suturing techniques. It is important to ensure that there is no twist in the small bowel before and after the anastomosis. This can be accomplished by following the cut edge of the mesentery all the way from the terminal ileum staple line to the transverse colon staple line. The abdomen is carefully examined for bleeding or signs of mesenteric torsion, after which the fascial defects are closed as mentioned above.

   We prefer an extracorporeal approach to resection and anastomosis of the specimen for several reasons. First, due to the fact that the specimen must be delivered from the abdomen in both approaches, the fascial incision length is nearly the same. Thus, the possible benefit of a smaller incision with the intracorporeal approach is lost. In addition the extracorporeal approach is faster and technically easier, saving valuable time in the operating room, and the mesenteric defect can be closed quickly and easily.

B.   Sigmoid and Left Hemicolectomy—Surgical Technique

1.   Port Placement/Placement of Hand-Assist Devices

A 30° or flexible laparoscope is required for a left-sided colectomy. Trocars are inserted in an anchor-shaped pattern after placement of a 10/12 mm trocar in the periumbilical region as previously described. A variety of hand-assist ports are available that provide the advantage of allowing the surgeon to use his or her hand for retraction, dissection, and palpation. Hand-assist posts also provide the surgeon with a small (7 cm) incision through which the specimen can be extracted, dissection can be completed, and a stapled end-to-end anastomosis in the pelvis can be carried out quickly and efficiently. Most of the newer devices also have the added advantage of allowing placement of a 10/12 trocar through the device itself during the initial stages of the procedure before the surgeon will need to place a hand through the port to assist with splenic flexure mobilization. In addition, the skin incision required for placement of the hand-assist port can be oriented either vertically or transversely, the latter of which provides for a better cosmetic result as it can be hidden below a bikini line. The use of a hand-assist device requires placing the trocar that will hold the laparoscope several centimeters cephalad to the umbilicus in the midline. This allows the laparoscope to move freely without interfering with the hand of the intra-abdominal portion of the hand-assist device. Since hand-assist colectomy is only useful in resection of the left colon, sigmoid colon, and rectum, the suprapubic site is most advantageous as it provides access to the pelvis and the left paracolic gutter and acts as an extraction site. Targarona et al. recently published a prospective study designed to evaluate hand-assisted laparoscopic surgery (HALS) with respect to perioperative features, patient clinical response, effect on the inflammatory response, and oncological issues. They found that HALS was associated with a far lower conversion rate (7% vs. 23%) and immediate clinical outcomes, oncological features, and costs that were similar to standard laparoscopic surgery. Although they did note a significantly greater increase in IL-6 and C-reactive protein with HALS as compared to traditional laparoscopic techniques, they concluded that the benefit of lower conversion rate and simplification of difficult situations was obtained while still preserving the features of a minimally invasive approach.

2. Exposure

Positioning, exposure, and exploration of the abdominal cavity are similar to that described for a right hemicolectomy, except that the patient is tilted to the right and the viscera are subsequently swept to that side.

3. Dissection

Starting with the patient in steep Trendelenburg position and tilted to the right, the sigmoid colon is identified and retracted medially and cephalad by the assistant using an atraumatic clamp. The lateral and pelvic peritoneal attachments of the sigmoid colon are sharply incised with the curved cautery scissors (Fig. 13), after which the sigmoid and descending colon are mobilized along the white line of Toldt. As the colon is mobilized cephalad, the left ureter should be identified as it crosses the left iliac artery. If a ureteral stent was placed preoperatively, it can be palpated with an atraumatic clamp, or, if a hand-assist port is being used, the surgeon can place a hand in the abdomen and locate the ureter. After the left colon has been mobilized as far as possible from the lateral approach, the patient is placed in reverse Trendelenburg position and the splenic flexure and transverse colon are retracted caudally. It is at this point that, if a hand-assist port is in place, the surgeon will move between the patient's legs. The left hand is placed into the abdomen to aid in exposure and caudal retraction of the colon while the right hand is used to dissect with the cautery scissors through the left lateral port. In the event that a hand port is not used, the surgeon or the assistant will retract through the right lateral port using an atraumatic instrument. Dissection is carried out through the left lateral port by the surgeon from the same position between the patient's legs. The splenic flexure is then released from the lateral attachments and the lesser sac is entered from the left lateral side (Fig. 14). The gastrocolic omentum is then dissected free from the transverse colon in the avascular plane

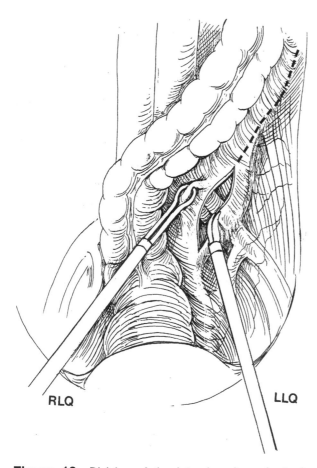

Figure 13 Division of the lateral peritoneal attachments of the sigmoid colon. The peritoneum is incised cephalad to facilitate mobilization of the left colon.

using the cautery scissors as described previously for a right hemicolectomy. The peritoneal attachments in the left upper quadrant that suspend the splenic flexure contain several arterial and venous branches from the hilum and inferior pole of the spleen. These vessels should be meticulously controlled using any of the techniques mentioned earlier (endoclips, staples, harmonic scalpel, or the LigaSure device). Although visualization during splenic flexure mobilization is often better during a laparoscopic case than in a traditional open procedure, tactile sensation is largely lost. Excessive downward traction on the colon can be a result of poor tactile sensation and may lead to splenic capsular injury. The fact that endoscopic instruments lack the tactile sensation that helps to prevent such injuries argues in favor of using a hand-assist approach in any case that will require splenic flexure mobilization.

After the sigmoid colon, left colon, and splenic flexure have been freed of their retroperitoneal attachments, attention is directed toward division of the arterial supply and venous drainage. The patient is returned to Trendelenburg position, and the sigmoid colon is grasped and suspended anteriorly. The peritoneum overlying the base of the mesocolon is then scored with the curved cautery scissors along the right side, anterior to the aorta

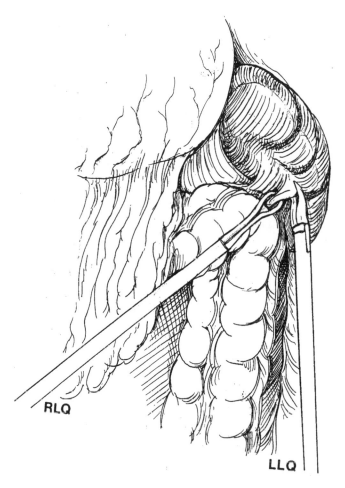

RLQ

LLQ

Figure 14 Division of the lateral attachments of the splenic flexure. After the flexure is mobilized, dissection is continued medially and the lesser sac is entered from a lateral approach.

from the pelvic brim cephalad. The left colon is then suspended from an atraumatic clamp placed behind the superior hemorrhoidal artery through the left lower quadrant port. The inferior mesenteric artery (IMA) is then identified and mobilized using blunt dissection techniques along the anterior aorta, after which it is divided either at the aorta or near the root of the mesentery, depending on the indications for resection (Fig. 15). Care should be taken to check the position of the left ureter prior to division of the mesentery to ensure that it is not inadvertently injured. The inferior mesenteric vein (IMV) is found cephalad from the IMA as it enters the splenic vein under the tail of the pancreas. The vein can be easily identified adjacent to the duodenum at the ligament of Treitz tethering the mesentery when the mobilized splenic flexure and left colon are retracted anteriorly toward the abdominal wall. The IMV is divided 2–3 cm from the inferior border of the pancreas. The base of the mesentery of the distal transverse colon may require further dissection if more splenic flexure mobility is needed. There will generally be a vessel in

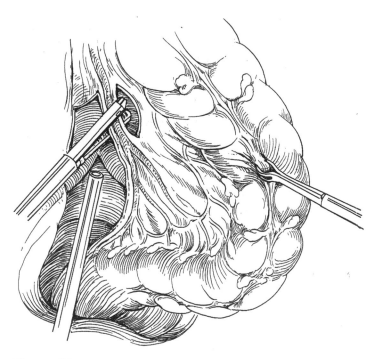

Figure 15   Division of the inferior mesenteric artery.

this otherwise thin mesentery, which will require management. The level of the planned proximal resection can be prepared by dividing the mesentery at right angles to the colon with cautery and clips to control the marginal vessel up to the colon wall. The proximal left and transverse colon are then grasped and brought to the pelvis to ensure that there is sufficient mobilization to allow for a tension-free anastomosis. Division of the left branch of the middle colic artery and further mobilization of the colon to the hepatic flexure are maneuvers that can be used to gain sufficient length.

The mesorectum and its vessels are controlled using harmonic scalpel, LigaSure, or staples at the level of the planned distal resection, which is generally at or just below the level of the sacral promontory. At this level the superior hemorrhoidal artery and vein still run together and can be divided as a single unit. In the case of a patient with diverticulitis the distal staple line must be on soft, pliable, tenia-free rectum regardless of the position relative to the sacral promontory.

4.   Resection and Anastomosis

Although the resection and anastomosis can be performed intracorporeally as described previously for a right hemicolectomy, we recommend the use of a stapled or hand-sewn extracorporeal end-to-end anastomosis after either an intracorporeal or extracorporeal transection of the colon. A double-stapled technique using a circular stapler has proven to be both quick and technically easier than other methods and has become our method of choice for an anastomosis at or near the sacral promontory. After the specimen is delivered, either through a previously placed hand port incision or through a separate incision extended from one of the port sites (usually the midline suprapubic), transection of the bowel is completed using a linear cutter/stapler. The proximal limb is then opened and the anvil of the circular stapler is inserted after a purse string stitch is placed. Once the purse string is secured around the post of the anvil, the proximal end of the colon is returned to the abdomen and the circular stapler is inserted into the anus and advanced carefully until it is snug against the staple line in the distal rectal stump. Through the suprapubic extraction incision the anvil is reinserted into the stapler to create a stapled end-to-end anastomosis. The bowel is carefully inspected prior to firing the stapler to ensure that the bowel has not been twisted during exteriorization or during the anastomosis. The completed staple line should be tested by occluding the bowel proximal to the anastomosis and submerging the staple line in saline while insufflating air into the rectum through the anus with a proctoscope. If an air leak is noted during insufflation, simple sutures should be placed to reinforce the staple line at areas of leakage. The ureters should be inspected carefully prior to closure of the minilaparotomy incision and port sites.

C. Low Anterior Resection—Surgical Technique

1. Port Placement/Placement of Hand-Assist Devices

Port placement and placement of hand-assist ports is carried out exactly as described for a left hemicolectomy. As mentioned in the previous section, the incision used for placement of a hand-assist port provides the surgeon with a site for specimen extraction. The hand-assist device incision site also gives the surgeon the option of completing the pelvic dissection in an open fashion.

2. Exposure and Dissection

Exposure and dissection of the left colon and sigmoid colon are identical to those described for a left colectomy. Rectal dissection should begin posteriorly in the avascular plane between the fascia propria of the rectum and the presacral fascia and be continued as far distally as possible (Fig. 16). During posterior dissection the sigmoid and rectum should be suspended over a 5 mm grasper or articulating retractor placed through the left lower port and retracted anteriorly toward the abdominal wall. This will allow the avascular dissection plane to open up and make it easier to identify and dissect with the cautery scissors. The avascular, areolar tissue plane is followed all the way to the pelvic floor around the entire enveloping fascia propria of the mesorectum (Fig. 17). The cautery scissors or harmonic scalpel is placed through the right lower quadrant port or suprapubic port if there is no hand access port present. The pelvic nerves and presacral veins are covered and protected by a presacral fascia, which is untouched during an appropriate dissection.

Dissection continues by scoring the peritoneal leaves on each side of the rectum down to the anterior peritoneal reflection. The surgeon directs the cautery scissors placed through the right lower quadrant or suprapubic port while a second atraumatic clamp is placed through one of the lateral ports and used to aid in retraction and exposure. Retraction by the opposite wall atraumatic clamp provides tension on the lateral ligaments as they are divided with controlled cautery. Division of the posteriorly positioned Waldeyer's fascia reflection in a transverse line allows final mobilization of the rectum all the way to the pelvic floor. Pushing the rectum posteriorly with a closed atraumatic clamp facilitates dissection of the rectovaginal or rectoprostatic septum as another grasper pushes anteriorly to expose the areolar tissue plane. The anterior lateral vascular pedicles

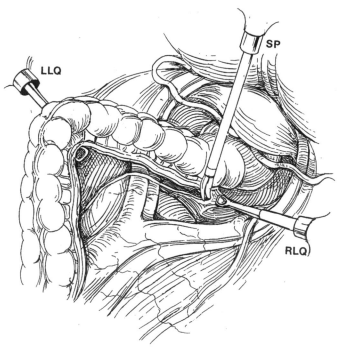

Figure 16 Posterior dissection of the rectum begins at the pelvic brim. The rectum is suspended from a grasper introduced through the LLQ port site. This aids in identification of the avascular plane posterior to the rectum.

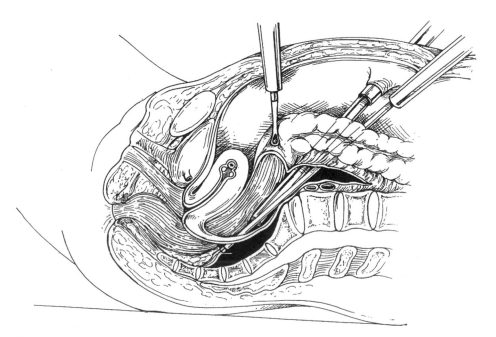

Figure 17 Dissection in the avascular plane should be carried as far as possible posteriorly.

containing the middle hemorrhoidal vessels can be divided either with cautery or harmonic scalpel (preferred).

A true low anterior resection removes all of the mesorectum and allows transection of the rectum at the top of the anal canal (3 cm proximal to the dentate line). At this level the rectum can easily be divided using a 30 mm stapling device placed either laparoscopically or through the suprapubic midline incision described for a left colectomy. If a hand port was previously placed, it can be removed at this point to allow open stapling and specimen extraction.

3. Resection and Anastomosis

After the lesion is resected in a laparoscopically assisted manner as described above, a conventional circular intestinal stapler is introduced through the anus. The proximal limb of the colon is delivered through the small fascial incision and the anvil of the stapling device is secured in the transected end with a purse-string suture. The anvil of the stapler is then seated securely into the stapling device (Fig. 18). Prior to firing the stapler, the proximal segment and its mesentery should be inspected to ensure that there has been no twisting during manipulation that could result in compromise of the blood supply. The anastomosis is inspected by submerging the colon under saline and gently insufflating air through the anus. All ports are removed, and the fascia is closed in the standard fashion.

D. Abdominoperineal Resection—Surgical Technique

1. Exposure, Port Placement, and Positioning

The patient positioning and equipment are set up exactly the same as for a low anterior resection and a left colectomy. A 30° or flexible laparoscope is required. Placement of the

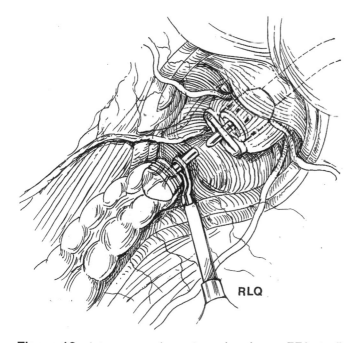

Figure 18 Intracorporeal anastomosis using an EEA stapling device.

trocars for an abdominoperineal resection is similar to that described previously for a left colectomy. The only variation on the standard anchor configuration is that the left lateral port site should be positioned at the desired colostomy site, usually in the left rectus muscle. A hand-assist port can be used, although the advantage of being able to use this incision for specimen extraction and anastomosis is lost. Since the specimen can be delivered through the perineal wound and no anastomosis needs to be performed, we prefer to attempt complete laparoscopic resection and avoid any incisions on the abdomen except for port sites and the colostomy site.

2. Dissection and Resection

The sigmoid colon, descending colon, and splenic flexure are mobilized as described for a left hemicolectomy. The rectal dissection is then approached as described above for a low anterior resection. After complete mobilization and division of the blood supply to the left colon and rectum, attention is directed toward proximal transection of the colon. The proposed site for proximal division of the colon is identified and grasped with an atraumatic clamp placed through the right lateral port. The colon is then brought to the left lateral port site to ensure that it will reach to the stoma site without tension. At this point, the colon can then be divided, either intracorporeally with a laparoscopic linear stapler (Fig. 19) or extracorporeally with a standard linear stapler. The distal limb is dropped back into the abdomen and the proximal end is brought out through the enlarged left lateral port site and matured as an end colostomy (Fig. 20).

The perineal dissection can be performed simultaneously with division of the colon and maturing of the stoma if the surgeon has a second team and wishes to perform the dissection with the patient in the lithotomy position. Another approach is to complete the stoma and close all of the port sites, after which the patient can be flipped into a prone jackknife position and the perineal dissection completed from that approach. The sigmoid and rectum, now completely mobilized from above and freed circumferentially from the levator muscles below, can be delivered through the perineal wound. Large suction drains can be placed from below lateral to the perineal wound, or from above through one of the port sites. The perineal wound is then closed in layers in the standard fashion.

E. Total Abdominal Colectomy and Total Proctocolectomy—Technique

Combining the techniques described above, the entire colon and rectum can be resected laparoscopically. The procedure begins with trocar placement and patient positioning as described for a right hemicolectomy. The umbilical trocar should be placed above the umbilicus if the placement of a hand-assist device is planned for dissection of the left colon. Once the right colon has been mobilized and the blood supply divided up to the middle colic artery, attention is directed toward dissection of the sigmoid and left colon. The sigmoid colon is first freed laparoscopically, after which a hand-assist device can be placed through a low midline incision extended from the suprapubic port site. The left colon is then dissected cephalad, around the splenic flexure as described previously. The dissection and division of the blood supply should continue up to the middle colic artery. The entire specimen is now tethered by the middle colic blood supply, which is left intact until any pelvic dissection that is deemed necessary is completed laparoscopically. The middle colic blood supply is then divided using the hand as a guide for the laparoscopic stapler placed through the right upper quadrant port. The fingers and thumb encircle the middle colic vessels, keeping the SMA and small bowel posterior to prevent inadvertent

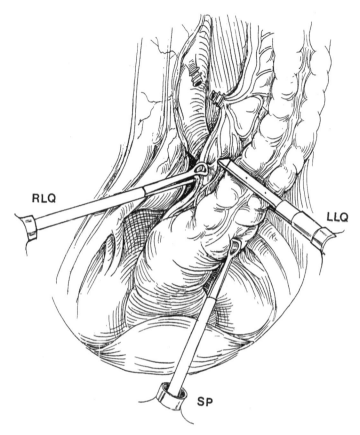

Figure 19 Intracorporeal division of the proximal sigmoid colon after completion of the rectal dissection.

stapling of the SMA. The entire specimen is delivered through the hand-assist device incision site or through an incision extended from the suprapubic trocar site incision if the entire dissection was completed without the aid of a hand-assist device. Anastomosis and, if necessary, completion of a pouch is carried out in a standard fashion through the limited (5–7 cm) lower midline incision.

F. Other Procedures—Technique and Discussion

A variety of other colon and rectal procedures can be performed laparoscopically using a combination of the techniques described above for various colonic resections. If a pneumoperitoneum can be safely established and the abdomen is relatively free of adhesions, it is possible to attempt almost any colon or rectal procedure from a laparoscopic approach.

1. Diverting Colostomy

A diverting colostomy may be performed for a variety of reasons including protection of a perineal wound and distal obstruction. Trocar placement and technique is similar to that described for a left colectomy. The sigmoid colon, left colon, and splenic flexure need to

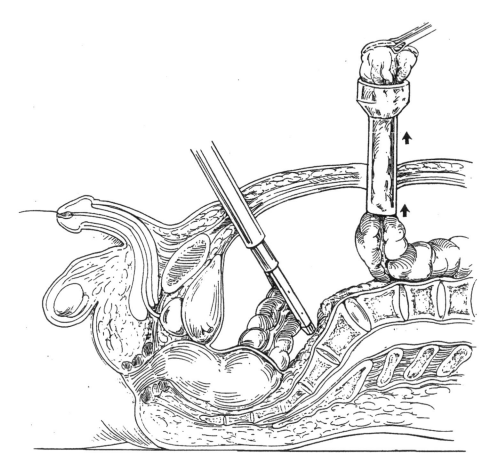

Figure 20   Delivery of the distal left colon through the LLQ port site for maturation as an end colostomy.

be mobilized to ensure that there will be enough length to easily reach to the abdominal wall, usually the left lower quadrant. As mentioned previously, when a stoma is planned, the lateral port on that side should be placed at the planned colostomy site. After mobilization, the vessels are left intact and the colon is grasped using an atraumatic clamp placed through the trocar located in the proposed colostomy site. The colon loop is then delivered through a slightly enlarged trocar site incision (to allow two fingers to pass through both fascia and skin) and divided with a linear cutter/stapler. The proximal colon is then matured as an end stoma while the distal limb is returned to the abdomen. If reestablishment of intestinal continuity is planned, the distal end may be tacked to the abdominal wall near the stoma site to aid in locating it at the time of takedown of the stoma.

2. Colostomy Takedown

An end descending colostomy is usually the result of a Hartmann's procedure performed for either distal obstruction or complicated diverticulitis. In either case, reestablishment of intestinal continuity should begin with a thorough exploration of the abdomen to ensure that a minimally invasive approach can be performed safely. Trocar placement is similar to that used for a low anterior resection except that the left lateral port site position may need to be altered due to the presence of the colostomy. If the original procedure was performed for benign disease, the goal of the pelvic dissection will be to identify and mobilize the rectal stump as described previously for a low anterior resection. The presence of an obstructing mass changes the approach in that the goal will be curative resection rather than simple mobilization of the rectum. In either scenario, pelvic dissection should be the initial step in the procedure. After the rectum has been sufficiently mobilized, attention is directed toward mobilization of the left colon and splenic flexure as described previously for a left hemicolectomy. Complete mobilization of the left colon will ensure a tension-free anastomosis in the pelvis. A surgeon performing the original Hartmann's procedure who is planning the subsequent laparoscopic takedown should mobilize the splenic flexure at the time of the original procedure and use adhesion barrier in the pelvis to cover the rectal stump. Takedown of the colostomy is approached extracorporeally in the standard fashion. Once the descending colon is completely freed from the surrounding fascia, the anvil of a properly sized circular stapler is secured into the end of the colon with a purse-string suture. Any specimen present can then be delivered intact through the old colostomy site and examined. The abdomen is again insufflated, and a standard end-to-end circular stapled anastomosis can be completed.

3. Rectopexy

The patient probably receives more benefit from a laparoscopic approach to this procedure than any of the other colon and rectal procedures described above. Since there is no specimen to deliver, incisions other than those used for the trocar sites are not necessary. In addition, there is no anastomosis and the entire blood supply is left intact, thus greatly reducing the risk of colonic leak or ischemia. Bowel manipulation is kept to a minimum, resulting in even quicker return of bowel function and eventual discharge.

Trocar placement is identical to that described previously for a low anterior resection. After placing the patient in steep Trendelenburg position, the rectum is completely mobilized to the pelvic floor. This dissection is necessary to bring the redundant rectum below the peritoneal refection into the peritoneal cavity and prevent recurrent prolapse. The rectum is then affixed to the sacrum either with sutures through the lateral rectal mesenteric peritoneum or with mesh stapled to the sacral promontory and secured to the anterior rectum with sutures.

Many authors advocate a perineal approach to the treatment of rectal prolapse in both young and old patients, arguing that it is less invasive than a transabdominal approach and provides nearly equal results with regard to function and recurrence. The use of laparoscopic techniques in the abdominal approach may eventually yield results superior to a perineal approach with respect to recovery and return of bowel function. However, a prospective trial is needed to answer those questions.

IV. POSTOPERATIVE CARE AND MANAGEMENT OF COMPLICATIONS

A. Postoperative Care

Gastric decompression is generally not needed postoperatively, and any gastric tube that was placed after induction of anesthesia can be removed either at the time of extubation or in the recovery room. If the procedure is completed early in the day, patients can be offered liquids by evening; otherwise, the introduction of liquids is delayed until the morning of postoperative day 1. In most cases bowel activity is evident within 24–36 hours after surgery, and the diet is then advanced as tolerated. Patients should have normal bowel function and be able to tolerate a normal diet by postoperative day 3. Activity is generally encouraged on the evening of surgery. Due to the limited fascial incisions normal activity can be resumed by the end of 2 weeks, with the exception of very heavy lifting. Oral analgesics are started as soon as the patient is tolerating any oral intake and are usually adequate for postoperative pain control beyond the early postoperative period. Intravenous narcotics are generally not required beyond 24 hours postoperatively. The average hospital stay after a laparoscopic colon resection is less than 5 days, with the most common reason for a prolonged hospital stay being a delayed return of bowel function.

B. Management of Complications

Some of the most common potential complications are listed in Table 3. Complications associated specifically with laparoscopic surgery are infrequent but do occur. They are not any more common, however, than complications associated specifically with open surgery, such as wound dehiscence or evisceration.

V. OUTCOMES AND DISCUSSION

The techniques described above can potentially be used in the treatment of a variety of both benign and malignant diseases affecting the colon and rectum. Despite the fact that the first reported laparoscopic colon resections appeared in the literature more than 10 years ago, the question of whether or not this approach will become the standard of care remains unanswered. Multiple studies have compared laparoscopic colon surgery to standard open procedures with respect to a variety of different parameters, but the primary question still remains: Does a laparoscopic approach to diseases of the colon and rectum provide a clear benefit without compromising the extent of resection or potential for cure of the patient with malignant or benign disease? The issues that prevent widespread acceptance of laparoscopic techniques in the treatment of colon and rectal cancer have largely centered on the lack of data regarding long-term survival and recurrence. Moreover, questions have recently been raised regarding the true benefit of minimally invasive procedures in the colon and rectal cancer population with regard to short- and long-term quality of life.

Studies reviewing short-term survival and recurrence rates after laparoscopic resection of colon cancer have been encouraging. Yamamoto et al. reviewed a group of 48 patients who underwent laparoscopic colectomy for advanced colon cancer and compared them to matched controls who underwent standard open resection during the same time period. They found that no port site recurrence occurred in the laparoscopic group, and the medium-term disease-free rate, overall survival rate, as well as the patterns of recurrence were comparable in the two groups. Similarly, Khalili et al. found that laparoscopic and open colectomy were therapeutically similar for treatment of colorectal cancer in terms of operative time, length of hospitalization, recurrence, lymph node yield, and survival rates. The laparoscopic approach was superior in blood loss and resumption of oral intake.

Initial concerns surrounding the issue of trocar site metastasis have largely been dispelled by recent data as well. There is consensus that trocar site implants usually occur because of tumor spillage if improper technique is used and the tumor is excessively

Table 3 All Reported Complications for Laparoscopic Colectomies

Complication	n	%
Wound infections	30	5.7
Respiratory	16	3.1
Cardiac	15	2.9
Hemorrhage	10	1.9
Anastomotic leaks	8	1.5
Urinary tract infections	3	0.6
Small bowel perforations	3	0.6
Port site herniation	2	0.4
Hematoma	2	0.4
Septicemia	1	0.2
Peritonitis	1	0.2
Anastomotic stricture	1	0.2
Anastomotic edema	1	0.2
Hypoxia	1	0.2
Acute renal failure	1	0.2
Discompensated renal insufficiency	1	0.2
Urinary retention	1	0.2
Deep venous thrombosis	1	0.2
Small bowel obstruction	1	0.2
Phlebitis	1	0.2
Intraabdominal abscess	1	0.2

Source: Chapman et al., 2001.

manipulated with instruments. Alternatively, Ramas et al., looking at trocar site and extraction site recurrences, concluded that recurrence may be attributable to the advanced nature of the disease rather than the laparoscopic technique itself. Wu et al. made observations in animal studies suggesting that peritoneal tumor bourdon, regardless of etiology, rather than peritoneal insufflation was the major factor in development of trocar site metastasis. More recent clinical studies by Cook et al. have also suggested that port-site recurrence may be related to serosal involvement with tumor. Zmora and Weiss concluded that port-site metastasis may not be an inherent detriment of laparoscopic colectomy, but rather an unfortunate sequelae of the learning curve of the application of laparoscopy for colorectal cancer. Paik et al. demonstrated in animal studies that laparoscopy does not increase the incidence of peritoneal tumor implantation, and Hofsetter et al. that carbon dioxide peritoneal insufflation has no effect on tumor growth.

Initial results of a laparoscopic approach to rectal cancer have also been encouraging. Fleshman et al. retrospectively reviewed 194 patients who underwent either laparoscopic (42) or open (152) abdominoperineal resection for rectal cancer. Although there were more perineal wound infections in the laparoscopic group, there was a significant decrease in hospital stay (7 vs. 12 days). The incidence of positive radial margins was almost identical (12 vs. 12.5%), and tumor recurrence and survival rates were similar (Fig. 21). The largest retrospective study published to date reviewed 372 patients treated laparoscopically for colon cancer by members of the Clinical Outcomes of Surgical Therapy (COST) Study Group prior to 1994. These early results revealed that a laparoscopic approach to colorectal cancer yields early outcome after treatment that is

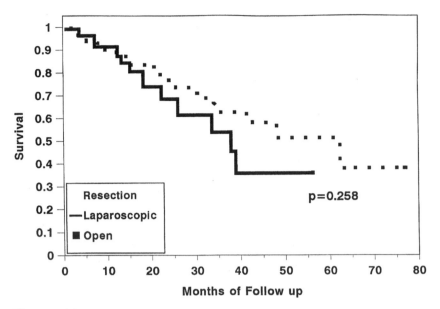

Figure 21 Overall survival rate of patients treated with laparoscopic or open abdominoperineal resection. *Source:* Fleshman et al., 1999.

comparable with conventional therapy for colorectal cancer. However, this study also concluded that a randomized trial is needed to compare long-term outcomes of open and laparoscopic approaches with colorectal cancer.

To address the risks and benefits of laparoscopic-assisted colectomy (LAC) for colon cancer, the National Cancer Institute funded the randomized controlled Clinical Outcomes of Surgical Therapy (COST) study, which was initiated by the North Central Cancer Treatment Group in 1994. The primary objective of this COST study was to compare the disease-free survival and overall survival following laparoscopic-assisted colectomy with open colectomy. The trial was also designed to test the hypothesis that laparoscopic-assisted colectomy is associated with superior quality-of-life (QOL) outcomes. Accrual of patients into this study was closed in August 2001, and final data regarding long-term survival and recurrence will not be available for several years. However, initial data regarding the extent of resection following laparoscopic approach compared to standard open techniques has been published by Nelson. At the time that this trial update data was published, over 800 patients had been enrolled and results were available for 408 patients: 203 open and 205 LAC. With regard to extent of resection, all parameters tested show no difference between the LAC and open cases (Table 4).

In addition to initial results regarding extent of resection from patients enrolled in the COST study, early results regarding QOL outcomes after surgery have also been published and yielded interesting results. In contrast to other studies that have compared laparoscopic surgery to standard open approaches with respect to some determined endpoint, such as analgesia requirements or length of hospital stay, this study focused on differences in patient QOL outcomes between the two groups. Patients were surveyed preoperatively and at 2 days, 2 weeks, and 2 months postoperatively with standardized instruments that had been previously validated in trials of cancer patients for assessing

Table 4 Extent of Resection Data for LAC Versus Open Colectomy—Initial Data from the COST Study

Parameter	LAC	Open colectomy
Total bowel length	26 cm	27 cm
Proximal margin	12 cm	11 cm
Distal margin	10 cm	12 cm
Total mesenteric length	9 cm	8 cm
Mean no. of lymph nodes	12	13

symptoms and QOL. Although the laparoscopically assisted colectomy group required less analgesia postoperatively and had a shorter hospital stay (0.8 days), the only statistically significant difference in QOL was seen at 2 weeks. In the immediate postoperative period and at 2 months after surgery, there was no significant difference in QOL between the two groups. Weeks et al. concluded that "the modest benefits in short-term QOL proxy measures we observed are not sufficient to justify the use of this procedure in the routine care setting until the safety and efficacy of the procedure in the treatment of cancer have been definitively established." Although these results do raise some interesting questions regarding the true benefit of laparoscopic surgery in the cancer population, it is important to point out that in this study patients were grouped by intention-to-treat and were analyzed by their assigned group, not by the procedure that was actually performed. Fifty-eight patients (25.7%) in the LAC group were converted to open colectomy and kept in the LAC group for data analysis. This may have skewed the overall QOL results for the laparoscopic group as the patients converted to open colectomy consistently reported poorer QOL assessments at all follow-up surveys.

In contrast to the treatment of malignant disease, the application of laparoscopic surgical techniques to the treatment of benign disease processes has been largely accepted without much debate. There is little question that in most cases patients recover faster and with less discomfort than with standard open techniques. Even in cases where there is no clear advantage with respect to patient recovery, many argue that cosmesis and improved postoperative body image alone are enough to argue in favor of minimally invasive techniques despite possible increased costs and operative times. This is especially true in the young patient population.

Current recommendations regarding the use of laparoscopic techniques in the treatment of diseases of the colon and rectum include the treatment of inflammatory bowel disease, diverticulitis, benign polyps not resectable by endoscopy, and those procedures described above such as diverting colostomy and rectopexy. Wu et al. looked at the treatment of patients with complicated ileocolic Crohn's disease using laparoscopic techniques and compared the results with patients treated with standard techniques. Forty-six patients had an attempted laparoscopic resection and were divided into three subgroups. Patients in Group 1 had an abscess or phlegmon treated with bowel rest before operation, Group 2 had recurrent Crohn's disease at the previous ileocolic anastomosis, and Group 3 had no previous operation and no phlegmon or abscess associated with their disease. These three groups were compared with a fourth group, all of whom had open resection of their disease. Group 4 had the longest hospital stay and operative time as well as the greatest degree of blood loss and morbidity. Only five of the original 46 patients in the LAC group required conversion to open resection, with Group 2 having the highest conversion rate. The authors concluded that a laparoscopic-assisted approach to Crohn's disease is feasible and safe with good outcomes. In addition, comorbid preoperative findings such as abscess, phlegmon, or recurrent disease at the previous ileocolic anastomosis are not contraindications to a successful laparoscopic-assisted ileocolic resection in select patients.

Similar success has been achieved with laparoscopy in the treatment of diverticular disease. As with Crohn's disease, Martinez et al. found that staged laparoscopic approach to diverticulitis is both safe and feasible and provides excellent immediate postoperative recovery. Our approach to the treatment of diverticulitis is to attempt to convert all cases except those with fecal peritonitis to an elective, one-stage procedure. We have found that cases with very large abscess or even free air at the time of initial presentation can be successfully managed with percutaneous drainage of any abscess present, antibiotics, and bowel rest. Once the initial inflammation has subsided, many of these patients can be managed laparoscopically, especially with the aid of a hand-assist device. Lauro et al. found that a laparoscopic approach to the surgical treatment of uncomplicated diverticulitis provides reduced postoperative pain, more rapid recovery of intestinal peristalsis and shorter postoperative stay. They felt that laparoscopic sigmoid colectomy should represent the treatment of choice for diverticulitis in uncomplicated cases.

Although the initial data from the COST study seems to show little QOL benefit in colon cancer patients resected laparoscopically, the same does not appear to hold true with patients resected for benign polyps. Young-Fadok et al. retrospectively reviewed a series of patients undergoing right hemicolectomy for unresectable benign polyps. They found that laparoscopic-assisted colectomy resulted in shorter postoperative ileus (time to flatus, 3.0 vs. 4.0 days, $p < 0.001$; time to bowel movement, 3.5 vs. 5.0 days, $p < 0.001$), earlier tolerance of regular diet (3.5 vs. 6.0 days, $p < 0.001$), and fewer days of narcotic administration (3.0 vs. 4.5 days, $p < 0.001$). The overall result was a significantly shorter length of hospital stay (4.0 vs. 7.0 days, $p < 0.001$) without a significant difference in the incidence of postoperative complications. Their conclusions were that laparoscopic right hemicolectomy has significant patient benefits that are apparent when procedures of equal complexity and equivalent indications are compared. In addition, they commented, "laparoscopic-assisted resection has become our preferred approach for polyps not amenable to colonoscopic polypectomy." The authors also noted that their conversion rate was 18.4% (7/38), 21.4% early in the series and 10% in later experience, which raises the issue of clinical competence with the procedure itself. As one might expect, operative times and conversion rates are expected to decrease as the surgeon gains experience. Zmora and Weiss estimated that the learning curve for laparoscopic colectomy is between 20 and 70 cases. Thus, the average general surgeon will not gain clinical expertise in these techniques for several years, even in a busy practice.

Although laparoscopic techniques can be applied to many disease processes affecting the colon and rectum, it is important that the surgeon and the patient understand the risks and benefits of these techniques in a given situation. After a review of recent literature it is clear that until final data regarding long-term survival and recurrence rates are available, laparoscopic techniques should not be offered to patients in the treatment of colon and rectal cancer outside of a controlled clinical trial. In addition, more clear-cut benefits to the patient need to be established in this population before alternative methods of resection are recommended. With respect to benign disease, established benefits to the patient are more forthcoming in the literature. According to Dunker et al., even issues such as patient perception as well as cosmesis and improved postoperative body image are outcomes that can be improved through laparoscopic techniques in the treatment of benign disease. Operative times and overall admission expenses will decrease as surgeons gain experience and conquer the steep learning curve associated with these procedures. Laparoscopic techniques have been shown by Peters and Fleshman and Tuech et al. to be safe and efficacious not only in otherwise healthy patients, but also in elderly and obese patient populations, respectively. Thus, without cost or safety issues to deter the surgeon from exploring laparoscopic options, minimally invasive techniques are certain to become standard of care in the treatment of benign diseases of the colon and rectum.

SELECTED READINGS

Bokey EL, Moore JW, Chapuis PH, Newland RC. Morbidity and mortality following laparoscopic-assisted right hemicolectomy for cancer. *Dis Colon Rectum* 1996;39(10 suppl):S24–S28.

Chapman AE, Levitt MD, Hewett P, Woods R, Sheiner H, Maddem GJ. Laparoscopic-assisted resection of colorectal malignancies: a systematic review. *Ann Surg* 2001;234(5):590–606.

Cook TA, Dehn TC. Port-site metastases in patients undergoing laparoscopy for gastrointestinal malignancy. *Br J Surg* 1996;83(10):1419–1420.

Dunker MS, Bemelman WA, Slors JF, van Duijvendijk P, Gouma DJ. Functional outcome, quality of life, body image, and cosmesis in patients after laparoscopic-assisted and conventional restorative proctocolectomy: a comparative study. *Dis Colon Rectum* 2001;44(12):1800–1807.

Fleshman JW, Nelson H, Peters WR, Kim HC, Larach S, Boorse RR, Ambroze W, Leggett P. Bleday R, Stryker S, Christenson B, Wexner S, Senagore A, Rattner D, Sutton J, Fine AP. Early results of laparoscopic surgery for colorectal cancer. Retrospective analysis of 372 patients treated by Clinical Outcomes of Surgical Therapy (COST) Study Group. *Dis Colon Rectum* 1996;39(10 suppl):S53–S58.

Fleshman JW, Wexner SD, Anvari M, LaTulippe JF, Birnbaum EH, Kodner IJ, Read TE, Nogueras JJ, Weiss EG. Laparoscopic vs. open abdominoperineal resection for cancer. *Dis Colon Rectum* 1999;42(7):930–939.

Hofstetter W, Ortega A, Chiang M, Brown B, Paik P, Youn P, Beart RW. Abdominal insufflation does not cause hematogenous spread of colon cancer. *J Laparoendosc Adv Surg Tech A* 2000;10(1):1–4.

Jones DB, Fleshman JW. Laparoscopic approaches to rectal cancer. In: Soper N, Problems in General Surgery. Philadelphia: Lippincott-Raven Pub, 1996; 135–145.

Khalili TM, Fleshner PR, Hiatt JR, Sokol TP, Manookian C, Tsushima G, Phillips EH. Colorectal cancer: comparison of laparoscopic with open approaches. *Dis Colon Rectum* 1998;41(7):832–838.

Lauro A, Alonso Poza A, Cirocchi R, Doria C, Gruttaduria S, Giustozzi G, Wexner SD. Laparoscopic surgery for colon diverticulitis. *Minerva Chir* 2002;57(1):1–5.

Martinez SA, Cheanvechai V, Alasfar FS, Sands LR, Hellinger MD. Staged laparoscopic resection for complicated sigmoid diverticulitis. *Surg Laparosc Endosc Perutan Tech* 1999;9(2):99–105.

Nelson H. Laparoscopic colectomy for colon cancer—a trial update. *Swiss Surg* 2001;7(6):248–251.

Paik PS, Misawa T, Chiang M, Towson J, Im S, Ortega A, Beart RW Jr. Abdominal incision tumor implantation following pneumoperitoneum laparoscopic procedure vs. standard open incision in a syngeneic rat model. *Dis Colon Rectum* 1998;41(4):419–422.

Peters WR, Fleshman JW. Minimally invasive colectomy in elderly patients. *Surg Laparosc Endosc* 1995;5(6):477–479.

Ramos JM, Gupta S, Anthone GJ, Ortega AE, Simons AJ, Beart RW Jr. Laparoscopy and colon cancer. Is the port site at risk? A preliminary report. *Arch Surg* 1994;129(9):897–900.

Simmang C, Jones DB. Wound implantation of cancer after laparoscopic colectomy clinical and basic research. In: Schoetz D, Seminars in Colon and Rectal Surgery. Philadelphia: W.B. Saunders, 1999; 1081–1089.

Tomita H, Marcello PW, Milsom JW, Gramlich TL, Fazio VW. CO2 pneumoperitoneum does not enhance tumor growth and metastasis: study of a rat cecal wall inoculation model. *Dis Colon Rectum* 2001;44(9):1297–1301.

Tuech JJ, Regenet N, Hennekinne S, Pessaux P, Duplessis R, Arnaud JP. Impact of obesity on postoperative results of elective laparoscopic colectomy in sigmoid diverticulitis: a prospective study. *Ann Chir* 2001;126(10):996–1000.

Wu JS, Birnbaum EH, Kodner IJ, Fry RD, Read TE, Fleshman JW. Laparoscopic-assisted ileocolic resections in patients with Crohn's disease: are abscesses, phlegmons, or recurrent disease contraindications? *Surgery* 1997;122(4):682–689.

Wu JS, Jones DB, Guo LW, Brasifeld EB, Ruiz MB, Connett JM, Fleshman JW. Effects of pneumoperitoneum on tumor implantation with decreasing tumor inoculum. *Dis Colon Rectum* 1998;41(2):141–146.

Yamamoto S, Watanabe M, Hasegawa H, Kitajima M. Oncologic outcome of laparoscopic versus open surgery for advanced colorectal cancer. *Hepatogastroenterology* 2001;48(41):1248–1251.

Young-Fadok TM, Radice E, Nelson H, Harmsen WS. Benefits of laparoscopic-assisted colectomy for colon polyps: a case-matched series. *Mayo Clin Proc* 2000;75(4):344–348.

Zmora O, Weiss EG. Trocar site recurrence in laparoscopic surgery for colorectal cancer. Myth or real concern? *Surg Oncol Clin North Am* 2001;10(3):625–638.

31

Splenectomy

EMILY R. WINSLOW and L. MICHAEL BRUNT

Institute for Minimally Invasive Surgery
Washington University School of Medicine
St. Louis, Missouri, U.S.A.

Laparoscopic splenectomy was first introduced in 1992 and has since become a widespread laparoscopic procedure. Because of the bulk and vascularity of the spleen, laparoscopic splenectomy is one of the more challenging laparoscopic procedures. Despite this, laparoscopic splenectomy has become the preferred method for resection in patients with normal-sized spleens. However, a wide variety of pathological conditions that affect the spleen and necessitate its removal also cause significant splenomegaly, which presents a further challenge to the laparoscopic surgeon. Laparoscopic techniques, especially with the addition of hand-assistance technology, have been used successfully to carry out splenectomy in selected patients with marked splenomegaly.

I. SPLENIC FUNCTION

In the normal physiological state, the spleen has two major functions. First, the spleen has several important hematological functions as part of the reticuloendothelial system. The red pulp of the splenic parenchyma serves as a filter for the removal of senescent erythrocytes (called culling) and the remodeling of healthy red cells, including removal of nuclear remnants, denatured hemoglobin, and iron granules (called pitting). The splenic macrophages and reticular cells then phagocytose these filtered particles. Another minor hematological function of the spleen is to serve as a reservoir for platelets. In certain diseased states (e.g., myelofibrosis) the adult spleen becomes a major site of extramedullary hematopoiesis.

Second, the spleen is a component of the body's immune system. The white pulp effectively serves as a nonspecific filter and removes bloodborne pathogens (bacteria and viruses) coated with complement. The spleen also participates in the specific immune response by producing antibody (primarily IgM), plasma cells, and memory cells in response to specific trapped antigens. Encapsulated bacteria are also effectively removed, likely via prolonged contact with macrophages in the splenic parenchymal cords where the transit time is slow. Finally, the spleen manufactures opsonins that circulate systemically. Although the spleen serves these and other functions as part of the hematological and immunological systems, there is clearly redundancy as splenectomy results in relatively few major alterations in the host, the most notable of which is an increased susceptibility to sepsis from encapsulated bacteria.

II. INDICATIONS FOR SPLENECTOMY

The primary therapy for most nontraumatic splenic disorders is medical. Splenectomy is generally warranted only after failure of medical therapy or as a palliative adjunct to therapy. Conditions in which splenectomy (either open or laparoscopic) plays a potential therapeutic role are listed in Table 1. Over time, the role of surgery in most of these disorders has fluctuated with the development of more effective diagnostic tools, better medical therapies, and improved understanding of the natural disease process. The intended outcome from splenectomy varies from diagnosis to cure, making it important for the surgeon to understand the patient's and hematologist's goals prior to undertaking an operative approach. In general, the goals of splenectomy can be grouped into the following categories:

Relief of symptomatic splenomegaly
Palliation of hypersplenism

Table 1   Indications for Splenectomy

Hematological splenic pathology
  Thrombocytopenias
    Immune thrombocytopenic purpura
    Thrombotic thrombocytopenic purpura
  Anemias
    Hereditary hemolytic anemias (hereditary spherocytosis)
    Acquired autoimmune hemolytic anemias
    Congenital hemoglobinopathies (sickle cell anemia)
  Myeloproliferative disorders
    Chronic myelogenous leukemia
    Polycythemia vera
    Myelofibrosis or myeloid metaplasia
    Myeloproliferative disorder not otherwise specified
  Lymphoproliferative disorders
    Chronic lymphocytic leukemia
    Hairy-cell leukemia
    Non-Hodgkin's lymphoma
    Hodgkin's lymphoma
  Neutropenias
    Felty's syndrome
Nonhematological splenic disorders
  Splenic abscess
  Splenic cyst/pseudocyst
  Storage diseases
Other disorders
  Trauma
  Incidental splenectomy
  Vascular problems (splenic artery aneurysm, splenic vein thrombosis)

Cure or palliation of hematological disease
Control of ongoing splenic bleeding
Diagnosis of splenic pathology

Massive splenomegaly can result in symptoms due to the mass effect of the spleen (including pain, early satiety, weight loss, and abdominal distention) and due to hypersplenism. For example, late in the course of myelofibrosis and other myelo-proliferative disorders, massive splenomegaly often produces bothersome symptoms that are not otherwise well palliated. For these patients, splenectomy serves only to palliate symptoms and does not impact on the underlying disease process. In contrast, in immune thrombocytopenic purpura (ITP), splenectomy is performed with curative intent. Because the spleen is the primary site for both production of platelet antibodies and of platelet destruction, splenectomy can eliminate the disease and restore platelet counts to normal. Complete remission is achieved by splenectomy in approximately 70–80% of patients with ITP. Patients with ITP that develops in association with systemic lupus erythematosus or human immunodeficiency virus (HIV) infection may also respond to splenectomy. The most common hemolytic anemias for which splenectomy is indicated are hereditary spherocytosis and autoimmune hemolytic anemia. Gallstones develop in 30–60% of these patients and should be screened for preoperatively with ultrasound. Concomitant laparoscopic cholecystectomy may be carried out if gallstones are present.

Splenectomy is occasionally indicated for patients with lymphoma for diagnostic reasons. Patients with chronic lymphocytic leukemia (CLL) and chronic myelogenous leukemia (CML) may also occasionally require splenectomy for symptomatic splenomegaly or refractory cytopenia. For patients with either secondary hypersplenism from CLL or myelofibrosis, splenectomy is not curative but can significantly palliate the disease in some patients by decreasing transfusion requirements and improving refractory cytopenias.

III. CONTRAINDICATIONS TO LAPAROSCOPIC SPLENECTOMY

Laparoscopic splenectomy is contraindicated in any patient with a general contra-indication to laparoscopic surgery (see Chapter 2). A number of potential contra-indications to laparoscopic splenectomy may also exist that are patient or disease specific. However, increasing experience and the availability of hand-assisted techniques have expanded the indications for attempting a minimally invasive approach to some conditions that were previously considered absolute contraindications. Currently, laparoscopic splenectomy is rarely performed for splenic trauma due to difficulties in managing ongoing bleeding and the possible need for using splenic salvage techniques and managing coexisting injuries elsewhere in the abdomen. It should not be attempted in the hemodynamically unstable patient with splenic trauma. Portal hypertension is also a contraindication because of the increased risk for major bleeding. The risk of hemorrhage may also be increased in patients with splenic vein thrombosis because of the associated gastric varices. Bulky splenic hilar adenopathy (usually found in patients with lymphomas or leukemias) may make the hilar dissection more treacherous. The presence of uncorrectable cytopenias is no longer considered a contraindication to laparoscopic splenectomy provided the surgeon is experienced and local splenic conditions are favorable. Morbid obesity increases the difficulty of the laparoscopic approach and may

Table 2 Contraindications to Laparoscopic Splenectomy

Absolute contraindications	Relative contraindications
Massive splenomegaly (>30 cm length)	Moderate splenomegaly (>20 cm)
Portal hypertension	Severe uncorrectable cytopenia
Splenic trauma, unstable patient	Splenic vein thrombosis
	Splenic trauma, stable patient
	Bulky hilar adenopathy

necessitate the use of additional port sites for exposure and retraction but is not itself a contraindication.

Splenomegaly complicates the laparoscopic approach because of the difficulty in manipulating the organ atraumatically and achieving adequate exposure of the ligaments and hilum. When the results of laparoscopic splenectomy for normal-sized and enlarged spleens are compared, it has been shown that splenomegaly is associated with longer operating times, more transfusions, and more frequent need for conversion to an open procedure [1,2]. In addition, because of the sheer bulk of the organ, accessory incisions may be necessary for extraction of the spleen at the end of the procedure [2,3]. Despite these difficulties, retrospective comparisons have shown that laparoscopic splenectomy for patients with splenomegaly is associated with less morbidity and a shorter hospital stay when compared with the open procedure [4].

The introduction of hand-assistance technology has pushed the limits of the spleen size feasible for a minimally invasive approach even further and may improve results as well. In one series of 56 patients with spleens that weighed over 700 g [5], the addition of hand-assisted technique shortened operative times, reduced hospital stay, and decreased the conversion rate fourfold when compared with the unassisted laparoscopic approach. This ability of the hand port to decrease conversion rates in the setting of splenomegaly has been confirmed by others [6]. Finally, it has been shown that with the selective addition of hand-assistance to laparoscopic splenectomy, the conversion and complication rates become equivalent in patients with normal-sized spleens and those with splenomegaly [7].

Although the size limits for attempting laparoscopic or laparoscopic-assisted splenectomy are still evolving, most patients with moderately enlarged spleens (< 1000 g weight or 15–20 cm in length) can be removed in a minimally invasive fashion, often without a hand port device. For spleens between 1000 and 3000 g, the use of a hand-port should be considered if the laparoscopic approach is attempted. Spleens > 28–30 cm in craniocaudal length or >3000 g should not be attempted laparoscopically, with rare exception, because of the low success rate. Considerable experience with laparoscopic splenectomy in nonenlarged spleens is advisable before this procedure is attempted in patients with splenomegaly.

IV. OPERATIVE PREPARATION

A. Patient Preparation

The decision to perform splenectomy should be made jointly by the surgeon and hematologist. All preoperative diagnostic tests and studies should be reviewed to ensure an accurate diagnosis. Routine imaging (either ultrasound or CT) is necessary in patients with malignancy, suspected splenomegaly, and to rule out gallstones in patients with symptoms or who are at high risk for developing gallstones (hemolytic anemias, sickle cell anemia).

The nature of and indications for laparoscopic splenectomy as well as potential risks and benefits of the procedure are discussed with the patient before surgery. The possible need to convert to an open splenectomy should be clearly explained. Preoperative counseling should include specific consideration of the potential for bleeding complications, particularly if there are disease-related cytopenias. Patients should also be counseled about transfusion risks and be given the opportunity to establish directed-donor units of blood products during the preoperative period if practical.

In the preoperative period, a type and screen should be obtained for all patients, and blood should be cross-matched for any patient with splenomegaly or preoperative anemia. Because it can be difficult to cross-match blood for patients with autoimmune disorders due to preexisting antibodies, the patient should have the type and screen done at least one day prior to the scheduled operation. In patients with marked thrombocytopenia, platelets should be available for transfusion intraoperatively, even though they are not often needed.

One essential part of the preoperative preparation prior to splenectomy is the administration of polyvalent pneumococcal vaccine (Pneumovax) and *Haemophilus influenza* type B vaccine (HIB) to reduce the risk of overwhelming postsplenectomy infection. Ideally, the vaccine should be administered 2–3 weeks before surgery. Vaccination against *Neisseria meningitidis* is recommended for children under 10 years of age if they were not vaccinated during infancy. Other important perioperative medical interventions include antibiotic coverage, usually with a first-generation cephalosporin, and stress-dose corticosteroids if the patient has had recent steroid treatment. Some surgeons recommend mechanical bowel preparation, but this has rarely been necessary in our experience.

The use of preoperative splenic artery embolization for patients with splenomegaly was advocated by some groups [8] early in the experience with laparoscopic splenectomy in order to decrease the risk of intraoperative hemorrhagic complications. Because this approach can lead to troublesome perisplenitis, is painful, and entails significant cost, it is rarely, if ever, used.

B. Operating Room Setup

Laparoscopic splenectomy is carried out under general endotracheal anesthesia. Sequential compression hose are placed on the patient's lower extremities to prevent deep venous thrombosis and a urinary catheter is inserted. Patients with splenomegaly should have two large-bore intravenous lines for rapid infusion of fluids and blood if major bleeding occurs. Patient positioning for laparoscopic splenectomy has evolved over time, with the supine position being the initial choice. Although preferences vary, most authors report the use of the lateral position [9]. We prefer a right semi-lateral decubitus position. Once the patient is placed in the semi-lateral decubitus position, the beanbag device is molded around the torso for stability. The patient must be secured to the operating room table with a well-padded beanbag mattress. All pressure points, including the axilla, hips and lower extremities, should be well padded to avoid nerve compression injuries. The operating table is then flexed approximately 30 degrees, and the table can be rotated to either the right or left to allow greater access anteriorly or posteriorly as desired. The

Table 3   Instruments Needed for Laparoscopic Splenectomy

Basic laparoscopic instrument set
5 mm blunt retractor
10 mm right-angled dissector
Trocars: 12 mm (1), 5 mm (3), 18 mm (1)
30° laparoscope
Endoscopic linear stapler (vascular loads)
Ultrasonic coagulation device
Laparoscopic suction irrigator
Endoscopic clips and clip applier
Extraction bag
Laparotomy set (available)
Hand-port (available)

---

prepared area should extend from the nipple line to the pubis and as far laterally as possible on both sides. The umbilicus should be left exposed so it can serve as a landmark during the placement of trocars.

The surgeon and camera operator stand on the patient's right side, and the first assistant is on the patient's left side. Video monitors are placed on either side of the patient's head in full view of all members of the surgical team. Irrigation, suction, and electrocautery connections are passed off the head of the table. Necessary instrumentation (Table 3) includes an angled laparoscope (30 or 45 degrees), electrocautery, scissors, a right-angled dissector, clip applier, an endovascular linear cutter stapler, and a sterile entrapment sack for removal of the spleen. An ultrasonic coagulator is used routinely for division of the splenic ligaments, especially the short gastric vessels. Because of the highly vascular nature of the organ and its dissection, a variety of ligation, suturing, and stapling devices should be available. A laparotomy set should be open on the back table in the event conversion to an open procedure is necessary. Finally, a hand-port device may be warranted in selected patients with splenomegaly.

C. Anatomical Relationships

The normal spleen weighs about 100 g and is suspended in the left upper quadrant by ligaments attaching it to the diaphragm, stomach, kidney, and splenic flexure of the colon. Peritoneal reflections in the region surrounding the spleen form the tough fibrous suspensory "ligaments" through which most of the principle vascular structures course (Fig. 1). The spleen is supported at its superior pole by the phrenosplenic ligament and at its inferior pole by the splenocolic ligament. These ligaments are relatively avascular, except in patients with portal hypertension, where the normally small vessels are dilated. Broad, leaf-like peritoneal attachments at the hilum include the gastrosplenic ligament anteriorly and the splenorenal ligament posteriorly. The short gastric and left gastroepiploic arteries are contained within the gastrosplenic ligament, and the splenic artery and its terminal branches are contained within the splenic hilum. The tail of the pancreas extends laterally to within 1 cm of the splenic hilum in most patients and is in direct contact with the pancreas in up to 30% of patients. The pancreas is partially invested in the leaves of the splenorenal ligament, just inferior to the contained splenic artery and its branches.

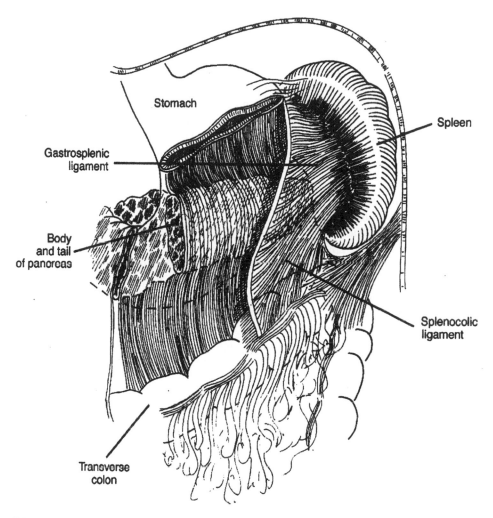

Figure 1   The peritoneal attachments of the spleen.

The rich and variable vascular anatomy and structural fragility of the spleen necessitates methodical laparoscopic dissection. The terminal vascularization of the spleen has been classified by some anatomists as either *distributive* or *magistral*, a classification that is relevant during laparoscopic splenectomy [10]. The distributive pattern, thought to be the more common anatomical configuration, is characterized by arborization of the main splenic trunk into 6–10 arterial branches that enter the hilum broadly over 75% of its surface area. The presence of splenic notching correlates clinically with a greater number of arteries entering the organ. The magistral configuration is characterized by a more dominant splenic artery that divides into a few small branches very close to the hilum and enters over a narrow, compact area, representing approximately 30% of the hilar surface area.

The major hazards and other potential anatomical pitfalls associated with laparoscopic splenectomy are:

1. Colonic injuries: Because of the close apposition of the left colon and the spleen, the splenic flexure must be taken down. Although rare, injuries to the colon may occur due to the use of cautery in this area during mobilization of the inferior splenic pole.

2. Pancreatic injuries: The pancreas is the most commonly injured contiguous organ during splenectomy because it lies adjacent to the splenic hilum and there is significant risk of injuring this organ when dissecting or transecting the splenic vessels. In one prospective study [11], 15% of patients demonstrated some degree of pancreatic injury, with splenomegaly being a significant risk factor for injury. Half had simple hyperamylasemia, while the others had more significant injuries (pancreatitis or pancreatic leaks) that prolonged the hospitalization.

3. Vascular injuries: Because the vascular pattern is variable, injury to a vascular structure, particularly an inferior polar vessel, during dissection is not uncommon. The splenic vein is often large and fragile and may be easily torn during dissection or by excessive traction. Significant variation may be encountered in the number, size, and length of the short gastric vessels that may be encountered when dividing the gastrosplenic ligament.

4. Accessory spleens: The identification of accessory spleens is important when splenectomy is undertaken for ITP or hypersplenism. The common locations of accessory spleens are illustrated in Figure 2. The most common sites are the splenic hilum, the gastrosplenic omentum, and along the tail of the pancreas. A methodical search in these locations should be undertaken prior to splenic dissection, so as not to obscure the tissue with blood or irrigant. Even if one accessory spleen is found, the search should continue as some patients have more than one accessory spleen.

V. SURGICAL TECHNIQUE

A. Port Placement

Laparoscopic splenectomy can be performed using three or four ports, depending on the splenic size and the difficulty of dissection. The precise port position should be chosen based upon the patient's body habitus and the size of the spleen. For most patients, the optimal configuration for the ports is in an arc that parallels the costal margin (Fig. 3a). Initial access can be obtained with a Veress needle just inferior to the left costal margin and medial to the anterior axillary line. A 5 mm trocar is then inserted at this site, and the remaining ports are placed under direct vision. A second 5 mm port is placed in the epigastric midline, and the third port (12 mm) is inserted in the left subcostal region about 5 cm lateral to the second port (Fig. 3b). The most lateral port is placed at about the mid-axillary line. For patients with a small body habitus and those with marked splenomegaly, initial access is best established at the umbilicus in the open fashion. The second and third trocars are placed so as to form a working triangle with the initial port at the umbilicus, usually one in the epigastrium and the other in a mid-left rectus position. Again, the fourth port is placed laterally in the mid-axillary line after mobilization of the colon.

After the insertion of the ports, attention should be directed to the identification of any accessory spleens within the greater omentum and splenocolic ligament. As the

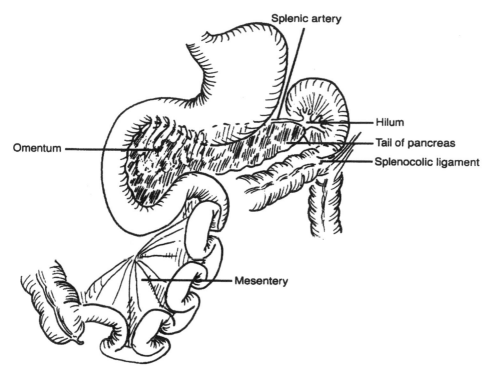

Figure 2 Sites of accessory spleens in decreasing order of frequency: the splenic hilum, the tail of the pancreas, the greater omentum, along the splenic artery, within the splenocolic ligament, within the mesentery of the colon or small intestine, and along the course of the gonadal vessels.

splenic ligaments are dissected later, the surgeon should continue to look for accessory splenic tissue in these locations.

B. Inferolateral Dissection

The patient is placed in the reverse Trendelenburg position to facilitate retraction of the stomach and colon inferiorly. The first maneuver is to free the inferior pole of the spleen. This is done by first dividing the adhesions between the spleen, colon, and the abdominal wall. The spleen should be carefully rotated anteriorly and superiorly by an assistant, using the shaft of a dissecting instrument or flexible retractor. Extreme care must be taken when manipulating the spleen laparoscopically, as its fragility and vascularity make it susceptible to fracturing from any pulling or shearing forces and the subsequent bleeding will interfere with laparoscopic visualization and dissection. The splenic flexure should be taken down with the use of ultrasonic cautery from medially to laterally, as shown in Figure 4. Small inferior polar vessels may be encountered during this part of the dissection and are usually controlled with the ultrasonic coagulator. After division of the splenocolic attachments, the splenorenal ligament may be divided along the entire craniocaudal length of the spleen (Fig. 5). The goal is to adequately free the spleen so it can be easily rotated medially to provide access to the hilum posteriorly. Alternatively, one may first proceed

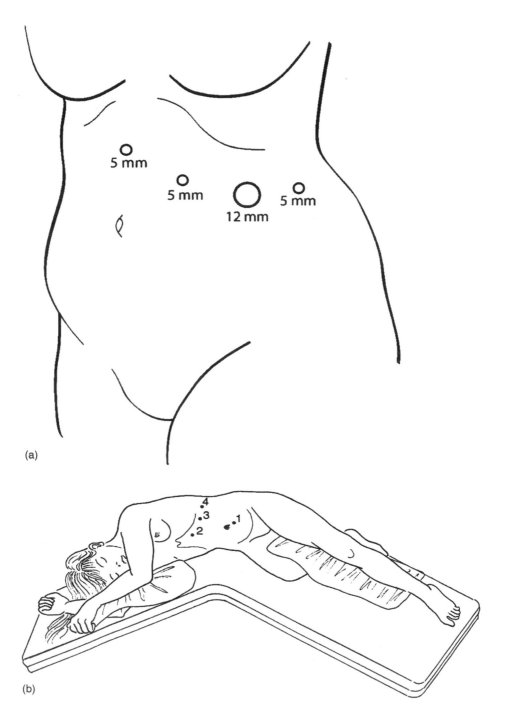

Figure 3 Patient positioning and port placement for laparoscopic splenectomy: (a) optimal positioning for majority of patients; (b) alternative configuration for patients with marked splenomegaly or thin body habitus.

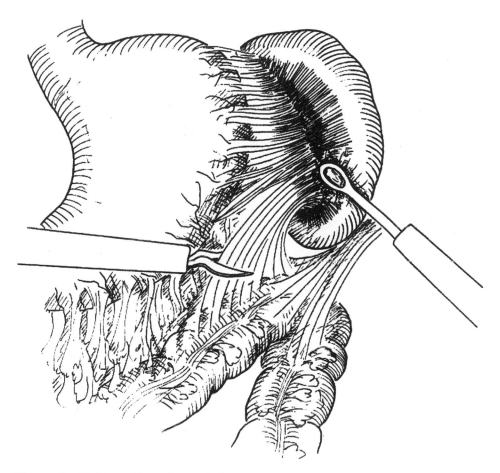

Figure 4 Division of the splenocolic ligament.

with the medial dissection of the gastrosplenic ligament before dividing the splenorenal ligament [12].

C. Medial Dissection

After the inferolateral attachments have been divided, attention is then turned toward the gastrosplenic ligament, looking for accessory splenic tissue as the dissection proceeds. The spleen is rolled back medially, and the ultrasonic coagulator is used to divide the ligament and the short gastric vessels within it (Fig. 6). Once the gastrosplenic ligament is taken, there is access to the lesser sac and the proximal splenic artery as it runs along the superior surface of the pancreas. In cases in which it is anticipated that the hilar dissection will be difficult or there is marked splenomegaly, or if the patient is markedly thrombocytopenic, our practice has been to isolate and ligate the splenic artery along the superior border of the pancreas proximal to the splenic hilum. This step can be accomplished using a right angle dissector and application of either a single clip or a suture. Once the splenic artery has been clipped and the short gastric vessels have been divided, all inflow to the spleen has been occluded. These maneuvers, therefore, should

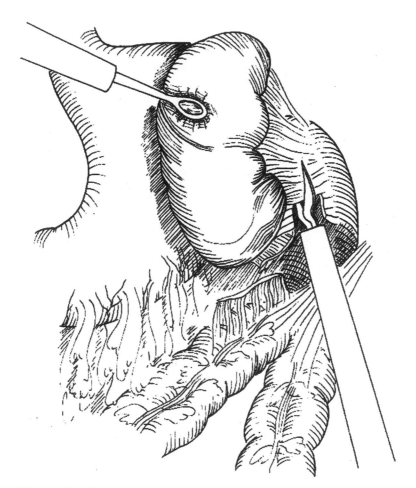

Figure 5   Division of the splenorenal ligament.

minimize the risk of significant hemorrhage during the subsequent hilar dissection and may allow some degree of autotransfusion for patients with enlarged spleens.

D.   Hilar Dissection

The hilar dissection can be carried out from either the anterior or posterior aspect, as dictated principally by the anatomical position of the hilar vessels. It is our preference to have all superior and inferior ligamentous attachments divided prior to the hilar dissection so that the spleen can be more easily elevated to better expose the hilum. As the assistant elevates the spleen, the hilum should be dissected so that the relationship of the vessels to the pancreatic tail can be precisely determined. The vessels can be controlled with either an endoscopic linear cutting stapler or clips. The most commonly used method involves using the endoscopic linear cutting stapler with a vascular load to staple across all hilar vessels. The advantages of this method are that it is fast, straightforward, and provides excellent and reliable hemostasis. Multiple applications (usually two to three) may be required to completely transect the hilum. If there is bleeding from the staple line, it can

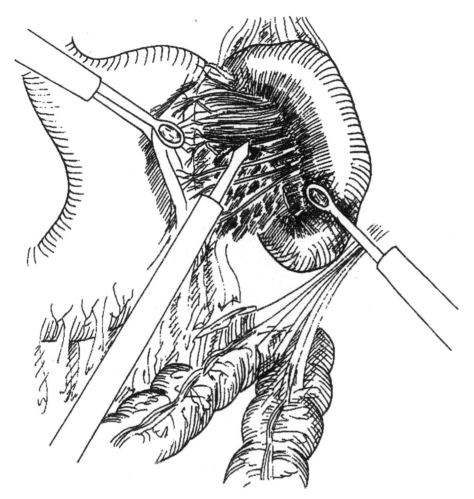

Figure 6 Division of the short gastric vessels.

usually be controlled with either application of a clip or by suture ligation. If the staple line only partially transects a major vessel, brisk bleeding can occur (although this can usually be controlled laparoscopically). Alternatively, the individual vessels can be dissected free with a right angle clamp and clips can be placed on each vessel (Fig. 7). Although some authors advocate this technique with the distributive vascular pattern [12], this technique is more time consuming and may be more likely to result in vascular injury or bleeding. In addition, the use of clips in the hilum prevents the subsequent use of a stapling device as a malpositioned clip can result in stapler misfire.

E. Specimen Retrieval

After transection of the vessels, the splenic bed should be inspected for any significant bleeding, which should be immediately controlled if present. The 12 mm port site is then exchanged for an 18 mm port through which a specimen retrieval bag can be delivered. Our preference is to use a bag preattached to an expandable ring (Endocatch II, US

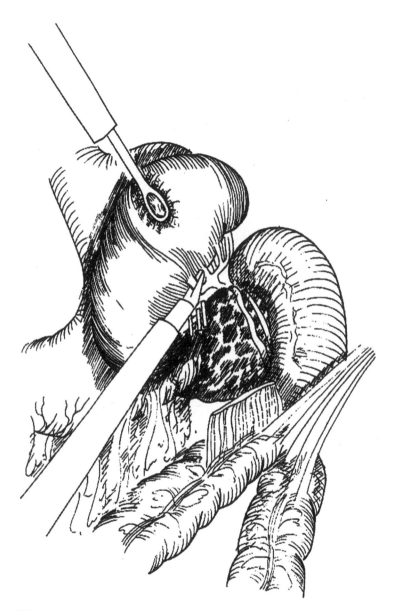

Figure 7   Hilar dissection and ligation of the splenic artery and vein with clips.

Surgical Corp., Norwalk, CT), although other entrapment sacs are available. Of primary importance is that the bag is of adequate strength to resist puncture so that intra-abdominal dissemination of splenic tissue and the resulting splenosis does not occur. The spleen is then scooped into the bag as it is deployed (Fig. 8). Once the spleen is completely inside the bag, it is closed by a pursestring suture at its apex, which is then externalized after removal of the 18 mm port. The spleen is then removed piecemeal with the digital fracture technique, being cautious to protect the wound from contamination with splenic tissue. A ring forceps is used to assist in removal of the splenic fragments (Fig. 9).

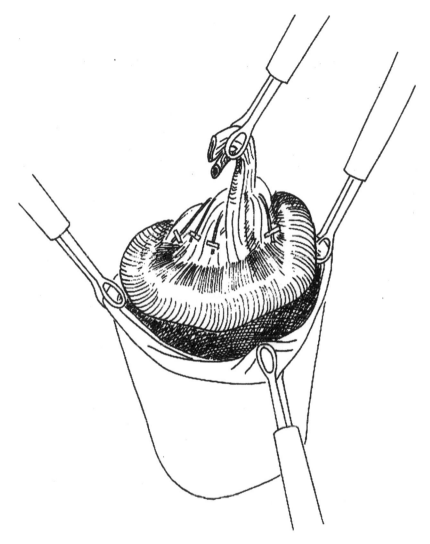

Figure 8 Placing the spleen within the entrapment sack.

F. Closure

The 18 mm port is reinserted, and the left upper quadrant is inspected for bleeding and irrigated thoroughly. A drain should be inserted if there is any concern that the pancreatic parenchyma has been violated or in patients who may be at increased risk for postoperative bleeding (e.g., splenomegaly). The abdomen is then desufflated and the fascia at all port sites ≥ 10 mm are closed. The skin incisions are closed subcutaneously and steri-strips are left in place. The beanbag is released and the patient is rolled supine and awakened from anesthesia.

G. Hand-Assisted Technique

The hand-assist device may be placed at a variety of locations depending on the patient's size and body habitus, the spleen size, and the preferred operating position of the surgeon.

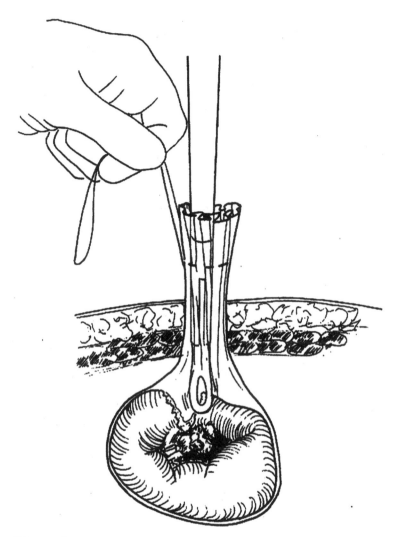

Figure 9 Extraction of the spleen from the abdomen.

The incision should be placed so that the surgeon can insert the non-dominant hand and use the laparoscopic instruments in the dominant hand (Fig. 10). The length of the incision should match the width of the surgeon's hand and should be placed so that one can reach the limits of the spleen superiorly. The hand-port device may be placed either as the initial peritoneal access or it can be inserted after laparoscopic inspection of the peritoneal cavity and assessment of splenic size. The surgeon's hand can then be used to facilitate exposure, retraction, and manipulation of the spleen and to tamponade bleeding vessels should it be necessary.

VI. POSTOPERATIVE CARE

The urinary catheter is usually removed the morning after surgery provided there is adequate urine output, and the diet is advanced as tolerated. All patients should have a

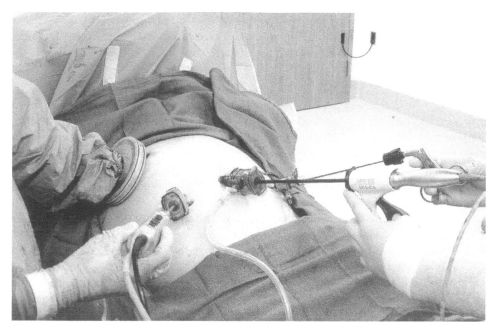

Figure 10 Use of the hand-port device during a laparoscopic splenectomy in a patient with splenomegaly.

complete blood count (CBC) done in the recovery room and the morning of postoperative day one. More frequent monitoring of the hematological status may be necessary depending on the preoperative levels and the specific underlying disease. Most patients with ITP can be discharged the day after surgery, providing the hematocrit is stable and their general medical condition allows. Patients who have undergone difficult splenectomies or who have had a hand-port incision usually require an additional 1–2 days of observation.

Complications after laparoscopic splenectomy appear to occur with less frequency than after open splenectomy [4,13,14], but few studies have addressed this issue prospectively. The most frequent operative complications appear to be hemorrhagic (wound hematoma, intra-abdominal bleeding) and infectious (pneumonia, wound infection), although, as discussed above, pancreatic injuries are not uncommon. Most of the well-known complications of abdominal surgery, including deep venous thrombosis, atelectasis, and ileus, have been described after laparoscopic splenectomy. Other more unusual complications, such as diaphragmatic perforation and portal vein thrombosis, have also been reported. It should be emphasized that any patient with an atypical course after laparoscopic splenectomy, including abdominal pain, fever, or leukocytosis, should be thoroughly evaluated (including abdominal imaging) to exclude operative complications. Although the complication rates vary widely (see Table 4) and depend on the vigor with which they are sought, the range appears to be on the order of 5–15%.

Using multivariate analysis, one group [15] reported that the principal predictors of complications after laparoscopic splenectomy were patient age, splenomegaly, and diagnosis of a malignant neoplasm. Others have shown that patients with a hematological malignancy have increased morbidity [3] and require longer hospital stays [6] than patients with benign disease. However, in a small series, one group [16] showed that patients with non-Hodgkin's lymphoma can be operated on safely and with equivalent outcomes to patients with benign hematological disease.

VII. OUTCOMES

Laparoscopic splenectomy has been shown to result in less postoperative pain, shorter length of hospital stay, and faster return to diet when compared retrospectively to open splenectomy [13–15]. In addition, it has resulted in less intraoperative blood loss and may be associated with lower overall hospital costs [14]. However, laparoscopic splenectomy has almost uniformly been associated with significantly longer operative times, especially early in a surgeon's experience [13–15]. Table 4 summarizes the results from several recent large series of laparoscopic splenectomies. The conversion rate for surgeons after the learning curve is on the order of 3% with an average operating time of 2–3 hours. Most patients are discharged by postoperative day 3, and the mortality rate is as low as 0.2%.

Another important outcome measure of splenectomy is its ability to reverse the underlying disease process, which is of particular concern for patients with ITP. In two studies [3,17] with 30–38 months mean follow-up, 78–82% of patients experienced long-term surgical cure (normal platelet counts and no medical therapy). This number is similar to the success rates after open splenectomy, but longer follow-up in larger numbers of patients will be required to draw firm conclusions. Of particular interest is the retrieval rate for accessory spleens, which has ranged from 12 to 18% in the series shown in Table 4. These results are similar to the rate of identification of accessory spleens in open splenectomy, although the experience of the surgeon undoubtedly plays a role.

VIII. CURRENT STATUS AND FUTURE INVESTIGATION

Presently, laparoscopic splenectomy is considered the preferred approach for patients with normal-sized spleens who require splenectomy. In the hands of experienced laparoscopic surgeons with a large volume of laparoscopic splenectomies, the indications for this approach are continuously expanding. With the introduction of hand-assisted techniques, even patients with significant splenomegaly are able to realize the benefits of a minimally invasive approach. Because the reversal or palliation of the underlying disease is an

Table 4   Results of Major Splenectomy Series

	Ref. 17	Ref. 3	Ref. 18	Ref. 19	Total
Number	103	111	204	100	518
OR time (min)	161	153	145	170	155
Conversion rate (%)	4	8	3	3	4
Accessory spleens (%)	17	14	12	13	14
ITP (%)	65	43	64	45	56
Mean spleen weight (g)	263	634	289	375	379
Length of stay (d)	2.5	4	2.7	3.3	3.0
Complications (%)	6	17	8.4	10	9.4
Mortality (%)	0	0	0	1	0.2

important outcome variable, the long-term outcomes for patients with hematological diseases will need to be carefully examined.

IX. TOP TEN SURGICAL TIPS

1. A semi-lateral decubitus position gives optimal access to and exposure of the spleen, as well as the rest of the abdominal cavity and facilitates conversion to open splenectomy if necessary.
2. Anesthetic preparation should include at least one large-bore peripheral intravenous (iv) line and a type and screen for blood (a type and cross-match and two iv lines for splenomegaly or any potentially difficult case).
3. Adequate mobilization of the splenic flexure of the colon is an important initial step and must be done carefully to avoid colonic injury.
4. Complete dissection of the splenorenal ligament facilitates medial rotation of the spleen and posterior exposure of the hilum.
5. The gastrosplenic ligament including the short gastric vessels should be divided to the diaphragm with an ultrasonic coagulator.
6. Isolation of the splenic artery in the lesser sac at the superior border of the pancreas should be considered in patients in whom a difficult hilar dissection is anticipated or patients with splenomegaly or marked thrombocytopenia.
7. Keep the field of dissection as free of blood as possible. If progress is significantly slowed, consider placing a hand-port device. If there is ongoing or uncontrolled bleeding, convert to an open operation.
8. Use a hand-port device to aid in the dissection for difficult cases or for patients with moderate splenomegaly (> 20 cm spleen).
9. Be prepared to suture if necessary to control contractile short gastric vessels, bleeding at the splenic hilum, or bleeding on the surface of the pancreas.
10. Leave a closed-suction drain if there is concern about injury to the tail of the pancreas or after difficult cases.

SELECTED READINGS

1. Terrosu G, Baccarani U, Bresadola V, Sistu MA, Uzzau A, Bresadola F. The impact of splenic weight on laparoscopic splenectomy for splenomegaly. Surg Endosc 2002; 16:103–107.
2. Targarona EM, Espert JJ, Balague C, Piulachs J, Artigas V, Trias M. Splenomegaly should not be considered a contraindication for laparoscopic splenectomy. Ann Surg 1998; 228:35–39.
3. Trias M, Targarona EM, Espert JJ, Cerdan G, Bombuy E, Vidal O, Artigas V. Impact of hematologic diagnosis on early and late outcome after laparoscopic splenectomy: an analysis of 111 cases. Surg Endosc 2000; 14:556–560.
4. Targarona EM, Espert JJ, Cerdan G, Balague C, Piulachs J, Sugranes G, Artigas V, Trias M. Effect of spleen size on splenectomy outcome: a comparison of open and laparoscopic surgery. Surg Endosc 1999; 13:559–562.
5. Targarona EM, Balague C, Cerdan G, Espert JJ, Lacy AM, Visa J, Trias M. Hand-assisted laparoscopic splenectomy (HALS) in cases of splenomegaly: a comparison analysis with conventional laparoscopic splenectomy. Surg Endosc 2002; 16:426–430.

6. Berman RS, Yahanda AM, Mansfield PF, Hemmila MR, Sweeney JF, Porter GA, M\Kumparatana M, Leroux B, Pollock RE, Feig BW. Laparoscopic splenectomy in patients with hematologic malignancies. Am J Surg 1999; 178:530–536.

7. Heniford BT, Park A, Walsh M, Kercher KW, Matthews BD, Frenetta G, Sing RF. Laparoscopic splenectomy in patients with normal-sized spleens versus splenomegaly: does size matter? Am Surg 2001; 67:854–858.

8. Poulin E, Mamazza J, Schlachta C. Splenic artery embolization before laparoscopic splenectomy. Surg Endosc 1998; 12:870–875.

9. Park A, Gagner M, Pomp A. The lateral approach to laparoscopic splenectomy. Am J Surg 1997; 173:126–130.

10. Katkhouda N, Hurwitz MB, Rivera RT, Chandra M, Waldrep D, Gugenheim Z. Laparoscopic splenectomy; outcome and efficacy in 103 consecutive patients. Ann Surg 1998; 228:568–578.

11. Chand B, Walsh RM, Ponsky J, Brody F. Pancreatic complications following laparoscopic splenectomy. Surg Endosc 2001; 15:1273–1276.

12. Katkhouda N, Mavor E. Laparoscopic splenectomy. Surg Clin North Am 2000; 80:1285–1297.

13. Brunt LM, Langer JC, Quasebarth MA, Whitman ED. Comparative analysis of laparoscopic versus open splenectomy. Am J Surg 1996; 172:596–601.

14. Park A, Marcaccio M, Sternbach M, Witzke D, Fitzgerald P. Laparoscopic vs open splenectomy. Arch Surg 1999; 134:1263–1269.

15. Targarona EM, Espert JJ, Bombuy E, Vidal O, Cerdan G, Artigas V, Trias M. Complications of laparoscopic splenectomy. Arch Surg 2000; 135:1137–1140.

16. Walsh M, Heniford BT. Laparoscopic splenectomy for non-Hodgkin lymphoma. J Surg Oncol 1999; 70:116–121.

17. Katkhouda N, Grant SW, Mavor E, Friedlander MH, Lord RV, Achanta K, Essani R, Mason R. Predictors of response after laparoscopic splenectomy for immune thrombocytopenic purpura. Surg Endosc 2001; 15:484–488.

18. Park A, Birgisson G, Mastrangelo MJ, Marcaccio MJ, Witzke D. Laparoscopic splenectomy: outcomes and lessons learned from over 200 cases. Surgery 2000; 128:660–667.

19. Brodsky JA, Brody FJ, Walsh RM, Malm JA, Ponsky JL. Laparoscopic splenectomy: experience with 100 cases. Surg Endosc 2002; 16:851–854.

20. Anglin B, Rutherford C, Ramos R, Lieser M, Jones DB. Immune thrombocytopenia purpura in pregnancy: laparoscopic treatment. JSLS 2001; 5:63–67.

32

Adrenalectomy

L. MICHAEL BRUNT

Institute for Minimally Invasive Surgery
Washington University School of Medicine
St. Louis, Missouri, U.S.A.

I. INTRODUCTION

Surgery is the primary treatment for adrenal masses that are hormonally functional or malignant. Adrenal disorders present with a wide variety of clinical manifestations, depending on the underlying pathophysiology. Specific indications for adrenalectomy are listed in the box. Over the last decade, laparoscopic adrenalectomy has become the procedure of choice for removal of most adrenal neoplasms. Factors to consider in choosing the best method of adrenalectomy for a given patient include the preoperative diagnosis, the size of the adrenal mass, the potential for malignancy, the occurrence of extra-adrenal or bilateral disease, invasion of adjacent structures, and individual patient characteristics. The traditional anterior transabdominal approach through a midline or bilateral subcostal incision is now used primarily for large primary adrenal malignancies or invasive adrenal tumors. The open posterior approach provides more limited access to each adrenal and has been almost completely replaced by laparoscopic adrenalectomy.

Laparoscopic adrenalectomy has several advantages over open adrenalectomy, including less postoperative ileus, decreased postoperative pain, a shorter hospitalization, and a faster return to full unrestricted activity. However, the surgeon performing laparoscopic adrenalectomy must be familiar with adrenal anatomy and the techniques for performing open adrenalectomy because of the potential for conversion to an open procedure. Before an adrenalectomy is performed, whether laparoscopic or open, the surgeon must confirm a correct preoperative diagnosis, exclude a pheochromocytoma, and localize the lesion to the correct adrenal gland. Specific tumors require specialized preoperative patient preparation for a successful surgical outcome as discussed below.

The indications for adrenalectomy are shown in Table 1.

Table 1   Indications for Adrenalectomy

Open anterior transabdominal approach
  Any locally invasive primary adrenal mass
  Adrenocortical carcinoma >6 cm
  Large tumor size (>10–12 cm)
Open posterior adrenalectomy
  Small (<5 cm) tumor with an existing contraindication to a laparoscopic approach
Laparoscopic Adrenalectomy
  Unilateral
    Cortisol-producing adenoma causing Cushing's syndrome
    Aldosteronoma
    Pheochromocytoma: familial or sporadic; bilateral adrenalectomy may be required in patients
      with hereditary pheochromocytoma and bilateral tumors
    Adrenal metastasis (isolated, well circumscribed)
    Nonfunctioning adrenal adenoma (>4 cm or atypical imaging characteristics)
  Bilateral
    Failed treatment of ACTH-dependent Cushing's syndrome
  Primary adrenal hyperplasia causing Cushing's syndrome
    Bilateral pheochromocytomas
  More difficult laparoscopic cases
    Large tumors
    Obese patients, especially patients with Cushing's syndrome
    Pheochromocytomas
    Adrenal metastases

II.   DIAGNOSIS AND PREOPERATIVE PREPARATION

A.   Pheochromocytoma

The diagnosis of pheochromocytoma is established by demonstrating elevated plasma levels of fractionated metanephrines or elevated 24-hour urinary catecholamines and metabolites and by radiographic localization with computed tomography (CT) or magnetic resonance imaging (MRI). MRI is the preferred imaging modality in most institutions because pheochromocytomas typically have a bright adrenal appearance on T2-weighted imaging. Once a pheochromocytoma is diagnosed, the main goal of preoperative management is to control hypertension and tachycardia. α-Adrenergic receptor blockade should be initiated by administering phenoxybenzamine, usually at a starting dose of 10 mg every 12 hours. The dose is increased over 5–7 days until blood pressure is controlled and paroxysms no longer occur. Postural hypotension usually develops with appropriate α-blockade, and symptomatic patients may require preoperative hospitalization and administration of intravenous fluids. Additional β-blockade is sometimes necessary for patients with persistent tachycardia, catecholamine-induced arrhythmias, or predominantly epinephrine–secreting tumors. β-Antagonists should be administered only after stable α-adrenergic blockade has been achieved to avoid unopposed α-receptor stimulation. Hypertensive crisis and sudden death have been reported in patients with undiagnosed pheochromocytomas and inadequate α-blockade who undergo invasive procedures, such as needle biopsy or surgery.

The metabolic effects of catecholamines and decreased perfusion from vasoconstriction often cause lactic acidosis. During the operative procedure, the electrocardiogram, pulse oximetry, and blood pressure (via an arterial line) are continuously monitored. Central venous lines and Swan-Ganz catheters are reserved for patients with significant associated cardiac abnormalities. Adequate fluid replacement is crucial. Intraoperative hypotension is managed with volume resuscitation and occasionally with intravenous administration of pressors. Acute episodes of hypertension and arrhythmia are most likely to occur during the induction of anesthesia, intubation, initial CO_2 insufflation, or manipulation of the tumor. Nitroprusside may be administered intravenously to control hypertensive exacerbations intraoperatively. Propranolol may be given for tachycardia or ventricular ectopy. These measures have substantially reduced the morbidity and mortality associated with surgical resection of pheochromocytoma.

B. Aldosteronoma

The diagnosis of primary aldosteronism is based on the clinical presentation (diastolic hypertension, hypokalemia) and by demonstration of elevated plasma aldosterone levels and suppressed plasma renin activity. The most common cause of primary aldosteronism is an aldosterone-secreting adenoma. These tumors are generally small (1–2 cm) and must be differentiated from bilateral idiopathic adrenal hyperplasia, which is treated medically rather than by adrenalectomy. Differentiation between an aldosteronoma and idiopathic adrenal hyperplasia can be achieved by abdominal CT that shows a unilateral adrenal mass (> 1 cm) and a normal contralateral adrenal. Patients with bilateral adrenal abnormalities or those who have microadenomas (< 1 cm) should undergo further testing with adrenal vein sampling to determine if the source of increased aldosterone production lateralizes to one adrenal. Spironolactone, an aldosterone antagonist, can be given preoperatively to facilitate correction of hypokalemia and hypertension. Clinical assessment for evidence of cardiac failure and renal insufficiency may be necessary in severe, long-standing cases.

C. Cushing's Syndrome

Cushing's syndrome may be caused by either primary adrenal or adrenocorticotropic hormone (ACTH)–dependent (pituitary Cushing's, ectopic ACTH production) sources. Adrenalectomy is indicated for primary adrenal sources of Cushing's syndrome and for patients who have failed treatment of ACTH-dependent Cushing's. The diagnosis of hypercortisolism is made by demonstrating elevated 24-hour urinary free cortisol levels or by failure to suppress plasma cortisol levels to lower than 3–5 µg/dL after administration of 1 mg of dexamethasone (overnight or low-dose dexamethasone suppression test). Once the diagnosis of hypercortisolism is established, ACTH-dependent causes of Cushing's syndrome should be differentiated from primary adrenal causes by measurement of plasma ACTH. If the plasma ACTH is low or suppressed, a primary adrenal source is likely and adrenal imaging with CT or MRI is the next step. All patients undergoing resection of an adrenal mass or cortical hyperplasia causing hypercortisolism are treated postoperatively with stress steroid doses since the hypothalamus-pituitary-adrenal is suppressed. Perioperative mineralocorticoid therapy is needed only when both adrenal glands are removed.

D. Adrenocortical Carcinoma

Adrenocortical cancers are rare tumors with an incidence of approximately 1 in 1.7 million. Cancer should be suspected in any adrenal cortical tumor larger than 6 cm in diameter, since the incidence of cancer increases with increasing tumor size. Smaller tumors causing Cushing's syndrome with concomitant evidence of virilization must also be regarded as suspicious for carcinoma. Adrenocortical cancers have an image intensity equivalent to the liver on T2-weighted MRI. Resection of all gross tumor with negative margins at the initial operation offers the best potential for cure. Complete abdominal exploration is essential, and invasion of adjacent organs including the kidney, liver, pancreas, bowel, or diaphragm necessitates resection of part or all of the involved tissues en bloc. Abdominal and chest CT, MRI, venacavogram, caval ultrasonography, bowel preparation, and confirmation of bilateral kidney function may be necessary preoperatively. At this time, the laparoscopic approach is contraindicated for primary adrenocortical tumors greater than 6 cm in size because of the high risk of malignancy and local invasiveness. Open adrenalectomy via a subcostal incision is the preferred approach.

E. Adrenal Incidentaloma

Unexpected adrenal masses are identified on approximately 0.4–4.0% of high-resolution abdominal CT scans obtained to evaluate extra-adrenal pathology. Although a great majority of incidentally discovered adrenal tumors are nonfunctioning benign adenomas that do not require adrenalectomy, hormonally functional or malignant adrenal tumors must be identified and resected. The patient with an adrenal incidentaloma should undergo a careful clinical history and examination to elicit possible signs and symptoms of excessive adrenal function. Most of these patients are asymptomatic, however, and, therefore, should undergo specific biochemical evaluation to exclude a functioning tumor. The biochemical evaluation should consist of an overnight dexamethasone test to exclude hypercortisolism, fractionated plasma metanephrines or urinary catecholamines and metabolites to rule out a pheochromocytoma, and for patients with hypertension and/or hypokalemia, plasma aldosterone, and renin concentrations. An elevated plasma aldosterone–to–renin ratio of greater than 20 should lead to further testing for primary hyperaldosteronism.

The size of the adrenal lesion as seen on imaging is an important factor in differentiating benign from malignant tumors, because the incidence of cancer in solid adrenal cortical lesions greatly increases as tumor diameter exceeds 6 cm. Adrenalectomy is indicated for large adrenal masses >4–5 cm in diameter or for lesions with suspicious imaging characteristics regardless of functional status. Radiographic imaging may provide additional information in distinguishing benign from malignant adrenal tumors. Cortical adenomas typically have low attenuation values (<10 Hounsfeld units) on unenhanced CT scans, whereas malignant lesions have higher attenuation values (>18 Hounsfeld units). On T2-weighted MRI, both primary adrenocortical and metastatic carcinomas have a signal intensity equivalent to or slightly brighter than the liver, and pheochromocytomas appear three times brighter than the liver, whereas adenomas appear darker than the liver. Benign adrenal adenomas, which have a greater lipid component than malignant lesions do, show a loss of signal intensity on MRI opposed-phase gradient echo images compared with in-phase images, whereas malignant lesions maintain similar signal intensities on both image types.

Fine needle aspiration (FNA) biopsy is rarely indicated in the diagnostic algorithm of an adrenal mass because of the inability to differentiate benign from malignant primary adrenal neoplasms. The principal role of FNA is in the evaluation of suspected adrenal metastases that are not amenable to surgical resection and in which a tissue diagnosis would effect a change in therapy. No adrenal lesions should ever be biopsied unless a pheochromocytoma has first been excluded biochemically because of the potential for triggering a life-threatening hypertensive crisis.

Patients with nonfunctioning adrenal adenomas <4 cm in size that have a benign radiographic appearance do not require adrenalectomy. Each patient should be reexamined for the development of clinical signs or symptoms of adrenal hyperfunction within 6 months. Adrenal CT should be repeated at 4 and 12 months to reassess the size of the mass; growth of the lesion mandates surgical resection. If the patient is asymptomatic and there is no change in the adrenal mass on CT at 12 months, further follow-up studies are not warranted.

F. Adrenal Metastases

The adrenal gland is a common site for metastases, most of which occur in the setting of obvious metastatic disease in other sites. Tumors that metastasize to the adrenal most often include carcinomas of the breast, lung, kidney, melanoma, and lymphoma. Resection of an adrenal metastasis is indicated only in the setting of a localized, solitary adrenal lesion and no extra-adrenal tumor. Laparoscopic adrenalectomy may be appropriate for carefully selected patients provided the tumor is not excessively large, it is well circumscribed, and the surgeon is highly experienced in the laparoscopic approach.

III. OPERATIVE TREATMENT

A variety of laparoscopic approaches to adrenalectomy have been described, including the transabdominal lateral flank approach, the anterior transabdominal approach, and the retroperitoneal endoscopic approach. Advantages of the transabdominal lateral flank approach include a large working space, easy access high within the retroperitoneum, and simplified exposure of the adrenal glands by gravity retraction of adjacent organs. Laparoscopic surgeons are most familiar with the view provided by the anterior transabdominal approach, but this approach requires placement of additional ports, may be associated with longer operating times, and requires more effort to retract adjacent organs for adequate exposure. The retroperitoneal endoscopic approach avoids entry into the peritoneal cavity but is limited by a smaller working space, which presents difficulties for patients with large tumors or large amounts of retroperitoneal fat. Our preferred operative approach to laparoscopic adrenalectomy is the transabdominal lateral flank approach, which will be described in detail.

A. Operating Room and Patient Setup

General anesthesia is induced with the patient in the supine position. An orogastric tube and a urinary catheter are inserted for gastric and bladder decompression. The patient is then placed in the lateral decubitus position with the affected side rotated upward (Fig. 1, top). This position, along with the subsequent tilting of the operating table in reverse Trendelenburg position, allows the intra-abdominal contents to fall away from the sites of port placement and the area of the dissection. A bean bag mattress is used to secure the patient to the operating table. Pressure points, especially the axilla, are well padded. The arm is positioned over the head and supported. The operating table is then flexed at the waist to allow greater access to the flank region for placement of laparoscopic ports. Monitors are positioned at the head of the table on each side. For right adrenalectomy, the surgeon stands at the patient's back, and the assistant and laparoscope operator generally stand on the abdominal side of the table.

For left adrenalectomy, the surgeon stands on the patient's right or abdominal side. The equipment and instruments required are:

One 10/11 mm and three 5 mm laparoscopic ports
30° laparoscope (5 mm)
Pressurized irrigation/suction cannula
5 mm atraumatic graspers
5 mm scissors
Hook electrocautery
10 mm curved or right angle dissector
9/11 mm clip applier
Atraumatic retractor (required for retraction of the right lobe of the liver during right adrenalectomy but optional for left adrenalectomy)
Impermeable entrapment sack for specimen removal
Ultrasonic coagulator (optional)
Laparoscopic ultrasound (optional)

B. Surgical Technique

1. Port Placement

A 5 mm incision is made just medial to the anterior axillary line, two fingerbreadths below the costal margin (Fig. 1, bottom). Initial access to the peritoneal cavity is usually achieved by a closed technique with a Veress needle inserted through this incision. Alternatively, an open insertion technique can be used with a Hasson-type cannula. After establishing pneumoperitoneum, a 5 mm port is placed into the peritoneal cavity at this site; a direct view optical trocar may be useful to view placement of this first trocar. The laparoscope is inserted through this port and the underlying viscera are visualized to assess for any injury. The laparoscope then guides placement of the remaining ports under direct vision in sequence from anterior to posterior. One port should be 10/11 mm to allow placement of the clip applier. It is important to allow at least 5 cm of space between the different port entry sites so that instruments may be maneuvered through the ports without impedance. On the left side, some dissection of the retroperitoneum and mobilization of the splenic flexure of the colon is required before the most dorsal or posterior port can be placed. The liver and upper abdomen should be inspected for evidence of other pathology. It is especially important to examine the liver in patients with pheochromocytomas and multiple endocrine neoplasia type 2 because of the potential for metastatic medullary thyroid carcinoma.

2. Exposure of the Retroperitoneal Space and Adrenal Glands

The right and left retroperitoneal spaces and each adrenal gland are exposed with the laparoscope placed in the second port, a grasper or retractor inserted through the most

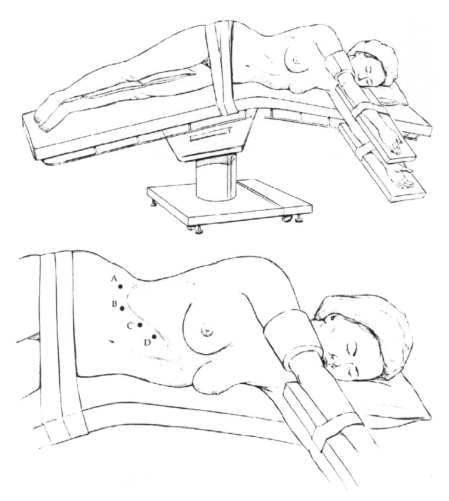

Figure 1 Positioning of patient for laparoscopic right adrenalectomy. (Top) The patient is placed in the lateral decubitus position with the affected side rotated upward and with the operating table flexed at the waist and in reverse Trendelenburg position. (Bottom) Port placement for laparoscopic adrenalectomy. Initial access is usually obtained at site C, and the other ports are then inserted under direct laparoscopic vision. Left adrenalectomy may be carried out using only 3 ports. (From Brunt LM. Laparoscopic adrenalectomy. In: Eubanks WS, Swanstrom LL, Soper NJ. *Mastery of Endoscopic and Laparoscopic Surgery*, Lippincott Williams & Wilkins, 2000; p. 324.)

medial port, and dissecting instruments manipulated through the more lateral ports. For right adrenalectomy, the initial step is mobilization of the right hepatic lobe by incising the triangular ligament all the way to the diaphragm (Fig. 2). It is rarely necessary to mobilize the hepatic flexure of the colon. Once the liver has been partially mobilized, a retractor is placed through the most medial port to retract the right hepatic lobe anteriorly and medially. Division of the hepatic ligaments with cautery continues while the liver is retracted medially away from the retroperitoneum. The right adrenal gland is identified in the perinephric fat posterolateral to the vena cava and superior to the right kidney.

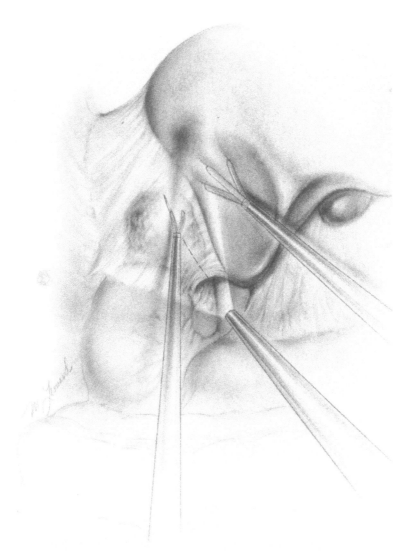

Figure 2 Exposure of the right adrenal gland. Access to the right retroperitoneum is gained by incising the triangular ligament lateral to the right lobe of the liver. (From Brunt LM. Laparoscopic adrenalectomy. In: Eubanks WS, Swanstrom LL, Soper NJ. *Mastery of Endoscopic and Laparoscopic Surgery,* Lippincott Williams & Wilkins, 2000; p. 325.)

The left adrenal gland is exposed by first mobilizing the left colon and spleen. The attachments of the splenic flexure of the colon are divided with either cautery scissors or an ultrasonic coagulator. With sufficient dissection, the colon falls away from the spleen and retroperitoneum. If needed, a more dorsal fourth port can then be safely inserted. The splenorenal ligament is next divided to the diaphragm using cautery, which allows the spleen to fall anteriorly and medially away from the retroperitoneum (Fig. 3). With adequate mobilization and proper positioning of the patient and table, minimal retraction of the spleen is required because it is displaced by gravity away from the adrenal gland.

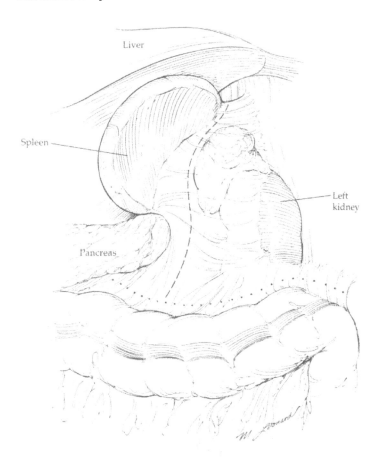

Figure 3 Exposure of the left adrenal gland. After the splenic flexure of the colon has been mobilized (dotted line), the splenorenal ligament (dashed line) is incised and divided all the way up to the diaphragm. Perinephric fat is visualized and the left adrenal gland is identified superior to the left kidney, in close association with the aorta, pancreas, stomach, kidney, and renal vessels. (From Brunt LM. Laparoscopic adrenalectomy. In: Eubanks WS, Swanstrom LL, Soper NJ. *Mastery of Endoscopic and Laparoscopic Surgery*, Lippincott Williams & Wilkins, 2000; p. 326.)

One should avoid dissecting posterior to the kidney to prevent the kidney from falling forward and interfering with the exposure. It is also usually necessary to mobilize the tail of the pancreas away from the renal hilum in order to expose the inferior aspect of the adrenal and gland and left adrenal vein. The left adrenal gland is buried in the perinephric fat, closely applied to the superior pole of the left kidney, near the aorta, pancreas, stomach, and renal vessels.

3. Dissection of the Adrenal Gland

Once the retroperitoneum is entered and the fourth port is placed, the perinephric fat superior to the kidney is dissected with electrocautery to uncover and identify the adrenal gland. Laparoscopic ultrasound may be useful in more precisely localizing the adrenal gland and tumor, especially the left adrenal in obese patients and those with Cushing's syndrome. Ultrasound is rarely needed to localize the right adrenal. When the adrenal gland is uncovered, an atraumatic grasping forceps are used to gently retract the gland and any associated mass by grasping the periadrenal fat or gently pushing the gland. One should avoid grasping the adrenal gland or tumor directly, because the gland is fragile, bleeds easily, and there is the potential for spillage of tumor.

The adrenal gland is bluntly dissected from surrounding tissues beginning at its medial margin and proceeding superiorly and inferiorly. On the right side, the connective tissue between the adrenal gland and inferior vena cava is dissected with the hook cautery, and the adrenal is gradually mobilized off the vena cava. One must be aware of the location of the vena cava at all times to avoid injury to it. The right adrenal vein is hidden at the gland's medial aspect, is short (approximately 1 cm long), and empties directly into the inferior vena cava (Fig. 4a). It should be carefully isolated with a right angle dissector and then gently clipped and divided with two clips on the vena cava side. Care should be taken to not dislodge the clips during the subsequent dissection, which could result in major hemorrhage from the vena cava. For the left adrenal, a single long vein lies at the inferomedial aspect of the gland and empties into the left renal vein; the inferior phrenic vein usually joins the left adrenal vein proximal to its junction with the renal vein (Fig. 4b). Clipping the adrenal vein early in the course of dissection may be desirable when one is resecting a pheochromocytoma, because manipulation of these tumors may result in catecholamine release into the systemic circulation and significant intraoperative hypertensive paroxysms and tachycardia.

Once the adrenal vein is clipped and divided, the numerous small arteries that enter the gland at its superior, medial, and inferior margins are either cauterized or divided with the ultrasonic coagulator as encountered. On the left side, arterial branches also enter the gland laterally along the superior pole of the kidney. Incomplete hemostasis of the small arteries may lead to a small amount of bleeding, which obscures vision under magnification of the laparoscope and greatly increases the difficulty of the dissection. Once freed from all retroperitoneal attachments, the gland is then placed into an impermeable entrapment sack for removal. After the incision is slightly enlarged, the sack containing the adrenal gland is withdrawn through the most medial port site. The operative bed is irrigated and hemostasis is confirmed. The adrenal vein pedicle should be visualized to ensure that the clips are securely in place. The fascia at all 10 mm port sites is then closed with absorbable sutures. The orogastric tube and urinary catheter are removed in the operating room after wound closure.

IV. POSTOPERATIVE CARE

Patients usually require only limited parenteral analgesic medications after laparoscopic adrenalectomy; most patients are taking oral pain medications only by the first postoperative day. A liquid diet is started when the patient is fully awake and is advanced as tolerated. Most patients can be discharged from the hospital by postoperative day 1 or 2.

Patients with an adrenal tumor causing Cushing's syndrome must receive glucocorticoids postoperatively but do not require mineralocorticoid replacement. Hydrocortisone should be administered at a maintenance dose of $12-15$ mg/m^2 each day. Glucocorticoid therapy is tapered when the hypothalamic-pituitary-adrenal axis recovers (based on symptoms and ACTH stimulation testing), which may not occur for up to $12-18$ months postoperatively. Patients who undergo bilateral adrenalectomy require lifelong

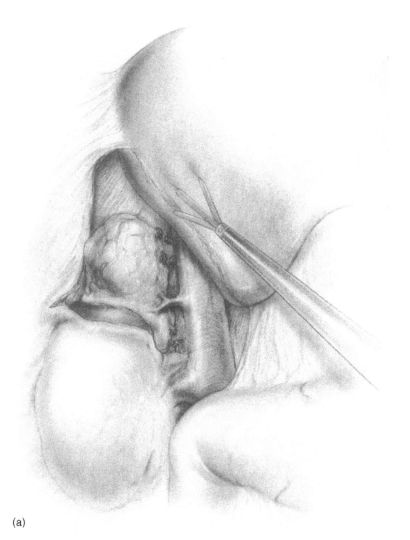

(a)

Figure 4   Adrenal dissection. Retroperitoneal fat is cleared by blunt and cautery dissection to uncover the adrenal gland. The adrenal is gently retracted laterally with atraumatic graspers as the gland is mobilized by blunt dissection, beginning at its medial edge. There are numerous small arteries that circumferentially penetrate the peripheral aspect of each gland, which must be cauterized or coagulated as encountered. Each gland has a single adrenal vein that should be doubly clipped and divided early in the course of dissection. (a) The medial border of the adrenal has been dissected away from the inferior vena cava to expose the right adrenal vein, which is short and is located at the gland's medial aspect. (b) The left adrenal vein is longer and courses along the anteromedial aspect of the gland to drain into the renal vein inferiorly. Note the inferior phrenic vein entering the left adrenal vein proximal to the latter's entry into the renal vein. Dissection continues circumferentially until the entire gland is freed. (From Brunt LM. Laparoscopic adrenalectomy. In: Eubanks WS, Swanstrom LL, Soper NJ. *Mastery of Endoscopic and Laparoscopic Surgery*, Lippincott Williams & Wilkins, 2000; pp. 325, 327.)

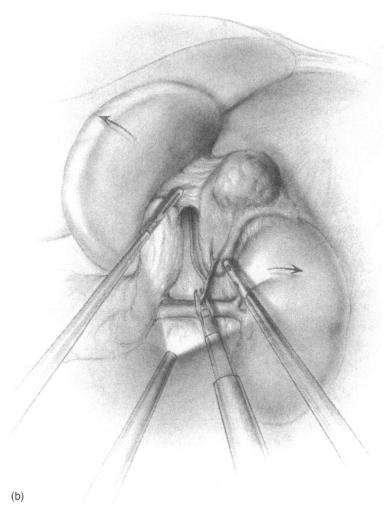

(b)

Figure 4 (*continued*)

mineralocorticoid (fludrocortisone 100 to 200 µg/dL) and glucocorticoid replacement. Patients with pheochromocytomas may require administration of large amounts of intravenous fluids postoperatively because of intravascular volume expansion as a result of the loss of α-receptor agonist activity. These patients are also at risk for developing hypoglycemia because of the loss of inhibition of insulin secretion by circulating catecholamines.

Close patient follow-up is required after resection of all adrenocortical tumors and pheochromocytomas. In patients with adrenocortical malignancies, hormone levels that are elevated preoperatively should be measured periodically. Local recurrences and metastases may be detected by CT or MRI. For pheochromocytomas, plasma fractionated metanephrine levels or 24-hour urinary catecholamine and metanephrine levels should be measured postoperatively and on a yearly basis thereafter. Surgical resection of localized or solitary recurrences or metastases may be indicated.

V. MANAGEMENT OF COMPLICATIONS

One of the principal benefits of the laparoscopic approach to adrenalectomy has been a reduction in the complication rate associated with adrenal surgery. In a recent meta-analysis, the incidence of complications after laparoscopic adrenalectomy was 10.9% compared to 25.2% after open adrenalectomy. This reduction in the complication rate was primarily due to fewer wound, pulmonary, and infectious complications and a decreased incidence of associated organ injury (primarily splenectomy) in the laparoscopic group. Only 3 deaths in over 1500 patients (mortality 0.3%) have been reported following laparoscopic adrenalectomy. The most common complication of laparoscopic adrenalectomy is bleeding, which is also the most common reason for conversion to open adrenalectomy. The incidence of this complication should decrease with increasing operative experience and attention to dissection technique and hemostasis strategies as listed in Table 2. Adrenal vein or vena cava hemorrhage occurs uncommonly, and if laparoscopic control cannot be gained promptly, the patient should be converted to open adrenalectomy without delay. Of the 97 patients treated by laparoscopic adrenalectomy at our institution, there were no emergent conversions to open procedures for uncontrollable hemorrhage; 3 cases were converted (conversion rate 3%) either because of minor bleeding that interfered with the dissection or violation of the adrenal capsule near the tumor.

Other potential sequelae specific to this procedure are listed in Table 2. Hypertensive crises may occur in patients with pheochromocytoma if the diagnosis was not made preoperatively or if the patient did not receive adequate α-adrenergic receptor blockade. Adrenal insufficiency may occur in patients undergoing bilateral adrenalectomy or after

Table 2 Complications of Laparoscopuic Adrenalectomy

Potential complication	Possible prevention
Bleeding	Thorough knowledge of adrenal anatomy and surgical landmarks
	Good exposure, meticulous dissection technique, and hemostasis
	Careful support and retraction of large adrenal masses
	Precise isolation and ligation of the adrenal vein
Hypertensive crisis from pheochromocytoma	Biochemical evaluation preoperatively with plasma fractionated catecholamines or urinary catecholamines/metanephrines
	Preoperative α-receptor blockade in preparation for surgery
Acute postoperative adrenal insufficiency	Exclude subclinical hypercortisolism preoperatively
	Postoperative administration of stress doses of glucocorticoids postoperatively in at-risk patients
Tumor recurrence	Extracapsular dissection of adrenal and tumor
	Open approach for large (>6 cm) adrenal malignancies

resection of a cortisol-producing tumor. Adrenal insufficiency is easily treated once diagnosed but potentially fatal if unrecognized. Symptoms include weakness, fever, leukocytosis (eosinophilia), hypotension, nausea, vomiting, and abdominal pain. A high index of suspicion is necessary to make the diagnosis, and acute adrenal insufficiency should always be included in the differential diagnosis of hypotension postadrenalectomy. All patients with adrenal cortical tumors should be screened for subclincial hypercortisolism preoperatively to avoid this complication. Treatment consists of prompt administration of stress doses of hydrocortisone.

Isolated cases of local and/or disseminated tumor recurrence have recently been reported after laparoscopic adrenalectomy, even for apparently benign lesions, including both adrenal cortical tumors and pheochromocytomas. The extent to which the laparoscopic approach contributed to this complication is not entirely clear, since most of these lesions were removed intact and the recurrences may have been due to the biological behavior of the tumor rather than the dissection technique. In some cases, however, violation of the tumor capsule or tumor disruption occurred during the dissection. These reports emphasize the importance of extracapsular dissection of the gland, removal of an intact specimen, and, in the absence of more extensive long-term follow-up data, selecting an open approach in patients with large, potentially malignant or invasive adrenal tumors.

VI. OUTCOMES AND COSTS

In early series, operative times for laparoscopic adrenalectomy have averaged 2–3 hours and have been significantly longer than that for either open transabdominal or open posterior retroperitoneal adrenalectomy. However, operative times have decreased with increasing laparoscopic experience. Bilateral laparoscopic adrenalectomy is a significantly longer procedure because entirely separate operative approaches and patient repositioning are required for each adrenal gland. Short-term follow-up indicates that laparoscopic adrenalectomy for the resection of small adrenal tumors may be accomplished safely and with less operative blood loss, decreased parenteral pain requirements, less postoperative morbidity, more rapid hospital discharge, and a shorter rehabilitation period when compared with traditional open adrenalectomy procedures. Laparoscopic adrenalectomy also appears equivalent in cost to open posterior adrenalectomy and is somewhat less expensive than open transabdominal adrenalectomy. Prospective analyses of outcomes and costs comparing the laparoscopic and open approaches for adrenalectomy have not been done. Costs should also decrease with decreasing operative times and shortened hospitalizations.

VII. CURRENT STATUS AND FUTURE INVESTIGATION

Laparoscopic adrenalectomy has supplanted open adrenalectomy as the procedure of choice for most patients with adrenal tumors. This approach has many advantages for these patients, including a reduction in the complication rate. Current issues of controversy include the size limitation for attempting laparoscopic adrenalectomy and the role of this procedure in removing well-circumscribed lesions that appear malignant or have malignant potential. Surgeons who undertake laparoscopic adrenalectomy should be intimately familiar with adrenal anatomy, should understand the pathophysiology, clinical presentation, and diagnostic evaluation of functional tumors, and should be skilled in advanced laparoscopic skills.

VIII. TOP TEN SURGICAL TIPS

1. Ensure a correct preoperative diagnosis with complete biochemical work-up and precise tumor localization.

2. Select patients carefully for a laparoscopic approach according to surgeon experience and tumor characteristics. Avoid difficult cases early in one's laparoscopic experience. Use open adrenalectomy for large primary adrenal malignancies or locally invasive tumors.

3. Establish proper perioperative pharmacological management: provide stable α-adrenergic blockade and adequate volume replacement for pheochromocytoma; administer stress doses of steroids perioperatively for patients with hypercortisolism.

4. Use the transabdominal lateral flank approach with the table flexed and pad all pressure points.

5. Allow adequate space between the port entry sites and the costal margin so that instruments may be maneuvered freely; use an angled laparoscope for better visualizaton and use 5 mm ports for all sites except the one 10 mm port for placement of the clip applier.

6. Use a laparoscopic ultrasound probe to assist in localizing the adrenal gland and tumor and adjacent vascular structures in difficult cases.

7. Expose the retroperitoneum adequately by dividing the triangular ligament on the right side and the splenorenal ligament on the left.

8. Meticulously ensure hemostasis and maintain extracapsular dissection of the adrenal gland and tumor throughout the procedure. Carefully dissect and apply clips securely to the adrenal vein.

9. Retract the adrenal gland gently and support large adrenal masses carefully to prevent tearing the adrenal vein or disrupting the adrenal parenchyma.

10. Remove the specimen in an entrapment bag; close the fascia at all 10 mm port sites.

SELECTED READINGS

Bonjer H, Berends F, Kazemier G, Steyerberg E, de Herder W, Bruining H. Endoscopic retroperitoneal adrenalectomy: lessons learned form 111 consecutive cases. Ann Surg 2000; 232:796–803.

Brunt LM, Moley JF. Adrenal incidentaloma. World J Surg 2001; 25:905–913.

Brunt L. The positive impact of laparoscopic adrenalectomy on complications of adrenal surgery. Surg Endosc 2001; 16:252–257.

Brunt LM, Bennett HF, Teefey SA, Moley JF, Middleton WF. Laparoscopic ultrasound imaging of adrenal tumors during laparoscopic adrenalectomy. Am J Surg 1999; 178:490–495.

Brunt LM, Doherty GM, Norton JA, Soper NJ, Quasebarth MA, Moley JM. Laparoscopic compared to open adrenalectomy for benign adrenal neoplasms. J Am Coll Surg 1996; 183:1–10.

Brunt LM, Moley JM, M. DG, Lairmore TC, DeBenedetti MK, Quasebarth MA. Outcomes analysis in patients undergoing laparoscopic adrenalectomy for hormonally active adrenal tumors. Surgery 2001; 130:629–635.

Foxius A, Ramboux A, Lefebvre Y, Broze B, Hamels J, Squifflet J-P. Hazards of laparoscopic adrenalectomy for Conn's adenoma. Surg Endosc 1999; 13:715–717.

Gagner M, Lacroix A, Bolte E, Pomp A. Laparoscopic adrenalectomy: the importance of a flank approach in the lateral decubitus position. Surg Endosc 1994; 8:135–138.

Gagner M, Pomp A, Heniford B, Pharand D, Lacroix A. Laparoscopic adrenalectomy: lessons learned from 100 consecutive cases. Ann Surg 1997; 226:238–247.

Heniford BT, Ianniti DA, Hale J, Gagner M. The role of intraoperative ultrasonography during laparoscopic adrenalectomy. Surgery 1997; 122:1068–1074.

Henry J-F, Defechereux T, Raffaelli M, Lubrano D, Gramatica L. Complications of laparoscopic adrenalectomy: results of 169 consecutive cases. World J Surg 2000; 24:1342–1346.

Imai T, Kikumori T, Phiwa M, Mase T, Funahashi H. A case-controlled study of laparoscopic compared with open lateral adrenalectomy. Am J Surg 1999; 178:50–54.

Li ML, Fitzgerald PA, Price DC, Norton JA. Iatrogenic pheochromocytomatosis: a previously unreported result of laparoscopic adrenalectomy. Surgery 2001; 130:1072–1077.

Thompson G, Grant C, van Heerden J, Schlinkert R, Young WJ, Farley D. Laparoscopic versus open posterior adrenalectomy: a case-control study. Surgery 1997; 122:1132–1136.

33

Pancreatic Surgery

EMILY WINSLOW and L. MICHAEL BRUNT

Institute for Minimally Invasive Surgery
Washington University School of Medicine
St. Louis, Missouri, U.S.A.

JUSTIN S. WU

University of California, San Diego
California, U.S.A.

I. INTRODUCTION

Laparoscopic staging of pancreatic cancer was first described almost two decades ago [1], but the application of laparoscopic techniques to pancreatic surgery has developed slowly. Because of the location of the pancreas and the nature of the pancreatic tissues, advanced laparoscopic skills are required for all laparoscopic pancreatic procedures. As laparoscopy has matured, several new technologies have allowed for a broader application of the minimally invasive approach to diseases of the pancreas. The most important is the use of intraoperative ultrasound with Doppler flow, which has allowed for detection of small lesions in the absence of palpation and for appreciation of the relationship between a mass and the ductal system. More recently, the development of hand-assist devices has encouraged the application of laparoscopy to more involved procedures and has provided a middle ground between laparoscopy and open surgery.

The field of laparoscopic pancreatic surgery is still in its developmental phase despite an increasing number of case reports and small single-institution case series of laparoscopic pancreatic procedures. No prospective studies have been done that show an advantage of laparoscopic surgery in the treatment of pancreatic disease. Thus, the descriptions that follow reflect what has been reported as technically feasible, although the advantages of a laparoscopic approach over open surgery for pancreatic disease remain under evaluation.

II. INDICATIONS

A. Staging of Pancreatic Cancer

Laparoscopic staging has become an important part of the assessment of resectability of pancreatic cancer. The dilemma for the pancreatic surgeon is that although resection is the only chance for cure in pancreatic cancer, only a small proportion of patients have resectable tumors. Although the ability to determine resectability has improved with the development of high-resolution spiral computed tomography (CT) scanning, a significant number of patients still undergo laparotomy for what turns out to be unresectable disease. It is this subgroup of patients who have benefited from the adoption of laparoscopic staging prior to laparotomy for pancreatic cancer. It has been demonstrated that laparoscopic staging with intraoperative ultrasound will spare 38–44% [2,3] of patients an unnecessary laparotomy. A recent study from our institution [4] demonstrated that the yield of laparoscopic staging depends on the location of the tumor. Of patients with cancer of the head and uncinate process deemed resectable by traditional preoperative workup (including high-resolution CT scanning), 31% were found to have unresectable or metastatic disease at laparoscopic staging with ultrasound and were spared a laparotomy. In contrast, only 17% of patients with cancer in the body and tail of the pancreas had the planned laparotomy aborted.

B. Pancreatic Neuroendocrine Tumors

Many pancreatic neuroendocrine tumors are potentially amenable to laparoscopic excision, provided they are not invasive and can be localized preoperatively. Because one of the principal causes of morbidity of pancreatic resection is related to the trauma of traditional abdominal access, laparoscopic enucleations and distal pancreatectomies for these tumors are increasing in frequency. The ideal tumor for laparoscopic resection is the solitary, benign insulinoma located in the pancreatic body or tail. Glucagonomas are rare tumors that often present as a large mass (> 5 cm) in the body or tail of the pancreas and are often malignant. Laparoscopic resection of gastrinomas may be carried out in carefully selected patients; however, the tumors in these patients are often extrapancreatic and may be malignant. Nonfunctioning neuroendocrine tumors can also be resected depending on the location and tumor size. Before embarking on the resection of a neuroendocrine tumor, it is important to differentiate sporadic tumors from those that occur in patients with multiple endocrine neoplasia type 1 (MEN 1). The management of patients with MEN 1 is more difficult because their tumors tend to be multiple and small, and thus the application of the laparoscopic approach in these patients is unclear.

C. Cystic Pancreatic Lesions

Cystic lesions of the pancreas may also be removed laparoscopically in selected patients. The treatment of benign cystadenomas (both serous and mucinous) with laparoscopic distal pancreatectomy has been reported by several groups [5,6]. However, this approach remains somewhat controversial given that some seemingly benign lesions may prove to be malignant cystadenocarcinomas on pathological examination. For this reason, any suspicion of malignancy, such as large, bulky tumors, adherence to the splenic vessels, or evidence of infiltrative properties on ultrasound during a laparoscopic pancreatic resection, should be an indication for conversion to an open procedure. Some groups have suggested that mucinous ductal ectasia can be resected laparoscopically, but there are very few case reports of this type. Finally, the use of laparoscopic exploration with ultrasound and biopsy of cystic lesions of unclear etiology has been reported [7] and can be a useful tool in planning the subsequent management.

D. Complications of Pancreatitis

Laparoscopic distal pancreatectomy for chronic pain in patients with pancreatitis has been described in a small number of reports. The selection of patients for this procedure must be limited to those whose gross pathology is confined to the pancreatic body and tail, that is, those with proximal strictures and calculi. Unlike patients with neuroendocrine and cystic tumors, this group of patients usually will have a densely scarred retroperitoneum with associated lesser sac inflammation that virtually precludes splenic salvage. Although a limited number of favorable early reports have been published [5,8,9], the long-term results in terms of pain relief are unknown.

A second application of laparoscopic surgery in this setting is in the management of complications of pancreatic pseudocysts by laparoscopic cystgastrostomy or cystenterostomy. Minimally invasive approaches such as radiologically guided external drainage and endoscopic procedures have been criticized for high rates of cyst recurrence and postprocedure bleeding. The laparoscopic approach offers the benefits of minimal access while potentially providing a more durable drainage procedure with a decreased rate of postoperative bleeding. Three different techniques have been described. First, intragastric creation of a cystgastrostomy with the aid of a gastroscope has been described [10], but the limited space available may make suturing of the anastomosis technically challenging and the anterior port gastrostomies must be repaired. A second approach is laparoscopic anterior gastrotomy with performance of a stapled or handsewn cystgastrostomy [11]. The third and more recent approach is a lesser sac or infracolic approach to the cyst with the construction of either a stapled cystgastrostomy [12] or handsewn cystjejunostomy [13], depending on the location of the cyst and surgeon preference. The preliminary results of this latter procedure, although limited in number, have been promising, and the use of laparoscopy for this indication is likely to grow.

A final application of laparoscopy in the setting of pancreatitis is the performance of necrosectomy and drainage of infected pancreatic necrosis from acute pancreatitis. Several different techniques have been reported as this new procedure has evolved. One group [13] performed laparoscopic infracolic pancreatic necrosectomy with placement of drains for continuous irrigation in the lesser sac. This approach allows for complete necrosectomy of the lesser sac and for postoperative continuous or selective irrigation. A second approach has been laparoscopic intracavitary debridement of necrosis in which patients who fail percutaneous drainage have trocars inserted over the drains and undergo blind laparoscopic debridement with jet irrigation followed by reestablishment of drainage [14]. This approach was modified by Horvath and associates [15], who used a laparoscopic retroperitoneal approach along the drain track to debride the cavity and break up loculations that were preventing drainage in patients who failed to improve with percutaneous drainage, a technique they termed "laparoscopic-assisted percutaneous drainage." In these case series, laparotomy was avoided in a small number of critically ill patients. The latter group is now undertaking a prospective phase II study to identify the patients most likely to benefit from laparoscopic-assisted debridement.

III. DIAGNOSTIC IMAGING

The development of high-resolution CT scanning with 3–4 mm cuts through the pancreas has significantly improved the detection rate of pancreatic lesions. The nature of the lesion (solid or cystic), its relationship to important vascular structures (inferior mesenteric vein, portal vein, superior mesenteric artery), and the presence of metastatic disease can all be assessed. Therefore, in most situations involving a pancreatic mass, the initial diagnostic test should be a dedicated pancreatic CT scan with intravenous and oral contrast.

Endoscopic retrograde cholangiopancreatography also plays an important role in the diagnosis of pancreatic disorders. The clear depiction of the ductal system and the presence or absence of stones and strictures is important in the evaluation of patients with chronic pancreatitis. Recent improvements in endoscopic ultrasound have also aided the pancreatic surgeon in localizing small pancreatic lesions. With ultrasound technology, pancreatic head and uncinate process masses can be more easily detected and even biopsied if needed.

The initial imaging test for suspected neuroendocrine tumors should be a CT scan, both to localize the tumor and to exclude metastatic disease. Other localization tests that can be helpful include endoscopic ultrasound, radionuclide-labeled octreotide scanning, and calcium-stimulated angiography with hepatic venous sampling. Laparoscopic ultrasound has proven useful intraoperatively in localizing small lesions and defining their relationship to other structures, such as the pancreatic duct.

IV. OPERATIVE TREATMENT

A. Preoperative Preparation

The benefits and risks of laparoscopic pancreatic surgery must be discussed with the patient, including the limited experience and outcome data available for these procedures. Such risks include pancreatic fistula and a higher rate of conversion to an open laparotomy than with many other laparoscopic procedures. Because these may be prolonged procedures, patients must be medically able to tolerate 3–4 hours of anesthesia and pneumoperitoneum. Patients with apparent or suspected cardiopulmonary disease should be subjected to objective testing prior to proceeding with the operation.

Preoperatively, patients for whom distal pancreatectomy is planned should receive Pneumovax and *Haemophilus influenzae* type B vaccines because of the potential for splenectomy. Even if a spleen-preserving procedure is planned, the patient should be adequately prepared in case the spleen needs to be taken due to unexpected intraoperative findings (bleeding, adherence, invasion). The use of preoperative octreotide to decrease the incidence of pancreatic fistula postoperatively is controversial, but is used in some centers. Mechanical bowel preparation should be carried out in patients in whom the gastrointestinal tract will be entered as part of the procedure.

B. Operating Room and Patient Setup

The patient can be positioned in one of two ways: modified lithotomy with the surgeon standing between the legs or supine with the surgeon standing on the patient's right side. The patient should be on a padded bean bag mattress so that the table can be placed in reverse Trendelenburg position and rolled from side to side to facilitate exposure. For distal pancreatectomy, there should be some degree of elevation of the left side (e.g., with a sandbag) and the assistant should be on the patient's right side. The camera holder and scrub nurse are positioned on the patient's left side with two video monitors at the top of the table. The bladder should be decompressed with a catheter, and preoperative antibiotics should be administered. The patient should have at least one large-bore intravenous line should significant bleeding be encountered during the dissection. The equipment required is listed below.

> 30 degree laparoscope
> Atraumatic graspers
> Endoscopic linear stapler
> Ultrasonic coagulator (ultrasonic scalpel)
> Laparoscopic ultrasound probe and machine
> Standard monopolar electrosurgery curved scissors
> Suction/irrigation device
> Ring forceps (spleen morcellation)
> Curved dissectors
> Endoscopic clip applier
> Needle holder and suture material
> Entrapment sack
> Laparotomy set (in room)
> Hand-assist device (available)
> Fibrin sealant (optional)
> Closed suction drain

C. Port Placement

The precise placement of the ports for pancreatic surgery varies depending on the indication for surgery and location of the pathology. In general, four to five ports are needed. The 12 mm port needed for the endoscopic linear stapler must be positioned far enough away from the pancreas to facilitate easy positioning and transection. The camera is best positioned at the umbilicus. One port is needed in the left lateral subcostal position to facilitate dissection of the splenic attachments should a splenectomy be necessary. One possible port configuration used for distal pancreatectomy is shown in Figure 1.

D. Pancreatic Exposure

After pneumoperitoneum is achieved and all ports have been placed, inspection of the peritoneal surfaces and liver should be the first step to rule out previously undetected metastatic deposits. The first step is entry into the lesser sac through the gastrocolic omentum. The greater curvature of the stomach should be grasped and elevated in a cephalad direction with atraumatic graspers. At a point halfway up the greater curve, just below the gastroepiploic arcade, a window should be created into the lesser sac. The gastrosplenic omentum should be divided up to the short gastric vessels such that the pancreas is fully exposed (Fig. 2). This step is facilitated by the use of the ultrasonic shears. If adhesions are present between the liver and stomach from prior surgery, these should not be taken down as they can help keep the stomach elevated. Patients with lesser sac inflammation will require careful dissection of the adhesions from the posterior stomach to the pancreas. Dense adhesions between a pancreatic mass and the posterior stomach or colon suggest malignant disease, and consideration should be given to

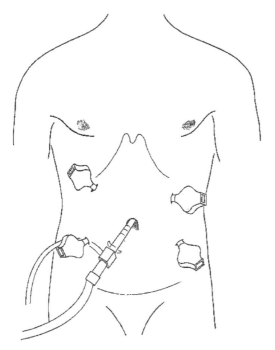

Figure 1   One possibility for port placement during distal pancreatectomy.

converting to an open procedure. For distal pancreatectomy, some surgeons advocate leaving the short gastric vessels intact if splenic preservation is planned, but they may need to be divided to ensure adequate exposure. For exposure of tumors in the pancreatic head, a complete Kocher maneuver should be performed, which is facilitated by rotating the table to the left side.

After adequate pancreatic exposure, an ultrasonic examination should be performed. The many advantages of this imaging modality include precise localization of a given lesion, determination of its proximity to the ductal system and relationship to the major vessels, exclusion of previously undiagnosed lesions, and exclusion of invasive properties suggestive of malignancy. Only after this type of information is obtained can the determination be made to proceed laparoscopically and the type and extent of resection be planned.

V.   DISTAL PANCREATECTOMY WITH SPLENECTOMY

If distal pancreatectomy with splenectomy is planned, the next step is to mobilize the splenic flexure of the colon, as this will allow for better access to the retroperitoneum and will be a necessary step in freeing the spleen. The short gastric vessels should be divided with the ultrasonic coagulator. The posterior peritoneum overlying the superior and inferior border of the pancreatic body and tail should then be incised. With blunt dissection and gentle elevation of the pancreas, the gland should be freed from the retroperitoneal fat posteriorly. The dissection should be carried medially to the inferior mesenteric vein (IMV). Any small tributaries between the vessels and the pancreatic parenchyma should

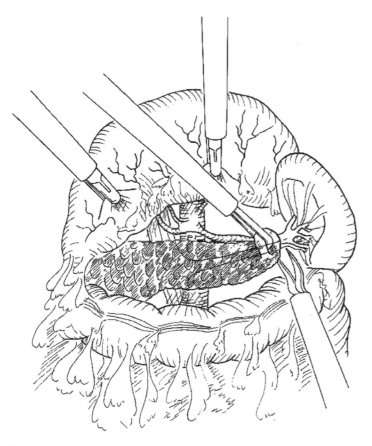

Figure 2   Exposure of the pancreas after opening the lesser sac.

be clipped or sealed with the ultrasonic scalpel. The splenic artery is then identified along the superior border of the pancreas and should be isolated using a right angle dissector. The splenic artery is then divided at the planned line of transection by clips, ligatures, or vascular staplers. Our preference is to use large clips and a pretied suture loop for the proximal end. After the artery has been divided, the pancreatic parenchyma and splenic vein must then be divided (Fig. 3). The ideal method for division of the pancreatic parenchyma during laparoscopic distal pancreatectomy has not yet been determined. Most groups have carried this out using an endoscopic linear stapler cutter placed across the neck of the pancreas. However, in many cases the pancreas is thicker than ideal for application of a stapler, and postoperative fistula rates of 20% have been reported with this technique [12]. Other options for division of the pancreas include the LigaSure bipolar electrocautery system (Valleylab, Boulder, CO) or use of a hand-assisted technique. With either technique, an attempt should be made to identify and suture ligate the pancreatic duct with nonabsorbable suture. If a stapler is used, the pancreatic parenchyma should be sutured closed as well. If a stapler is to be used, it must be passed carefully behind the pancreas under direct vision in order to prevent inadvertent damage to the IMV and portal vein. Depending on the location of the entry of the IMV into the portal system and the planned location of transection, the IMV may need to be ligated separately. The splenic

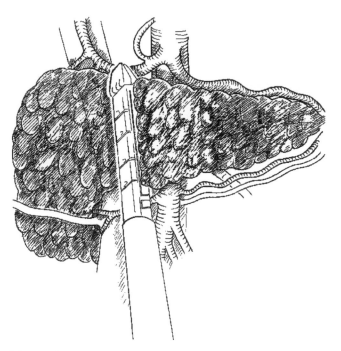

Figure 3   Transection of the pancreatic parenchyma with an endoscopic stapler.

vein may be transected with an endovascular stapler. After transection of the artery, vein, and pancreatic parenchyma has been accomplished, the distal pancreas can then be mobilized from medial to lateral. This can best be done by applying superior traction on the pancreas and carefully dividing any remaining bridging vessels. When the pancreas is completely freed, attention should be turned to the remaining splenic attachments, specifically the lateral and diaphragmatic attachments. These should be taken down, freeing the specimen completely. When the lesion is located in the pancreatic tail, it may be most convenient to first free the splenic attachments, and then using a "suspended pedicle" type technique, the pancreatic dissection can proceed from lateral to medial. When freed, the entire specimen should then be placed in a bag and the spleen morcellated digitally and with ringed forceps prior to extraction (Fig. 4). The sac should then be pulled through an enlarged trocar site with the pancreatic part of the specimen intact. The proximal pancreatic stump should next be carefully inspected for hemostasis. A fibrin sealant (Tisseel, Baxter, Inc.) is usually applied to the pancreatic stump to seal any small-caliber ducts. After adequate irrigation and hemostasis, a closed suction drain should be placed with the tip overlying the pancreatic stump. The trocars should be removed and the port sites closed in the standard fashion.

VI.   DISTAL PANCREATECTOMY WITH SPLEEN PRESERVATION

After adequate exposure is obtained, the posterior peritoneum inferior to the pancreas is incised and the dissection proceeds between the retroperitoneum and posterior aspect of the pancreas until the splenic vein is reached. The peritoneum superior to the pancreas should also be incised and the splenic artery dissected completely, so that the artery can be

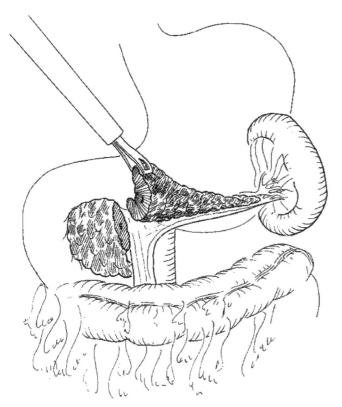

Figure 4   Removal of the resected distal pancreatic specimen.

easily ligated should significant bleeding occur. The tail of the pancreas is then retracted to expose the branches of the splenic artery and vein that supply the pancreatic parenchyma, and these are taken with either the ultrasonic coagulator, LigaSure electrocautery unit (Valleylab, Boulder, CO), or between clips. Care should be taken not to injure the splenic artery or vein in this process, as significant bleeding is difficult to control without ligation, which precludes spleen preservation if the short gastric vessels have been taken. The pancreas should be freed until the planned point of transection. The linear stapler should then be carefully placed and the pancreatic parenchyma transected. The specimen should be extracted in a bag through an enlarged port site. The pancreatic stump and conclusion of the procedure are handled as outlined above.

VII.   ENUCLEATION OF PANCREATIC TUMORS

Small pancreatic neuroendocrine tumors may be appropriate for enucleation. After adequate exposure has been obtained, the location of the lesion should be confirmed using intraoperative ultrasound. A laparoscopic Kocher maneuver is required to visualize the pancreatic head. Placement of a hand-assist device may be necessary if palpation is required to localize the tumor or to facilitate exposure. Once the lesion is located, it must then be determined if it is suitable for enucleation. Only those tumors that are on the anterior surface have a distinct capsule, and are clearly away from the ductal system should be enucleated. The dissection begins between the tumor and the normal parenchyma and proceeds around the tumor circumference. There may be small feeding vessels, which should either be clipped or sealed with the harmonic scalpel. The dissection itself can be done with a standard electrocautery hook/scissors or the ultrasonic scalpel. If the border of the tumor is unclear at any point during the dissection, ultrasound should be used to assure an adequate resection. Once the tumor is free, it should then be placed in an entrapment sac and removed. The resection bed is then irrigated and carefully examined for adequate hemostasis. Fibrin sealant is applied to the enucleation site and a closed-suction drain is inserted, as fistula formation is a potential complication of this procedure.

VIII. CYSTGASTROSTOMY OR CYSTJEJNOSTOMY

Four different techniques can be used to establish cyst-enteric drainage laparoscopically in patients with chronic pseudocysts. The first approach involves transgastric intraluminal creation of a cystgastrostomy [4]. This is accomplished by placing radially expanding trocars directly through the anterior gastric wall. With the aid of a gastroscope, the posterior gastric wall is then incised overlying the cyst, creating a cystotomy. The cyst's contents are aspirated and the anastomosis is sutured to aid in hemostasis. Because of the limited intragastric space in which to suture, this is a technically demanding procedure. The second approach entails creation of a cystgastrostomy via a laparoscopic anterior gastrostomy [11]. With this technique, trocars are placed in the peritoneal cavity and a longitudinal anterior gastrotomy is performed under direct vision with the electrocautery. Once access to the stomach is obtained, a posterior cystgastrostomy is fashioned as above. Although this approach allows for easier suturing, it adds the need for repair of the anterior gastric wall and the potential for peritoneal contamination.

The third approach to cystgastrostomy is via the lesser sac [11]. Entry into the lesser sac can be difficult and requires careful dissection given the previous pancreatitis in these patients. After the lesser sac has been entered, the pancreatic cyst can be seen to bulge out of the retroperitoneum. The nature of the cyst can then be delineated with ultrasound to determine if a significant solid component exists. After selection of the proper location, a cystotomy is made and the fluid aspirated immediately. The cyst is then copiously irrigated and explored with the laparoscope. A biopsy of the cyst wall should be taken with any pseudocyst drainage procedure to rule out a cystic neoplasm. A posterior gastrotomy is then made in close proximity to the cystotomy. An endoscopic GIA stapling device is then used to create the anastomosis. The remaining opening is then closed with a running suture. After adequate irrigation, a closed suction drain is placed at the anastomosis and the procedure concluded.

The fourth and final approach to a pseudocyst is the creation of a cystjejunostomy via the infracolic approach [13]. This procedure commences with elevation of the transverse colon to expose the root of the transverse mesocolon. If a large pseudocyst can be seen to bulge out at the root of the mesentery just to the left of the middle colic vessels, then the overlying peritoneum is incised to expose the thickened wall of the most dependent part of the cyst. Ultrasound can be used in a fashion similar to that described above. The cyst is then opened just enough to allow placement of the suction irrigator into the cavity and the space is aspirated and irrigated copiously. The fibrous wall of the sac is then opened a distance of 3–4 cm allowing for adequate visualization of its contents. A Roux Y loop of jejunum is then brought up and a 3 cm enterotomy is made on the antimesenteric surface. Either a single-layer hand-sewn or stapled anastomosis can then be fashioned. The enterotomy is closed and the jejunal-jejunal anastomosis is completed in a similar fashion. Adequate irrigation and hemostasis are assured, and a closed suction drain is left next to the cyst-jejunal anastomosis.

IX. PANCREATIC NECROSECTOMY AND DRAINAGE

Three different minimally invasive techniques designed to drain pancreatic necrosis have been described. The first [13] is to establish access to the lesser sac via the infracolic approach as described above (for cystenterostomy). Once the cavity is entered, a necrosectomy is performed with Babcock type graspers and the pancreatic slough is then placed in a protection bag for extraction. Two large drains (both for inflow and outflow) are placed within the lesser sac and the defect closed around them, allowing for effective postoperative irrigation. A second approach [14] that has been proposed for patients who have failed to resolve with percutaneous drainage involves utilization of the previously established percutaneous drain tract. A trocar is advanced over the drain into the cavity and the drain is then removed. A suction-irrigator is then placed into the cavity, which is washed. After the fluid is clear of debris, the cavity is insufflated and a scope is placed to assess the degree of residual necrosis in the cavity. The difficulty with this approach is that the necrosectomy is performed blindly and that multiple "wash-outs" have been required in the patients reported to date. The final approach to the patient with failed percutaneous drainage has been reported by the group at the University of Washington, Seattle [15]. With this technique, a 4–5 cm flank incision is made so that the entry into the retroperitoneum is in proximity to the undrained cavity and the preexisting drain tracts. Two 12 mm trocars (with blunt tips) are placed into this incision side by side, and the cavity is then insufflated. Pneumoperitoneum is maintained using a combination of towel clips and moist laparotomy pads. With the aid of a 30° laparoscope, the cavity is then debrided and irrigated under direct vision. The goal of the intervention is not to completely clean the cavity of debris, but rather to facilitate further percutaneous drainage. A red rubber catheter and two soft rubber drains arc brought out through the flank incision and are used for postoperative lavage. This approach has the advantage of debridement under direct vision, but still requires blind placement of the initial trocar. It is important to emphasize that only a small number of these procedures have been reported and the technical details of the procedure are still evolving.

X. POSTOPERATIVE CARE

The nasogastric tube is usually removed either at the end of the case or on the first day postoperatively. When the patient is ready to attempt oral intake, a trial of liquids should be given and the diet advanced as tolerated. The output and character of drainage from the closed suction drain should be observed during diet advancement, and the amylase content of the fluid should be checked once the patient is on a regular diet. The drain should not be removed until the output is clear and the amylase level is normal. It is not our practice to administer octreotide postoperatively, although some surgeons use it selectively in this setting. Blood glucose levels should be closely monitored postoperatively if pancreatic resection has been performed as these patients may require insulin. Other routine measures include the use of compression stockings until the patient is fully ambulatory, the use of H_2-blockers until the patient tolerates a diet, and administration of peri-operative antibiotics.

Table 1   Conversion Rates and Complications

	Ref. 5	Ref. 16	Ref. 17	Ref. 12	Ref. 18	Ref. 9
Number	19	13	10	5	6	14
OR time (hr)	4.4	3.5	3.0	5.0	5.0	4.5
Conversions (%)	11	NS	40	NS	33	7
Total comp. (%)	26	46	50	NS	NS	21
Panc fistula (%)	16	38	20	20	33	7
LOS (days)	6	5	7	4.9	25.6	6.4

NS = not specified; comp. = complications.

XI. OUTCOMES

An assessment of the results and complications of laparoscopic pancreatic surgery is difficult due to the limited number of case series published and the diversity of the patient populations, surgical techniques, and use of prophylactic measures (fibrin glue, octreotide). A summary of conversion rates and complications from the major reported series is given in Table 1. The most common complication is pancreatic fistula, which appears to be more common after enucleation than after distal pancreatectomy. The incidence of this complication depends on how it is defined and how carefully it is searched for; however, it may occur in up to 20% of patients. Nearly half of the patients with fistulas included in the series listed in Table 1 were managed conservatively with continued drainage until spontaneous resolution. Some patients have required initiation of parenteral nutrition and a prolonged hospital stay, but only one patient required operative repair. Although the existing data are limited, it would appear that patients with an uncomplicated course derive all the standard benefits of a laparoscopic approach, including faster return to normal activity and less postoperative pain.

XII. CURRENT STATUS AND FUTURE INVESTIGATIONS

Currently, the most common laparoscopic pancreatic procedures include laparoscopic staging of pancreatic cancer and enucleation of neuroendocrine tumors. Less commonly, distal pancreatectomy is performed for removal of benign pancreatic lesions. The other indications discussed above are much less common and are mostly carried out by groups of advanced laparoscopic surgeons with a special interest in this area. Further clinical trials in larger numbers of patients are needed to evaluate the safety, efficacy, and benefits of a laparoscopic approach to the various pancreatic lesions.

XIII. TOP TEN SURGICAL TIPS

1. High-resolution dedicated pancreatic CT scan with intravenous and oral contrast is the test of choice to characterize pancreatic lesions.
2. Assure preoperatively that the patient can tolerate 3–4 hours of anesthesia and pneumoperitoneum.
3. Place the patient on a padded bean bag mattress to facilitate safe changes in patient position during the procedures.
4. Use intraoperative ultrasound to define the relationship between the pancreatic lesion, vessels, and pancreatic ductal system.

5. Be prepared to perform a splenectomy in conjunction with distal pancreatectomy.
6. Use a hand-assist device when the laparoscopic dissection is difficult.
7. Attempt to identify and suture ligate the pancreatic duct (with nonabsorbable suture) after distal pancreatectomy.
8. Convert to an open procedure if there is evidence of invasion into adjacent organs or ultrasonic characteristics of malignancy.
9. Use fibrin sealant on pancreatic enucleation bed or transection stump.
10. Place a closed suction drain after all pancreatic resections to identify and control postoperative fistulas.

SELECTED READINGS

1. Warshaw AL, Tepper JE, Shipley WU. Laparoscopy in the staging and planning of therapy for pancreatic cancer. Am J Surg 1986 1986;151:76–80.
2. Callery MP, Strasberg SM, Doherty GM, Soper NJ, Norton JA. Staging laparoscopy with laparoscopic ultrasonography: optimizing resectability in hepatobiliary and pancreatic malignancy. J Am Coll Surg 1997;185:34–41.
3. Conlon KC, Dougherty EM, Klimstra DS, Coit DG, Turnbull AD, Brennan MF. The value of minimal access surgery in the staging of patients with potentially resectable peripancreatic malignancy. Ann Surg 1996;223:134–140.
4. Vollmer CM, Drebin JA, Middleton WD, Teefey SA, Linehan DC, Soper NJ, Eagon CJ, Strasberg SM. Utility of staging laparoscopy in subsets of peripancreatic and biliary malignancies. Ann Surg 2002;235:1–7.
5. Patterson EJ, Gagner M, Salky B, Inabner WB, Brower S, Edye M, Gurland B, Reiner M, Pertsemlides D. Laparoscopic pancreatic resection: single institution experience in 19 patients. J Am Coll Surg 2001;193:281–287.
6. Schachter PP, Aavni Y, Gvirz G, Rosen A, Czerniak A. The impact of laparoscopy and laparoscopic ultrasound on the management of pancreatic cystic lesions. Arch Surg 2000;135:260–264.
7. Strasberg SM, Middleton WD, Teefey SA. Management of diagnostic dilemmas of the pancreas by ultrasonographically guided laparoscopic biopsy. Surgery 1999;126:736–741.
8. Cuschieri A, Jajimowicz JJ, van Spreeuwel J. Laparoscopic distal 70% pancreatectomy and splenectomy for chronic pancreatitis. Ann Surg 1996;223(3):280–285.
9. Cushieri A, Jakimowicz JJ. Laparoscopic pancreatic resections. Sem Laparosc Surg 1998;5:168–179.
10. Mori T, Abe N, Sugiyama M, Atomi Y, Way LW. Laparoscopic pancreatic cystgastrostomy. J Hepat Bil Panc Surg 2000;7:28–34.
11. Smadja C, Badawy A, Vons C, Giraud V, Franco D. Laparoscopic cystogastrostomy for pancreatis pseudocyst is safe and effective. J Laparoendosc Adv Surg Tech 1999;9:401–403.
12. Park A, Schwartz R, Tandan V, Anvari M. Laparoscopic pancreatic surgery. Am J Surg 1999;177:158–163.
13. Cuschieri A, Jajimowicz JJ. Laparoscopic infracolic approach for complications of acute pancreatitis. Sem Laparosc Surg 1998;5:189–194.
14. Alverdy J, Vargish T, Desai T, Frawley B, Rosen B. Laparoscopic intracavitary debridement of peripancreatic necrosis: preliminary report and description of the technique. Surgery 2000; 127:112–114.

15. Horvath KD, Kao LS, Ali A, Wherry KL, Pellegrini CA, Sinanan MN. Laparoscopic assisted percutaneous drainage of infected pancreatic necrosis. Surg Endosc 2001; 15:677–682.

16. Fernandez-Cruz L, Herrera M, Saenz AM, Pantoja JP, Astudillo E, Sierra M. Laparoscopic pancreatic surgery in patients with neuroendocrine tumors: indications and limits. Best Prac Res Clin Endocrinol Metab 2001;15:161–175.

17. Berends FJ, Cuesta MA, Kazemier G, van Eijik CHJ, de Herder WW, van Muiswinkel JM, Bruining HA, Bonjer HJ. Laparoscopic detection and resection of insulinomas. Surgery 2000; 128:386–391.

18. Vezakis A, Davides D, Larvin M, McMahon MJ. Laparoscopic surgery combined with preservation of the spleen for distal pancreatic tumors. Surg Endosc 1999;13:26–29.

34

Gynecology

THOMAS J. HERZOG

Washington University School of Medicine
St. Louis, Missouri, U.S.A.

EDWARD R. KOST

Brooke Army Medical Center
Ft. Sam Houston, Texas, U.S.A.

ROBERT L. COLEMAN

Center for Minimally Invasive Surgery
University of Texas Southwestern Medical Center
Dallas, Texas, U.S.A.

I. BRIEF HISTORY

Operative laparoscopy is a well-know modality in the efficacious treatment of gynecological lesions. Gynecologists were among the first surgical specialists to embrace laparoscopy in the United States in the early 1980s. Initial uses were primarily diagnostic, but as skills and equipment improved, operative techniques became widely employed. Hysterectomy, performed either abdominally or vaginally, is one of the most common gynecological operations performed in the United States. Reich et al. reported the first laparoscopic hysterectomy in the United States in 1989. Since that time, the laparoscopic approach to hysterectomy and oophorectomy has gained increasing popularity in some centers in the United States and Europe and has been used for a wide range of conditions. Although multiple variations have been described, including total laparoscopic supracervical hysterectomy with morcellation and laparoscopic removal of the uterus, the more common procedure involves combining laparoscopically directed dissection of the adnexa and upper uterine attachments with vaginal hysterectomy—a laparoscopic assisted vaginal hysterectomy (LAVH). Considerable controversy exists concerning appropriate indications for LAVH versus the standard traditional vaginal hysterectomy.

Traditionally laparotomy, a major surgical procedure, has been advocated as the technique of choice for treatment of adnexal masses. However, recently several series have shown that properly selected patients can be treated by laparoscopic salpingo-oophorectomy. One potential concern with the laparoscopic approach is rupture of a malignant mass with resultant dissemination of malignant cells. The introduction of laparoscopic bags has greatly aided in the laparoscopic removal of ovarian neoplasms without intraoperative rupture. Currently laparoscopic tubal ligation is the most common approach, accounting for over 50% of procedures. With the advent of bipolar cautery, a lower incidence of bowel injury has been seen in comparison with unipolar technique.

II. PREOPERATIVE PREPARATION

A detailed patient history is obtained as well as appropriate laboratory studies and a current Pap smear. The patient is maintained on clear liquid diet for 24 hours prior to surgery and NPO after midnight the evening prior to surgery. We recommend a mechanical bowel preparation for all major laparoscopic procedures both to decompress the small bowel and colon and as a precaution in the event of bowel surgery. Once in the preanesthesia area, a peripheral IV is started and cephalosporin antibiotics are administered 30 minutes prior to the procedure. Compression stockings should be used routinely as prophylaxis against thromboembolic disease. The compression stockings should be applied prior to the induction of anesthesia.

III. OPERATING ROOM AND PATIENT SET-UP

The operating room set-up is shown in Figure 1. Two monitors are generally employed such that both the surgeon and the co-surgeon have a comfortable view of the operation. The laparoscopy cart with insufflator, light source, and monitor will be at the foot of the table opposite the surgeon so that the surgeon may easily view the intra-abdominal pressure and flow rates at all times. The other lines coming onto the table should be situated on the same side as the person who will be using that particular piece of equipment. Thus, the camera cables, insufflator tubing, and suction irrigation tubing should come off the co-surgeon's side of the table; the electrosurgical cable (i.e., for the monopolar or bipolar cautery) should come off the surgeon's side of the table.

Once in the operating room, a naso- or orogastric tube and pneumatic compression stockings are placed and a urethral catheter is inserted. The patient is placed in a dorsal lithotomy position with her legs in conventional or Allen stirrups. The arms are tucked and protected by the patient's sides. Cane stirrups offer the advantage of easy repositioning intraoperatively, allowing access to both the abdomen and later the perineum for the vaginal phase of the procedure. The entire abdomen and vaginal vault should be prepped and draped. Various uterine manipulation devices are used transvaginally so that the uterus can be manipulated to improve access to the cul-de-sac, bladder, and ovaries.

IV. LAPAROSCOPIC HYSTERECTOMY

A. Port Placement

The patient is placed in the Trendelenburg position. Approximate trocar placement for laparoscopic hysterectomy is shown in Figure 2. A 10–12 mm trocar is placed and

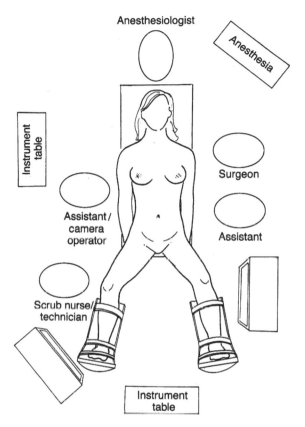

Figure 1 Operating room set-up.

anchored in the umbilical location. A 10 mm diagnostic laparoscope with video camera is inserted and the peritoneal contents are identified. A high-flow insufflator is used to establish a pneumoperitoneum to an internal pressure of 15 mmHg. After assuring the presence of a functioning Foley catheter, a 10–12 mm trocar is placed in the lower midline under direct visualization, just superior to the symphysis pubis. Two 5 mm trocars are then placed lateral to the inferior epigastric vessels, once again using direct visualization.

B. Dissection and Operation

Initially a complete laparoscopic examination of the pelvis and entire abdomen is performed. If either or both ovaries are to be harvested as part of the procedure, the appropriate infundibulopelvic ligament is isolated. Prior to ligation of this ligament, the ureter must be clearly identified. We strongly recommend opening the retroperitoneum and identifying the ureter as it crosses the pelvic brim and courses into the pelvis. This can be performed safely and easily in the following fashion: the surgeon stands on the opposite side of the pelvic sidewall to be explored. The camera is placed through the umbilical port and is held by the assistant. The assistant also uses a grasper placed through the ipsilateral lateral port. The surgeon uses a grasper through the lower midline port and scissors with monopolar cautery through the contralateral port. The assistant provides lateral

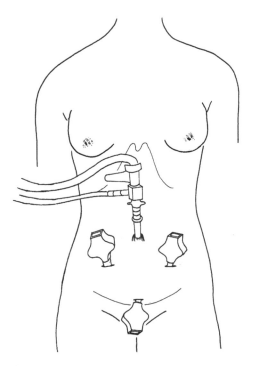

Figure 2   Position of trocars for laparoscopic hysterectomy.

countertraction while the surgeon incises the round ligament and the peritoneum over the psoas muscle between the round ligament and the ovarian vessels (Fig. 3). The pelvic side wall structures are exposed, including the external iliac and hypogastric vessels and the ureter (Fig. 4). If the uterus is to be left in place, tenting and incising the peritoneum just cephalad to this ligament can spare the round ligament. If difficulty arises in identification of the ureter on the medial left of the peritoneum, the dissection is carried cephalad along the external iliac vessels until the bifurcation of the common iliac vessels is encountered. The ureter is easily identified in the retroperitoneal space as it crosses the bifurcation of the internal and external iliac vessels. A window is then made under the ovarian vessels using the scissors with monopolar cautery. An endo-GIA stapling device is then placed through the 10–12 mm lower midline port, and the instrument is placed around the ovarian vessels (Fig. 5). Prior to engagement of the instrument, both the anterior and posterior surfaces of the blades are inspected to ensure that the intended staple line does not entrap the ureter. Alternatively, suture material may be employed to doubly ligate the infundibulopelvic ligament followed by monopolar scissor transection. Suture material can be in the form of previously tied knots, or intra- or extracorporeal knots may be employed. With the use of scissors with monopolar cautery and graspers, the ovary and fallopian tube are mobilized and retracted medially. This is easily performed by excising the broad ligament peritoneum superior and parallel to the ureter (Fig. 6). If a laparoscopic pelvic lymphadenectomy is to be performed, the previous dissection allows development of the paravesical and pararectal spaces (Soper et al., 1994).

Two options are available to the surgeon at this point in the operation. Having freed the ovaries, fallopian tubes, and round ligaments from their pelvic attachments, the

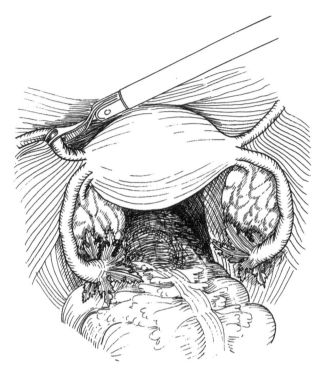

Figure 3 Transection of the round ligament.

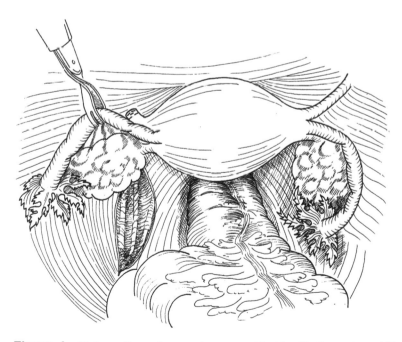

Figure 4 Retroperitoneal space is exposed to identify the external iliac and hypogastric vessels and the ureter.

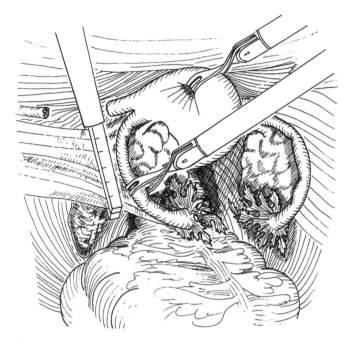

Figure 5   Endo-GIA stapler is placed around the ovarian vessels.

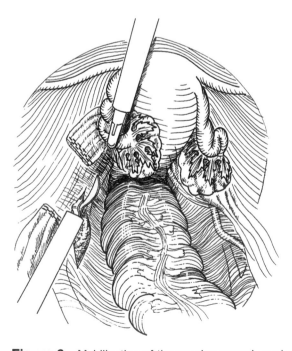

Figure 6   Mobilization of the ovarian vessels and ovary.

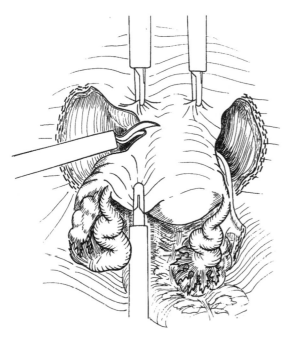

Figure 7 Development of the bladder flap using scissors with monopolar cautery.

surgeon can proceed with the vaginal phase of the procedure, essentially performing a standard vaginal hysterectomy (Saye and Espy, 1994). Alternatively, the majority of the hysterectomy may be completed laparoscopically (Phipps, 1993).

If the operation is to continue laparoscopically, attention is subsequently turned toward skeletonization of the uterine vessels. Using scissors with monopolar cautery and graspers, the avascular peritoneal reflections and fibrovascular tissue surrounding the uterine arteries are carefully dissected so that the uterine arteries are clearly identified as they enter the lower uterine segment. As part of this step, the bladder flap is developed. The vesicouterine peritoneal fold is elevated with graspers and the bladder is dissected off the lower uterine segment using scissors with monopolar cautery (Fig. 7). After the uterine vessels have been skeletonized and the bladder flap developed, the uterine vessels are divided using the endo-GIA stapler (Fig. 8). The uterus is deviated to the opposite side of uterine vessel ligation using graspers via the contralateral port and the vaginal uterine manipulator. The endo-GIA stapler is passed through the lower midline 10–12 mm port and positioned as medially as possible and parallel to the lower uterine segment to avoid incorporation of the ureter in the uterine pedicle. At this point the major blood supply to the uterus has been cut, and the relatively avascular cardinal and uterosacral ligaments remain to be transected.

The operation may be completed laparoscopically by transection of the cardinal and uterosacral ligaments by application of large titanium clips followed by transection using monopolar scissors. Alternatively, the division of these supporting ligaments may be performed during the vaginal phase of the procedure. All major supporting structures of the uterus have now been transected. In the final step the surgeon completes the circumcision of the vaginal mucosa from the cervix using scissors with monopolar

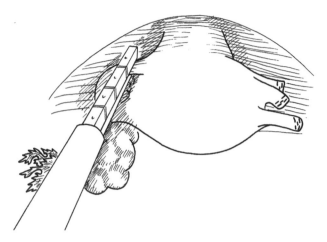

Figure 8   Uterine vessels are divided using endo-GIA stapler.

cautery, endoscopic stapling device, or fiber optic laser system. The surgical specimen is removed through the vagina, and the vaginal cuff is closed using figure-of-eight stitches and an extracorporeal pelviscopic tie (Fig. 9). Once the vagina is entered laparoscopically, the surgeon must place a 50 cc balloon into the vagina to prevent loss of the pneumoperitoneum.

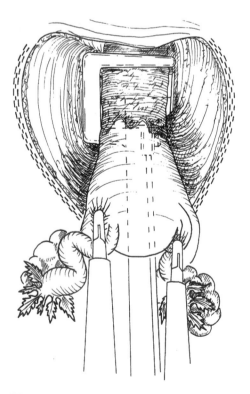

Figure 9   Vaginal cuff closure after removal of the uterus.

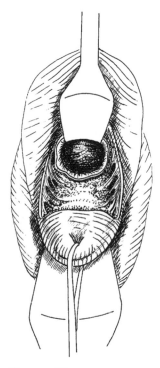

Figure 10 Anterior colpotomy.

LAVH, unlike the previously described "complete" laparoscopic hysterectomy, involves only the laparoscopic excision of the uterus from the superior aspect to the uterine vessels. Ligation and division of the uterine vessels are performed during the vaginal phase of the procedure. The laparoscopic instruments are removed from the pelvis, but the trocars are left in place. The pneumoperitoneum is evacuated, and attention is turned to the vaginal phase. We perform the vaginal portion of the procedure using the Heaney technique. Briefly, anterior colpotomy is performed after dissection of the plane between the bladder and uterus (Fig. 10). Anterior colpotomy may be facilitated if the bladder flap has previously been developed during the laparoscopic phase of the hysterectomy. Posterior colpotomy is performed in the standard fashion, and the uterosacral ligaments are divided and ligated (Figs. 11, 12). The uterine vessels and cardinal ligaments are clamped, divided, and ligated, and the specimen is delivered. The uterosacral ligaments are ligated, the peritoneum closed, and the vaginal mucosa reapproximated.

Attention is returned to the peritoneal cavity. After reestablishing pneumoperitoneum, the pelvis is irrigated and examined thoroughly and hemostasis is obtained using electrocautery or endoscopic clips. The trocars are removed under direct visualization to minimize the possibility of failing to diagnose an occult injury to a major anterior wall blood vessel. The fascia underlying the 10–12 mm trocar incisions is closed with delayed absorbable suture to minimize the chance of incisional hernias. Subcuticular stitches are used for skin closures.

C. Postoperative Care

At the conclusion of the procedure, a Foley catheter is left in place until the patient is fully ambulatory. The pneumatic compression stockings remain in place until the patient

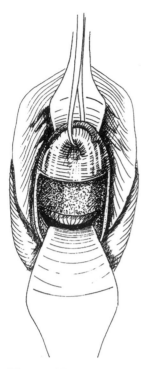

Figure 11   Posterior colpotomy.

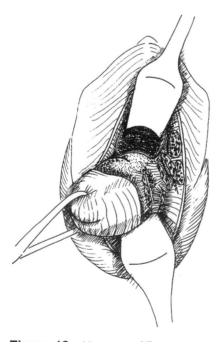

Figure 12   Uterosacral ligaments are divided and ligated.

reaches an ambulatory status. Patients are usually observed overnight and receive IV fluids and appropriate analgesia. A hematocrit level is obtained the morning after surgery. Once patients are tolerating a regular diet, they are discharged, usually within 24 hours of their surgery. Selective earlier discharge on the same day of surgery is possible on an individual basis.

D. Indications and Contraindications

Until recently the gynecologist had only two methods of removing the uterus: vaginal or abdominal hysterectomy. The gynecological surgeon now has several options available to perform the above operation using the laparoscopic method for either one or several phases of the operation. These new operative techniques need full evaluation, and the fact that they are technically feasible is no indication that they offer an advantage over the standard abdominal or vaginal approaches. In fact, there is considerable controversy regarding the usefulness of LAVH compared to standard vaginal hysterectomy. Performing a LAVH when the procedure can be accomplished vaginally alone is inappropriate and unnecessarily costly. (The indications and contraindications for laparoscopic hysterectomy are listed in Tables 1 and 2).

V. LAPAROSCOPIC SALPINGO-OOPHORECTOMY

A. Dissection and Operation

The preoperative preparation, operating room, and patient set-up for laparoscopic salpingo-oophorectomy are generally the same as described for laparoscopic hysterectomy. Placement of the trocars is similar to that shown in Figure 2. Either one or two lateral trocars may be employed, depending on the degree of adhesiolysis and difficulty of dissection. The blood supply to the ovary and tube include the ovarian vessels (the infundibulopelvic ligament) and the anastomosing ascending branches of the uterine artery. Prior to ligation of the infundibulopelvic ligament the ureter is identified in the retroperitoneal space (Fig. 4). The ligament is then divided with the endoscopic GIA or suture and monopolar cautery, and the ovary and fallopian tube are mobilized as described previously (Figs. 5, 6). Attention is then directed to the medial attachment of the adnexa, the utero-ovarian ligament. The endo-GIA is then placed on the utero-ovarian ligament

Table 1 Indications for Laparoscopic Hysterectomy

Probable adhesions (entero-uterine)
Bilateral salpingo-oophorectomy is coindicated prophylactic oophorectomy
   Age >45 years
   Nonmalignant ovarian abnormality
   Chronic pelvic pain (endometriosis, pelvic inflammatory disease, etc.)
   Stage I adenocarcinoma of the endometrium
   Poor vaginal access
   Narrow pubic arch
   Lack of descensus
   Limited vaginal space secondary to soft tissue
   Uterine leiomyomata

Table 2 Contraindications for Laparoscopic Hysterectomy

Relative
  Severe adhesions
  Uterus larger than 16-week size
  Vaginal removal of uterus precluded
  Ovarian or cervical cancer
  Endometrial adenocarcinoma beyond stage I disease
  Inflammatory bowel disease
  Severe bleeding abnormalities
  Intolerance of anesthesia

Absolute
  Massive hemorrhage
  Ruptured tubo-ovarian abscess with sepsis
  Complete bowel obstruction
  Pregnancy

midway between the ovary and the corneal portion of the uterine fundus (Fig. 13). Firing of the endo-GIA will allow the adnexa to be separated from the uterus. Suture or monopolar cautery can be employed to accomplish utero-ovarian ligament transection as well.

Several methods have been proposed for removing the adnexal from the peritoneal cavity, which include placement in plastic bags and then removal of the bag via posterior

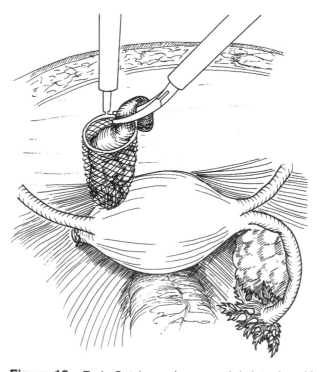

Figure 13 Endo Catch specimen pouch is introduced into pelvis.

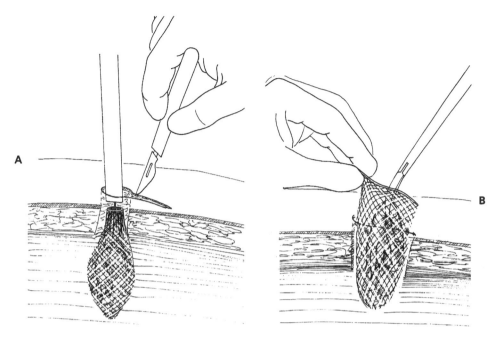

Figure 14 (A) Pouch is exteriorized and (B) contents extracted with clamp.

colpotomy or extraction of the bag through the lower midline 10–12 mm trocar, which can be extended as necessary. One such disposable specimen pouch is made by Auto Suture, Endo Catch. As shown in Figure 14, the Endo Catch specimen pouch is introduced into the pelvic cavity via the lower midline port, and the pouch is unrolled using graspers. The specimen is placed in the pouch with care not to inadvertently rupture the mass (Fig. 15). The pouch is exteriorized via the port, and the contents are extracted with a Kelly clamp (Fig. 16).

B. Postoperative Care

The patient's hemodynamic status, blood pressure, and pulse are monitored in the recovery room. If blood loss is a concern, serial hematocrit levels can be checked. The patient is then observed in the recovery area until she has recovered sufficiently from anesthesia to be fully ambulatory. She should have no nausea and vomiting and be able to tolerate oral fluids. Prior to discharge the patient is given precautions for increasing abdominal pain, fever and chills, and lack of bowel function.

C. Indications and Contraindications

Laparoscopic oophorectomy alone has been performed for a wide range of indications to include prophylactic oophorectomy, the removal of ovarian cysts or suspected ovarian malignancies, and more recently in conjunction with hysterectomy and lymph node dissection in the laparoscopic staging of endometrial cancer.

Contraindications to laparoscopic oophorectomy relate mainly to the removal of suspected ovarian malignancies and sequela of rupture. Even benign masses such as

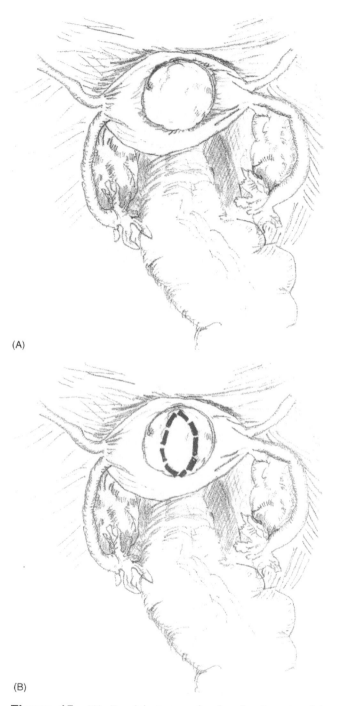

(A)

(B)

Figure 15 (A) Fundal myoma is visualized and pelvic anatomical relationships are restored prior to dissection. (B) Bold marking outline the intended myometrial incisions. These are made in the thinnest layer over the myoma. (C) Following fulguration of the overlying myometrium, dissection is made circumferentially along the pseudocapsule. (D) Traction is used along with electrocautery to eviscerate the myoma. (E) Closure of the myometrial defect is made using delayed absorbable suture.

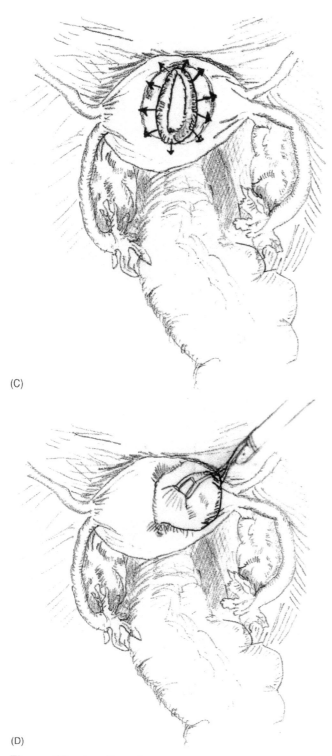

(C)

(D)

Figure 15 (*continued*)

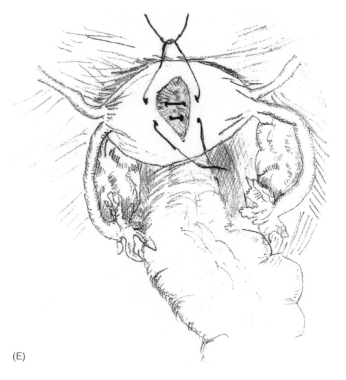

(E)

Figure 15 *(continued)*

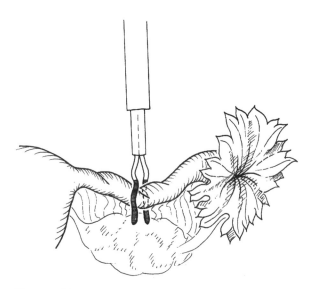

Figure 16   Mid-ampullary portion of tube is grasped with Kleppinger bipolar forceps.

mature cystic teratomas (dermoids) may result in a severe chemical peritonitis upon rupture during removal. In general, adnexal masses suspicious for malignancy should not be approached laparoscopically unless frozen section capabilities are available to allow for immediate laparotomy and proper staging, preferably by a gynecologic oncologist, in the event a malignancy is discovered. Traditional teaching has restricted laparoscopic resection to those masses that could be removed intact. Intraoperative rupture of an ovarian malignancy changes the surgical stage from Ia to Ic and allows cells to be disseminated into the upper abdomen, which theoretically could implant and result in stage III ovarian cancer. Although there is debate concerning the significance of intraoperative rupture on overall prognosis, in general, if the ovarian neoplasm is densely adherent to the bowel or pelvic structures, laparotomy should be performed. Proposed criteria for the laparoscopic management of cystic adnexal masses in postmenopausal women include ultrasonographic findings of a cystic adnexal mass < 10 cm with distinct borders and no evidence of irregular solid parts, thick septa, ascites, or matted bowel, and a normal serum CA 125 value (< 35 U/mi) (Parker and Berek, 1988).

VI. MYOMECTOMY

A. Preoperative Preparation

While the removal of uterine myomata using laparoscopic techniques is technically feasible, it is a procedure for which the surgeon should be prepared for laparotomy conversion (0–40%) and one for which strategic planning must be outlined prospectively. Preoperative planning begins with history and physical examination. Pertinent details that should be investigated include the presence of menorrhagia or metrorrhagia, constitutional symptoms of anemia, and history of infertility. Such information will help delineate the location, extent, and outcome measure of myomata resection. Radiographic workup with transvaginal and transabdominal ultrasound is essential to outline the number, size, and location of targeted lesions. In this manner, uterine masses that appear to encroach or invade the uterine cavity should be further evaluated with hysteroscopy. This approach helps to distinguish submucous myomata from polyps and adenomyomas. In cases of infertility, evaluation of tubal patency and uterine cavity morphology by hysterosalpingo-graphy and/or hysteroscopy should be performed. Comparison of findings from examination, radiographic studies, and, if performed, hysteroscopy are used to develop an operative strategy.

Since myomectomy is a procedure often associated with bleeding, some authors have advocated the use of gonadotropin-releasing hormone (GnRH) agonists, preoperatively. This treatment has the end result of reducing estrogen stimulation, which reduces growth rate and size of uterine masses. Such intervention has also been associated with less intraoperative blood loss. However, several other investigators have reported that the practice makes intraoperative dissection more difficult, increases the risk of laparotomy conversion, and may augment the risk of recurrence by hiding smaller foci. The treatment appears most applicable to the anemic patient undergoing preoperative resuscitation before surgery.

B. Dissection and Operation

The procedure, as with myomectomy at laparotomy, is associated with bleeding, primarily from release of the compressed peritumoral vasculature. This observation has caused some surgeons to consider local injection of vasoconstricting medications, such as pitressin; others have advocated tamponade of the uterine vessels. In either event, strict and meticulous hemostasis is crucial to reduce postoperative adhesions and to insure a strong and stable scar capable of pregnancy. In general, the following principles are followed for laparoscopic myomectomy:

> Trocar placement mimics that described above for laparoscopic hysterectomy (Fig. 2). We prefer to place the lateral ports (5 mm) outside the distribution of the inferior epigastric vessels (equivalent to McBurney's point) on either side. The central trocar (generally 10–12 up to 20 mm) is placed suprapubically or in another place strategic to the myoma location where traction, morsellation, and extraction can occur.
>
> Fine and atraumatic manipulation of the tissues around the myoma will reduce intraoperative bleeding. Traction from a variety of devices can be more rigorous on the myoma once exposed.
>
> Incision is made with electrocautery over the thinnest section of myometrium. Generally a separate incision is made for each myoma (Fig. 17). Once the myoma is reached, dissection proceeds along the plane of the pseudocapsule (Fig. 18). Facilitated by monopolar electrocautery on a curved scissors, the mass can be enucleated circumferentially. Caution is made as extensive use of electrocautery has been associated with weak scar formation and should be avoided.
>
> Extraction is aided with the "traction/countertraction" principle (Fig. 19). Traction with a heavy endoscopic grasper (or myoma screw) and countertraction with the intrauterine manipulator help to provide appropriate exposure and operative field for dissection.
>
> Closure of the uterine defect is accomplished with intra- or extracorporeal suturing with absorbable materials (Fig. 20). The closure should be full thickness and may occasionally require more than one layer. Prevention of hematoma formation in the scar will allow for a stronger closure. Interrupted suture placement with single or figure-of-eight passes are effective for hemostasis.

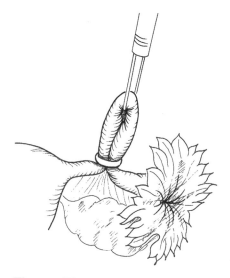

Figure 17   Silastic band (Falope ring) is pushed over a knuckle of tube.

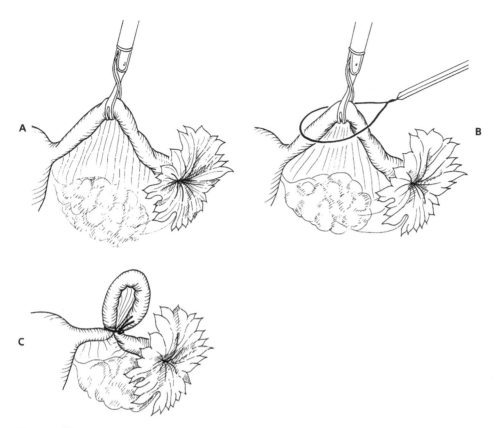

Figure 18 Segmental resection of tube (Pomeroy method).

Prevention of adhesion formation begins and centers around meticulous hemostasis. Some authors have advocated various other adjuvants to reduce adhesion formation (Seprafilm, Interceed, Hyskon). Their effectiveness is unknown at this time.

Small myomata are removable through the larger center trocar. Larger lesions, however, require some form of morsellation. There are several devices available which are quite effective in reducing the myoma for extraction. In these cases the myoma is cut by a circular blade and passed through the instrument to the outside. Alternative extraction sites are the abdominal wall via mini-laparotomy or vaginally, through a posterior colpotomy. In the latter case, a specialized vaginal tube manipulator (C.C.L. vaginal extractor, Karl Storz, Germany) maintains the pneumoperitoneum during morsellation. In cases where exposure is limited, such as myomata in the posterior uterus, broad ligament, and anterior lower uterine segment, consideration of assisted techniques (e.g., mini-laparotomy and hand-assist sleeve) can facilitate successful extirpation.

C. Postoperative Care

Careful attention to serial blood counts will enable rapid response to postoperative hemorrhage, should it occur. Hematoma formation may also occur in the expandable potential space bordered by the broad ligament. This is a particular concern in cases where the broad ligament was dissected or if the myoma was para-uterine and received its blood supply from the uterine vessels. Long-term treatment strategies, particularly for those patients considering pregnancy, include consideration of a second-look procedure to reduce adhesions, address missed lesions, and assess the uterine scar and hysterosalpingogram, to assess the uterine and tubal morphology.

D. Indications/Contraindications

Myomata are ubiquitous in women and seldom are a distinct reason for surgical evaluation. However, hemorrhage unable to be controlled hormonally, pain, infertility, uterine growth, and, rarely, infection all influence the decision to resect these uterine tumors. Consideration of the laparoscopic approach is entertained when the number is limited (usually fewer than three), the size is not too large as to inhibit exposure (usually <8–10 cm), and the location is accessible. Myomata outside these parameters are challenging and increase significantly the rate of conversion to laparotomy. Lesions that involve the endometrium are generally handled to some extent by hysteroscopy. However, it is probably unwise to approach such lesions both laparoscopically and hysteroscopically, as distention of the uterus by the latter procedure will promote in-field bleeding during the laparoscopic hysterotomy.

VII. TUBAL LIGATION

A. Preoperative Preparation

A pregnancy test should be performed immediately prior to the procedure. Before any tubal sterilization procedure, it is imperative that informed consent be obtained from the patient that emphasizes alternative birth control methods, potential surgical complications, and possible failure of sterilization with resultant pregnancy including ectopic pregnancy. A considerable number of patients will request reversal of the tubal sterilization at a later time (30/1000 women in the United States). It is important to stress to the patient that the procedure is intended to be permanent sterilization. One key to successful laparoscopic tubal ligation is certain differentiation between the round ligament and the fallopian tube. The overall incidence of intraoperative or postoperative complication is 1.7 per 100 laparoscopic tubal occlusion procedures performed. Complications include intraoperative bleeding, ureteral injury, and thermal injury to the bowel. Pregnancy rates following laparoscopic procedures are as follows: Falope ring, 0.5%; Hulka clip, 0.7%; and bipolar cautery, 0.4%.

B. Dissection and Operation: Bipolar Electrocautery Technique

A 5 mm trocar is inserted through a subumbilical incision. A second 5 mm trocar is inserted through a suprapubic incision under direct visualization. A 5 mm laparoscopic is introduced via the subumbilical port, while a blunt probe is passed via the suprapubic port. After examination of the pelvic organs and removal of the blunt probe, the mid-ampullary portion of the fallopian tube is grasped with a pair of bipolar forceps (Kleppingers). The tube is grasped such that the flat, duckbill portion of the tips contacts the full thickness of the tube and contacts the mesosalpinx (Fig. 21). The tube is coagulated for a distance of at least 2–3 cm. Prior to coagulation, the tube is elevated and care is taken to avoid thermal injury to the surrounding structures, such as the small intestines and the colon.

C. Silastic Band and Spring-Loaded Clip Techniques

The laparoscopic technique for Falope ring and Hulka clip placement is the same as that for the electrocoagulation procedure. First, each fallopian tube is visualized by identifying the distal fimbriae. For placement of Falope rings, the tongs of the band applicator are then extended and one tube is grasped at the ampulloisthmic junction and brought into the applicator. The band is pushed over a knuckle of tube, the tongs are released, and the tube is dropped (Fig. 22). The spring-loaded Hulka clip consists of two small serrated Silastic jaws held together by a metal clip. Teeth at the end of the jaws lock the clip in place. The clip is attached to the fallopian tube with an applicator.

D. Segmental Resection Technique (Pomeroy Method)

In this procedure the mid-portion of the fallopian tube is grasped with an endo-Babcock clamp. A 0 chromic endo-loop is passed over the knuckle of fallopian tube and the loop is cinched down. With the use of monopolar scissors the knuckle of fallopian tube is excised and the tubal segment removed and sent to pathology (Fig. 23). This technique will require the placement of three trocars: subumbilical (5 mm), suprapubic (5 mm), and lower lateral (5 mm).

E. Postoperative Care

The patient's hemodynamic status, blood pressure, and pulse are monitored in the recovery room. If blood loss is a concern, serial hematocrit levels can be checked. The patient is then observed in the recovery area until she has recovered sufficiently from anesthesia to be fully ambulatory. She should be able to tolerate oral fluids without nausea and vomiting. Routine discharge orders for precautions and activity level are given.

F. Indications and Contraindications

Undesired fertility in a patient who has had proper informed consent (see preoperative preparation) serves as the primary indication for a laparoscopic tubal sterilization procedure. Contraindications include the usual contraindications for laparoscopy (Saye and Espy, 1994), as well as a suspicion of acute salpingitis or pelvic inflammatory disease.

VIII. COMPLICATIONS AND THEIR MANAGEMENT

Penetrating injuries during laparoscopic hysterectomy generally occur during placement of the initial trocar. Direct trauma to the bowel, bladder, vessels, and other pelvic organs is well recognized. Catheterization of the bladder and pelvic examination under anesthesia to exclude an unexpected pelvic mass reduces such risk of injury. Prior abdominal surgeries with resultant adhesions predispose to bowel perforation injuries. In such cases an open technique may be used for trocar insertion. Furthermore, several reports describe initial lateral trocar placement with a 5 mm or smaller diameter laparoscope. After initial trocar placement is accomplished, all subsequent trocars are placed under direct view. One-wall puncture of the bowel may be recognized by the red rugae of the inside of the bowel wall with no intra-abdominal organs visualized. Through and through bowel injuries are recognized by the fact that the trocar point is contaminated with bowel contents. This type of injury may be difficult to visualize if the bowel is tightly adherent to the anterior abdominal wall. If concern exists about a bowel injury during subumbilical port placement, the camera should be placed via one of the inferior ports to allow direct visualization. The method of repair will depend on the experience of the surgeon; however, through and through bowel injury should generally be repaired by open laparotomy. Another potential area of bowel injury is thermal injury during dissection with the endo-shears (monopolar cautery) or at the time of laparoscopic tubal fulguration with the Kleppinger paddles (bipolar cautery). Small burns on the serosa of the small or large bowel do not ordinarily require special therapy; however, when there is a question of the extent of the injury, it is important to realize that the actual area of thermal damage to the bowel is about five times greater than it appears to be on inspection. The damaged segment of bowel should be resected rather than oversewn, and no attempt should be made to excise only the perforation site. The site is drained and antibiotic therapy is employed. Obviously preoperative bowel preparation is mandatory in all major laparoscopic surgical procedures in which the potential exists for bowel injury. Prevention of bowel injury is facilitated through steep Trendelenburg positioning as well as meticulous lysis of large and small bowel adhesions to pelvic structures prior to initiation of the laparoscopic surgical procedure.

Injury to the large vessels may be immediately apparent because of a blood-filled abdomen or a rapidly developing retroperitoneal hematoma. Trocar removal can result in rapid vascular collapse, and if possible the trocar should be left in place providing temporary tamponade. Immediate laparotomy is performed and pressure applied to the site of injury. Consultation with a vascular surgeon should be obtained. Injury to the great vessels can be prevented by understanding the anatomical relationship of the umbilicus to the aortic bifurcation by confining the plane of the trocar on first entry to the midline and 45 degrees from horizontal.

During the laparoscopic hysterectomy the most common site of intraoperative hemorrhage is between the uterine artery pedicle, which is secured laparoscopically, and the utero-sacral and cardinal ligaments, which are divided and ligated vaginally. Small arterial branches which are not incorporated into the uterine artery pedicle are avulsed as downward traction is placed on the uterus during the vaginal phase of the operation. If hemostasis cannot be obtained through the conventional vaginal approach, as when small vessels retract into the loose areolar tissue of the parametria, hemostasis may have to be achieved laparoscopically via diathermy electrocautery, bipolar cautery, titanium clips, or laparoscopic suturing techniques. Injury to the pelvic side wall or pelvic floor venous system can result in rapid, life-threatening hemorrhage, and control should not be attempted by the random placement of clips or suture, as this will often result in worsening of the injury. Furthermore, when attempting to control bleeding from an incompletely ligated infundibulopelvic ligament, care must be taken to avoid injury to the underlying ureter.

Penetration into the bladder is recognized by the laparoscopic appearance of the inside of the bladder with its smooth urothelium and the urethral catheter. Bladder injury should also be suspected if gas or blood is noted in the Foley bag. The bladder is mainly vulnerable to injury at two stages during laparoscopic hysterectomy: first, when the peritoneum of the uterovesical pouch is divided and the bladder dissected free from the anterior surface of the uterus and cervix, and second, when the uterine artery pedicle is stapled laparoscopically, without prior mobilization of the bladder. The first type of injury can be avoided by carefully placing the peritoneum and extravesical tissue on stretch with the graspers and dissecting with the scissors with cautery close to the uterine surface. The second type of injury is avoided by developing the bladder flap prior to ligation of the vessels via sharp dissection and skeletonization of the vessels prior to ligation. If injury is suspected, the bladder should be instilled with indigo carmine and carefully inspected for leakage of blue urine. A tear in the bladder wall can be repaired either laparoscopically or via laparotomy in a standard two-layer closure with absorbable suture. In either case cystoscopy should be performed to identify the ureteral orifices bilaterally. If the injury is near the ureter, a stent should be placed. Security of the bladder closure can be checked by reinstallation of indigo-carmine. The bladder is drained postoperatively for 4–14 days, depending upon the location of the injury. Penetrating injury of the bladder can be largely avoided by assuring that the bladder is completely drained prior to the onset of the procedure.

Ureteric injury may occur at two phases of the laparoscopic hysterectomy: the division of the ovarian vessels and the division of the uterine vessels. In each phase prior identification of the ureter as previously described can eliminate ureteral injury. If ureteral injury is suspected the patient is given intravenous indigo carmine dye and the ureter inspected for leakage of dye. If complete transection of the ureter is suspected (i.e., from incorporation of the ureter in the endo-GIA stapler), no leakage of dye will be seen. If the injury is not apparent, either cystoscopy or cystotomy can be performed and the ureteral orifices are observed for blue jets of urine. The method of repair of the ureteral injury is beyond the scope of this discussion; however, consultation with either a gynecological oncologist or urologist is warranted.

Postoperative infection following laparoscopic surgery may arise in the abdominal wounds, pelvis, chest, or urinary tract. The use of prophylactic antibiotics has been shown to significantly reduce morbidity in women undergoing vaginal hysterectomy. On this basis, prophylactic antibiotics are advocated for all laparoscopic hysterectomies, although prospective studies have not been performed.

IX. OPERATIVE LAPAROSCOPY IN GYNECOLOGICAL ONCOLOGY

A. Overview

The role of laparoscopy in the field of gynecological oncology has expanded tremendously in the last decade. Previously many gynecological oncologists had considered laparoscopy as an inadequate technique in properly staging and removing pelvic tumors. Both advances in skill and equipment have facilitated rapid adoption of novel minimally invasive techniques at many centers, both in the United States and throughout the world. Numerous reports, heretofore focusing upon complication rates and feasibility, now report both efficacy and survival data for each of the three major gynecological malignancies. Thus, the role of laparoscopy in cervical, endometrial, and ovarian cancer is continually emerging. Results of larger prospective studies replete with outcome data including cost and quality of life assessment are forthcoming. Certainly, the robust enthusiasm for laparoscopy in gynecological malignancies remains tempered by the need for thorough and cost-effective staging and tumor removal. Continued advances, however, have made attainment of these goals feasible, at least by highly trained individuals in specialized centers. Unbiased research and the continual development of optical and surgical technologies will ultimately define the expanding role of minimal-access surgery in gynecological oncology (AC0G Technical Bulletin, 1988).

B. Cervical Cancer

Pioneered largely outside of the United States, laparoscopy has played a significant role in the treatment of cervical malignancies. Procedures have ranged from simple laparoscopic lymphadenectomy for nodal assessment in advanced stage patients to complete execution of radical hysterectomies accomplished entirely laparoscopically including the removal of lymph nodes in patients with earlier stage disease (Chi and Curtain, 1999). Dargent was the first to describe an endoscopic approach using laparoscopically assisted radical vaginal hysterectomy and found that this technique was feasible (Dargent, 1993). An expanded role for lymphadenectomy was examined in a study by Querleu et al. (1991) in which laparoscopy was employed transperitoneally for pelvic lymph node removal. Thus, radical hysterectomy can be performed both vaginally or laparoscopically assisted in combination with laparoscopic lymphadenectomy in either case. A more novel approach for women who wish to preserve fertility with early-stage cervical cancer has incorporated radical resection of the cervix and is termed radical trachelectomy (Dargent, 2001). Both vaginal and curiously abdominal routes have been reported. The Gynecologic Oncology Group (GOG) has enrolled patients on a prospective clinical trial assessing laparoscopic lymphadenectomy for early stage cervical cancer (Schlaerth, et al., 2002). A total of 73 women were enrolled, only 40 of whom were completely evaluable. The mean number of lymph nodes removed from each site equaled or exceeded those from open procedures based on historical controls. Just over 10% of the evaluable patients were judged to have incomplete resections laparoscopically.

C. Endometrial Cancer

Almost 75% of patients with endometrial cancer have disease confined to the uterus at the time of diagnosis as most patients present with postmenopausal bleeding. Nonetheless, there is a growing body of evidence suggesting that lymphadenectomy, even in apparent early stage disease, may be the most cost-effective and efficacious mode of treatment for this disease. With lymphadenectomy, patients can be properly triaged to receive or avoid radiation based upon complete surgical staging information. Certainly the ability to remove the lymph nodes in a thorough manner laparoscopically would allow patients to then undergo vaginal hysterectomy and avoid a laparotomy incision. Washings can be obtained through the scope, and removal of the adnexa as well as visual inspection for metastatic disease can all be accomplished via laparoscopy. Certainly one of the major impediments to laparoscopic surgery for patients with endometrial cancer is the clear association between increased body mass index (BMI) with the development of endometrial cancer due to increased endogenous estrogen exposure. The patients with large BMI are technically challenging, especially laparoscopically. Feasibility of this approach has been reported by numerous authors, first by Childers et al. (1993) and then Boike et al. (1994).

The GOG has an ongoing Phase III trial assessing the ability to perform laparoscopic lymphadenectomy and washings combined with a vaginal hysterectomy with BSO. Cost, adequacy of staging, complications, and quality of life data are currently pending. Certainly this large trial will be an important contributor to the literature; however, the results may be somewhat limited by the fact that the majority of patients enrolled thus far have been from only a few centers in the United States that have taken a particular interest in laparoscopic procedures. The data thus may not be applicable to other cancer centers that have not focused upon minimally invasive surgery as a primary initiative. A recent study examined survival after laparoscopy in women with endometrial cancer, finding that 100 women who underwent laparoscopy failed to show any impairment in 2- and 5-year recurrence-free survivals in comparison to historical laparotomy controls (Eltabbakh, 2002). These results are reinforced by a report by Holub et al. (2002) examining 177 women who had undergone laparoscopic-assisted surgical staging. They found a shorter length of stay, a longer operating time, but no difference in complications, recurrence, or survival in the laparoscopic cohort.

D. Ovarian Cancer

Laparoscopy has certainly been shown to be feasible for staging of apparent early stage ovarian cancer with no gross disease spread throughout the peritoneal cavity. Adequate assessment of the lymph nodes, omentum, and peritoneal biopsies, as well as diaphragm surface can be readily accomplished laparoscopically. A number of reports have confirmed this assessment. The greatest challenge for the clinician is discerning which pelvic masses lend themselves best to laparoscopic removal. Certainly for the less experienced laparoscopist, they should limit their laparoscopic removal criteria to masses that appear to be benign, such as those of simple cysts < 6 cm in diameter. For masses > 6 cm in diameter or that are complex, laparoscopic challenges are certainly increased and the risk of injury to surrounding organs such as the ureter are enhanced. One should be equipped and prepared to do full surgical staging for a resection of any mass thought to be potentially malignant. Pelvic washings are taken initially for cytology, and this is also readily accomplished through the laparoscope. Frozen section should be obtained after the mass is removed, and every effort should be made to remove the mass intact to prevent any spill of potential malignant cells. Many clinicians will convert to a laparotomy at the time of positive frozen section for malignancy; however, some skilled laparoscopists would continue to perform the staging fully laparoscopically as noted above. Once again, GOG data may be helpful in that this organization is evaluating the ability of laparoscopy to stage patients who were incompletely staged at the time of initial laparotomy, at which time ovarian cancer was diagnosed.

The role of the second-look operation has been an area of contention in the treatment of ovarian cancer. Laparoscopy has served as a surrogate for exploratory laparotomy in this setting, and a number of reports have studied this issue. The general trend in the literature has been that early studies have demonstrated a significant concern with procedure adequacy, at which time both training and instrumentation was more primitive. More recent data have suggested that laparoscopy can be safely and effectively performed in substitution for second-look laparotomy in terms of both safety and efficacy.

E. Future Directions for Laparoscopy in Gynecological Oncology

A number of gaps in our current database exist with regards to a thorough understanding of the role of laparoscopy in gynecological oncology. Certainly the emerging data in terms of survival with endometrial cancer need to be duplicated in other disease sites. Furthermore, economic, long-term survival, and quality-of-life parameters require further study in patients who undergo laparoscopy for treatment of gynecological malignancies. One challenge that needs to be met for treating patients with endometrial cancer is the ability to operate on patients who have a quetelet index exceeding 28. Another concern with treating patients with endometrial cancer is the reported increased incidence of positive peritoneal cytology due to possible uterine manipulation during the procedure. Similar findings have been reported after hysteroscopy performed for the diagnosis of endometrial cancer. Confirmation that these findings are of clinical importance and actually impact survival is required. Similarly, study of port site recurrences and their prevention is an important issue that will likely influence the choice of insufflation media, port site material, and prophylactic measures. The evolving and ever-expanding role of sentinel node identification will likely further complement laparoscopy and perhaps greatly enhance the ability of minimally invasive surgery to play a more dominant role in the management of patients with gynecological malignancies.

X. EQUIPMENT AND INSTRUMENTATION (SPECIALIZED)

1. Suction-irrigation unit
2. Atraumatic grasper, spoon forceps, traumatic graspers
3. Insulated curved scissors with unipolar cautery
4. Bipolar cautery (e.g., Kleppinger)
5. Multifire clip applicator
6. Multifire endoscopic stapler
7. Laparoscopic endo-loop device
8. Laparoscopic needle driver
9. Disposable endoscopic specimen pouch

XI. SURGICAL TIPS

1. Proper preparation with adequate mechanical bowel preparation and steep Trendelenburg positioning facilitate removal of the bowel out of the surgical field. Care should be taken to carefully position and pad the patient's legs, shoulders, and arms to avoid postoperative neuropathies.
2. Pelvic sidewall dissection is performed using endoscopic scissors with unipolar cautery. The surgeon performs the dissection from the contralateral side of the table, with the graspers passed through the lower midline port and the scissors passed through the contralateral port.
3. The ureter is identified in the retroperitoneal space at the start of the case.
4. During dissection of the bladder from the lower uterine segment upward, traction is applied on the bladder peritoneum and careful dissection is performed with the endoscopic scissors with unipolar cautery.
5. If the uterine vessels are divided via the laparoscopic approach, care should be taken to apply the endoscopic stapler as parallel to the uterus as possible to avoid ureteral damage.
6. During the vaginal phase of the hysterectomy, care must be taken to assure that the upper vaginal pedicles meet the laparoscopic staple lines.
7. At the completion of the procedure, the pneumoperitoneum must be reestablished and hemostasis assured.
8. If any question exists as to ureteral injury, a thorough intraoperative evaluation is performed as previously described.

9. A guiding principle in laparoscopic surgery is to perform the procedure as much as possible as an open procedure with attention to traction and countertraction, good exposure, and proper identification of anatomical landmarks.

XII. COMPLICATIONS

Penetrating injury from port placement (great vessels, anterior abdominal wall vessels, bowel, and bladder)
Ureteral transection or ligation
Hemorrhage from uterine artery or ovarian vessels
Thermal injury to the bowel
Gas emboli (supportive therapy)
Subcutaneous emphysema (expectant management)

SELECTED READINGS

ACOG Technical Bulletin—Sterilization, No. 113, Feb 1988.

Boike G, Lurain J, Burke J. A comparison of laparoscopic management of endometrial cancer with tradition laparotomy (abst). Gynecol Oncol 52:105, 1994.

Chi D, Curtain J. Gynecologic cancer and laparoscopy. Obstet Gynecol Clin North Am 26(2):201–215, 1999.

Childers JM, Brzechffa PR, Hatch KD, et al. Laparoscopically assisted surgical staging (LASS) of endometrial cancer. Gynecol Oncol 51:33–38, 1993.

Dargent D. Laparoscopic surgery and gynecologic cancer. Curr Opin Obstet Gynecol 5:294&–300, 1993.

Dargent D, 569437 Lyon: Radical Trachelectomy: Vaginal. Bull Acad Natl Med 185(7):1295–1304. 2001.

Eltabbakh GH. Analysis of survival after laparoscopy in women with endometrial carcinoma. Cancer 1:95(9):1894–1901, 2002.

Holub Z, Jabor A, et al. Laparoscopic surgery for endometrial cancer: long-term results of a multicentric study. Eur J Gynaecol Oncol 23(4):305–310, 2002.

Jones DB, Simmang CL, Coleman R. The emerging role of laparoscopy in bowel surgery. In Gershenson DM, ed. Operative techniques in gynecologic surgery. W.B. Saunders; 2001, 6(2):105–112.

Parker WH, Berek JS. Management of selected cystic adnexal masses in postmenopausal women by operative laparoscopy: a pilot study. Am J Obstet Gynecol 1990;163:1574–1577.

Phipps JH. Laparoscopic Hysterectomy and Oophorectomy. New York, Churchill Livingstone, 1993.

Querleu D, Leblanc E, Castelain B. Laparoscopic pelvic lymphadenectomy in the staging of early carcinoma of the cervix. Am J Obstet Gynecol 1564:578–581, 1991.

Saye WB, Espy GB. Laparoscopic Döderlein hysterectomy. In: Surgical Rounds. Lousiana: A Romaine Pierson Publication, June 1994, pp 415–425.

Schlaerth JB, Spirtos NM, Carson LF, Boike G, Adamed T, Stonebraker B. Laparoscopic retroperitoneal lymphadenectomy followed by laparotomy in women with cervical cancer: A GOG study. Gynecol Oncol 85(1):81–88. 2002.

Soper NJ, Odem RR, Clayman RV, McDougall EM. Essentials of Laparoscopy. St. Louis: Quality Medical Publishing, Inc., 1994.

35

Urological Procedures

JEFFREY A. CADEDDU

University of Texas Southwestern Medical Center
Dallas, Texas, U.S.A.

RALPH V. CLAYMAN

University of California, Irvine Medical Center
Orange, California, U.S.A.

Laparoscopic urological procedures began with exploration for the undescended testicle and have expanded to the point where almost all open urological procedures have been done successfully by a laparoscopic approach. Over the years, some laparoscopic procedures that were once popular have been abandoned as they failed to show benefit over their open counterparts, e.g., bladder neck suspension and varicocelectomy. On the other hand, many other procedures have come to the fore and are commonly practiced at many major medical centers, e.g., nephroureterectomy, renal biopsy, ureterolysis, and radical prostatectomy. In addition, even cystectomy and diversion have now been successfully done laparoscopically. In this chapter we will focus on two of the more commonly done laparoscopic procedures, one ablative (nephrectomy) and one reconstructive (pyeloplasty).

I. NEPHRECTOMY

In 1869, the first nephrectomy was performed by Simon for a ureterovaginal fistula. Since that time dramatic changes in anesthesia, surgical technique, and medical management have reduced the morbidity of the procedure and allowed nephrectomy to become a useful and safe tool in the practicing urologist's armamentarium against renal disease. However, for over a century little change with regard to the actual performance of a nephrectomy occurred.

In June 1990, Clayman et al. were the first to apply transperitoneal laparoscopic technology to the removal of a large, nonhollow organ. A 190 g tumor-bearing kidney was removed laparoscopically using a specially developed entrapment sack and high-speed electrical tissue morcellator. Subsequently, in 1991, the same authors performed the first totally retroperitoneal laparoscopic nephrectomy. Initially, problems with exposure made the retroperitoneal route less desirable; however, in 1993, Gaur et al. described the use of a balloon technique to rapidly and atraumatically expand the retroperitoneal space. Accordingly, the retroperitoneal approach has become very popular for the removal of small (i.e., <100 g) benign kidneys and in some centers (e.g., Cleveland Clinic) even for the removal of tumor-bearing kidneys. To date, several thousand laparoscopic nephrectomies for benign or malignant renal disease have been performed worldwide. In addition, in 1995, Kavoussi and colleagues at Johns Hopkins reported the first successful laparoscopic donor nephrectomy. Over the past 7 years, laparoscopic donor nephrectomy has become the standard of care at many major transplant centers; indeed, over 2000 cases of laparoscopic donor nephrectomy have now been done.

A. Clinical Presentation and Indications

Benign renal disease is a common disorder. Persistent flank pain, recurrent urinary tract infection, and suspected renovascular hypertension are only a few of the signs or symptoms that lead physicians to investigate the kidney as a possible source of pathology. When the patient has a nonfunctioning or poorly functioning noncancerous kidney, any of these signs or symptoms are an indication for laparoscopic nephrectomy. The only benign condition that remains a relative contraindication to laparoscopic nephrectomy is xanthogranulomatous pyelonephritis. These patients commonly present with flank pain and low-grade fevers. The urine culture commonly produces a *Proteus* species; however, if the process has resulted in total obstruction of the affected renal unit, then the urine culture can be sterile. Radiographic studies reveal the presence of a renal calculus, poor or nonfunction of the kidney, and a "mass" effect. The computed tomography (CT) scan may show extension of the inflammatory process into the perirenal fat, psoas muscle, or adjacent organs. These kidneys are still, in general, best removed via an open approach.

Most renal cell cancers today present serendipitously on an ultrasound or CT scan obtained for nonrenal reasons. The classic triad of flank pain, mass, and gross hematuria has become exceedingly rare. While the indications for laparoscopic nephrectomy in benign disease are clearcut, the indications for laparoscopic nephrectomy in malignant disease initially raised some questions. While it is well documented in every series that the convalescence, use of pain medications, time to ambulation, and hospital stay are all reduced with the laparoscopic approach, there are several areas of concern, specifically the effectiveness, efficiency, and cost of the procedure. Major studies have now shown that the effectiveness of the laparoscopic radical nephrectomy with regard to cancer-specific survival and recurrence is identical to that achievable with an open approach. These follow-up data are now out to 4.5 years. The efficiency of the procedure has improved with experience. In many centers, the overall operative time for a transperitoneal laparoscopic nephrectomy is down to 3–4.5 hours, while the retroperitoneal approach is down to 2.5 hours. By improving the efficiency of the procedure, the cost of the laparoscopic approach has been reduced below that of open nephrectomy. Recently Cadeddu and associates demonstrated that once the laparoscopic operative time fell below 4.7 hours with operative expenses of <$5500 and a hospital stay of <5.8 days, the laparoscopic procedure saved over $1000 versus open nephrectomy. Indeed, in most centers the operative time is under 4 hours and the hospital stay is 3 days or less. Other concerns with regard to laparoscopic radical nephrectomy centered about morcellation versus intact removal. At present, morcellation is now done mechanically via a 20 mm incision; hence, accurate clinical staging along with grade can now be obtained. Concerns over tumor seeding due to morcellation have been largely unfounded. Indeed, after a decade of laparoscopic radical nephrectomy there are only three cases of seeding of the trocar site, with two of them coming from the same institution with fewer than 30 cases performed. In the latter circumstance, the morcellation had been done in a plastic sack rather than in the specialized nylon/plastic sack specifically designed for morcellation. With intact removal there have been no cases of seeding of the trocar site. This method of removal has become even more popular with the advent of hand-assisted nephrectomy. Accordingly, today for all T1, T2 or T3a lesions (i.e., 4–10 cm), a laparoscopic nephrectomy is the preferred method of removal at many major medical centers. The laparoscopic approach has also been applied to renal tumors affecting the renal vein and in a couple of cases to renal tumors with minimal caval involvement. Likewise, renal tumors invading the renal vein or just into the inferior vena cava (T3b) have been successfully removed, as have tumors as large as 15 cm.

B. Diagnostic Tests

For patients with benign disease, a functional radiographic study, usually a nuclear renal scan, is done to document poor function of the affected kidney and satisfactory function of the contralateral kidney. A CT scan if the primary process is inflammatory; this is done to assess for possible xanthogranulomatous pyelonephritis. For patients with renal cancer, a full metastatic evaluation is obtained: chest radiograph, serum liver function tests, serum calcium, CT of the abdomen, and, if the patient has an elevated calcium, alkaline phosphatase, and/or bone pain, a bone scan. The CT should confirm the size of the tumor, assess if there is renal vein or inferior vena caval involvement, rule out liver involvement, assess the status of the ipsilateral adrenal gland, confirm the presence of a normal contralateral adrenal gland, and alert the urologist to any hilar or regional lymphadenopathy.

C. Operative Treatment

Surgical therapy for the diseased benign kidney removes the kidney itself without necessarily including the surrounding fat and fascia (i.e., simple nephrectomy). In patients with malignant disease confined to the kidney, the nephrectomy includes all of the perirenal fat and all but the superior portion of Gerota's fascia (i.e., total nephrectomy excluding the ipsilateral adrenal). In patients where the ipsilateral adrenal is abnormal on CT scan, all of the perirenal fat within an intact Gerota's fascia, including the ipsilateral adrenal, is removed (i.e., radical nephrectomy).

   Absolute contraindications to a laparoscopic nephrectomy include inability to tolerate general anesthesia or the presence of an uncorrectable coagulopathy. Patients with severe obstructive pulmonary disease are difficult to manage laparoscopically due to hypercarbia; however, use of helium as the insufflant can still allow even these patients to have a laparoscopic approach. Similarly, even massive obesity is no longer considered a contraindication for a laparoscopic nephrectomy. Finally, a history of extensive abdominal surgery or prior retroperitoneal surgery (e.g., abdominal aortic aneurysm repair or prior renal surgery) is a relative contraindication to laparoscopic nephrectomy, because scarring and adhesion formation will distort much of the anatomy and render the dissection more difficult.

Specific contraindications to a laparoscopic nephrectomy are few. Patients with the rare condition of xanthogranulomatous pyelonephritis are better treated by an open nephrectomy. However, even patients with large benign kidneys, such as those associated with autosomal dominant polycystic kidney disease, can be done laparoscopically, especially with a hand-assist approach. For renal cancer, patients with tumors > 13 cm or with venal caval involvement are, in general, considered not to be candidates for a laparoscopic approach.

D. Preoperative Preparation

The expectations and risks of a laparoscopic nephrectomy are discussed with the patient. These include but are not limited to life-threatening hemorrhage and injury to the bowel, spleen, liver, and pancreas. Patients are counseled that if at any point during a laparoscopic operation a major complication occurs or suitable exposure becomes unattainable, the operation will be converted to an open approach.

Healthy patients are admitted the day of surgery. Preoperative preparation such as 1 day of a clear liquid diet, an evening cleansing enema, or a bottle of magnesium citrate is optional. The patients are routinely typed but not crossmatched unless this is early in the surgeon's experience with laparoscopic nephrectomy. Because this is an elective procedure, all patients are offered the option of banking autologous blood or directed donor units. Just before transfer to the operating room, the patient is given a single dose of a broad-spectrum antibiotic (e.g., cefazolin, 1 g) intravenously.

During the initial experience with laparoscopic nephrectomy, renal artery embolization was performed. Today this practice has been largely abandoned. It is only used in a suspected case of xanthogranulomatous pyelonephritis or when a very large renal cancer is being approach (i.e. > 10 cm). This allows the surgeon to take the renal vein first and may also decrease some of the collateral venous flow associated with a large tumor. In this regard, the embolization should be performed on the morning of the planned procedure so that the post-embolization syndrome of pain and fever is avoided.

E. Equipment for Transperitoneal Nephrectomy: Standard*

Disposable equipment:
5 mm Endoshears (U.S. Surgical)
12 mm Multifire EndoGia—vascular and tissue staple with reloads available (U.S. Surgical)
10 mm Ligasure device (Valleylab)
Trocars—12 mm (3) (axially dilating clear ports-Ethicon)
5 × 8 and 8 × 10 inch LapSacs (Cook Urological)
Veress needle (150 mm) (U.S. Surgical)
CO_2 insufflation tubing
10 sponges (Raytex)
5 mm harmonic scalpel (curved jaws) (Ethicon)

Nondisposable equipment:
Trocars—5 mm (2) (Endotip—Storz)
Endoholder [Codman (division of Johnson and Johnson)]

*Equipment listed in this section as used at University of California, Irvine.

Suction irrigator, extra long, 5 mm (Nezhat system: Storz)
Laparoscope: 10 mm, 0° lens and a 10 mm, 30° lens and a 5 mm, 0° lens (Storz)
3 atraumatic, nonlocking 5 mm smooth tip (duckbill) grasping forceps (Storz)
4 traumatic (toothed), locking, 5 mm grasping forceps (Storz)
LapSac introducer (Cook)
Electroshield device to attach to electrocautery for active electrode monitoring
    (Encision)
5 mm hook electrode (Encision)
5 mm and 10 mm PEER retractors (J. Jamner Inc.)
5 mm Needleholders (J. Jamner, Inc. and Storz)
10 mm soft curved angled forceps (Maryland dissector) (Storz)
10 mm right angle dissector (Storz or J. Jamner)
5 mm diamond-shaped "snake" retractor (Genzyme)
Carter Thomason needle suture grasper and closure cones (Inlet Medical)

Available but not opened equipment:
Disposable roticulating endoshears (U.S. Surgical)
Endostitch and all types of suture used (0,2-0,4-0, Polysorb, Polydac, and Prolene)
    (U.S. Surgical)
Disposable Hasson trocar 12 mm Blunt Tip (U. S. Surgical)
3-0 cardiovascular silk (RB-1 needle) and 0-Vicryl suture for fascial closure
Lapra-ty clips and 10 mm Laparo-Ty clip applier (Ethicon)
Gauze rolls (5) (Carefree Surgical Specialties)
10 mm Satinsky clamp with flexible port (Acsculap)
10 mm clip appliers with 9 mm and 11 mm clips (Ethicon)

F. Equipment for Transperitoneal Nephrectomy: Hand-Assist

Disposable equipment:
GelPort (Applied Medical)
5 mm Endoshears (U.S. Surgical)
12 mm Multifire EndoGia—vascular and tissue staple with reloads available (U.S.
    Surgical)
10 mm Ligasure device (Valleylab)
Trocars—12 mm (2) (axially dilating clear ports-Ethicon)
5 × 8 and 8 × 10 inch LapSacs (Cook Urological)
CO_2 insufflation tubing
10 sponges (Raytex)
5 mm harmonic scalpel (curved jaws) (Ethicon)

Nondisposable equipment:
Trocars—5 mm (1) (Endotip Storz)
Suction irrigator, extra long, 5 mm (Nezhat system: Storz)
Laparoscope: 10 mm, 0° lens and a 10 mm, 30° lens and a 5 mm, 0° lens (Storz)
3 atraumatic, nonlocking 5 mm smooth-tip (duckbill) grasping forceps (Storz)
4 traumatic (toothed), locking, 5 mm grasping forceps (Storz)
Electroshield device to attach to electrocautery for active electrode monitoring
    (Incision)

5 mm hook electrode (Incision)
5 mm and 10 mm PEER retractors (J. Jamner Inc.)
5 mm needleholders (J. Jamner, Inc. and Storz)
10 mm soft curved angled forceps (Maryland dissector) (Storz)
10 mm right angle dissector (Storz or J. Jamner)
Carter Thomason needle suture grasper and closure cones (Inlet Medical)

Available but not opened equipment:
Same as with standard transperitoneal approach

G.   Equipment for Retroperitoneal Nephrectomy

Disposable equipment:
12 mm trocar-mounted balloon distension device (Bluntport, US Surgical)
5 mm endoshears (U.S. Surgical)
12 mm Multifire EndoGia—vascular and tissue staple with reloads available (U.S. Surgical)
10 mm clip appliers with 9 mm and 11 mm clips (Ethicon)
Trocars—12 mm (2) (axially dilating clear ports—Ethicon)
5 × 8 and 8 × 10 inch LapSacs (Cook Urological)
CO_2 insufflation tubing
10 sponges (Raytex)
5 mm harmonic scalpel (curved jaws) (Ethicon)

Nondisposable equipment:
Trocars—5 mm (2) (Endotip—Storz)
Endoholder [(Codman (division of Johnson and Johnson)]
Suction irrigator, extra long, 5 mm (Nezhat system: Storz)
Laparoscope: 10 mm, 0° lens and a 10 mm, 30° lens and a 5 mm, 0° lens (Storz)
3 atraumatic, nonlocking 5 mm smooth-tip (duckbill) grasping forceps (Storz)
4 traumatic (toothed), locking, 5 mm grasping forceps (Storz)
Electroshield device to attach to electrocautery for active electrode monitoring (Incision)
5 mm hook electrode (Incision)
5 mm and 10 mm PEER retractors (J. Jamner Inc.)
5 mm needleholders (J. Jamner, Inc. and Storz)
10 mm soft curved angled forceps (Maryland dissector) (Storz)
10 mm right angle dissector (Storz or J. Jamner)
Carter Thomason needle suture grasper and closure cones (Inlet Medical)

Available but not opened equipment:
Same as with standard transperitoneal approach

H.   Surgical Technique

1.   Transperitoneal Approach: Standard

Operating Room and Patient Setup.   With the patient lying supine, the operating room personnel and equipment are arranged with the surgeon on the side contralateral to the

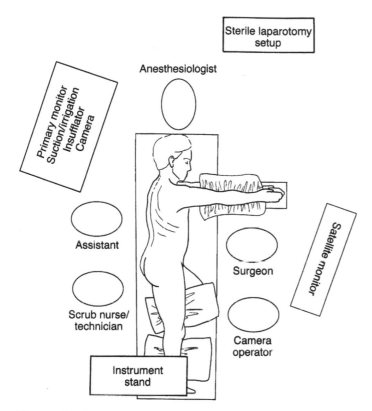

Figure 1 Operating room setup for laparoscopic transperitoneal nephrectomy.

surgical dissection (Fig. 1). The camera operator also stands on this side, just below the surgeon. The first assistant stands opposite the surgeon on the ipsilateral side of the table. The scrub nurse stands just opposite or below the camera operator. Equipment is arranged with the primary monitor viewed by the surgeon placed on the surgical assistant's side of the table, just above his or her shoulder. A satellite monitor for the assistant is placed on the surgeon's side of the table, just above the surgeon. Suction/irrigation lines, the insufflator line, and the camera cords are brought off the head of the table on the assistant's side. The electrosurgical cord, cord to the harmonic scalpel, and cord for the Ligasure device are brought off the foot of the table on the assistant's side. The sterile instrument table is placed behind the nurse, and an instrument stand is placed across the foot of the table. The anesthesiologist with all appropriate critical monitoring equipment is at the head of the table, behind the sterile ether screen.

As with any laparoscopic surgery, a full sterile laparotomy setup, including vascular clamps, must be available in the operating room should emergency conversion to an open procedure become necessary.

Once the patient is in the operating room, general endotracheal anesthesia is established and a nasogastric tube and Foley catheter are placed. Thigh-high elastic TED stockings and pneumatic sequential compression stockings are placed to prevent deep venous thrombosis. The patient is turned from a supine into a lateral decubitus position. The use of orthopedic "hip huggers" is helpful to maintain the flank position; these are placed at the shoulder and hip and further padded with foam "egg crate." The kidney rest is positioned beneath the contralateral iliac crest and then raised. The table is flexed. Appropriate measures should be taken to avoid patient injury in this position, including placement of two or three pillows between the upper and lower portion of the legs such that the upper leg is nearly level with the iliac crest, flexion of the lower leg to 30 degrees at the knee and hip, extension of the upper leg, support of the upper arm by an elevated arm board, padding of the lower arm and axilla with a gel pad to protect the brachial plexus, and appropriate padding of all dependent bony prominences (e.g., downside hip, knee, and ankle) to prevent undesired bruising or irritation to the unprotected skin. Additional security may be obtained with appropriately placed padded sandbags and padded straps. A full flank and abdominal surgical scrub follows.

Pneumoperitoneum and Port Placement.   In the lateral decubitus position a 12 mm incision is made approximately two fingerbreadths above and three fingerbreadths over from the ipsilateral superior iliac spine; there is a natural hollow that can usually be palpated in this area. The external oblique aponeurosis is identified and secured with two clamps. A small fascial incision is made and the Veress needle is passed. A pneumoperitoneum is established at 25 mmHg. Alternatively, an open Hasson approach, described elsewhere in this text, can be used.

After establishing an adequate pneumoperitoneum, a 12 mm noncutting port is passed usually under endoscopic control with a 0 degree lens. Next, the 30 degree laparoscope is inserted and the intra-abdominal pressure is reduced to 10–15 mmHg. The abdominal cavity and its contents are thoroughly inspected. All subsequent ports are placed under direct endoscopic control: an upper 12 mm midclavicular line subcostal noncutting port and a supraumbilical pararectus 12 mm noncutting port. The first two ports are usually used by the surgeon, whereas the supraumbilical port is used for the laparoscope. During the procedure, a 5 mm noncutting port is placed in the anterior axillary line, subcostal. For a right nephrectomy, an optional 5 mm noncutting upper midclavicular line port may be placed subcostally to aid retraction of the liver.

Entering the Retroperitoneum.   Once transperitoneal access is safely achieved, exposure of the affected kidney requires incision of the ipsilateral lateral colonic peritoneal reflection (i.e., the white line of Toldt). This line of demarcation is often readily visible, with the patient in a full lateral position as gravity displaces the colon away from the abdominal side-wall (Fig. 2). The surgeon, working through the lower 12 mm anterior axillary line port, grasps the line of Toldt with atraumatic forceps and retracts the peritoneum medially. With the line of Toldt elevated and on stretch, the surgeon passes a harmonic shears or electrosurgical scissors through the upper 12 mm anterior axillary line port and incises the peritoneal fold. Incision of the line of Toldt is continued inferiorly to the level of the common iliac artery and superiorly above the hepatic or splenic flexure.

With the colon moved medially, the 5 mm anterior axillary line port is placed . This port is primarily reserved for the assistant or for use of the Endoholder for retracting the kidney. For a *right* nephrectomy, medial retraction of the ascending colon and its hepatic flexure reveals the underlying duodenum. (For a radical nephrectomy, the posterior coronary ligament of the liver is incised from lateral to medial, thereby further freeing Gerota's fascia and providing exposure to the supra-adrenal portion of the inferior vena cava. In addition, the triangular ligament of the liver is incised.) A Kocher maneuver is subsequently performed as the duodenum is reflected medially, thereby uncovering the underlying vena cava.

The approach to the right kidney is dependent upon the type of nephrectomy that is indicated. For a simple nephrectomy, a triangle is created in which one side is the line of

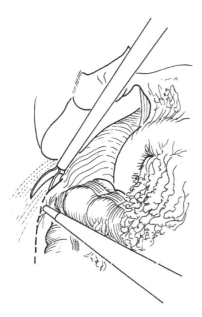

Figure 2   Incision of the line of Toldt.

Toldt. The other two sides are created at the upper and lower poles of the kidney, after the colonic reflection and duodenum have been mobilized medially. At this time an incision is made through the pararenal fat, Gerota's fascia, and the perirenal fat, to come directly on to the renal capsule. The apex of this triangle is created at the point of insertion of the right renal vein into the vena cava. In contrast, on the right side, for a radical nephrectomy, a geometric wedge is created whereby the line of Toldt and triangular ligament of the liver serve as the thin edge of the wedge and the colonic reflection medially, the Kocher maneuver on the duodenum, and the dissection directly on the inferior vena cava create the broad opposite or medial portion of the wedge. The sides of the wedge consist of the colonic reflection inferiorly and the incision in the posterior coronary hepatic ligament superiorly. This approach assures a broad dissection of the kidney intact within Gerota's fascia as well as inclusion of the adrenal gland.

For a *left* nephrectomy, careful dissection must be undertaken at the level of the splenic flexure, because the phrenicocolic, lienocolic, and lienorenal ligaments may be quite thick. The assistant must be vigilant so that no traction is placed directly on the spleen to avoid injury of the spleen. The surgeon must be fastidious in thoroughly coagulating these ligaments as they are incised. Furthermore, careful dissection must be done to separate the colon and colonic mesentery off of the underlying Gerota's fascia; it is essential to identify the natural occurring plane between these two structures or else the surgeon may enter the mesentery of the colon. Additionally, both surgeon and assistant must be constantly aware of the close proximity of the pancreas to the upper anterior surface of the left kidney. Dissection in this area must be meticulous and bloodless.

The approach to the left kidney is likewise dependent upon the type of nephrectomy that is indicated. For a simple nephrectomy, a triangle is created in which one side is the line of Toldt. After reflection of the colon and the colonic mesentery, the other two sides are created at the upper and lower poles of the kidney. An incision is made through the pararenal fat, Gerota's fascia, and the perirenal fat, to come directly on to the renal capsule. As the colon is reflected medially, the apex of this triangle is created at the level of the renal hilum. In contrast, for a left radical nephrectomy, an inverted cone is created (i.e., a "water-scooper"). The elongated lateral border of the cone (i.e., the handle of the "water-scooper") consists of the incision in the line of Toldt and the incision of the spleno-phrenic attachments. The opposite side of the cone is created where the surgeon "V's" off of the line of Toldt caudally to begin to separate the colon and colonic mesentery from the underlying Gerota's fascia. This line begins at the most caudal point of the incision in the line of Toldt and proceeds cephalad; as it progresses over the anterior surface of Gerota's fascia covering the kidney, it moves more medially. The line ends superiorly as the surgeon approaches the spleen, thereby completing the upper broader medial end of the cone. The upper portion or opening of the cone (i.e., mouth of the "water-scooper") consists of the freeing of the splenic flexure of the colon and the spleno-colic attachments (i.e., anterior portion of the cone) and the release of the splenorenal ligament which forms the posterior portion of the cone. This approach assures a broad dissection of the kidney within Gerota's fascia along with the adrenal gland.

Isolating the Ureter.   Once the retroperitoneum has been adequately exposed, attention is turned to isolation of the ureter. The ureter typically lies directly posterior to the gonadal vessels and medial to the medial edge of the psoas muscle. As such, the gonadal vein is first identified, dissected, secured with four clips, and cut. The ureter should lie directly

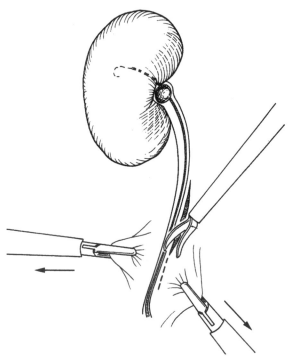

Figure 3   Exposing the ureter. Note the critical traction/countertraction between the surgeon's and assistant's instruments.

posterior. The ureter can then be dissected (Fig. 3); it can be secured with clips and cut at this point or later in the procedure. The former maneuver may facilitate the subsequent hilar dissection.

Dissecting the Kidney. Once the ureter has been freed superiorly to the level of the ureteropelvic junction (UPJ), attention may be turned to the task at hand—freeing up the kidney. Pararenal fat (i.e., outside Gerota's fascia) around the lower pole and lateral surface of the kidney typically clears easily with blunt dissection.

If a nephrectomy is being performed for benign disease, Gerota's fascia is sharply incised and the pararenal fat is cleared from the lower pole, lateral, anterior, and upper pole surfaces of the kidney. In this regard, it is most helpful to make a cross-shaped incision in Gerota's fascia along the anteromedial aspect of the kidney (horizontally) and along the middle of the anterior surface of the kidney (vertically). This will make later access to the renal hilum a bit more straightforward.

For nephrectomies undertaken for renal cancer, it must be remembered that Gerota's fascia should remain intact. The only exception is if the adrenal is to be spared, in which case the upper end of Gerota's fascia can be entered and the renal surface identified.

On the right side, dissection of the upper pole of the kidney is complicated by the overlying liver. The camera operator may help in this situation by placing a "snake" or PEER retractor through the 5 mm port or through an additional 5 mm subcostal midclavicular line port. On the left side, the spleen poses less of an impediment; however, retraction of this organ must be undertaken with great care to avoid a splenic laceration. The "snake" retractor is preferred for this purpose as it lies flat against the underside of the liver or spleen, whereas the legs of the PEER retractor can present a potential problem. Retraction of either the liver or spleen is most safely done by placing the retractor along the underside of the incised peritoneal reflection (i.e., posterior coronary ligament of the liver or lienocolic ligament of the spleen) closest to the liver or spleen and retracting cephalad. As such, the organ is protected by the intervening layer of peritoneal tissue and fat. To prevent inadvertent injury while retracting either organ, it is advisable to place a mechanical holder (e.g., Endoholer) on the opposite side of the table and then affix it to the retractor to keep the retractor in place.

Dissecting the Renal Hilum. The role of the assistant or the mechanical holder during this stage is to provide constant lateral retraction of the kidney in order to put traction on the renal hilum. This is best done with a 5 mm PEER retractor opened such that its legs straddle the hilum; the retractor is then deflected laterally to put the hilum on stretch. Again, affixing this retractor to the mechanical holder is the safest way of maintaining reliable, safe traction during the ensuing dissection. The surgeon begins the hilar dissection on the right side by identifying the inferior vena cava and tracing it to the main renal vein. On the left side, the surgeon can follow the gonadal vein cephalad until it joins the main renal vein. On the left side, the anterior leaflet of Gerota's fascia seems thicker than on the right side; nevertheless, it must be incised in order to access the underlying hilar vessels. On the right side, the renal vein is usually a single structure with no branches; on the left side, the adrenal, ascending lumbar, and gonadal branches of the renal vein must all be identified, separately dissected, and occluded. While this is usually done with four 9 mm clips, of late the Ligasure bipolar device has been found to be very effective and efficient for securing and dividing these venous tributaries. The renal vein and renal artery are then dissected until a 360-degree window is established around each vessel. The artery is typically occluded and transected first; a total of five 9 mm clips are placed on the artery: three proximal and two distal. The vein is then simultaneously occluded and transected using a 12 mm Endo GIA *vascular* stapler. Recently, the 12 mm Endo GIA vascular stapler has been also used to secure the renal artery; the closure obtained is rapid and secure.

Dividing the Ureter.   With vascular control of the renal hilum achieved, the kidney is bluntly dissected from the retroperitoneal tissues. Hemostasis is maintained with electrocautery. If not previously divided, this leaves the ureter as the final attachment of the kidney to the retroperitoneum.

Two pairs of 9 mm clips are placed and the ureter is incised. The kidney is suspended by the ureter at the level of the UPJ with 5 mm traumatic, *locking* grasping forceps passed through the 5 mm upper anterior axillary line port (Fig. 4). The kidney is then displaced above the liver on the right or above the spleen on the left, its final resting place before removal.

The pneumoperitoneum is reduced to 5 mmHg. A careful check for hemostasis is completed. Special attention is given to the ipsilateral renal hilum and the area around the ipsilateral adrenal gland.

Introducing the Entrapment Sack.   If morcellation is planned, then an 8 × 10 inch LapSac with a pre-threaded Terumo guidewire around its lip (i.e., threaded in and out of each of the holes through which the drawstring has been passed) is neatly rolled onto its metal two-pronged introducer. Both tines of the introducer remain outside the sack. The drawstrings and ends of the guidewire should run parallel to the handle of the introducer. The uppermost 12 mm port is removed. The introducer and sack are passed through the 12 mm incision and are endoscopically directed toward the most inferior reaches of the pelvis. The assistant provides downward drag on the bottom of the sack with an atraumatic grasper.

The introducer is removed and the 12 mm port is replaced. Using two blunt atraumatic 5 mm graspers, the sack is unfurled in the abdomen. Now the laparoscope is

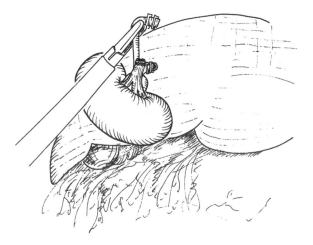

Figure 4   Grasping the kidney. Through the 5 mm upper midaxillary line port, the kidney is suspended by the ureter at the level of the UPJ with 5 mm traumatic locking graspers.

moved to the 12 mm upper port. To open the mouth of the sack, two 5 mm traumatic locking graspers are introduced via the remaining ports and each is used to securely grasp two opposite tabs on the mouth of the sack. The tabs are pulled in different directions to open the sack. Looking straight down into the mouth of the sack, the laparoscope is introduced into the sack and moved in ever-widening concentric circles, thereby further opening the sack. The Terumo guidewire further facilitates the broad opening of the neck of the sack.

Organ Entrapment. Once the sack is in place, the assistant, holding the forceps in which the ureter is secured, now guides the kidney from its superior location into the mouth of the sack (Fig. 5). It is helpful to guide the upper midaxillary line grasper such that it is directed at the superior tab of the sack, thereby helping the kidney to clear the lower edge of the sack. With downward pushing of the kidney deeper into the sack by the assistant and upward pulling of the *lower* lip of the sack by the surgeon via the lower grasper on the lip of the sack, the kidney is deposited deep within the sack. Once entrapment is visually confirmed, the Terumo guidewire is pulled out and the drawstring is snared by a grasper and cinched closed.

Alternatively, if the specimen is to be removed intact, the surgeon may choose to use one of the readily expandable plastic sacks (e.g., EndoCatch or EndoPouch). The 15 mm device can be passed through the upper 12 mm port, opened beneath the liver or spleen, and the kidney can then be rolled off of the liver or spleen and deposited in the widely

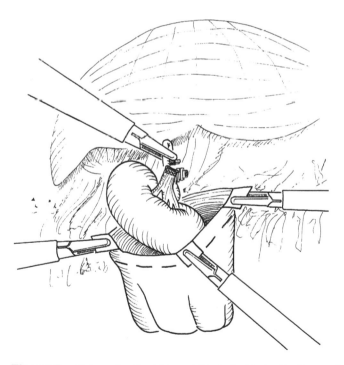

Figure 5 Entrapping the kidney. This is facilitated by the assistant guiding the kidney deep into the sack; once the lower pole of the kidney lies over the lower lip of the sack, the surgeon can raise the lower lip upward, thereby curling the lower lip of the sack over the lower pole of the kidney and pushing the kidney deeper into the sack.

opened sack. The metal band on the lip of these plastic sacks makes opening and closing of the sack very easy. Also, the metal band provides a stiffness to the lip of the sack which facilitates organ entrapment.

At this time, if the nephrectomy was undertaken for cancer, a pericaval or periaortic node dissection may be performed in the area of the ipsilateral renal hilum if so desired by the surgeon. Simple blunt dissection of the lymph nodes around the hilum, as opposed to a formal pericaval or periaortic node dissection, should be sufficient to provide the pathologist with adequate specimen to determine nodal status of the patient. Meticulous hemostasis should be maintained with electrocautery and surgical clips. The nodal specimen is delivered separately and sent for pathology.

Removal of the Kidney: Intact Versus Morcellation.　The laparoscope is returned to the middle 12 mm port. The sack is regrasped by the drawstring and pulled into the 12 mm upper port. With the neck of the sack pulled snugly into this port, the pneumoperitoneum can be maintained. The drawstring and 12 mm upper port are pulled through the abdominal wall as a single unit, thereby delivering the neck of the sack onto the surface of the abdominal wall. The port itself is removed.

A decision is made at this time whether to deliver the kidney intact with the sack through a 5–7 cm transverse subcostal laparotomy or to morcellate the kidney in situ in the sack. In cases of renal malignancy, intact removal is commonly performed; care must be taken not to incise the entrapment sack while extending the fascial incision. Basic surgical principles dictate a two-layer closure of the small laparotomy.

Morcellation can presently be accomplished only mechanically. Mechanical morcellation can be done in the sack with a ring forceps. This is quite effective and inexpensive. This is most easily done by expanding the port to 20 mm. The neck of the sack in all cancer cases is triply draped: nephrostomy drape, towel drape, and a plastic adhesive drape. The morcellation process is endoscopically monitored to make sure the sack is not perforated. Throughout the morcellation procedure, the neck of the sack must be pulled up taut so that folds do not develop in the sack; this precludes any possible injury to the wall of the sack due to inadvertent grasping of the sack by the ring forceps. After all pieces have been removed from the sack, the sack is pulled from the abdominal cavity. Throughout the process, the camera operator maintains an endoscopic view of the sack to alert the surgeon to any sign of perforation (e.g., loss of pneumoperitoneum, blood dripping from the sack). At the end of the morcellation process, the surgeon and first assistant regown and reglove. The morcellation site is swabbed in betadine and the 12 mm port is replaced.

Exiting the Abdomen and Closure.　At the end of the operation, the pneumoperitoneum pressure is lowered to 5 mmHg and a careful check for hemostasis is again performed. The 10 mm laparoscope is replaced with a 5 mm laparoscope passed through the 5 mm port. If intact removal has been performed, then a standard two-layer closure is performed. If the specimen was morcellated, then the morcellation site is closed usually with two 0 absorbable sutures placed with a Carter Thomason device. The other port sites, since they were nonbladed and not through the midline, do not require fascial closure. Similarly the 5 mm port site does not require a fascial closure. The skin is closed using running subcuticular 4-0 absorbable sutures for the 12 mm ports. Adhesive strips are applied to all skin incisions.

2. Transperitoneal Approach: Hand-Assist

Operating Room and Patient Setup. With the patient lying supine, the operating room personnel and equipment are arranged in the same manner as the standard transperitoneal approach. As with any laparoscopic surgery, a full sterile laparotomy setup, including vascular clamps, must be available in the operating room should emergency conversion to an open procedure become necessary.

The patient is placed supine on the operating room table. General endotracheal anesthesia is established and a nasogastric tube and Foley catheter are placed. Thigh-high elastic TED stockings and pneumatic sequential compression stockings are placed to prevent deep venous thrombosis. The planned incision site for the placement of the hand-assist device is drawn on the skin with an indelible marker. The patient is turned from a supine into a lateral decubitus position. The kidney rest is positioned beneath the contralateral iliac crest and then raised. The table is flexed. As with the standard transperitoneal approach, appropriate measures should be taken to avoid patient injury in this position. A full flank and abdominal surgical scrub follow.

Hand Port Placement and Pneumoperitoneum. With this technique, the incision and placement of the hand port device occurs first. Two second-generation hand-ports are most commonly employed: the Gelport (Applied Medical) and Omniport (Ethicon). Both allow the surgeon to place his or her hand into the abdomen without the need for using a special sleeve. The Omniport has a smaller profile but allows gas to escape when the hand is removed while the Gelport maintains the seal when inserting or removing the hand but is larger and can be cumbersome in small patients. The incision for the hand port is positioned according to which is the surgeon's dominant hand and which kidney is being removed. For right-handed surgeons, the hand port is placed in the right lower quadrant or infraumbilically for a right nephrectomy. For a left nephrectomy, the hand port incision is made supraumbilically. For a left-handed surgeon, the locations are reversed as the goal is for the surgeon to use the nondominant hand for finger dissection. Once the device is in position, the abdomen may be insufflated through the device itself, the laparoscope inserted through the device, and the procedure commenced. Two or three additional 12 mm ports are then placed. For a right-handed surgeon and right nephrectomy, a camera port is generally placed at or above the umbilicus and a second trocar is placed midway between the xyphoid and umbilicus. For a left nephrectomy, a 12 mm trocar is placed just below the umbilicus (camera) and another in the left lower quadrant lateral to the rectus muscle. At this point, the abdominal cavity and its contents should be thoroughly inspected.

Entering the Retroperitoneum. Once transperitoneal access is safely achieved, exposure of the affected kidney requires incision of the ipsilateral lateral colonic peritoneal reflection (i.e., the white line of Toldt). The entire technique mirrors that of the standard transperitoneal approach except that the inserted hand replaces an instrument to facilitate dissection (see description in Sec. I.H.1).

Isolating the Ureter. See Sec. I.H.1.

Dissecting the Kidney. See Sec. I.H.1.

Dissecting the Renal Hilum. The role of the hand during this stage is to provide constant lateral retraction of the kidney in order to put traction on the renal hilum and to palpate the renal hilum to assist with renal artery identification. This is accomplished with fingers placed such that they straddle the hilum and move laterally to put the hilum on stretch. Alternatively, the surgeon can create a "C" with the thumb and index finger and work within the confines of this area, while using the thumb and index finger to provide exposure and traction/countertraction on the tissues to be dissected. The surgeon begins the hilar dissection on the right side by identifying the inferior vena cava and tracing it to the main renal vein. On the left side, the surgeon can follow the gonadal vein cephalad until it joins the main renal vein. On the right side, the renal vein is usually a single structure with no branches; on the left side, the adrenal, ascending lumbar, and gonadal branches of the renal vein must all be identified, separately dissected, and occluded. While this is usually done with four 9 mm clips, of late the Ligasure bipolar device has been found to be very effective and efficient for securing and dividing these venous tributaries. The renal vein and renal artery are then dissected until a 360-degree window is established around each vessel. The artery is typically occluded and transected first; a total of five 9 mm clips are placed on the artery: three proximal and two distal. The vein is then simultaneously occluded and transected using a 12 mm Endo GIA *vascular* stapler. Recently, the 12 mm Endo GIA vascular stapler has been also used to secure the renal artery; the closure obtained is rapid and secure.

Dividing the Ureter.   See Sec. I.H.1.

Introducing the Entrapment Sack.   In hand-assisted laparoscopic nephrectomy, the kidney is not morcellated. Rather it is entrapped in one of the readily expandable plastic sacks (e.g., EndoCatch or EndoPouch). The 15 mm device can be passed through the upper 12 mm port, opened beneath the liver or spleen, and the kidney can then be manually deposited in the widely opened sack. The metal band on the lip of these plastic sacks makes opening and closing of the sack very easy. Also, the metal band provides a stiffness to the lip of the sack, which facilitates organ entrapment. The sack is then closed, disconnected from the delivery handle and manually pulled through the hand-assist device. If the specimen is too large to fit through the device, the device should be removed and the incision retracted or extended as necessary.

Exiting the Abdomen and Closure.   At the end of the operation and prior to kidney removal, the pneumoperitoneum pressure is lowered to 5 mmHg and a careful check for hemostasis is performed. The traditional port sites, since they were nonbladed, do not require fascial closure, unless they were placed through the midline. Similarly, any 5 mm port site does not require a fascial closure. The fascia of the hand port incision is closed in one or two layers in standard fashion. The skin is closed using a running subcuticular 4-0 absorbable suture for the hand and 12 mm ports.

3.   Retroperitoneal Approach

This approach is reserved for removal of a benign, small (< 100 g) noninflamed kidney, as might occur in reflux nephropathy or renal artery stenosis. However, some surgeons have successfully extended this approach to include radical nephrectomy with intact removal.

Operating Room and Patient Setup.   The operating room personnel and equipment are arranged in a *mirror image* configuration of the transperitoneal approach setup: the surgeon stands on the ipsilateral side of the table relative to the side of surgical dissection

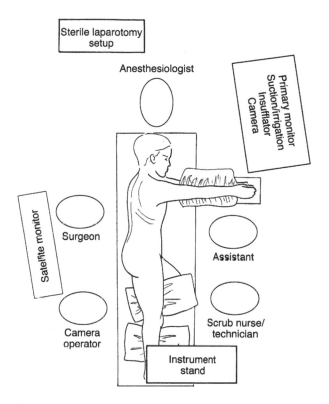

Sterile laparotomy setup

Anesthesiologist

Primary monitor
Suction/irrigation
Insufflator
Camera

Satellite monitor

Surgeon

Assistant

Camera operator

Scrub nurse/ technician

Instrument stand

Figure 6 Operating room setup for laparoscopic retroperitoneal nephrectomy.

(Fig. 6). The camera operator also stands on this side, below the surgeon. The first assistant stands opposite the surgeon, on the contralateral side of the table relative to the side of surgical dissection. The scrub nurse stands opposite the camera operator.

Equipment is arranged with the primary monitor viewed by the surgeon placed on the surgical assistant's side of the table, just above his or her shoulder. A satellite monitor for the assistant is placed on the surgeon's side of the table, between the surgeon and the camera operator. Suction/irrigation, insufflator, and camera lines are brought off the head of the table on the assistant's side. The electrosurgical, harmonic, and Ligasure cords are brought off the foot of the table on the surgeon's side. The sterile instrument table is placed behind the nurse and an adjustable instrument stand is placed across the foot of the table. The anesthesiologist, with all appropriate critical monitoring equipment, is at the head of the table, behind the sterile ether screen.

Once in the operating room, the patient is placed supine and general endotracheal anesthesia is established and a nasogastric tube and Foley catheter are placed. Elastic thigh-high TED stockings and pneumatic sequential compression stockings are placed to prevent deep venous thrombosis. The patient is turned from a supine into a lateral decubitus position. The kidney rest is positioned beneath the contralateral iliac crest and then raised. The table is flexed. Appropriate measures should be taken to avoid patient injury in this position, including placement of two or three pillows between the upper and lower portion of the legs such that the upper leg is nearly level with the iliac crest, flexion of the lower leg to 30 degrees at the knee and hip, extension of the upper leg, support of the upper arm by an elevated arm board, padding of the lower arm and axilla with a gel pad to protect the brachial plexus, and appropriate padding of all dependent bony prominences (e.g., downside hip, knee, and ankle) to prevent undesired bruising or irritation to the unprotected skin. Additional security may be obtained with appropriately placed padded sandbags and padded straps. A full surgical scrub of the patient's abdomen and ipsilateral flank from the umbilicus to the vertebral column is performed

Dilation of the Retroperitoneal Space and Creation of a Pneumoretroperitoneum. The essence of extraperitoneal laparoscopy is active creation of approximately an 800 cc working space via balloon dilation. Because of the fat-filled nature of the retroperitoneal space, traditional insufflation is inadequate to create a suitable operative field. Instead, dilation with a balloon catheter is used to physically establish a working space within the retroperitoneal fat. Several instruments have been fashioned to perform this task; however, the simplest to use is the 800 cc dilating balloon that comes with a blunt port which has a laparoscopic 12 mm cannula that can be sealed on the inside (via a balloon) and outside (via a foam cuff) to the retroperitoneal wall (i.e., Bluntport; U.S. Surgical) (Fig. 7).

Retroperitoneoscopy begins with a 2 cm incision just posterior to the tip of the 12th rib. Under direct vision the incision is deepened until the lumbodorsal fascia is incised and the retroperitoneal space is sharply entered. The surgeon should be able to see the retroperitoneal fat through this incision. An examining finger is then passed through the incision; the psoas muscle should be easily palpated, and fat in this area can be gently swept away thereby creating a space. With the retroperitoneum satisfactorily entered, the dilating balloon catheter is inserted. The balloon is inflated with 40 pumps to approximately an 800 cc size. Following dilation, the balloon is deflated and removed. The blunt port is then placed; the inner balloon on the 12 mm cannula is inflated with 20–30 cc of air and then the outer cuff is snugged down on the skin, thereby compressing the

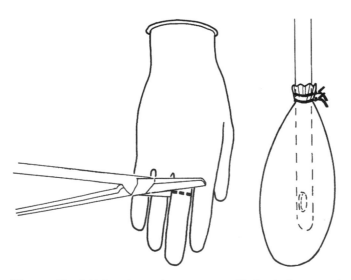

Figure 7 A high-volume, low-pressure dilating balloon can be fashioned by the surgeon from the middle finger of a size 8 Triflex surgeon's glove finger tied over the end of 16 Fr red rubber catheter.

abdominal wall between the balloon and the foam cuff. This effectively creates a tight seal and precludes the development of subcutaneous emphysema during the case.

Port Placement. The laparoscope is passed through the bluntport and the retroperitoneum is inspected. At this point visualization of the psoas muscle, genitofemoral nerve, Gerota's fascia, and occasionally the ureter is possible. All subsequent ports are placed under direct vision.

Three additional ports can then be placed: an upper 12 mm subcostal port posterior to the initial port, which enters the retroperitoneum just above the psoas muscle, an upper 5 mm port in the anterior axillary line two fingerbreadths below the costal margin, and a lower 12 mm port two fingerbreadths above the anterior, superior iliac crest. This creates a "T" array of ports; other arrays are either an "I" (the first three ports are placed alone) or "W" array in which there are two additional inferior ports added to the aforedescribed "I" array. The laparoscope is deployed usually through the initial port behind the tip of the 12th rib or via the port just above the iliac crest.

Dissection. Initial attention is turned to the psoas muscle. Its antero-medial surface is dissected free of overlying fatty tissue. The medial dissection on the psoas must continue until the medial border of the psoas muscle is clearly identified. Now as the surgeon moves cephalad along the psoas, the pulsations of the renal hilum can usually be appreciated. Gerota's fascia is identified and entered sharply. The resulting access provided the surgeon is excellent for immediate dissection of the posterior and lateral surfaces of the kidney. Dissection proceeds inferiorly and then superiorly directly along the renal capsule (Fig. 8).

Due to the retroperitoneal approach, the renal artery is encountered prior to the renal vein on both sides. The renal artery is dissected and secured with 5 clips and cut such that 3 clips remain on the stump side; similarly, an Endo-GIA stapler or 3 hemo-lok clips can be used (2 on the artery's stump). The renal vein can then be dissected. On the left side the three key branches of the renal vein are individually secured: the adrenal, ascending lumbar, and gonadal. This can be done nicely with a Ligasure device or with 4 clips for each vein. Of note, with the retroperitoneal approach, it appears that the renal vein is not as closely applied to the renal artery as one sees with the transperitoneal approach. The renal vein must be carefully dissected free of all surrounding tissue. The renal vein is taken with an Endo-GIA stapler.

Now the ureter is identified. It is secured with 4 clips and cut. The upper part of the ureter is secured with a 5 mm traumatic, locking grasper passed through the upper medial 5 mm axillary line port. The kidney, now freed of all retroperitoneal attachments, is delivered to the uppermost part of the retroperitoneum and held in place for later entrapment.

Entrapment and Removal. Through the upper 12 mm port, a medium size plastic entrapment sack or a 4 × 6 inch LapSac is introduced into the retroperitoneum; the former is opened directly, whereas the latter needs to be unfurled with an atraumatic instrument. The retroperitoneum is somewhat restricting in size, and this can present difficulty in unfurling and opening the sack; nevertheless, entrapment has been successful in all retroperitoneal cases in which the kidney has been smaller than 100 g. The sack with the entrapped kidney is delivered through the initial 2 cm incision; if a LapSac has been used the specimen can be morcellated. Alternatively, the specimen can be pulled out intact with the plastic sack or the incision can be increased in size.

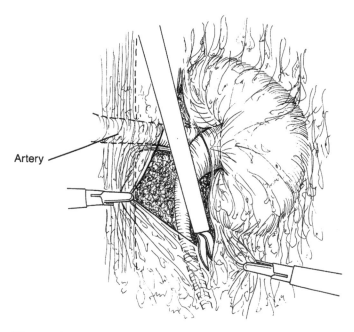

Artery

Figure 8 Transretroperitoneal dissection of the renal hilum. Note the superficial lie of the renal artery with respect to the renal vein that occurs with a retroperitoneal approach.

If one has done a renal cell cancer in this manner, then the large size of the specimen mandates a larger incision for intact tumor extraction without entrapment. Entrapment in these cases usually requires the surgeon to laparoscopically incise the peritoneum in order to gain access to the larger peritoneal space in which the sack can then be manipulated and the specimen entrapped.

Exiting the Retroperitoneum.   The pneumoretroperitoneum is reduced to 5 mmHg and the surgical field and port sites are carefully examined to rule out bleeding. Ports are removed under direct vision. No fascial closure is needed except on the initial 2 cm incision. The skin sites are closed as previously described for the transperitoneal approach.

I. Postoperative Care

The patient undergoing laparoscopic nephrectomy requires no postoperative stomach decompression; the nasogastric or orogastric tube is removed at the end of the procedure. The patient is begun on a clear liquid diet on the evening of surgery and is advanced as tolerated to a regular diet. The Foley catheter is removed at midnight, and on the first postoperative day the patient is ambulated. Intravenous antibiotic therapy is continued for 24 hours postoperatively. Pain control is achieved with patient-controlled parenteral morphine sulfate or a nonsteroidal anti-inflammatory on the evening of surgery and is changed to oral pain medication as the diet is advanced. By postoperative day 1 or 2, any incisional pain should be well controlled with oral analgesics and the patient should be ready for discharge. The only discharge medication is a nonnarcotic analgesic. Full nonstrenuous activity can be resumed after 1 week.

J. Management of Complications

Despite good postoperative outcomes, laparoscopic nephrectomy involves unique risks to the patient. These risks are very much dependent upon whether a simple nephrectomy for an uncomplicated problem (e.g., renovascular hypertension, nonfunctioning kidney secondary to ureteropelvic junction obstruction) is being done or whether the nephrectomy is for a large renal cancer or for a complicated problem such as a preoperatively undiagnosed xanthogranulomatous pyelonephritis. Accordingly, the conversion rate for simple nephrectomy is only 3%, whereas for radical nephrectomy it may be as high as 16% early in one's experience. Conversion is usually undertaken for one of three major reasons: failure to progress, bowel injury, or vascular injury. In addition, overall rates of complications intraoperative and postoperative complications for laparoscopic ablative renal surgery are both in the 5% range.

Complications specific to nephrectomy are myriad. The most common complications are intraoperative bleeding and postoperative ileus. Intraoperative bleeding can successfully be avoided by careful dissection techniques. The most commonly injured vessels are renal hilar and the inferior vena cava (during right nephrectomy). Special care must also be taken to avoid injury or erroneous occlusion of the splenic artery or superior mesenteric artery during a left nephrectomy. Any suspected "renal" artery needs to be carefully traced to the kidney before it is clipped and divided. Ileus is not uncommon after a transperitoneal approach. In general, many surgeons elect to avoid use of postoperative morphine analgesia in an effort to not exacerbate this problem. Significant ileus, requiring nasogastric drainage, should prompt one to become concerned about a possible occult bowel injury; a CT scan of the abdomen with and without oral contrast would be indicated.

The most disconcerting postoperative complication is that of a bowel injury. The resulting clinical scenario can be quite confusing. In general, when there is a laparoscopically induced bowel injury it is most commonly secondary to electrosurgical current. These injuries have a tendency to present usually several days to upwards of 2 weeks after the procedure. Symptoms may include localized tenderness or mild peritoneal signs. Often the patient is afebrile. The key tipoff is that a patient who was fine on postoperative day 1 appears to be worse on postoperative day 2 or 3. The major laboratory finding is either a mild leukocytosis or even leukopenia, but always with a marked left shift. The diagnosis is confirmed by a CT scan with oral contrast showing extravasation of contrast; delayed scans may be necessary in order to diagnose the problem. Indeed, the authors have seen one case in which the problem was diagnosed only at the time of a repeat CT scan. The threshold for proceeding with a CT scan in these patients should be very low. Treatment consists of exploration and repair, either open or laparoscopic.

Also, paresthesias due to the lateral decubitus position have been reported; these problems include nerve palsies of the brachial plexus, lateral popliteal, or lateral femoral cutaneous nerves of the thigh and stretch injury to the sciatic nerve. Additionally, as with open surgery, during a left radical nephrectomy the spleen is particularly vulnerable to injury. However, by widely incising the splenic attachments this can be avoided; in the rare case of a splenic capsular laceration, the use of argon beam coagulation or fibrin glue has been effective. Lastly, special attention to fluid balance during laparoscopic procedures is important. There is a tendency to fluid overload these patients because of two reasons: their urine output is markedly decreased due to the pneumoperitoneum and their insensible loss is much less than one would expect with a typical open surgical procedure.

For the elderly patient, this problem may lead to iatrogenic fluid overload with resultant congestive heart failure and hemodilution, requiring transfusion.

K. Top Ten Surgical Tips

1. As with any laparoscopic surgery, a full sterile laparotomy setup, including vascular clamps, must be available in the operating room should emergency conversion to an open procedure become necessary.
2. Appropriate measures should be taken to avoid nerve injury or bruising in the lateral decubitus position, including placement of two or three pillows between upper and lower legs, flexion of the lower leg to 30 degrees at the knee and hip, extension of the upper leg, support of the upper arm by an elevated arm board, padding of the lower arm axilla with a gel pad to protect the brachial plexus, and appropriate padding of all dependent bony prominences (e.g., downside hip, knee, and ankle).
3. For a *left* nephrectomy, careful dissection must be undertaken at the level of the splenic flexure, because the splenophrenic attachments, lienocolic ligament, and lienorenal ligament may be quite thick. The assistant must be vigilant so that no traction is placed directly on the spleen, and the surgeon must be fastidious in thoroughly electrocoagulating these ligaments as they are incised. The surgeon and assistant also must be constantly aware of the close proximity of the tail of the pancreas to the upper anterior surface of the left kidney. Also, on the left side, the gonadal vein is the key to finding the renal vein; it should be found caudal and traced upward to its junction with the main renal vein.
4. In isolating the ureter, it is prudent to recall that the ureter typically lies directly posterior to the gonadal vessels and medial to the medial edge of the psoas muscle. Thus the gonadal vein is first identified, dissected, secured with four clips, and cut. The ureter should lie directly posterior. Additionally, the ureter is most easily detected just above the level of the iliac vessels.
5. For a right nephrectomy, dissection of the upper pole of the kidney is complicated by the overlying liver. The assistant can help by placing a diamond "snake" or fan retractor through the 5 mm lateral subcostal port to push the liver cephalad or by placing a sixth port (5 mm subcostal midclavicular line) to be used for retraction; in either case, the retractor should be secured in place with an Endoholder. Retraction of the liver is most safely done by placing the retractor along the underside of the incised peritoneal reflection (i.e., the posterior coronary ligament of the liver) and retracting cephalad. Thus the organ is protected by the intervening layer of peritoneal tissue and fat.
6. Dissection of the renal hilum is greatly facilitated if the assistant provides constant lateral retraction of the kidney and ureter/lower pole to put the hilum "on stretch."
7. The pneumoperitoneum is reduced to 5 mmHg at the end of the procedure to check for hemostasis, especially around the ipsilateral renal hilum and the area around the ipsilateral adrenal gland. All port sites are also inspected at 5 mmHg as each trocar is withdrawn.

8. In opening the entrapment sack (i.e., LapSac), it is helpful to guide the upper midaxillary line grasper that is holding the kidney via the ureter so that it is directed at the most superior tab of the sack, thereby helping the kidney to clear the lower edge of the sack. With downward pushing of the kidney deeper into the sack by the assistant and upward elevation of the *lower* lip of the sack by the surgeon, the kidney can be deposited deep within the sack. Use of the nitinol guidewire is very helpful in facilitating the opening of the mouth of the LapSac.

9. During tissue morcellation, care is taken not to allow any redundancy to develop in the sack wall; the sack on either side is constantly pulled tautly upward by the assistant. The neck of the sack is triply draped if one is morcellating a renal tumor.

10. The essence of retroperitoneal laparoscopy is active creation of an 800 cc space through balloon dilation. If need be, the balloon can be deflated and inflated at a different position in the retroperitoneum to create an even larger working space.

L. Outcomes and Costs

Preliminary reports with short-term follow-up after the laparoscopic nephrectomy have been encouraging. Patients have significantly less postoperative pain, shorter hospitalization, and faster recovery after a laparoscopic nephrectomy than after an open nephrectomy. Operative time for the transabdominal approach for nephrectomy was originally 5.5 hours, however with experience these times have come down to under 4.5 hours. With the retroperitoneal approach, Gill and Abbou have reported times under 3 hours. In most hospitals today, the postoperative stay after laparoscopic nephrectomy is usually only 1–2 days. Cost analysis has shown that once the procedural time drops below 4.7 hours and the hospital stay is less than 5.8 days along with operative costs limited to $5500, the overall savings for the laparoscopic approach are just over $1000.

M. Current Status and Future Investigation

Over the past 12 years, laparoscopic nephrectomy has proven to be a highly effective and now cost-efficient means of kidney removal. The procedure's efficacy is similar to that of open nephrectomy, and laparoscopic patients experience less pain, shorter hospitalization, faster convalescence, and improved cosmesis. For these reasons, laparoscopic simple and radical nephrectomy (for T1, T2, and T3a disease: 4–10 cm tumors) have become the standard of care at many major medical centers, replacing open nephrectomy.

II. PYELOPLASTY

Ureteropelvic junction (UPJ) obstruction is an uncommon condition whereby urine flow between the renal pelvis and ureter is impaired. The etiology is either congenital or acquired (stone disease or postoperative stricture). Until the 1980s this condition was traditionally corrected by open surgery, termed a pyeloplasty. Then with the advent of endourology, endoscopic techniques largely replaced open surgery as the standard of care. Since the mid-1990s laparoscopic pyeloplasty has become increasingly popular as an approach which combines the advantages of minimally invasive surgery with the high success rate ($\backsim$ 95%) of traditional pyeloplasty.

A. Clinical Presentation and Indications

The vast majority of patients with UPJ obstructions present as an infant or child with pyelonephritis, pain, and/or loss of renal function. They are generally treated with an open dismembered pyeloplasty due to their small size and medical condition.

In the adult patient, the classic presentation of UPJ obstruction is episodic flank or abdominal pain, commonly after a fluid challenge. Others may present with pyelonephritis or hematuria associated with minor trauma. Rarely, a thin patient may have a palpable mass, which is the distended renal pelvis. The four indications for surgical intervention are pain secondary to obstruction, deteriorating renal function, urinary tract infection, or development of renal calculi.

B. Diagnostic Tests

A UPJ obstruction is generally diagnosed with either an intravenous pyelograms (IVP) or by CT. In either case, a gross overall assessment of the renal parenchyma, collecting system, and function of the kidney results. However, a diuretic renal scan with furosemide washout is mandatory to determine the degree of obstruction and measure the percentage of renal function. In general, the half-life of the tracer washout should exceed 19 minutes (>19 = obstruction; <12 = not obstructed; $12-19$ = equivocal). If the affected renal unit contributes less than 20% of the overall renal function, it is usually not deemed salvageable since surgical correction in these cases is often successful and the repaired kidney in the adult only rarely shows any improvement in function.

If the distal ureter is not demonstrated on IVP, then a retrograde pyelogram should be performed prior to correction to ensure that the remaining ureter is patent. Particularly in the case of secondary UPJ obstructions, a CT angiogram or endoluminal ultrasound is recommended to diagnose the presence of a UPJ crossing vessel, which may contribute to the obstruction. These may be difficult to identify during laparoscopic repair of a secondary UPJ obstruction due to periureteral fibrosis. Indeed, in many primary UPJ cases, the spiral CT angiogram with 3D reconstruction is obtained prior to any procedure in order to determine the presence of crossing vessels. When crossing vessels are present, the laparoscopic approach is often chosen as it has a higher success rate than endopyelotomy under these circumstances. Also, the degree of hydronephrosis is important as patients with grade 3–4 hydronephrosis have a poorer outcome with endopyelotomy; the laparoscopic approach allows the surgeon to both reduce the size of the renal pelvis as well as repair the UPJ obstruction: a dismembered reduction pyeloplasty.

C. Operative Treatment

The patients best suited for laparoscopic pyeloplasty are those who have failed a previous endoscopic procedure and those with a large redundant renal pelvis and/or segmental crossing vessel thought to obstruct the UPJ. Absolute contraindications to a laparoscopic pyeloplasty include inability to tolerate general anesthesia or pneumoperitoneum and an uncorrected coagulopathy. Relative contraindications include prior open renal surgery, prior laparoscopic pyeloplasty, or history of renal trauma.

D. Preoperative Preparation

The expectations and risks of laparoscopic pyeloplasty are discussed preoperatively, and the patient is counseled that if at any point the procedure cannot be continued safely, the operation will be converted to an open approach. Potential complications specific to laparoscopic pyeloplasty include bowel injury, bleeding, segmental renal parenchymal infarction (if a crossing artery is injured), prolonged urine leak, re-obstruction, possible nephrectomy, and deterioration of kidney function.

Patients are admitted the day of surgery after completion of a mechanical bowel preparation and are given a single dose of a broad-spectrum antibiotic (cefazolin). Preoperative urine cultures are mandatory and, if positive for bacteria, antibiotics are given until a sterile urine culture is obtained.

E. Operating Room and Patient Setup

The surgeon stands on the side of the table opposite the side of dissection with the camera holder/assistant standing next to him or her. The video monitor, insufflator, and light source are positioned opposite the surgeon at the level of the patient's chest. The scrub nurse with instrument stand should be positioned just below the monitor across from the surgeon. It is mandatory that a sterile laparotomy setup be available in the operating room should an emergent conversion become necessary.

If the patient does not already have an indwelling ureteral stent, then this is usually placed first with the patient in the lithotomy position. Fluoroscopic guidance and confirmation of placement is mandatory. Either an indwelling or external stent can be placed; in the latter circumstance, at the end of the procedure, the external stent is exchanged under fluoroscopic guidance for an indwelling ureteral stent. Alternatively, no stent can be placed at the outset of the procedure; instead, the stent is placed during the laparoscopic procedure in an antegrade fashion after the backwall of the ureteropelvic anastomosis has been completed. In this case, a check fluoroscopy is done at the end of the case to confirm proper stent position in the renal pelvis and bladder.

Pneumatic sequential compression stockings are placed for deep venous thrombosis prophylaxis. All pressure points (hip, knee, ankle, and shoulder) are well padded. An orogastric tube and Foley catheter are placed. An anesthetic regimen that excludes nitrous oxide is recommended to avoid bowel dilatation.

The patient is positioned in a modified flank position similar to that for laparoscopic transperitoneal nephrectomy. The use of orthopedic "hip huggers" is helpful to maintain the flank position; these are placed at the shoulder and hip and further padded with foam "egg crate." The kidney rest is positioned beneath the contralateral iliac crest and then raised. The table is flexed. Finally, the patient should be secured to the operating room table with 3-in.-wide cloth tape padded restraints at the shoulder, hips, and knees to prevent movement when the table is rotated. Generally the table is rotated maximally toward the surgeon after positioning such that the flank is in a full upright position. Full rotation away from the surgeon is utilized only if open urgent conversion is required.

F. Equipment for Laparoscopic Pyeloplasty*

Disposable equipment:
5 mm endoshears (U.S. Surgical)
5 mm clip appliers (U.S. Surgical)
Trocar—12 mm (1) (Step system U.S. Surgical)

*Equipment listed used at University of Texas Southwestern Medical Center.

Trocar—12 mm Visiport (U.S. Surgical)
Trocar—5 mm Versaport (U.S. Surgical)
Veress needle (150 mm) (U.S. Surgical)
CO_2 insufflation tubing
Suction irrigator, 5 mm (ACMI)
1 5 mm closed suction drain
1 EndoStitch 4-0, Polysorb suture

Nondisposable equipment:
Laparoscope: 10 mm, 0° lens and a 10 mm, 30° lens and a 5 mm, 0° lens (Storz)
1 atraumatic, nonlocking 5 mm smooth curved-tip grasping forceps (Storz)
1 5 mm electrosurgical scissors (Storz)
5 mm needleholders (Storz)
10 mm soft curved angled forceps (Maryland dissector) (Storz)
10 mm right angle dissector (Storz)
Carter Thomason needle suture grasper and closure cones (Inlet Medical)
1 Lapra-Ty applicator with rack of Lapra-Tys (Ethicon)
5 mm Pott's scissors

G. Surgical Technique

The procedure is generally performed via the transperitoneal approach. Though retroperitoneal techniques have been reported, there is greater experience with the transperitoneal approach, which is technically easier due to the larger working space.

Pneumoperitoneum and Port Placement.   With the bed rotated away from the surgeon, a 12 mm incision is made above the umbilicus and the Veress needle is inserted into the abdomen. A pneumoperitoneum is established at 25 mm Hg. Alternatively, an open Hasson approach, described elsewhere in this text, can be used.

After establishing an adequate pneumoperitoneum, a 12 mm trocar using a Visiport device or a visual blunt trocar is passed. The laparoscope is inserted and the intra-abdominal pressure is reduced to 10–15 mmHg. The abdominal cavity and its contents are thoroughly inspected. All subsequent ports are placed under direct vision through the laparoscope: an upper 12 mm midline port midway between the umbilicus and xyphoid and a midclavicular line 5 mm port in the ipsilateral lower quadrant. The umbilical port is used for the laparoscope. For a right pyeloplasty, an optional 5 mm upper midclavicular line port may be placed subcostally to aid the retraction of the liver. Also, a 5 mm port may be placed subcostally in the anterior axillary line to help with following the suture during the anastomosis or for retraction during the UPJ dissection.

Entering the Retroperitoneum.   Once transperitoneal access is safely achieved, exposure of the affected kidney requires incision of the ipsilateral lateral colonic peritoneal reflection (i.e., the white line of Toldt). This line of demarcation is often readily visible, with the patient in a full lateral position as gravity displaces the colon away from the abdominal side wall. In addition, the dilated, redundant renal pelvis is often identifiable through the peritoneal surface lateral to the colon. Incision of the line of Toldt is continued inferiorly to the level of the common iliac artery and superiorly above the hepatic or splenic flexure. The hepatic or splenic flexure is likewise incised to allow the colon to fall medially away from the kidney. On the right side, a Kocher maneuver on the duodenum is also sometimes necessary.

After reflection of the colon, the proximal ureter is identified in the retroperitoneum. It is generally posterior and lateral to the gonadal vessels. The ureteral stent is palpated and the renal pelvis is identified by following the ureter cephalad. Alternatively, dissection can begin on the renal pelvis and proceed caudal to identify the UPJ and the proximal ureter; in this case, care must be taken to not injure any crossing vessels. A crossing vessel is encountered approximately 50% of the time. Arterial vessels should be preserved to avoid infarction of renal parenchyma. Most of the renal pelvis, UPJ, and proximal 3–5 cm of ureter are freed from adjacent structures and tissues by a combination of blunt and sharp dissection. Extensive dissection of the proximal ureter should be avoided to preserve the periureteral vascular supply. Use of clips to control bleeding near the UPJ should be avoided as they could migrate into the reconstructed anastomosis. In this regard, use of the harmonic shears can be quite helpful as one can obtain excellent hemostasis with the least chance of damage to surrounding tissues.

Dismembered Pyeloplasty. In performing a dismembered pyeloplasty (Fig. 1) the renal pelvis immediately above the obstructed UPJ is incised circumferentially. The proximal end of the stent is removed from the renal pelvis and, if there is a crossing anterior vessel, transposed anteriorly. The ureter below the obstruction is then incised circumferentially (without cutting the stent) and the resected UPJ is removed from the end of the proximal stent. The proximal ureter is then spatulated laterally with laparoscopic scissors for 1–1.5 cm. Care is taken not to spiral this incision. Alternatively, the second incision on the ureter can be deleted, in which case the spatulation traverses the former area of obstruction and continues caudal for another 1–2 cm; in this fashion, there is never any concern about having sufficient ureteral length to reconstruct the UPJ.

If a redundant pelvis exists, it can be excised (Fig. 9). If renal stones exist, they can be extracted under direct vision with a laparoscopic forceps or a flexible nephroscope can be inserted through the upper 12 mm trocar for direct intrarenal inspection and stone removal.

Suture Completion of Pyeloplasty. Polyglycolic acid suture (4-0) is utilized for all suturing. Suturing and stitch placement at the anastomosis can be performed free-hand or with the Endo-Stitch device. This depends on surgeon comfort and sewing experience. The initial stitch in a dismembered pyeloplasty is placed outside-in on the renal pelvis, at the proper orientation with the ureteral spatulation, and then inside-out on the ureter at the apex of the spatulated ureter (Fig. 1). All tied square knots are external to the urinary tract. The posterior anastomosis is completed first in either a running fashion or with 2–4 interrupted sutures. The ureteral stent is then positioned in the renal pelvis prior to completing the anterior anastomosis or if an external stent was used, then this is done at the end of the procedure. If no stent were placed, then a Terumo guidewire can be advanced into the ureter via the upper 12 mm port; the guidewire is advanced until it seems to be well coiled in the bladder. Over the guidewire and through the 12 mm port, a 28 or 30 cm 7F indwelling ureteral stent is advanced until the surgeon is comfortable that it too is well in the bladder. With a pusher holding the stent in place, the guidewire is withdrawn. Filling of the bladder via the Foley catheter should confirm proper placement of the stent in the bladder, as the irrigant should clearly reflux up the stent and into the abdomen. The upper coil of the stent is then positioned in the renal pelvis. Again, interrupted or a running suture

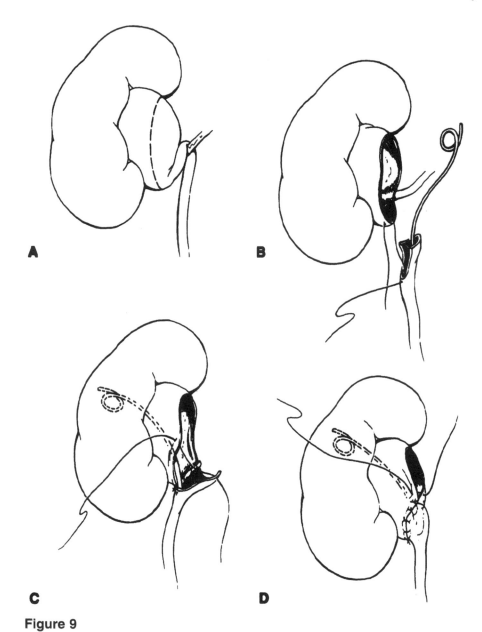

A

B

C

D

Figure 9

may be utilized to close the anterior portion of the ureteralpelvic anastomosis. The remaining pyelotomy is closed with a running 4-0 suture. To facilitate knot tying at the end of a running suture (only), a Lapra-Ty polydioxanone absorbable clip may be placed as long as it is external to the urinary tract.

Foley Y-V Pyeloplasty and Fengerplasty. A Foley Y-V plasty procedure is indicated when the obstructed UPJ is associated with a high ureteral insertion (Fig. 10). The incision in the UPJ forms a "V," the point of which is then carried caudal as an extension into the

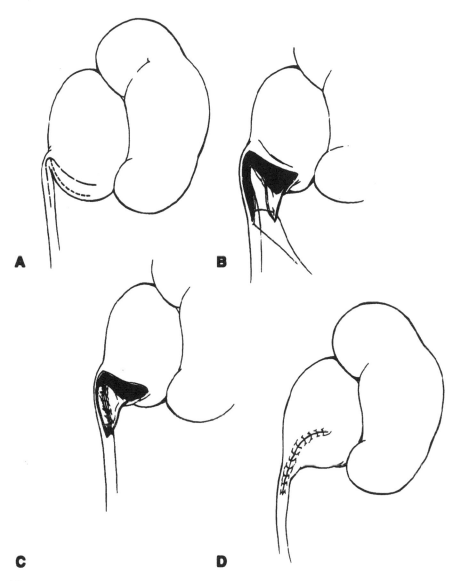

Figure 10

proximal ureter for 1 cm, hence creating a "Y" incision. Now, the point of the original "V" in the renal pelvis is advanced down the lower limb of the "Y" and sewn into the apex of the ureteral spatulation, thereby creating a new "V." The incision on either side is then closed by taking close bites on the flap side and broader spaced bites on the pelvis side to make up the disparity in length between the flap and the remaining renal pelvis.

A Fengerplasty is occasionally employed when there is a short intrinsic UPJ obstruction and no crossing vessel. This technique consists of a longitudinal full-thickness incision through the obstructed segment from 0.5 cm above the stricture to 0.5 cm below. The incision is then closed transversely, creating a widened UPJ.

Suturing of the Foley Y-V pyeloplasty or Fengerplasty is similar to the dismembered closure. All suture material and knot-tying techniques are the same except that all sutures placed should be of the interrupted variety.

Completing the Procedure.   A closed suction drain is placed dorsal and lateral to the reconstructed UPJ and brought out through a lateral incision. The drain should not abut the anastomosis and, if possible, should not traverse the peritoneum, but rather exit through the flank. It is secured to the skin with a 2-0 silk or nylon suture. If a 5 mm port was placed subcostal, then the drain is placed through this site. The colon should be replaced over the operative site and the fascia of 12 mm trocar sites inspected and closed with suture if the defect is greater than 5–8 mm. Alternatively, others prefer to close the fascia of any midline 12 mm port site.

H. Postoperative Care

Before the patient is transferred from the operating room, the orogastric tube is removed. The Foley catheter stays in place and is removed on the second postoperative day if there is minimal drain output (<50 cc in 24 hours). The drain is removed approximate 6 hours after the Foley catheter if there is no increased output. The patient may begin a clear liquid diet immediately after surgery, and the diet can be advanced as tolerated. Usually by the first morning the patient is eating a regular diet. The patient should ambulate the evening after surgery. Additional postoperative doses of a parenteral broad-spectrum antibiotic are administered before the patient is discharged home, usually on postoperative day 2, on a broad-spectrum antibiotic that is maintained until the ureteral stent is removed (4–6 weeks postoperatively).

Adequate analgesia during the postoperative period can often be achieved with 650 mg or 1000 mg of acetaminophen and parenteral ketorolac. The patient may require parenteral narcotic analgesics during the first 12 hours postoperatively. The need for narcotic pain medications beyond the first day may be the first indication of an underlying bowel injury or other postoperative complication.

As stated, the ureteral stent is removed 4–6 weeks after surgery. Thereafter, the adequacy of the repair is evaluated quarterly both clinically and radiographically. An IVP or renal scan is routinely obtained 1–6 weeks after the stent is removed and then renal scans are obtained 6, 12, and 18 months after surgery. Late failures beyond 12 months are very rare after laparoscopic pyeloplasty.

I. Management of Complications

The potential complications of laparoscopic pyeloplasty mirror those incurred with open pyeloplasty. Bleeding, infection, recurrence of the UPJ obstruction, and persistent urine leak can occur with both techniques. A urinoma can be treated with percutaneous drainage of the collection and a nephrostomy tube, although often placement of the nephrostomy tube by itself is sufficient.

Injury to adjacent intraperitoneal organs is unique to laparoscopic pyeloplasty as the open technique is generally performed via a retroperitoneal approach. If recognized intraoperatively, a bowel injury should be repaired immediately.

J. Top Ten Surgical Tips

1. As with any laparoscopic surgery, a full sterile laparotomy setup, including vascular clamps, must be available in the operating room should emergency conversion to an open procedure become necessary.
2. Appropriate measures should be taken to avoid nerve injury or bruising while the patient is in the lateral decubitus position. These precautionary measures include placement of two or three pillows between the upper and lower legs, flexion of the lower leg to 30 degrees at the knee and hip, extension of the upper leg, support of the upper arm by an elevated arm board, padding of the lower arm axilla with a gel pad to protect the brachial plexus, and appropriate padding of all dependent bony prominences (e.g., downside hip, knee, and ankle).
3. In isolating the ureter, it is prudent to recall that the ureter typically lies directly posterior to the gonadal vessels and medial to the medial edge of the psoas muscle. Thus the gonadal vein is first identified. The ureter should lie directly posterior. Additionally, the ureter is most easily detected just above the level of the iliac vessels but should only be mobilized 3–5 cm distal to the UPJ.
4. In cases of secondary UPJ obstruction, a vascular study such as a three-dimensional CT angiogram is recommended to assess for a crossing vessel. In these cases there may be extensive periureteral fibrosis due to the previous failed endopyelotomy making identification of a crossing vessel difficult. Knowledge of its existence and precise location preoperatively is helpful.
5. For surgeons who perform laparoscopic suturing infrequently, practice in a pelvic trainer with free-hand techniques and the Endo-Stitch will greatly facilitate the procedure and reduce operative time.
6. The renal pelvis must be mobilized extensively, both posteriorly and anteriorly. Anteriorly, care must be taken to identify the renal vein and artery. Often the renal vein is flattened across the distended renal pelvis.
7. The pneumoperitoneum is reduced to 5 mmHg at the end of the procedure to check for hemostasis, especially around the ipsilateral renal hilum and anastomosis. All port sites are also inspected at 5 mmHg as each trocar is withdrawn.
8. When spatulating the proximal ureter, the surgeon must avoid spiraling the incision. Laparoscopic Pott's scissors may help with this maneuver.
9. A long ureteral stent where the proximal curl lies in the upper pole or upper renal pelvis facilitates suturing. If the curl is at the anastomosis, it may place undue tension on the sutures and result in prolonged urine leakage.
10. If the patient has an indwelling nephrostomy tube preoperatively, it should be removed intraoperatively under direct visualization or, if left postoperatively to maximize drainage, it should be removed under fluoroscopic visualization to ensure removal of the nephrostomy tube does not dislodge the ureteral stent.

K. Outcomes and Costs

Patients have significantly less postoperative pain, shorter hospitalization, and faster recovery after a laparoscopic pyeloplasty than after an open pyeloplasty. Operative times are reasonable. Long-term success rates mirror that of open surgery and exceed those of antegrade or retrograde endopyelotomy. However, cost analysis has shown that laparoscopic pyeloplasty is more costly than the endoscopic approaches but advantageous when compared to open surgery (Yair Lotan, personal communication).

L.   Current Status and Future Investigation

Over the past 7 years, laparoscopic pyeloplasty has proven to be a highly effective and efficient means of UPJ obstruction repair. The procedure's efficacy is similar to that of open pyeloplasty, and laparoscopic patients experience less pain, shorter hospitalization, faster convalescence, and improved cosmesis. For these reasons, laparoscopic pyeloplasty has become the standard of care at many major medical centers, replacing open pyeloplasty.

SELECTED READINGS

Nephrectomy

Bishoff JT, Allaf ME, Moore RG, et al. Laparoscopic bowel injury: Incidence and clinical presentation. J Urol 161:887–890, 1999.

Clayman RV, McDougall EM. Laparoscopic renal surgery: nephrectomy and renal cyst decortication. In Clayman RV, McDougall EM, eds. Laparoscopic Urology. St. Louis: Quality Medical Publishing, 1993, pp 272–308.

Dunn MD, Portis AJ, Shalhav AL, et al. Laparoscopic vs open radical nephrectomy: a 9-year experience. J Urol 2000; 164:1153–1159.

Gill IS, Kavoussi LR, Clayman RV, et al. Complications of laparoscopic nephrectomy in 185 patients: a multi-institutional review. J Urol 1995; 154:479–483.

Gill IS, Schweizer D, Hobart MG, et al. Retroperitoneal laparoscopic radical nephrectomy: The Cleveland Clinic Experience. J Urol 2000; 163:1665–1670.

Kavoussi LR, Kerbl K, Capelouto CC, McDougall EM, Clayman RV. Laparoscopic nephrectomy for renal neoplasms. Urology 42:603–610, 1993.

McDougall EM, Clayman RV. Laparoscopic nephrectomy, nephroureterectomy, and partial nephrectomy. In: Das S, Crawford ED, eds. Urologic Laparoscopy. Philadelphia: WB Saunders, 1994, pp 127–144.

McDougall EM, Clayman RV, Fadden PT. Retroperitoneoscopy: The Washington University Medical School experience. Urology 43:446–452, 1994.

Nakada SY, Clayman RV. Laparoscopic nephrectomy and nephroureterectomy. In Marshall FF, ed. Operative Urology. Philadelphia: WB Saunders, 1996, pp 107–132.

Ming PU, Chau SO, Shwu LC, et al. Complications and recommended practices for electrosurgery in laparoscopy. Am J Surg 2000; 179:67–73.

Portis AJ, Yan Y, Landman J, Chen C, Barrett PH, Fentie DD, Ono Y, McDougall EM, Clayman RV. Long-term follow-up after laparoscopic radical nephrectomy. J Urol 167:1257–1262, 2002.

Rassweiler J, Fornara P, Weber M, et al. Laparoscopic nephrectomy: the experience of the laparoscopy working group of the German Urologic Association. J Urol 1998; 160:18–21.

Strup SE, Trabulsi EJ, McGinnis, ED, et al. Complications of hand-assisted laparoscopic nephrectomy: a review of 118 consecutive cases. J Urol 2002; 167 (suppl):168.

Wolf JS Jr, Marcovich R, Gill IS, et al. Survey of neuromuscular injuries to the patient and surgeon during urologic laparoscopic surgery. Urology 2000; 55:831–836.

Pyeloplasty

Bauer JJ, Bishoff JT, Moore RG, et al. Laparoscopic versus open pyeloplasty: assessment of objective and subjective outcome. J Urol 1999, 162:692–695.

Frauscher F, Janetschek G, Klauser A, et al. Laparoscopic pyeloplasty for UPJ obstruction with crossing vessels: contrast-enhanced color Doppler findings and long-term outcome. Urology 2002, 59:500–505.

Janetschek G, Peshcel R, and Bartsch G. Laparoscopic Fenger-plasty. J Endourol 2000, 889–893.

Jarrett TW, Chan DY, Charambura TC, et al. Laparoscopic pyeloplasty: the first 100 cases. J Urol 2002, 167:1253–1256.

Pattaras JG, Moore RG. Laparoscopic pyeloplasty. J Enodurol 2000, 14:895–904.

36

Minimally Invasive Vascular Surgery

MARK R. JACKSON

Greenville, South Carolina, U.S.A.

The development of catheter-based techniques has caused a similar degree of change to the practice of vascular surgery as did laparoscopy with general surgery. Gone are the days when the vascular surgeon's tools consisted entirely of an open surgical approach for the direct repair or bypass of an aneurysmal or occluded artery. Now, many abdominal aortic aneurysms are treated with endovascular stent grafts. By 2002, two FDA-approved devices were approved and other devices will likely become readily available. Arterial occlusive disease, traditionally treated with surgical bypass or endarterectomy, in many cases can be treated with balloon angioplasty and stenting, particularly for aortoiliac occlusive disease. This chapter will focus on these newer endovascular techniques. Additional information regarding laparoscopic-assisted vascular surgery is also included.

I. ENDOVASCULAR REPAIR OF ABDOMINAL AORTIC ANEURYSM

Since the mid-1950s, the standard surgical repair of abdominal aortic aneurysm (AAA) has required surgical celiotomy with direct aortic replacement using a prosthetic graft conduit. This has been a durable, time-tested approach that remains today the gold standard against which all new therapies are compared. Since this standard approach requires extensive surgical dissection of the retroperitoneum and aortic cross-clamping, the morbidity and mortality of the operation have rendered it too risky for some elderly patients and those with substantial comorbidities. Previous aortic surgery and presence of abdominal stomas also complicate the standard open approach.

In 1991, Parodi described the first use of a catheter-based, endoluminal, stent-supported graft delivered by a transfemoral approach for the treatment of AAA. Since then, there has been an explosive development of newer, commercially prepared endovascular devices for this application. In 1999 the U.S. Food and Drug Administration (FDA) approved two devices—Guidant Ancure and Medtronic AneuRx—for AAA. Other devices are in development and have been submitted for FDA approval.

II. CLINICAL PRESENTATION AND RISK OF RUPTURE

Unfortunately, most AAAs are diagnosed at time of rupture or during an abdominal imaging test performed for another indication. Men over the age of 60 with atherosclerotic risk factors have a 5–8% prevalence of AAA, yet widespread screening programs are uncommon. Unless mass screening programs are instituted, this is unlikely to change.

The risk of AAA rupture is directly related to aneurysm diameter. The risk appears to be linearly related for aneurysms between 4 and 6 cm in diameter and exponentially related for larger diameter aneurysms. The risk of AAA rupture for aneurysms smaller than 5.5 cm does not appear to be as great as has been generally accepted. In a recently published study from Veteran's Affairs medical centers, the annual risk of rupture for aneurysms between 4.0 and 5.5 cm was only 0.6%, and there was no survival advantage to immediate surgery over observation in this size category. Of note, 61% of the patient randomized to observation had undergone aneurysm repair by the end of the study period. All repairs were performed with conventional open surgery; endovascular stent grafts were not performed. Similar findings were recently reported in the United Kingdom Small Aneurysm Trial in which patients with an AAA between 4.0 and 5.5 cm were randomized to surgical repair or ultrasound surveillance. The 30-day surgery mortality rate of 5.5% led to an early survival advantage with observation. The survival curved crossed at 3 years, and at 8 years mortality in the early surgery group was 7.2% lower. In a separate report of patients in the VA study with AAA diameter over 5.5 cm and who were either unfit for surgery or who refused surgery, the one-year incidence of AAA rupture was 9.4%. For aneurysms between 6.5 and 6.9 cm, the risk was 19%, and the risk was 32% for aneurysms 7.0 cm and larger. From these studies it can be concluded that aneurysm repair should only be offered to relatively younger, low-risk patients for aneurysms smaller than 5.5 cm. Whether an endovascular repair should be offered at a lower threshold for small aneurysms has not been determined. This is particularly true for aneurysms smaller than 5.0 cm. Clearly, aneurysms of 6.0 cm and larger represent a significant risk of rupture and death and should always be considered for repair in the absence of overwhelming medical risk or terminal illness.

III. DIAGNOSTIC TESTS AND PREOPERATIVE IMAGING

Large aneurysms can often be palpated on physical exam, often enough that this should be a routine component of the physical exam in elderly patients with atherosclerotic risk factors. Unfortunately, the negative predictive value of a "normal" abdominal exam is likely low, particularly in high-prevalence groups. For those in high-risk groups and for those in whom the exam is suspicious for the presence of a AAA, abdominal ultrasound is the preferred imaging modality. It is relatively inexpensive and requires no radiation or use of contrast agents.

The role of computed tomography (CT) scanning for AAA has evolved greatly with the advent of endovascular stent grafts. For those patients with an AAA identified by ultrasound and who are being considered for endovascular repair, spiral CT with three-dimensional reconstruction has emerged as the preferred imaging modality for operative planning (Fig. 1). In fact, the CT angiogram component of the study is usually of sufficient quality that conventional angiography is seldom required. This results in cost savings and is much more convenient for the patient. For AAA stent graft planning, images from the superior mesenteric artery to the femoral bifurcation are obtained with and without

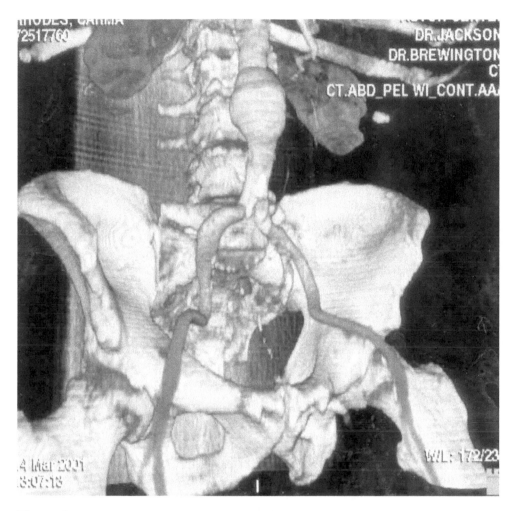

Figure 1   Three-dimensional CT angiogram rendering of AAA.

contrast, then reformatted on a 3-D workstation. This allows for true length and diameter measurements that are corrected for aortic angulation and tortuosity. Even with "straight" aortic necks, there is generally about 20 degrees of AP angulation of the aorta due to lumbar lordosis. Without 3-D corrections, the AAA diameter in the AP dimension will be overestimated. 3-D corrected length measurements are essential for selection of the appropriate length stent graft device and ancillary components. This cannot be done on standard axial CT images and, in our experience, is less accurate when performed using marker catheters and conventional angiography. Furthermore, CT images provide useful information regarding aortic plaque morphology and thrombus that is quite helpful for planning the endovascular stent graft deployment. The computer hardware and software for such image analysis is generally only available in the radiology departments of large medical centers. Alternatively, a commercial service that provides such images suitable for viewing on a PC exists and is another alternative for obtaining this vital information (Medical Media Systems, West Lebanon, NH).

Approximately 50% of patients with AAA have anatomy that is suitable for the two currently available AAA stent graft devices. The primary reason for exclusion is an inadequate proximal aortic neck, the "normal" part of the infrarenal aorta within which the device must seat and provide an effective seal. The main components related to proximal neck evaluation are length, diameter, and angulation. For currently available devices, it is recommended that there be at least 15 mm of length between the lowest renal artery and the beginning of the aneurysmal segment of the aorta. This allows a suitable length of a "seal zone" for effective exclusion of the aneurysm. The acceptable maximum aortic neck diameter is limited by the maximum diameter of the currently available devices, which is 26 mm for the Guidant device and 25 mm (allowing for oversizing of the self-expanding nitinol exoskeleton) for the Medtronic device. Aortic neck angulation is also a problem if there is significant tortuosity from the proximal neck into the aneurysm or from the suprarenal aorta into the proximal neck. Ideally, this angulation should be less than 30 degrees. Angulation over 60 degrees should be considered an absolute contraindication.

Preoperative conventional angiography is relegated to the minority of cases in which greater intraluminal detail must be obtained (some cases of iliac or renal occlusive disease) or when adjunctive measures such as internal iliac artery embolization must be performed. A standard contrast arteriogram is generally performed during endovascular repair, although sometimes this is only a completion study. Conventional angiography is sometimes performed as a preoperative study in centers without access to sophisticated 3-D CT equipment. In such cases, the aortogram is generally performed using a 5F catheter that has 20 1 cm marks for determining device length. These catheters, however, tend to follow the "shortest path" through the iliacs aorta and do not follow the true "center line" of the arteries. This can result in an underestimate of the device length.

IV. EQUIPMENT

The equipment needs for the operating room that enable performance of endovascular procedures can be focused upon four primary components: (1) fluoroscopy imaging equipment, (2) a radiolucent OR table, (3) a contrast injector, and (4) an inventory of catheters, guidewires, sheaths, stents, and other devices for endovascular interventions.

Most vascular surgeons who perform intraoperative endovascular procedures such as AAA stent graft placement use portable C-arm fluoroscopy for these cases. Although a fixed imaging dedicated angiography suite will generally allow for superior image quality, the image quality of modern digital portable fluoroscopy is quite good and is generally more than sufficient for AAA stent grafts. Perhaps the greatest advantage of fixed overhead fluoroscopy units is that they cannot be "borrowed" and unavailable. Portable fluoroscopy C-arm units can be more easily moved out of the way during parts of the case that only require open surgery. Such portable units now have digital subtraction and road-mapping capability for use during arterial interventions. It is essential that the portable units have a 12-inch image intensifier in order to provide sufficient field of view for AAA stent graft procedures.

If the purpose of the room is to primarily enable the performance of standard percutaneous endovascular procedures, such as arteriography, in addition to procedures that require both open surgery and catheter-based interventions, then a fixed imaging suite, with its inherently higher quality imaging, can be justified. A portable C-arm is not ideal for bilateral lower extremity arteriography. The disadvantage of the dedicated angiography suite is principally cost ($1.5 million dollars and up). Also, if open surgery is performed in this room, the large image intensifiers and x-ray tubes take up precious OR real estate and can get in the way. Biplanar imaging equipment, for example, is very useful for arteriography but presents two sets of x-ray tube and image intensifier to take up space in the room. The angiography tables that accompany this equipment are often poorly suited to use as an operating room table. Special consideration and space for cooling equipment for the x-ray tube must be provided. Fixed imaging also requires that the room be lead-lined for radiation safety. These limitations can be addressed, but it is imperative that such facilities be designed from the onset for use with open surgery and not be constructed like a typical angiography suite.

Standard OR tables are not sufficiently radiolucent for endovascular procedures. The side rails and section hinges are metal and will obscure fluoroscopic imaging. Even the so-called "fluoro-compatible" OR tables generally do not provide sufficient length of radiolucent material for imaging of the torso and legs. Also, most available fluoro-compatible OR tables do not allow for 4-way movement, or "float" of the table top as is the case with angiography tables. This 4-way float feature is important for precise positioning of the area of interest by the operator in order to minimize movement of the C-arm. The ability of the operator to move the table top in small, precise increments results in less use of fluoroscopy. There are now tables available that provide the 4-way table top movement of an angiography table, while retaining the classic functionality of an OR table (Trendelenburg positioning, side-to-side tilt, attachment sites for fixed retractor systems).

Hand injection of contrast agents can be satisfactory for imaging small, low-flow arteries such as those of the lower extremity, but a rapid, high-volume injection is necessary for imaging of the aorta. In order to provide an adequate volume (20–40 mL) of contrast at a sufficient rate (15–20 mL/s), a specialized contrast injector must be used. This is particularly the case with AAA stent graft procedures where accurate, precise imaging of the juxtarenal aorta is critical to a successful and safe outcome.

The fluoroscopy source, the table, and the contrast injector are the three key "enabling" pieces of equipment, but without an adequate supply of expendable catheters, guidewires, sheaths, and other related devices, it would not be possible to do any endovascular procedure. In some circumstances it might be feasible to borrow this equipment from the interventional radiology suite, but for a variety of reasons this is not generally a workable situation. The ability to perform endovascular procedures in conjunction with emergency vascular operations virtually mandates that the OR stock a separate inventory of catheters and related equipment for these cases. A basic inventory is presented in Table 1.

V. STENT GRAFT DEVICES

In September 1999 the FDA approved two aortic stent graft devices for the treatment of AAA. Both devices are available as bifurcated systems for aortobi-iliac deployment. Neither company manufactures a tube graft for straight aortic deployment. Earlier studies indicated that these tube grafts eventually develop leaks at the distal end of the aorta due to continued aortic dilation and relatively short-length distal attachment sites. For this reason, currently available AAA devices are primarily used in the bifurcated configuration. The Guidant graft is now available in an aorto-monoiliac configuration, which must be used in concert with a standard femoral-femoral bypass for contralateral limb perfusion. The salient features of each device is summarized below.

Table 1 Basic Catheter Inventory for Endovascular Procedures

1. Diagnostic catheters
   Straight and Omni Flush, Pigtail
   Verterbral (Berenstein or Kumpe)
   Visceral (Sos, Cheung B)
2. Guidewires (180 cm and 300 cm lengths, 0.035, 0.018, 0.014)
   3 mm J-wire
   Bentson wire
   Hydrophilic wires for crossing lesions
   Stiff exchange wires (Amplatz, Meier)
3. Introducer sheaths
   5–6F short
   6–8F bright tip, 11, 25, 55 cm lengths
   9–12F for WallGrafts
   12F, 16F, 22F, 24F for aortic stent grafts
4. Balloon angioplasty catheters
   7–12 mm diameter × 2–4 cm length for iliac artery PTA
   4–6 mm diameter for infrainguinal, renal PTA
   2–3.5 mm for tibial, renal branch PTA (require 0.018 or 0.014 wires)
5. Stents
   Self-expanding (5–14 mm diameters, assorted lengths)
   Balloon—expandable (4–9 mm, 8–12 mm, 10–25 XL)
6. Miscellaneous items
   Balloon inflators
   Insertion needles
   Flow switches and stopcocks
   10–25 mm gooseneck snares
   Tuohy-Borst and Y-adapters
   Torque devices, dilators, radiopaque marker strips

A. Medtronic AneuRx® Device

The Medtronic AneuRx device is a modular, externally supported stent graft that is deployed through its integrated 21F delivery system (Fig. 2). There are no hooks for aortic or iliac artery attachment, rather, the nitinol stent exoskeleton provides a friction fit within the aorta. The graft is intentionally oversized by approximately 15% to allow for adequate sealing and friction fit. A minimum of two graft components are needed for deployment: the main body and the contralateral limb. Additional components are used for lengthening of the iliac limbs and extending the proximal aortic body.

The diameter range of the aortic component is 20–28 mm. The corresponding iliac limb diameters are 12–16 mm, respectively. The main body comes in two lengths: 13.5 and 16.5 mm. Considerable variation in limb lengths can be accommodated using the various accessory limb extenders. The larger aortic cuffs come in the same diameters as the main body (20–28 mm) but are all of equal length—3.75 cm.

The contralateral limb is placed from the common femoral artery through a 16F sheath. In order to position the contralateral limb, it is first necessary to cannulate the opening in the main body of the graft within which the limb must lie. There are radio-opaque markers on the graft body to facilitate this. This is generally performed using a

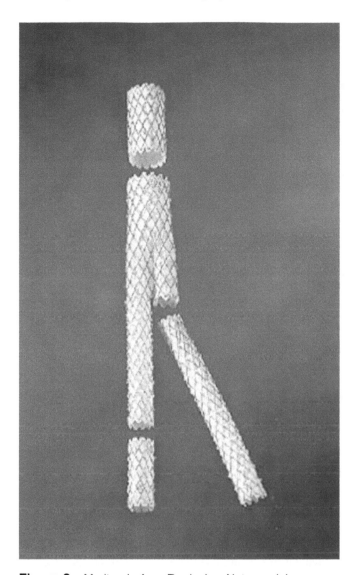

Figure 2 Medtronic AneuRx device. Note modular components.

hydrophilic guidewire and an angled catheter. One must confirm coaxial positioning of the guidewire within the main body limb opening in order to prevent inadvertent deployment of the contralateral iliac limb outside of the graft body.

The graft components are self-expanding, so it is not necessary to perform balloon angioplasty within the graft for apposition to the arteries or within other graft components. Since the graft components are placed coaxially, it is imperative to achieve sufficient overlap of the junctions in order to prevent subsequent separation and endoleak. For some deployments, multiple graft components are necessary, particularly when the iliac artery distal "landing zones" are wider than the largest iliac limb. In such circumstances it is possible to seal these larger iliac attachment sites using the 3.75-cm-long cuffs that are designed for extending the proximal aortic part of the stent graft. These cuffs come in diameters ranging from 20 to 28 mm and can be used to "bell-bottom" the distal end of the graft.

B. Guidant Ancure™ Device

The Ancure device is a bifurcated, unibody device that is deployed in an aortobi-iliac configuration (Fig. 3). Recently, a straight aorto-monoiliac device has become available, which is used in conjunction with a conventional cross-femoral bypass. The principal differences of this device in comparison to the AneuRx are (1) fixation hooks at the aortic and iliac ends of the device, (2) absence of external reinforcing stents, (3) unibody design (i.e., no multiple graft components), and (4) a significantly larger diameter delivery device, which typically requires a large introducer sheath.

The presence of fixation hooks is a significant advantage. This virtually eliminates distal device migration as can occur with the AneuRx device. Unfortunately, the use of metal hooks comes at a price—more bulk of the delivery device with a consequent need for a larger diameter delivery system. Furthermore, the Ancure device generally, but not always, requires the use of a 24F introducer sheath. This has a 9 mm outer diameter, which is too large for placement through some external iliac arteries. In such cases, surgical adjuncts such as suturing a graft extension onto the common iliac artery using retroperitoneal exposure can circumvent this limitation, but at the expense of added complexity and a less "minimally invasive" overall approach.

The lack of externally supporting stents on the body of the Ancure device also renders it more susceptible to external compression and kinking, which can ultimately lead to limb occlusion. This limitation is addressed by a more aggressive use of self-expanding stents within the graft limbs at the time of original stent graft deployment if the completion arteriogram indicates this problem.

VI. OPERATIVE TECHNIQUE

The technical detail of stent graft deployment is unique to the particular device. An in-depth description of all steps of deployment is beyond the scope of this text. The manufacturers of each device require a 2-day hands-on training class during which the technical details of the particular device are covered. There are common elements that pertain to aortic stent graft deployment in general, and these issues will be addressed.

General anesthesia is often used as this facilitates breath holding during abdominal imaging, but regional and even local anesthesia can be used and may be advantageous in high-risk pulmonary patients. We prep from the chest to the toes and leave the arms up for access to the anesthesiologist. In some cases the left arm is also prepped if use of a brachial artery catheter or guidewire is desired. Room layout is an issue since the imaging equipment, contrast injector, and table extensions for the long guidewires and devices require much more space than a conventional open AAA repair. Also, there are often multiple operators when different specialists collaborate on these procedures (e.g., vascular surgeon and interventional radiologist).

Open surgical access is required for insertion of the stent graft delivery device since they range in diameter from 21F to 24F. In most cases, the delivery device is placed through a transverse arteriotomy in the common femoral artery. If the common femoral is small, the distal external iliac artery can be used for access. Access to the contralateral common femoral artery is also required for deployment of the contralateral device

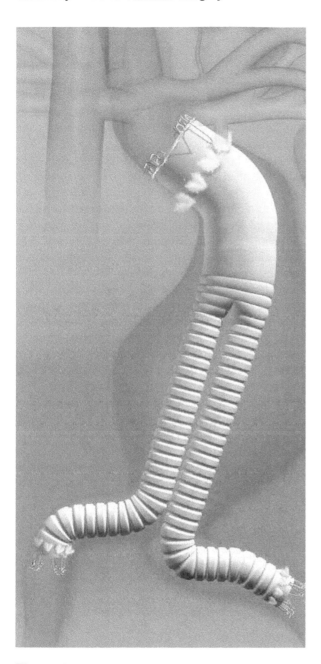

Figure 3   Guidant Ancure Device.

component (Medtronic) or manipulation of the contralateral graft limb (Guidant). It is possible to use a percutaneous access with an arterial closure device for the contralateral (smaller) component, but this is not generally recommended.

   An essential aspect of the procedure is accurate deployment immediately distal to the lowest renal artery. In order to facilitate this, an arteriogram of the juxtarenal aorta is performed prior to proximal deployment. The graft is then positioned to just below the renal using the digital roadmapping function of the C-arm, or the screen is simply marked with a marking pen to indicate the position of the renal arteries. The C-arm is placed in approximately 20 degrees of cranial angulation in order for the image to be perpendicular to the axis of the juxtarenal aorta. Even if there is no angulation of the aneurysm or its neck, there is generally about 15 degrees of angulation off the horizontal plane due to lumbar lordosis. Greater degrees of angulation can exist and must be considered when positioning the C-arm during this critical part of the procedure.

Deployment of the iliac limbs requires the operator to know the location of the iliac bifurcation in relationship to the distal end of the iliac limbs in order to prevent covering the internal iliac arteries. This can result in pelvic ischemia or inadequate distal exclusion of the aneurysm such that retrograde flow from the internal iliac continues to pressurize the aneurysm sac. Accurate preoperative arterial length measurement, preferably using CT angiography, is essential for precise deployment of the graft proximal to the iliac bifurcation. Intraoperative arteriography of the pelvis using a contralateral oblique can facilitate location of the iliac bifurcation and precise deployment.

At the completion of the procedure, a final arteriogram is performed to evaluate the following issues: patency of the renal arteries, patency of the endograft, extrinsic compression or kinking of the endograft, patency of the internal and external iliac arteries, and evidence of contrast flow within the aneurysm sac (Fig. 4). This last issue, residual flow within the aneurysm sac, is called an endoleak. More information is presented later on endoleaks, but in general, a delayed contrast blush indicates retrograde filling through side branches (lumbar arteries, inferior mesenteric) or graft porosity and generally is self-limiting. A more rapid contrast blush is indicative of a leak at a graft attachment site, and efforts should be made during the initial operation to find its source and to correct it. Continued flow and arterial pressurization of the aneurysm sac results in ineffective exclusion and risk of delayed rupture.

The femoral arteriotomies are closed with 5-0 prolene sutures. If general anesthesia is used, extubation is performed in the operating room. Postoperative monitoring in the

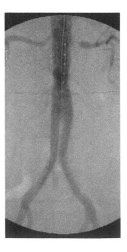

Figure 4 Completion arteriogram after AAA stent deployment.

standard recovery room and discharge within 24–48 hours is routine. Unless there are active cardiac or pulmonary problems, ICU care is not necessary.

VII. PATIENT FOLLOW-UP

Since hospital discharge is early, the initial follow-up is for the groin wounds. An early set of conventional abdominal x-rays is performed and repeated at least annually to provide complimentary imaging data to that derived from follow-up CT scanning. The plain x-rays can detect fractures in the metallic components and hooks that are not as readily seen on CT scan. CT scanning using the three-dimensional CTA protocol as with preoperative imaging is performed at one month for a baseline and then at 6-month intervals lifelong. The presence of endoleaks is noted by contrast opacification within the excluded aneurysm sac. The source of the endoleak, in our experience, can generally be identified using the CTA protocol. Other parameters to track sequentially are the maximum aortic sac diameter, the sac volume (which is computed from the three-dimensional CTA data set), and the distance of the proximal graft stent from the lowest renal artery as a measure of potential stent graft migration.

VIII. MANAGEMENT OF COMPLICATIONS

Despite the broad appeal of a minimally invasive approach to AAA repair, most contemporary series have not documented a reduction in 30-day mortality in comparison to the standard technique, which is approximately 5%. Comparison is made difficult by selection bias, whereby patients with severe comorbidities are offered stent graft repair but not open repair. There are other complications that are unique to endovascular stent graft deployment. Wound complications are more common with stent graft deployment since the devices are usually placed using open exposure of the common femoral arteries in the groins. In comparison, open AAA repair generally does not require femoral anastomoses and groin incisions are avoided. More problematic are the complications that are unique to the devices. The most significant limitation of any stent graft device is that of endoleak. Endoleak is persistent arterial flow within the aneurysm sac despite the presence of an endograft. This results in continued pressurization of the aneurysm and risk of delayed rupture. In fact, delayed rupture of the AAA after endograft deployment has now been reported in at least 25 patients, primarily all AneuRx devices. Some of this risk may now be reduced with a subsequent refinement of the device, rendering the proximal body less stiff, and a greater awareness of proper patient selection, especially when the proximal aortic neck is marginal.

Endoleaks are classified according to their source. A Type I endoleak results when the graft attachment site does not seal and there is persistent flow into the aneurysm. This can also present in a delayed fashion if there is any distal migration of the proximal endograft body. This Type I endoleak is considered the most dangerous and must be fixed if at all possible during the initial deployment if noted on the completion arteriogram. Measures such as aortic balloon dilation within the proximal graft or placement of additional stent graft components might be needed. Large-caliber balloon expandable stents are also sometimes used to address this problem. A Type II endoleak occurs if there is persistent flow within the aneurysm sac from aortic side branches such as patent lumbar arteries or the inferior mesenteric artery (IMA). Most of these Type II endoleaks spontaneously thrombose and are not considered to present a significant risk for delayed aneurysm rupture. An exception to this is the case of an endoleak that has established a flow pattern from a lumbar or the IMA with outflow through an accessory renal artery. These endoleaks can remain patent due to the low resistance outflow bed of the accessory renal. The presence of accessory renal arteries within the aneurysm sac must be noted on preoperative imaging. If the artery supplies a small portion of renal blood flow, consideration should be given to preoperative embolization to prevent such endoleaks. We do not routinely embolize other aortic side branches, since, as noted above, most will spontaneously resolve. Prolonged Type II endoleaks that are still present at one year are unlikely to spontaneously occlude, so consideration should be given to embolization of the offending side branch. This appears to be most effectively accomplished by a translumbar, direct approach to the aortic sac, which is itself also embolized with coils after selectively embolizing the offending side branch(es). Type II endoleaks associated with AAA sac enlargement should also be embolized regardless of their duration. Type III endoleaks are the result of flow through the stent graft itself, either at a junction of modular components or through a graft defect. These are dangerous and result in an aneurysm that has not been treated, so the Type III endoleaks must be treated. Often this can be performed by balloon dilation of the component junctions or placement of an additional component to seal the leak. A Type IV endoleak is continued pressurization of the AAA sac in the absence of any demonstrable contrast on imaging studies. It is unclear what significance and risk these Type IV, or "pressure endoleaks" pose. Since the fabric of the stent graft devices are not coated, the porosity of the Dacron can allow some flow just as with a non pre-clotted, non-coated, knitted Dacron conventional aortic graft. It is believed that most Type IV endoleaks will spontaneously seal and therefore do not pose a great risk for delayed aneurysm rupture.

More recently, commercially made covered stents, or stent grafts, have been used to treat complex occlusive lesions of the iliac arteries. These devices are not specifically FDA-approved for this purpose and generally have an approval for either tracheobronchial or biliary use. Nonetheless, it is possible to use these devices "off-label" in appropriate circumstances. The use of these devices is particularly appealing for medically high-risk patients in whom the iliac occlusive disease is extensive and diffuse, rendering conventional balloon angioplasty and stenting alone relatively ineffectual.

Unlike the PTFE-Palmaz stent device as described earlier, the newer covered stents are delivered in much the same way as a conventional stent. The covered stents are generally larger and require a larger introducer sheath. One such device, the Boston Scientific WallGraft™, comes in diameters ranging from 6 to 14 mm and lengths from 30 to 70 mm. Again, this device is not FDA-approved for arterial use. We have used this device in 15 high-risk patients with extensive iliac occlusive disease with good short-term results.

Since the introducer sheaths required for this device are large (as large as 12F for a 12 or 14 mm device), and since the occlusive disease frequently extends to the inguinal ligament, we have used an open approach to the distal common femoral or proximal superficial femoral artery for insertion. This allows control of the femoral vessels during deployment and predeployment angioplasty of long segment occlusions in order to reduce the risk of distal embolization. The open approach allows an insertion site distal to the extent of the external iliac disease and facilitates arterial closure of the large introducer sheath site.

From a technical standpoint, deployment of the WallGraft is very similar to that of a WallStent. Since the device is packaged within its delivery sheath in an elongated, constrained configuration, it tends to remain elongated, and not fully expanded, if it is

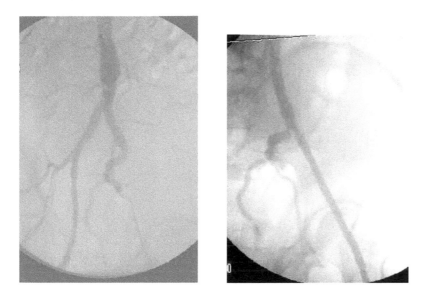

Figure 5   External iliac artery occlusion treated with WallGraft stent graft.

deployed within a severely stenotic artery. To overcome this, balloon dilation of the iliac artery deployment site to a diameter of 8–9 mm will help the WallGraft expand upon its deployment. Once deployed, the graft is expanded with a balloon angioplasty catheter. The final deployed diameter of the WallGraft should be at least 7 mm in the external iliac artery and 8 mm or larger in the common iliac artery (Fig. 5).

37

Endoscopic Plastic Surgery

ROD J. ROHRICH AND AMANDA GOSMAN

University of Texas Southwestern Medical Center
Dallas, Texas, U.S.A.

I. INTRODUCTION

The use of minimal access incisions in endoscopic surgery is ideally suited for the aesthetic objectives of plastic surgery. However, the creation of an optical cavity is essential for endoscopic surgery. The absence of naturally occurring optical cavities in the subcutaneous tissue initially limited the applications of endoscopy in plastic surgery. Over the past decade, plastic surgeons have developed endoscopic techniques that utilize surgically created optical cavities between tissue planes to facilitate visualization and dissection. The most popular applications of endoscopy in plastic surgery have been the forehead lift and augmentation mammaplasty. The use of endoscopy continues to expand into other common procedures of plastic surgery, including midface lift, abdominoplasty, and muscle flap harvest.

II. FOREHEAD LIFT

The objective of the forehead lift is the functional repositioning of the eyebrows. This is accomplished by resection of the brow depressor muscle group, release of the brow at the supraorbital rim, and brow repositioning with cephalad fixation. Indications for forehead lift are brow ptosis, transverse forehead furrows, glabellar frown lines, and transverse rhytids at the nasal root [1].

A. Procedure Selection

The decision to perform an open versus an endoscopic forehead lift is based on several factors, including the amount of skin excess, the need for skin resection, and the position of the hairline [1–2]. The open approach utilizes a lengthy bicoronal incision and soft tissue traction with skin resection for brow elevation and fixation [3]. The endoscopic technique utilizes multiple small incisions and depends upon skin retraction to maintain brow position [4]. Therefore the endoscopic approach is best for younger patients without

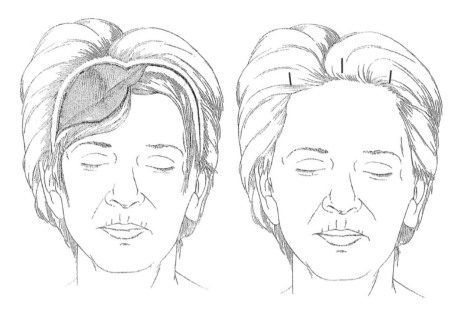

Figure 1 Position of scalp incisions for open (right) and endoscopic (left) forehead lift. (From Ref. 6.)

significant skin excess and with normal skin thickness and elasticity. The endoscopic approach has the advantages of small access incisions and magnified visualization of critical structures while avoiding the alopecia and scalp numbness associated with an extensive coronal incision (Fig. 1).

B. Surgical Technique

Endoscopic forehead lift may be performed under general anesthesia or local anesthesia with sedation. The patient is positioned supine with the surgeon at the head (Fig. 2) (Table 1). The brow and scalp are infiltrated with local anesthetic and epinephrine prior to the procedure. Multiple small (0.5–1 cm) access incisions are placed 1–2 cm posterior to the hairline. Typically there is one midline incision and two paramedian incisions at the mid-pupillary level. The initial dissection is done blindly to establish an optical cavity in either the subperiosteal or subgaleal plane, depending on surgeon preference. Before reaching the supraorbital ridge, a rigid 30 degree 4 mm endoscope is placed through the central port, and the dissection is continued under direct visualization.

  The supraorbital and supratrochlear neurovascular bundles are identified and carefully preserved. The brow depressor muscle group, which includes the procerus, depressor supercilli, corrugator, and medial orbicularis oculi, are identified and resected or weakened with grasping forceps. The brow is released from the supraorbital rim in either the subgaleal or subperiosteal plane [4]. The temporal dissection is performed lateral to medial in the plane between the superficial and deep temporal fascia down to the level of the orbital rim and the superior edge of the zygomatic arch (Fig. 3).

  Once the brow has been completely released and the depressor muscles modified, the brow is repositioned and fixated. Tension-free fixation is essential for up to 3 months, when wound healing is complete [5]. Many fixation methods have been described,

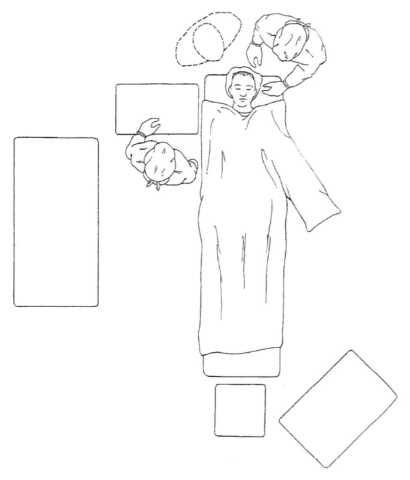

Figure 2 Operating room setup and patient positioning for endoscopic forehead lift. (From Ref. 6.)

Table 1 Equipment for Endoscopic Forehead and Midface Lift

Light source
4 mm 30 degree endoscope
Video monitor
Endoscopic instruments:
   Endoretractor
   Blunt and sharp forceps
   Dissecting scissors
   Clip appliers
   Suction irrigator
   Hook cautery
Power drill (optional)

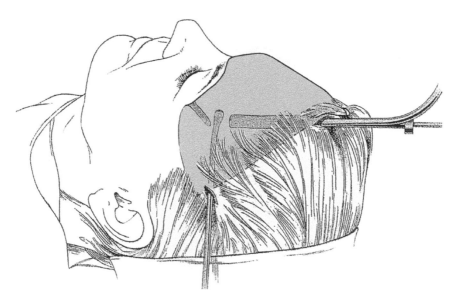

Figure 3   Endoscopic forehead lift. (From Ref. 6.)

including permanent and absorbable suture suspension, cortical tunnels, tissue adhesives, percutaneous screws, internal screw and plate fixation, mitek anchors, K-wires, and external bolster dressings [4,6–8] (Figs. 4 and 5). Rohrich and Beran classified fixation methods into 2 categories: endogenous and exogenous—the latter includes all methods utilizing permanent hardware fixation [4]. As a group, the exogenous methods are very precise but carry the risk of dural injury with the use of power equipment [4]. The endogenous methods are, in general, safer but less precise and have a higher risk of relapse [4]. Currently, the author's preferred methods of fixation are the use of cortical tunnels for vertical brow fixation and temporal spanning sutures for lateral brow fixation.

C.   Results

The endoscopic forehead lift is the most commonly performed endoscopic plastic surgery procedure. Favorable results of this procedure for forehead rejuvenation have been reported in the literature. Hamas and Rohrich reported 43 of 47 successful endoscopic forehead lifts based on brow elevation as demonstrated objectively in preop and postop photos and subjectively based on patient opinion [9]. Ramirez reported a 1 in 300 rate of reoperation for his endoscopic forehead procedures [8]. Hamas published a description of endoscopic corrugator resection for treatment of glabellar frown lines [10]. He reported a series of 35 patients followed for up to 1.5 years in whom maximal conscious frowning was successfully reduced to 50% of preop level and subconscious frowning was reduced to 20% of preop level [10]. Reported complications of the endoscopic forehead lift are rare and include relapse or redescent, hematoma, seroma, temporary sensory loss, facial nerve paresis, and hairline elevation [8–9]. Hamas and Rohrich reported 7 minor self-limited complications in their series of 47 patients. The endoscopic forehead lift is effective in

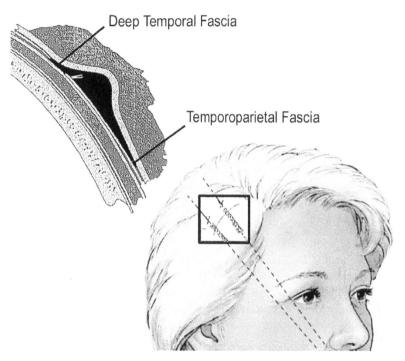

Figure 4 Temporal spanning sutures. (From Ref. 4.)

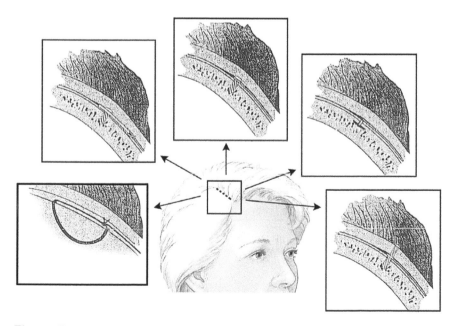

Figure 5 Cortical tunnel (below, left), internal screw with Gortex tab (above, left), internal screw (above, center), Mitek anchor (above, right), external screw (below, right). (From Ref. 4.)

achieving the aesthetic goals of forehead rejuvenation with decreased morbidity and improved patient acceptance when compared to the traditional open technique.

III. MIDFACE LIFT

Aging and the effects of gravity on the deep facial structures can be detected in the anatomical changes of the midface or malar region. Indications for midface rejuvenation include malar fat pad ptosis with loss of malar prominence, prominent nasolabial folds, tear trough, and jowl formation [11-13]. The objectives of midface rejuvenation procedures are repositioning of the malar fat pad, SMAS (superficial musculoaponeurotic system) tightening, and skin redraping [11].

A. Procedure Selection

The open midface lift is typically approached through preauricular, retroauricular, and lower lid incisions. These access incisions are needed for skin resection in patients with significant skin excess but they are frequently complicated by visible scars, hypoesthesia, increased postop pain and swelling, and longer recovery period compared to the endoscopic approach [11]. The endoscopic midface lift is ideal in patients with normal skin thickness and elasticity, who require subcutaneous and muscular corrections rather than skin excision [11].

B. Surgical Technique

The endoscopic midface lift can be approached in a subcutaneous plane, a subperiosteal plane, or both and is often performed in combination with a forehead lift or a full face lift. The midface lift can be done under general or local anesthesia with sedation. Operating room setup, patient positioning, and endoscopic equipment are the same as for the endoscopic forehead lift (Fig. 2) (Table 2). The face and scalp are infiltrated with local anesthetic and epinephrine. The forehead dissection is typically done first, followed by the midface, when these rejuvenation procedures are performed in combination. The midface lift is approached through a temporal incision 4–6 cm in length, 1–2 cm behind and parallel to the hairline extending superiorly from the above the helical rim (Fig. 6). The subcutaneous approach proceeds lateral to medial with subcutaneous dissection of the midface to the level of the malar fat pad, at which point the dissection is continued in a deeper plane under the fat pad. This dissection extends medially to the nose between the

Table 2 Equipment for Endoscopic Augmentation Mammaplasty

Light source
10 mm 30 degree endoscope
Video monitor
Endoscopic instruments:
   Endoretractor
   Blunt forceps
   Dissecting scissors
   Suction cautery
Saline implants

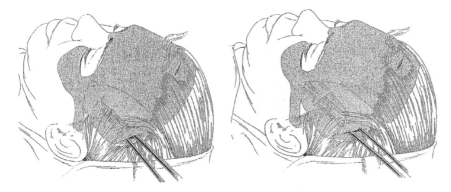

Figure 6 Endoscopic midface dissection. (From Ref. 11.)

fat pad and the zygomaticus muscles to elevate the malar fat pad attached to the skin flap. Once this flap is elevated, the SMAS layer is exposed laterally for placement of plication sutures. A lower lid incision is used for the subperiosteal approach, and for variations of the subcutaneous approach which include elevation of the orbicularis oculi muscle with the malar fat pad and skin in a composite flap.

The subperiosteal approach utilizes the lower lid incision to elevate the periosteum off of the inferior and lateral orbital rim, the zygomatic arch, and the maxilla, with careful preservation of the infraorbital nerve. This dissection is facilitated by the previous forehead dissection. The subperiosteal dissection is less commonly approached through a gingivobuccal incision. The endoscope is used during the procedure through either incision to visualize the plane of dissection, nerves, vessels, and suspension suture placement. Once dissection is complete, the malar soft tissue flap is suspended with sutures in a superiolateral direction to the temporal fascia or galea. The lower lid incision can be used for a lateral canthopexy or blepharoplasty if indicated and is usually closed last.

Byrd describes a unique multiplanar approach to the midface as a component of his endoscopically assisted "extended browlift" procedure [14]. This technique begins with subgaleal dissection of the forehead with release of the fibrous retinaculum, which attaches the orbicularis oculi to the orbital rim to free the brow. The temporalis fascia is incised laterally, and the dissection of the temple and lateral orbital rim is continued in the plane under the superficial temporal fascia to the level of the zygomatic arch. At the zygomatic arch the periosteum is incised and the plane of dissection over the arch to its junction with the zygoma is subperiosteal. The dissection plane over the medial zygoma changes to the level above the periosteum but below orbicularis oculi. The retinacular attachments of the orbicularis oculi to the inferior orbital rim are incised to free the lower lid. The zygomatic cutaneous ligament above the zygomaticus major is identified and transected. The zygomatic cutaneous ligament is the primary retaining ligament of the malar complex and contains attachments from the zygomaticus major, masseter, malar fat pad, zygoma, and skin. Release of this ligament results in a mobile cheek and malar complex. The zygomatic cutaneous ligament is repositioned and suture fixated to the fascia of the lateral orbital rim. The superficial temporal fascia is advanced and fixated over the deep fascia. The brow is fixated (with Gortex tabs), and lastly the temporal skin is advanced and fixated to the temporalis fascia. This technique emphasizes release of the soft tissue retaining attachments to the orbital rim and successfully repositions soft tissue with minimal resection [14].

C. Results

Prospective comparisons of the different techniques of the midface lift do not exist, but different authors report different rationale for each specific technique. Ramirez recommends the subperiosteal approach because the periosteum is a more rigid structure and has less tendency to descend than more superficial tissues [15–16]. Other advantages of the subperiosteal plane are that it provides a better optical cavity, orientation to critical structures, vascularity, and its dissection can be done safely and quickly [16]. De la Fuente recommends the subcutaneous approach with SMAS plication because of persistent orbitomalar edema in his patients who have undergone subperiosteal endoscopic midface lift [12]. The subperiosteal dissection may also have a greater incidence of transient facial nerve deficits [11]. The multiplanar approach described by Byrd consolidates the benefits of the superficial and deep dissection techniques [14]. In his series of 42 patients who underwent the extended browlift, Byrd reported two complications of transient forehead weakness [14].

Celik reported results in a series of 72 patients who underwent endoscopic upper and midface rejuvenation: 51 had excellent, 16 had good, and 5 had unsatisfactory results as determined by 4 plastic surgeons' evaluations of the preop and postop photos [13]. Patient satisfaction was evaluated by questionnaire: 63 were satisfied and 9 were not satisfied [13]. Reported complications of the endoscopic midface lift are temporary alopecia, temporary numbness, rare hematoma, lid retraction, midface widening, and preauricular skin folds if skin is too lax [12–13,16]. The endoscopic midface lift has several advantages over the open technique, including smaller scars, less alopecia, less sensory disruption, less incisional pain, less swelling, less bleeding, more vascularized flaps, and decreased recovery time [11].

IV. AUGMENTATION MAMMAPLASTY

Endoscopic breast augmentation has several advantages over traditional techniques, including smaller less conspicuous incisions, improved visualization, improved hemostasis, and more precise control of the inframammary crease and implant positioning [17–20]. Transaxillary, inframammary, periareolar, and transumbilical approaches have been described for endoscopic breast augmentation. The transaxillary approach is the safest and most successful approach. Indications for breast augmentation include bilateral mammary hypoplasia, atrophy, and asymmetry. Patients with mild degrees of breast ptosis can be treated successfully with an endoscopic approach. Patients with moderate to severe ptosis usually require open mastopexy in addition to augmentation and therefore are not good endoscopic candidates [17–18].

A. Procedure Selection

Implants can be positioned in a submammary, subpectoral, and subfascial position. Most plastic surgeons recommend the subpectoral position because implants feel more natural and sensation is preserved. Muscle coverage also minimizes problems of rippling and palpability and may even decrease the incidence of capsular contracture [18–20]. Subfascial positioning is a recent advancement and reportedly has the advantages of a submuscular position but does not have the disadvantages of implant movement and inferior pole flattenening with muscle contraction [18]. Experience with this technique is limited at this time.

Smooth or textured implants can be used for augmentation. Smooth implants are easier to position using the endoscopic approach but have a higher incidence of capsular contracture. Textured implants were designed to decrease capsular contracture, but they are thicker, more difficult to manipulate, more palpable, and create more visible rippling, especially in thin patients [17,19–20].

The transaxillary placement of a subpectoral implant is the most popular endoscopic augmentation technique. Traditionally augmentation through an open axillary approach was a blind procedure, but with endoscopic assistance it can be done under direct visualization through smaller incisions. Endoscopically assisted augmentation results in a more accurate placement of the implant and the inframammary crease.

B. Transaxillary Technique

The transaxillary technique is typically performed under general anesthesia with the patient in a supine position (Fig. 7) (Table 2). Local anesthetic and epinephrine are injected at the incision site. A 2 cm transverse incision is placed in the axilla posterior to the anterior axillary fold. Dissection is performed lateral to medial in a superficial plane to the lateral border of the pectoralis major and continues medially under the pectoralis through the fascia into the subpectoral space. This space is dissected with gentle blunt dissection to avoid bleeding. Once this space is developed, a 10 mm rigid endoscope mounted on an endoretractor is inserted and medial release of the pectoralis 1–2 cm from its origin at the level of the superior areola is performed using electrocautery (Fig. 8). The pectoralis is released from medial to lateral at the level of the new inframammary crease, which is marked 1–2 cm below the original crease preoperatively. When dissection is completed, the endoscope is removed and the implant is inserted into the pocket and expanded with saline. Position and symmetry are confirmed with the patient in an upright position.

C. Results

Endoscopic augmentation mammaplasty offers patients better results and less morbidity because of better visualization, more controlled dissection, and smaller incisions. Eaves et al. reported lower morbidity with the endoscopic approach based on a series of 70 patients who underwent endoscopic subpectoral transaxillary breast augmentation [20]. There were no reports of hematoma, seroma, or capsular contracture in their series [20]. Howard compared implant malpositioning in a series of 92 patients who underwent open transaxillary augmentation and a series of 58 patients who underwent endoscopic transaxillary augmentations [19]. The rates of implant malposition were 8.6% in the open series and 2.0% in the endoscopic series [19]. He concluded from this analysis that endoscopic technique improves position [19]. Graf et al. reported a series of 62 patients, followed for up to 3 years, who underwent endoscopic transaxillary breast augmentation. They reported only 3 complications: 1 hematoma and 2 implant malpositions that required secondary procedures [18].

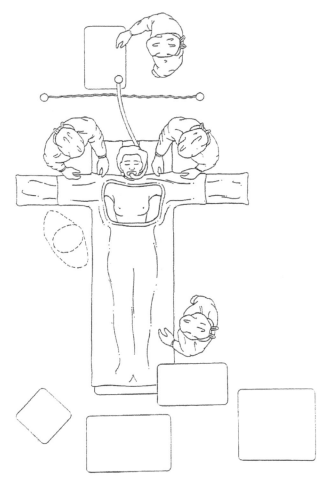

Figure 7 Operating room setup and patient positioning for transaxillary approach to endoscopic augmentation mammaplasty. (From Ref. 17.)

V. ABDOMINOPLASTY

Abdominoplasty techniques are used to improve the contour of the abdominal wall. Individual anatomical variations determine whether a patient will require dermolipectomy, liposuction, or fascial plication to achieve an improvement in abdominal wall contour [21]. Abdominoplasty is typically performed using a long transverse abdominal incision, which may be complicated by hypertrophic scar formation or skin necrosis. Endoscopic abdominoplasty, with or without liposuction, is indicated in a select group of patients with diastasis recti that require abdominal wall plication without skin excision [21–23]. The advantages of this endoscopic technique include reduced perioperative pain and morbidity, small incisions, and shortened recovery time [21–24]. The endoscopic approach utilizes suprapubic and/or periumbilical access incisions.

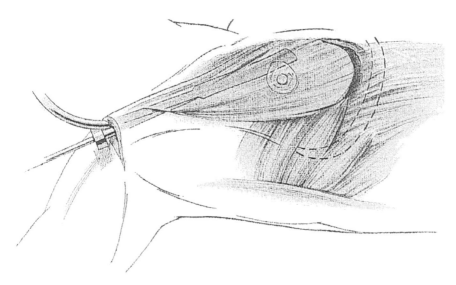

Figure 8 Transaxillary approach to endoscopic augmentation mammaplasty. (From Ref. 17.)

A. Surgical Technique

Preoperative markings are used to indicate the margins of the anterior rectus sheath for plication and areas that will require liposuction. The procedure is performed under general anesthesia with the patient in the supine position (Fig. 9) (Table 3). The abdominal wall is infiltrated with a tumescent solution of dilute lidocaine and epinephrine. Deep plane suction lipectomy is performed first and assists in the subsequent development of an optical cavity [21]. A 2–3 cm suprapubic incision is placed in the hair-bearing area and dissection continues to the anterior rectus sheath in an open manner until an optical cavity can be established. The endoscope mounted on the endoretractor is inserted, and using laparoscopic scissors, the dissection continues cephalad in the plane above the anterior fascia (Fig. 10). Dissection may proceed up to or beyond the umbilicus depending on the patient's anatomical indications. Hemostasis of the cavity is obtained prior to suture plication. Superior to inferior fascial plication may be performed with interrupted or continuous permanent sutures and is facilitated by the use of a long endoscopic needle holder (Figs. 11 and 12). After fascial plication is completed, the umbilicus is sutured to the midline, a drain is placed, and the suprapubic incision is closed. Additional superficial suction lipectomy will assist in final recontouring and promote skin retraction.

B. Results

Endoscopic abdominoplasty is an effective treatment of diastasis recti and abdominal wall lipodystrophy in a carefully selected patient population. This procedure is most applicable to patients with postgestational abdominal wall deformities without a need for skin excision [22–23]. Good skin quality and the use of liposuction result in satisfactory skin contraction over the fascial plication. In select patients, endoscopic abdominoplasty may be successfully performed in combination with uncomplicated ventral hernia repair [22].

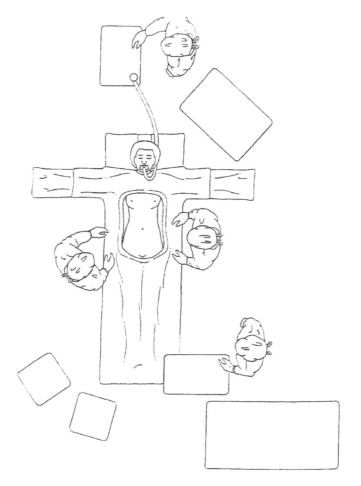

Figure 9   Operating room setup and patient positioning for endoscopic abdominoplasty. (From Ref. 21.)

Table 3   Equipment for Endoscopic Abdominoplasty

Light source
10 mm 30 degree endoscope
Video monitor
Tumescent solution
Liposuction equipment
Endoscopic instruments:
  Endoretractor
  Dissecting scissors
  Suction cautery
  Endoscopic needle holder

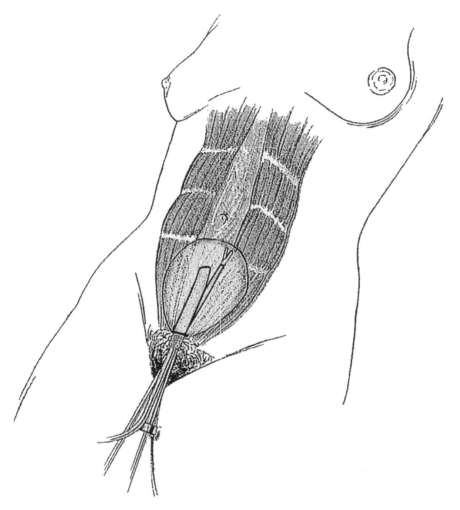

Figure 10 Endoscopic abdominoplasty. (From Ref. 21.)

VI. LATISSIMUS DORSI FLAP HARVEST

The latissimus dorsi flap is the most widely used muscle flap in reconstructive surgery [25]. It is a versatile flap and has been successfully used for breast, chest wall, head and neck, and lower extremity reconstruction. Latissimus harvest traditionally requires a lengthy incision (20–30 cm) and is associated with significant donor site complications, including seroma and hypertrophic scar formation [26–27]. Endoscopic harvest of this muscle flap has been pursued in an attempt to reduce donor site complications [25–26,28–35]. Balloon-assisted endoscopic harvest is an alternative technique that is gaining popularity with some reconstructive surgeons [30–31]. The traditional endoscopic harvest and the balloon-assisted techniques are described below.

A. Traditional Surgical Technique

Endoscopic latissimus harvest is performed under general anesthesia with the patient in a lateral decubitus or prone position (Fig. 13) (Table 4). The surgeon is positioned on the

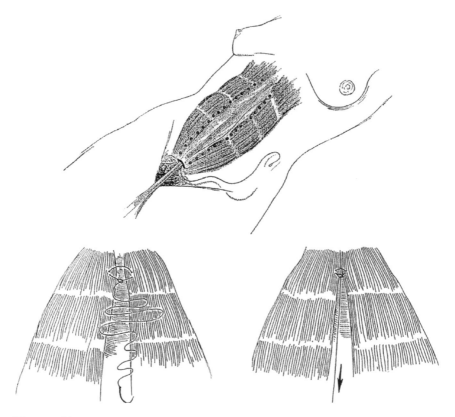

Figure 11   Endoscopic abdominoplasty: suture placement. (From Ref. 21.)

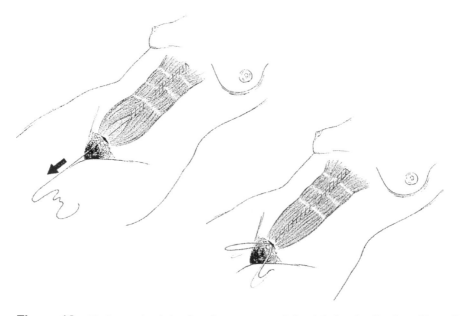

Figure 12   Endoscopic abdominoplasty: rectus abdominis fascia plication. (From Ref. 21.)

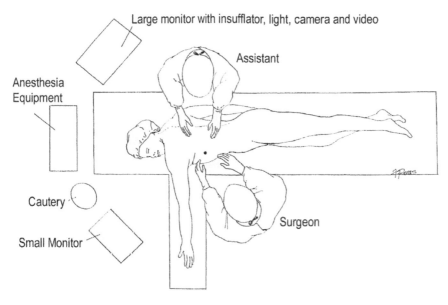

Large monitor with insufflator, light, camera and video

Assistant

Anesthesia Equipment

Cautery

Small Monitor

Surgeon

Figure 13 Operating room setup and patient positioning for endoscopic latissimus dorsi muscle harvest. (From Ref. 28.)

same side as the muscle to be harvested. Video monitors are placed on either side of the patient's head. For breast reconstruction the mastectomy incision may be sufficient for pedicled muscle harvest, and additional access incisions may be added if necessary during the course of the dissection [26]. For free flap harvest a 5–6cm incision is made along the posterior axillary line. The latissimus is identified and dissected off the chest wall under direct visualization until an optical cavity is created and direct vision is no long possible. The vascular pedicle is carefully identified and partially dissected under direct visualization. The endoscope and endoretractor are inserted into the optical cavity and the endoscopic dissection continues both above and below the muscle using blunt

Table 4 Equipment for Endoscopic Muscle Harvest

Light source
10mm 30 degree endoscope
Video monitor
CO_2 insufflator
Endoscopic instruments:
  10mm and 5mm ports
  Blunt and sharp forceps
  Dissecting scissors
  Clip appliers
  Suction irrigator
  Hook cautery
2 Dissecting balloons 750–2500cc (optional) (General
  Surgical Innovations Corp., Palo Alto, CA)

dissection and electrocautery. The optical cavity is maintained by use of external retraction or insufflation. Hemoclip ligation of perforating vessels is used to maintain hemostasis during the dissection. The harmonic scalpel is also a useful instrument for the endoscopic dissection of the muscle flap and ligation of the perforating vessels [34]. Once the muscle is elevated off the chest wall and back, it is divided from its lumbar and iliac attachments. A separate paramedian back incision may be needed to facilitate this difficult portion of the dissection. Once the muscle is freed from its origin, the pedicle dissection is completed under direct visualization. A drain is placed in the large optical cavity. Fixation sutures may be used for donor site closure to increase skin flap adherence and reduce seroma formation [25].

B.   Balloon-Assisted Technique

The patient position is the same as with the traditional technique. A 5 cm axillary incision is used to dissect the pedicle. Two additional 1 cm port incisions are made to facilitate the endoscopic dissection utilizing triangulation technique, one at the mid-lateral and one at the superior-medial border of the latissimus in the auscultatory triangle [27,30] (Fig. 14). The muscle dissection is started using the lighted retractor, cautery, and dissecting scissors. A 1500–2500 cc dissecting balloon is then inserted in the supramuscular plane through the auscultatory triangle incision and inflated with saline or water. This balloon is

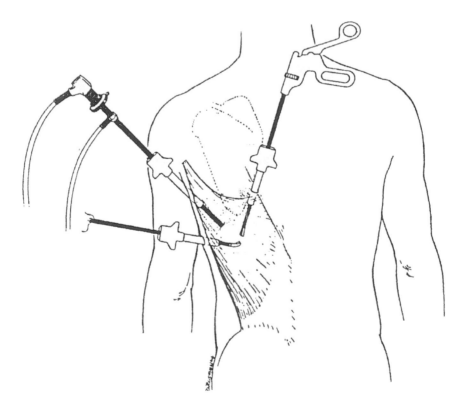

Figure 14   Location of ports for balloon-assisted endoscopic latissimus dorsi muscle harvest. (From Ref. 30.)

removed and a 750–1500 cc balloon dissector is placed in the submuscular plane and inflated. The balloon is removed after it is expanded, and the optical cavity is maintained with insufflation or retractors and the endoscopic camera is inserted. The segmental intercostal perforator vessels which have been dissected and stretched by the balloon are then ligated or cauterized under endoscopic visualization. The balloon completes up to 95% of the dissection [30]. The distal and medial margins of the muscle need to be sharply dissected beyond the margin of the balloon dissector to complete the muscle harvest. The distal margin is then transected and the muscle falls into the optical cavity and can be removed through the axillary incision. The pedicle dissection is then completed, a hemovac drain is placed, and the incisions are closed after hemostasis is achieved.

C. Results

Successful endoscopic latissimus harvest has been reported for a variety of reconstructive procedures [25–26,28]. Cho et al. reported a series of 10 patients who underwent endoscopic latissimus harvest for lower extremity reconstruction [25]. There were no donor site complications in this series, and although the harvest time was longer than for an open procedure, there was no total time difference when the time for donor site closure was included [25]. Ramakrishnan et al. reported a series of 12 patients with "high-risk chest walls" that underwent breast reconstruction with endoscopically harvested latissimus harvest and tissue expander placement [29]. A total of 5 complications were reported in this series and included 2 anterior chest wall hematomas, 1 expander loss due to infection, 1 wound infection, and 1 skin flap necrosis [29]. No seromas were reported; the authors attribute this to the magnified visualization of lymphatic and vascular structures, which facilitates more effective cauterization of these structures [29]. Masuoka et al. reported one complication of donor site seroma in a series of 7 patients undergoing breast reconstruction with endoscopically harvested latissimus flaps and tissue expanders [33].

Lin et al. compared donor site morbidity between endoscopically assisted and traditional harvest of free latissimus dorsi flaps. No statistically significant difference in donor site morbidity was demonstrated between the 22 endoscopically harvested and the 26 traditionally harvested patients. The incidence of seroma formation in the two groups was 9.1% and 11.5%, respectively. The only statistically significant finding was a higher level of overall satisfaction with the procedure and the resultant scar in the endoscopic group.

Variations of the endoscopic technique including the use of a harmonic scalpel and the balloon-assisted technique may have an important impact on the incidence of postoperative complications. Inaba et al. published a study that demonstrated less histological muscle damage and decreased wound infections with use of the harmonic scalpel in the harvest of canine latissimus dorsi flaps [34]. There is no published comparison of the morbidity of the balloon-assisted and traditional endoscopic technique. However, published reports of the balloon-assisted technique have rates of seroma formation that are similar to the traditional techniques. Karp et al. reported a series of 6 balloon-assisted flap harvests; 1 patient developed a donor site seroma [30]. Van Buskirk et al. published a series of 6 patients who underwent balloon-assisted endoscopic latissimus harvest for reconstruction with no reported donor site morbidity in a 6-month follow-up period [31].

The balloon-assisted technique has several important advantages, including decreased surgeon fatigue, steep learning curve, and less blood loss because vessels are stretched and frequently thrombosed prior to ligation [30]. Disadvantages to the balloon technique include difficult dissection over the curvature of the back with the inflexible balloon introducer and inability to harvest more than 80% of the muscle [30]. The balloon-assisted technique is not preferred for huge defects, which require every millimeter of flap. Although there are no statistically significant data that demonstrate that these minimally invasive techniques have a lower incidence of donor site morbidity, the results are encouraging, and success is expected as experience with these techniques continues to grow. The significant reduction in scar length and risk of hypertrophic scar formation is attractive to both the reconstructive surgeon and patient.

VII. RECTUS ABDOMINUS FLAP HARVEST

The rectus abdominis muscle is a popular reconstructive flap because it has a large surface area, it is reliable, and it has a wide arc of rotation [36]. The rectus abdominis can be used as an inferiorly or superiorly based pedicle flap or as a free flap. The disadvantages of the rectus flap are primarily due to its donor site complications, including seroma, wound infection, large incision with poor cosmesis, abdominal wall weakness, and hernias. Techniques of endoscopic rectus abdominis harvest have been investigated in cadaver and porcine models [28,37–38]. Recent clinical case reports support the practical application of endoscopic harvest techniques [36,39].

A. Surgical Technique

The endoscopic equipment used is the same as for the latissimus dorsi muscle harvest (Table 4). The patient is positioned supine with the surgeon on the same side as the rectus to be harvested and the assistant on the opposite side of the table. Video monitors are placed on both sides of the patient's head. There is no standard surgical technique for the endoscopic rectus harvest. Early investigations differentiated between transperitoneal and extraperitoneal approaches [28]. The transperitoneal utilized a standard intra-abdominal laparoscopic approach to harvest the rectus by incising the posterior sheath. This technique has been largely abandoned due to the increased morbidity of entering the peritoneal cavity. The extraperitoneal approach has been described using several different port site configurations. The most common configuration utilizes one 10 mm port site placed midline over the sheath at the superior or inferior aspect of the rectus and two 5 mm ports placed at the medial and lateral edge of the rectus sheath. The anterior rectus sheath is opened through the 10 mm incision, a 10 mm port and camera are inserted through the muscle fibers but not through the posterior sheath. The optical cavity is created using CO_2 insufflation up to 10 mmHg. The rectus muscle is dissected from the posterior sheath using a balloon dissector, an optical dissector, blunt and sharp dissection under endoscopic visualization, or a combination of these techniques [28,36–39] (Fig. 15). Perforating vessels and the superior and inferior vascular bundles are visualized and divided between clips. After the posterior sheath dissection is completed, the anterior sheath is dissected from the muscle. This requires careful dissection of the tendinous inscriptions to avoid unnecessary bleeding and damage to the rectus sheath or muscle. Some surgeons advocate harvest of the anterior rectus sheath with the muscle to avoid the difficult dissection around the tendinous inscriptions [37,39]. Removal of the anterior rectus sheath, especially below the arcuate line, will leave a fascial defect that may be difficult to close and predispose to abdominal wall hernia formation. Once the muscle flap is dissected from its sheath, it can

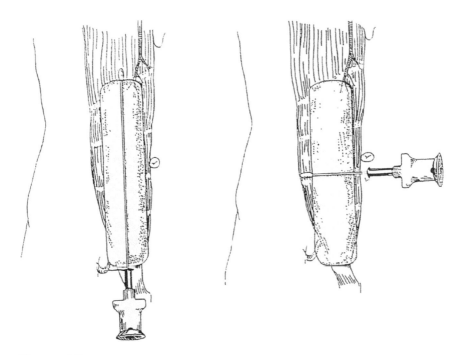

Figure 15 Balloon assisted rectus abdominis harvest: (left) axial balloon orientation; (right) perpendicular balloon orientation. (From Ref. 52.)

be harvested as a pedicled or free flap and the appropriate insertion or origin (or both) are transected and the flap is rotated or removed through the transverse incision. A drain is placed in the rectus sheath, and the sheath and skin incisions are closed.

B. Results

There are only two published clinical case reports of endoscopic rectus abdominis harvest. Sawaizumi et al. report 2 patients who had endoscopically harvested rectus flaps; both were superiorly based pedicled flaps, one for chest wall and one for breast reconstruction [39]. The technique described in this series harvests a spindle-shaped slip of anterior rectus sheath with the muscle flap. Both patients were young women and had satisfactory results without complications 1 year after the operation [39]. Dabb et al. report a series of 5 patients who underwent endoscopic harvest of superiorly based rectus flaps for sternal defects [36]. All patients had resolution of their sternal infections and "long-term" flap survival over an unspecified period of time. There were no reported hernias or other complications. The time of operation decreased significantly between the first and last patient in this series. The success of these clinical reports suggests that endoscopic rectus harvest is a successful technique with low morbidity and a steep learning curve.

VIII. ENDOSCOPIC SURAL NERVE HARVEST

Autogenous nerve grafting is an important component of surgical reconstruction. Sural nerve autografts are frequently used for reconstruction of peripheral nerve lesions.

Traditionally, the sural nerve has been harvested through a single long incision along the course of the nerve or multiple step ladder incisions. Endoscopic-assisted sural nerve harvest is performed through minimal incisions and eliminates the long scars associated with the traditional technique. The use of small access incisions decreases the risks of wound-healing problems.

A. Surgical Technique

The patient is positioned supine with the hip and knee flexed at 45 degrees and the surgeon stands near the ipsilateral foot (Fig. 16) (Table 5). The patient may be positioned prone for bilateral sural nerve harvest. The limb is exsanguinated with a tourniquet after the patient is under general anesthesia. A 3 cm incision is made posterior to the lateral malleolus. The nerve is identified and dissected in an open manner for several centimeters to establish the optical cavity. An endoscope mounted on an endoretractor is inserted and the nerve is

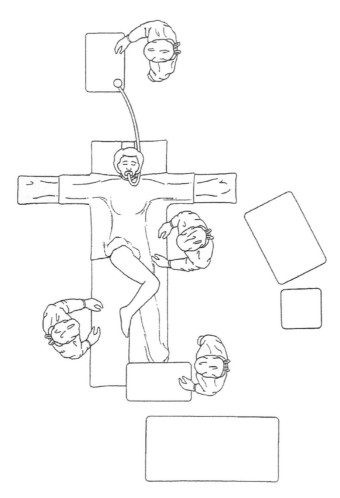

Figure 16 Operating room setup and patient positioning for endoscopic sural nerve harvest. (From Ref. 26.)

Table 5 Equipment for Endoscopic Sural Nerve Harvest

Light source
5 mm 30 degree endoscope
Video monitor
Tourniquet
Endoscopic instruments:
  Dissecting scissors
  Nerve retractor/dissector
  Clip applier
Optional: 16 Fr Foley, endoscopic vein harvest set

dissected proximally under endoscopic visualization using endoscissors or a nerve dissector. Alternative dissection techniques include balloon-assisted dissection and use of endoscopic vein harvest systems. The balloon dissection technique uses a 16 Fr foley catheter, which is sequentially inflated and advanced in the loose connective tissue surrounding the nerve [40]. Endoscopic vein harvest technique will be discussed in the next segment. The dissection becomes more difficult at the point where the nerve dives under the deep fascia to ascend between the heads of the gastrocnemius muscle. The fascia may need to be divided to facilitate proximal dissection. After the appropriate length of nerve is fully dissected, it is removed through the access incision. The tourniquet is then deflated and hemostasis is obtained at the access incision prior to closure. An elastic dressing is applied to the leg for 2 days postoperatively.

B. Results

The primary advantage of endoscopic harvest is the short access incision, which results in less postoperative pain and fewer wound-healing complications. There are currently no long-term follow-up studies comparing traditional and endoscopic nerve harvest techniques. Preliminary reports from small series of patients have been encouraging [26,40]. The endoscopic harvest time is longer than open harvest, but this can be offset by the decreased time for wound closure [41]. Microscopic examination of an endoscopically harvested nerve did not demonstrate intraneural injury or hemorrhage [26]. However, long-term evaluation of nerve function after endoscopic harvest still needs to be investigated.

IX. ENDOSCOPIC SAPHENOUS VEIN HARVEST

Vein harvest is required for some microvascular reconstruction procedures. Similar to endoscopic nerve harvest, endoscopic vein harvest has the potential to decrease wound-healing complications by avoiding long access incisions. The benefits of endoscopic vein harvest have been primarily investigated by vascular and cardiothoracic surgeons. Endoscopic vein harvest is particularly beneficial in vascular and cardiothoracic surgery patients who usually suffer from atherosclerotic disease and diabetes and therefore have a higher incidence of wound-healing problems. Reconstructive surgery patients are a younger population but frequently have traumatic comorbidities and benefit from the decreased donor site morbidity of endoscopic vein harvest.

A. Surgical Technique

Endoscopic vein harvest can be performed under general or regional anesthesia. The patient is positioned supine in a frog leg position (Fig. 17) (Table 6). A 1.5–2.5 cm incision is made on the medial thigh just above the knee. Guidant Corporation (Cardiac and Vascular Surgery, Menlo Park, CA) markets endoscopic vein harvest equipment. Their Vasoview Uniport System provides a vein dissector and flexible bipolar scissor, which can be used through a 12 mm trocar at the access site. The vein is identified through the access incision, the trocar is introduced and CO_2 insufflation is used to create an optical cavity for vein dissection. The vein is dissected proximally to the groin. Side branches are clipped or cauterized with the bipolar. Once dissection is complete, an additional incision is made in the groin to remove the transected vein. The vein is carefully inspected, side branches are ligated, and repairs made with 7-0 prolene as needed. The wound is inspected for hemostasis, the incisions are closed, and an elastic dressing is applied.

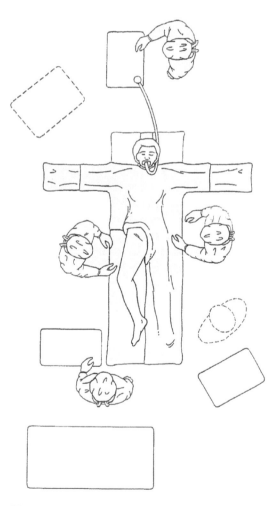

Figure 17 Operating room setup and patient positioning for endoscopic saphenous vein harvest. (From Ref. 26.)

Table 6   Equipment for Endoscopic Saphenous Vein Harvest

Light source
10 mm endoscope
Video monitor
CO_2 insufflator
Endoscopic instruments:
   Dissecting scissors
   Bipolar cautery
   Clip applier
VasoView Uniport
   or
VasoView Balloon Dissection System (Guidant Corp., Cardiac and
   Vascular Surgery, Menlo Park, CA)

An alternative harvest technique utilizes a balloon dissection cannula. The VasoView Balloon Dissection System (Guidant Corp.) includes a tapered-tip balloon dissector, which transmits an image to the video monitor. The balloon dissector is placed on the anterior surface of the vein through the access incision at the medial malleolus. The balloon dissector is sequentially advanced and inflated to form a perivascular endoscopic tunnel. Once the balloon dissection is completed, the dissector is removed, a trocar is placed into the access incision, and the tunnel is insufflated with CO_2 up to 15 mmHg. A 10 mm diameter endoscope is inserted into the trocar, and a counterincision is made at the proximal end of the tunnel. A trocar is sewn into this incision, and endoscissors are used to dissect the vein under visualization from the camera in the distal trocar. The vein side braches are ligated with a clip applier. This dissection technique can be continued proximally onto the thigh with an additional counterincision in the groin. The vein is transected and removed after dissection is completed. The vein graft is repaired if needed. The incisions are closed and an elastic bandage is applied to the leg.

B. Results

Traditionally, the saphenous vein is harvested through a long continuous incision. The incidence of wound complications from open harvest may be as high as 40% [42]. Wound complications such as hematoma, dehiscence, drainage, cellulitis, skin necrosis, neuralgia, edema, and infection contribute significantly to the morbidity of procedures that utilize vein graft. Endoscopic vein harvest reduces donor site morbidity. Vrancic et al. reported a 8.9% morbidity rate in a series of 179 patients who underwent endoscopic vein harvest for coronary bypass operations [43]. Marty et al. reported significantly less postoperative pain and better cosmetic results after endoscopic vein harvest compared to traditional open harvest [44]. Allen et al. published a prospective randomized trial comparing endoscopic and open vein harvest and reported wound complication rates of 4% for endoscopic harvest and 19% for open harvest [45]. In a comparision study of wound complications and vein quality, Crouch et al. reported a decreased incidence of wound complication for endoscopic harvest (5%) versus open harvest (14.2%) [46]. Microscopic examination did not identify any histological differences between the endoscopic and open harvest veins [46]. Meyer et al. also compared histology of endoscopic and open harvest vein specimens and found no significant difference in vein quality [47]. Endoscopic vein harvest is clearly associated with a decreased incidence of wound complications, and although current studies do not identify any significant histological differences, long-term patency of endoscopically harvested grafts still needs evaluation.

X. ENDOSCOPIC NASAL AIRWAY SURGERY

Nasal endoscopy has become a routine part of the evaluation of nasal airway problems. It is a versatile tool that is applied in the office for diagnosis and monitoring of nasal airway problems. An endoscopic examination of nasal anatomy is used as an extension of the physical exam. A 30 degree rigid nasal endoscope can be used to evaluate the septum, turbinates, osteomeatal complex, and the posterior pharynx [48]. Nasal endoscopy is also applied in the operating room to increase the precision and accuracy of nasal airway surgery. It has the ability to convert previously blind procedures into those done under direct visualization and magnification. Nasal endoscopy can be used in the treatment of sinus disease, exophthalmus, dacryocystostenosis, and epistaxis [48]. It can also improve the precision of septoplasty, nasal dorsum alterations, and inferior turbinate resection [48–50].

A. Inferior Turbinate Surgery

Inferior turbinate hypertrophy is a common cause of nasal airway obstruction The treatment of inferior turbinate hypertrophy is turbinate resection. Different techniques of turbinate resection have been described, and most techniques may be augmented by the use of endoscopy for direct visualization of the anatomy. Since many patients with inferior turbinate hypertrophy also have septal deviation, turbinate resection is frequently preceded by septoplasty and/or rhinoplasty to improve visualization of the inferior turbinate.

The endoscopically assisted partial anteroinferior turbinate resection is a commonly performed procedure for inferior turbinate hypertrophy (Table 7). A 30 degree nasal endoscope is inserted into the nose after septal reconstruction is completed. Under direct visualization endoscopic turbinate scissors are used to complete a full-thickness excision of the anterior turbinate (Fig. 18). An endoscopic cautery instrument is then used to cauterize the resected margin of the turbinate and to control excessive mucosal hypertrophy. The Boies fracture elevator is used to out-fracture the posterior portion of the turbinate. Surgicel (oxidized cellulose) and antibiotic ointment are placed along the

Table 7 Equipment for Endoscopic Inferior Turbinate Resection

Light source
4.5 mm 30 degree nasal endoscope
Video monitor
Endoscopic instruments:
  Endoscissors
  Cautery
Boies fracture elevator
Surgicel + antibiotic ointment
Intranasal splints

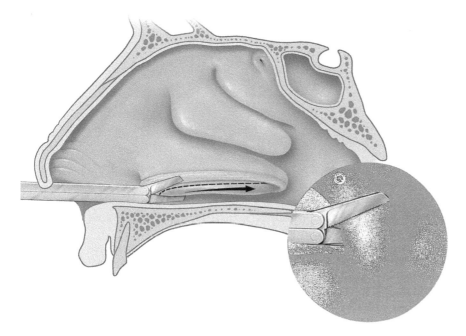

Figure 18   Endoscopically assisted inferior turbinate resection. (From Ref. 48.)

resection margin and intranasal splints are inserted. The precision of inferior turbinate resection is greatly enhanced by use of the endoscope.

B. Sinus Surgery

The ostia of the anterior ethmoids, maxillary, and frontal sinus all join to form the hiatus semilunaris of the middle meatus. Ethmoid sinus disease can result in persistent maxillary and frontal sinus disease due to obstruction of the osteameatal complex. Endoscopic sinus surgery can be used to perform anterior ethmoidectomy and enlarge the ostia of the involved sinuses to facilitate drainage of the diseased mucosa. Nasal endoscopy can also be used to treat frontal sinus trauma. Fractures involving the frontal sinus ostium have traditionally been treated with sinus obliteration to prevent the formation of a mucocele. The frontal sinus drains into the middle meatus via the frontal recess. Fronal sinus ostium reconstruction can be performed using endoscope-assisted anterior ethmoidectomy and clearance of the frontal recess [48]. Enlargement of the frontal recess improves outflow from the frontal sinus and decreases the risk of obstruction and mucocele formation. Complication rates for frontal sinusotomy with obliteration range from 18 to 42% and have encouraged surgeons to adopt endoscopic techniques to treat frontal sinus disease [51].

XI.   CONCLUSIONS

Compared to other surgical specialties, plastic surgery has been relatively slow to take advantage of endoscopic technology. In a field that places so much emphasis on aesthetics and scar minimalization, the applications of endoscopy are vast. The groundwork in endoscopic plastic surgery has focused on cosmetic procedures, and success with these techniques is now being applied to reconstruction. The challenge of creating an effective optic cavity in soft tissue planes will continue to diminish as new endoscopic technology and instrumentation are developed.

REFERENCES

1. Ramirez OM, Pozner JN. Endoscopic forehead lift. In: Evans GRD, ed. Operative Plastic Surgery. New York: McGraw-Hill, 2000:181–186.
2. Bostwick J, Nahai F, Eaves FF. Evaluation and planning for aesthetic surgery of the face and neck: an integrated approach. In: Bostwick J, Eaves FF, Nahai F, eds. Endoscopic Plastic Surgery. St. Louis: Quality Medical Publishing, 1995:136–163.
3. Isse NG. Endoscopic forehead lift: evolution and update. Clin Plast Surg 1995; 22:661–673.
4. Rohrich RJ, Beran SJ. Evolving fixation methods in endoscopically assisted forehead rejuvenation: controversies and rationale. Plast Reconstr Surg 1997; 100:1575–1582.
5. Romo T, Sclafani AP, Yung RT, McCormick SA, Cocker R, McCormick SU. Endoscopic foreheadplasty: a histologic comparison of periosteal fixation after endoscopic versus bicoronal lift. Plast Reconstr Surg 2000; 105:1111.
6. Nahai F, Eaves FF, Bostwick J. Forehead lift and glabellar frown lines. In: Bostwick J, Eaves FF, Nahai F, eds. Endoscopic Plastic Surgery. St. Louis: Quality Medical Publishing, 1995:164–229.
7. Guyuron B, Michelow B. Refinements in endoscopic forehead rejuvenation. Plast Reconstr Surg 1997; 100:154–160.
8. Ramirez OM. Anchor subperiosteal forehead lift: from open to endoscopic. Plast Reconstr Surg 2001; 107:868–873.
9. Hamas RS, Rohrich RJ. Preventing hairline elevation in endoscopic browlifts. Plast Reconstr Surg 1997; 99:10018–1022.
10. Hamas RS. Endoscopic management of glabellar frown lines. Clin Plast Surg 1995; 22:675–681.
11. Bostwick J, Nahai F, Eaves FF. Face and neck lift. In: Bostwick J, Eaves FF, Nahai F, eds. Endoscopic Plastic Surgery. St. Louis: Quality Medical Publishing, 1995:230–317.
12. de la Fuente A, Santamaria A. Endoscopic subcutaneous and SMAS facelift without preauricular scars. Aesthetic Plast Surg 1999; 23:119–124.
13. Celik M, Tuncer S, Buyukcayir I. Modifications in endoscopic facelifts. Ann Plast Surg 1999; 42:638–643.
14. Byrd HS. The extended browlift. Clin Plast Surg 1997; 24:233–246.
15. Ramirez OM. Endoscopic techniques in facial rejuvenation: an overview. Part I. Aesthetic Plast Surg 1994; 18:141–147.
16. Ramirez OM. Endoscopic subperiosteal browlift and facelift. Clin Plast Surg 1995; 22:639–659.
17. Eaves FF, Bostwick J, Nahai F. Augmentation mammaplasty. In: Bostwick J, Eaves FF, Nahai F, eds. Endoscopic Plastic Surgery. St. Louis: Quality Medical Publishing, 1995:356–399.
18. Graf RM, Bernardes A, Auersvald A, Damasio RCC. Subfascial endoscopic transaxillary augmentation mammaplasty. Aesthetic Plast Surg 2000; 24:216–220.
19. Howard PS. The role of endoscopy and implant texture in transaxillary submuscular breast augmentation. Ann Plast Surg 1999; 42:245–248.
20. Eaves FF, Bostwick J, Nahai F, et al. Endoscopic techniques in aesthetic breast surgery: augmentation, mastectomy, biopsy, capsulotomy, capsulorrhaphy, reduction, mastopexy, and reconstructive techniques. Clin Plast Surg 1995; 22:683–695.

21. Eaves FF, Bostwick J, Nahai F. Abdominoplasty. In: Bostwick J, Eaves FF, Nahai F, eds. Endoscopic Plastic Surgery. St. Louis: Quality Medical Publishing, 1995:421–463.

22. Core GB, Mizgala CL, Bowen JC, Vasconez LO. Endoscopic abdominoplasty with repair of diastasis recti and abdominal wall hernia. Clin Plast Surg 1995; 22:707–722.

23. Faria-Correa MA. Endoscopic abdominoplasty, mastopexy, and breast reduction. Clin Plast Surg 1995; 22:723–745.

24. Zukowski ML, Ash K, Spencer D, Malanoski M, Moore G. Endoscopic intracorporal abdominoplasty: a review of 85 cases. Plast Reconstr Surg 1998; 102:516–527.

25. Cho BC, Lee JH, Ramasastry SS, Baik BS. Free latissimus dorsi muscle transfer using endoscopic technique. Ann Plast Surg 1997; 38:586–593.

26. Jones GE, Eaves FF, Howell RL, Carlson GW, Lumsden AB. Harvest of muscle, nerve, fascia, and vein. In: Bostwick J, Eaves FF, Nahai F, eds. Endoscopic Plastic Surgery. St. Louis: Quality Medical Publishing, 1995:510–547.

27. Schwabeggar A, Ninkovic M, Brenner E, Anderl H. Seroma as a common donor site morbidity after harvesting the latissimus dorsi flap: observations on cause and prevention. Ann Plast Surg 1997; 38:594–597.

28. Miller MJ, Robb GL. Endoscopic technique for free flap harvesting. Clin Plast Surg 1995; 22:755–773.

29. Ramakrishnan V, Southern SJ, Tzafetta R. Reconstruction of the high-risk chest wall with endoscopically assisted latissimus dorsi harvest and tissue expander placement. Ann Plast Surg 2000; 44:250–258.

30. Karp NS, Bass LS, Kasabian AK, Eidelman Y, Hausman MR. Balloon assisted endoscopic harvest of the latissimus dorsi muscle. Plast Reconstr Surg 1997; 100:1161–1167.

31. Van Buskirk ER, Rehnke RD, Montgomery RL, Eubanks S, Ferraro FJ, Levin LS. Endoscopic harvest of the latissimus dorsi muscle using the balloon dissection technique. Plast Reconstr Surg 1997; 99:899–903.

32. Friedlander L, Sundin J. Minimally invasive harvesting of the latissimus dorsi. Plast Reconstr Surg 1994; 94:881–884.

33. Masuoka T, Fujikawa, Yamamoto H, Ohyama, Inoue Y, Takao T, Hosokawa K. Breast reconstruction after mastectomy without additional scarring: application of endoscopic latissimus dorsi muscle harvest. Ann Plast Surg 1998; 40:123–127.

34. Inaba H, Kaneko Y, Ohtsuka T, Ezure M, Tanaka K, Ueno K, Takamoto S. Minimal damage during endoscopic latissimus dorsi muscle mobilization with the harmonic scalpel. Ann Thorac Surg 2000; 69:1399–1401.

35. Lin C, Wei F, Levin LS, Chen MC. Donor-site morbidity comparison between endoscopically assisted and traditional harvest of free latissimus dorsi muscle Flap. Plast Reconstr Surg 1999; 104:1070–1077.

36. Dabb R, Wrye SW, Hall WW. Endoscopic harvest of the rectus abdominis muscle. Ann Plast Surg 2000; 44:491–494.

37. Friedlander LD, Sundin J. Minimally invasive harvesting of rectus abdominis myofascial flap in the cadaver and porcine models. Plast Reconstr Surg 1996; 97:207–211.

38. Bass LS, Karp NS, Benacquista T, Kasabian AK. Endoscopic harvest of the rectus abdominis free flap: balloon dissection in the fascial plane. Ann Plast Surg 1995; 34:274–280.

39. Sawaizumi M, Onishi K, Maruyama Y. Endoscope-assisted rectus abdominis muscle flap harvest for chest wall reconstruction: early experience. Ann Plast Surg 1996; 37:317–321.

40. Koh KS, Park S. Endoscopic harvest of sural nerve graft with balloon dissection. Plast Reconstr Surg 1998; 101:810–812.

41. Eich BS, Fix RJ. New technique for endoscopic sural nerve harvest. J Reconstr Microsurg 2000; 16:329–330.

42. DeLaria GA, Hunter JA, Goldin MD, Serry C, Javid H, Najafi H. Leg complications associated with coronary revasccularization. J Thorac Cardiovasc Surg 1981; 81:403–407.

43. Vrancic JM, Piccinini F, Vaccarino G, Iparraguirre E, Albertal J, Navaia D. Endoscopic saphenous vein harvesting: initial experience and learning curve. Ann Thorac Surg 2000; 70:1086–1089.

44. Marty B, Von Segesser LK, Tozzi P, Guzmann J, Frascarolo P, Muller X, Hayoz D. Benefits of endoscopic vein harvesting. World J Surg 2000; 24:1104–1108.

45. Allen KB, Griffith GL, Heimansohn DA, et al. Endoscopic versus traditional saphenous vein harvesting: a prospective, randomized allen trial. Ann Thorac Surg 1998; 66:26–32.

46. Crouch JD, O'Hair DP, Keuler JP, Barragry TP, Werner PH, Kleinman LH. Open versus endoscopic saphenous vein harvesting: wound complications and vein quality. Ann Thorac Surg 1999; 68:1513–1516.

47. Meyer DM, Rogers TE, Jessen ME, Estrera AS, Chin AK. Histologic evidence of the safety of endoscopic saphenous vein graft preparation. Ann Thorac Surg 2000; 70:487–491.

48. Pownell PH and Rohrich RJ. Nasal airway surgery. In: Bostwick J, Eaves FF, Nahai F, eds. Endoscopic Plastic Surgery. St. Louis: Quality Medical Publishing, 1995:319–338.

49. Hochberg J, Faria-Correa MA, Ramadam H. Development of an instrument for endoscopic nasal surgery. Clin Plast Surg 1995; 22:781–784.

50. Mitz V. Endoscopic control during rhinoplasty. Aesthetic Plast Surg 1994; 18:153–156.

51. Sillers MJ and Page EL. Endoscopic surgery of the frontal sinus. Clin Plast Surg 1995; 22:785–790.

38

Pediatric Surgery

KETAN M. DESAI

Washington University School of Medicine
St. Louis, Missouri, U.S.A.

MARK V. MAZZIOTTI

Houston Pediatric Surgeons
Houston, Texas, U.S.A.

In the early 1970s, Berci and Gans reported the application of laparoscopy to pediatric surgical practice. The laparoscopic approach was initially used to evaluate testicular feminization, gonadal dysplasia, and precocious puberty and to distinguish biliary atresia from neonatal hepatitis. Since that time, and particularly over the past decade, minimally invasive pediatric surgery has made great strides. Surgical procedures that once required large incisions are now being approached with laparoscopy and thoracoscopy. Improved technology in the form of better cameras, telescopes, and trocars has provided easier access into the abdominal cavity. As in adults, potential benefits include improved cosmesis, less postoperative pain, fewer adhesions, and a shorter hospital stay.

I. SPECIAL CONSIDERATIONS

Children are not just small adults. A number of differences in anatomy and physiology are present that must be clear in the operating surgeon's mind. The abdominal wall is thinner in a child, and thus much less force is needed to place a Veress needle or trocars into the peritoneal cavity. Differences in abdominal anatomy make the safe insertion of instruments more challenging. The liver in a child normally extends 1–3 cm below the right costal margin. The spleen tip is often palpable in the left upper abdomen, which is a rarity in adults. The stomach in children has a more horizontal orientation across the upper abdomen, so that a nasogastric tube should be used for decompression in every case. The bladder in the child is less contained in the bony pelvis, and therefore placement of a urinary catheter is essential.

The peritoneal cavity itself is much smaller in a child; thus, smaller gas volumes are required for adequate insufflation. Typically as little as 300 cc may be needed, depending on the size of the child. CO_2 insufflation pressures are kept less than 10 mmHg. Higher pressures can potentially result in decreased venous return to the heart and perfusion of visceral organs. This is in contrast to the commonly used insufflation pressure in adults of 15 mmHg, a value derived from studies in adults showing cardiovascular abnormalities with higher insufflation pressures.

II. OPERATING ROOM AND PATIENT SETUP

A. Laparoscopy

1. Patient Preparation

Before induction of general endotracheal anesthesia, the patient is placed supine on the operating room table and is restrained with either tape or gauze. A continuous pulse oximeter, cardiac monitor, automated blood pressure cuff, and end-tidal CO_2 monitor are used throughout the procedure. Preoperative bowel preparation is usually not needed. At the discretion of the operating surgeon, a preoperative dose of intravenous antibiotics to cover skin organisms is sometimes given prior to incision. A Foley catheter and nasogastric tube is placed and the skin is prepared with the surgeon's agent of choice. Pneumatic antiembolic stockings are usually used. In children who are too small for these devices, the legs can be wrapped with elastic bandages to prevent venous stasis and deep venous thrombosis.

2. Insufflation

Insufflation of the abdomen is carried out by one of two techniques: Veress needle placement or open insertion. We prefer the open technique in children to avoid visceral or vascular injury sometimes seen with the needle technique. An umbilical hernia does not preclude open insertion; in fact, the hernia site can be used to enter the abdomen, and it can then be repaired at the end of the procedure.

If a Veress needle is used, CO_2 insufflation should proceed at 1–2 L/min because of the small volume of gas needed in a child. Intra-abdominal pressure should not exceed 10 mmHg and must be monitored throughout the operation. The rise in end-tidal CO_2 in many patients is controlled by mild hyperventilation. Once the appropriate pressure has been achieved, the Veress needle is removed and a gloved finger or wet sponge is used to keep the CO_2 from escaping. A 5 mm port for the camera is inserted through the opening and into the distended peritoneal cavity.

For open insertion, a vertical or semicircular incision is made along the inferior aspect of the umbilicus. The subcutaneous fat is divided, the fascia incised, and the peritoneal cavity entered. Tacking sutures are placed in the fascia. The Hasson-type trocar is placed through the opening into the peritoneal cavity and attached to the fascia with tacking sutures. CO_2 insufflation is begun, and the camera is placed through the trocar.

The abdominal cavity is explored to identify any visceral injuries resulting from insufflation, and the remaining ports are placed under direct vision. A 0.25% bupivacaine solution is used to anesthetize the skin and underlying peritoneum. An incision is made through the anesthetized skin, and the trocar is passed under direct vision into the peritoneal cavity. Specific port placement and special instrumentation used vary according to the specific operation performed.

B. Thoracoscopy

1. Patient Preparation

General inhalational anesthesia is preferred, using a dual-lumen endotracheal tube or a bronchial blocker on the side to be operated on. If the child is too small, the contralateral mainstem bronchus can selectively be intubated. The patient is careflully monitored throughout the operation, as with laparoscopy. The small pleural space, more rapid respiratory rate, and less compliant pulmonary parenchyma of infants make anesthetic management for thoracoscopy potentially more difficult.

Positioning the patient for a thoracoscopic procedure is very important, since improper placement can make the operation impossible. The patient is placed in the lateral decubitus position, with the operative side up. Stabilization of the patient is important, using a bean bag and tape. The arm is placed over the patient's head or at a right angle, which helps to increase the distance between the ribs. The patient can be placed in a straight lateral or 30 degree anterolateral or posterolateral position, depending on which structures need to be reached.

The child is prepared and draped. Wide draping is employed so that the procedure can be readily converted to open thoracotomy if necessary. The intercostal spaces are identified, and a small incision is made over the rib at the fifth or sixth intercostal space in the mid or anterior axillary line, below the tip of the scapula. Dissection is carried out through the interspace, as if for chest tube insertion. The pleura is opened and the camera port is passed gently into the pleural cavity. The chest cavity is surveyed after allowing the lung to deflate, which should be complete if the endotracheal tube is properly positioned. Alternatively, insufflating the chest with carbon dioxide to a pressure of 5 or 6 mmHg effectively deflates the lung and creates an adequate working space. Additional ports can then be placed under direct vision. For many procedures, instruments can be passed directly through the chest wall without the need for trocars or ports.

III. TECHNIQUES COMMON TO BOTH CHILDREN AND ADULTS

A. General Considerations

Most operations performed on adults can be performed on pediatric patients, although sometimes the indications are different. Examples include diagnostic or staging laparoscopy, appendectomy, cholecystectomy, splenectomy, fundoplication, ovarian detorsion or cystectomy, lung biopsy, and pleural decortication.

Complex procedures that require the placement of four or more ports may be difficult in children because of the limited working space. However, the development of 2–5 mm trocars has made laparoscopic intervention on small children more practical. In general, smaller instruments are preferable, and pediatric surgeons routinely use a 5 mm camera.

B. Diagnostic or Staging Procedures

Laparoscopy is ideal for the evaluation of abdominal pain of unclear etiology. Most of these patients are adolescent girls with an atypical history and physical findings in whom noninvasive evaluation has been indeterminate. Insufflation is carried out as previously described, with the camera passed through the umbilical port. A second port may also be used to pass a blunt grasper or probe to facilitate exploration of the abdomen.

Laparoscopy is also valuable in the evaluation of abdominal tumors in children. Although the nature of the tumor can usually be appreciated by imaging studies, percutaneous biopsy, or bone marrow sampling, laparoscopy can be useful for evaluating intraperitoneal or nodal metastases. Visualization and biopsy of the liver can be expedited using laparoscopy, and expertise in laparoscopic ultrasound may be particularly helpful.

Laparoscopic techniques can be used for evaluation of suspicious abdominal and pelvic lymph nodes. In coordination with laparoscopic splenectomy and liver biopsy, staging for lymphoma can be accomplished entirely laparoscopically. Additionally, using a lateral port for the camera and the others for dissection and retraction provides safe and efficacious exposure to the retroperitoneal vessels from the aortic bifurcation to the pelvis.

Thoracoscopic techniques are ideal for the evaluation of both benign and malignant diseases of the pleural cavity. Patient positioning is of paramount importance for locating and resecting various chest lesions. Straight lateral position is less often used and is best for seeing posterior and some apical tumors. The 30 degree lateral position is ideal for viewing anterior, right middle lobe, or lingular lesions. The camera port is placed in the fourth or fifth intercostal space in the anterior axillary line for lesions in the pulmonary apex and pleural dome. Placement will be more lateral in the fourth or fifth intercostal space for anterior pulmonary lesions, those in the superior mediastinum, or mediastinal lymph nodes. Camera port placement is in the midaxillary line in the fifth or sixth intercostal space for access to the pericardium. Once the lesion has been located, a stapling device can be used to easily biopsy or resect pulmonary lesions.

C. Appendectomy

Appendicitis is relatively common in children, and approximately 50% of cases present with perforation. The technique used in children is similar to that for adults, with a 12 mm umbilical port used for the endostapler, a 5 mm suprapubic, midline port for instrumentation, and another 5 mm working port in the left lower quadrant. The largest port is used at the umbilicus because this is a "free" port site where scarring will not be as noticeable. The appendix can be divided either with a linear stapler or a loop ligature. If the stapler is used, a GI cartridge is used for the appendix, and a vascular reload is used for the mesentery.

Since appendectomy can be easily performed through a single small incision with very good results in young children, many pediatric surgeons reserve laparoscopy for obese children or in adolescent females, in whom the diagnosis may be in doubt. Potential advantages of the laparoscopic approach include complete exploration and irrigation of the abdominal cavity, a reduction in the incidence of postoperative adhesions, and a decreased incidence of postoperative wound infections.

D. Cholecystectomy

The incidence of gallbladder disease in the pediatric population is low compared with that in adults. However, there are certain groups of children in whom cholelithiasis and cholecystitis are more common. Patients with sickle cell disease and other hemoglobinopathies are predisposed to the formation of pigment (calcium bilirubinate) stones because of chronic hemolysis. Other risk factors for cholelithiasis include cystic fibrosis and long-term use of total parenteral nutrition. Because of the excellent results, high level of patient satisfaction, and low morbidity seen in adults, laparoscopic cholecystectomy has been applied to these infants and children, with the same benefits.

Present indications include children with cholelithiasis and biliary colic or those with hemoglobinopathy and asymptomatic gallstones. The latter patient population requires special consideration. These patients may be best managed by a preoperative transfusion regimen as described by Ware et al. Even if asymptomatic, these children require cholecystectomy because of the possibility of the complications of cholelithiasis, which may necessitate an emergency cholecystectomy in an unprepared higher-risk patient.

The operation is carried out in a similar fashion to that in the adult, with a few important differences. A 5 mm trocar may be used for the camera port in smaller children. The trocars are placed under direct vision four to five fingerbreadths below the right costal margin to avoid injury to the liver (Fig. 1). Typically, the largest port is 10 mm and is placed at the umbilicus, which is the site where the gallbladder is removed from the peritoneal cavity.

E. Splenectomy

Laparoscopic splenectomy in children can be performed safely and effectively using either the supine or the lateral approach (Fig. 2). Preoperative immunizations (pneumococcal and *Haemophilus influenzae* type B) are administered several weeks before splenectomy. Indications for spleen removal in children include medically refractory idiopathic thrombocytopenic purpura, hereditary hemoglobinopathies, and, rarely, staging for Hodgkin's disease. The hilum of the spleen is approached first and the individual vessels can be clipped and divided, or stapled, which is the preferred approach. The harmonic scalpel is useful in dividing the short gastric vessels as well as the ligamentous attachments of the spleen. The spleen is placed into a plastic pouch, where it is morcellated and removed through the largest port. Usually the larger endocatch bag (15 mm port) is

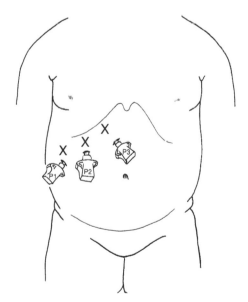

Figure 1 Port placement for laparoscopic cholecystectomy in childen. X = adult sites; P = pediatric sites.

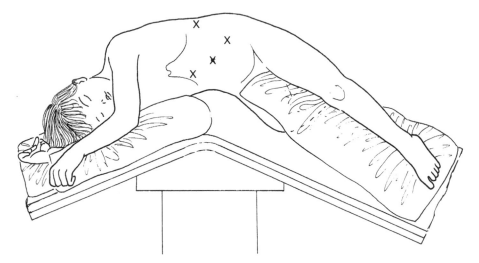

Figure 2   Port placement for a lateral approach to laparoscopic splenectomy in a child.

required because of the large size of the spleen being removed. Benefits of laparoscopic splenectomy over standard open splenectomy include a shorter hospital stay, improved cosmetic results, and less postoperative analgesia requirements.

F.   Fundoplication and Gastrostomy

Severe complications of gastroesophageal reflux disease (GERD) include aspiration pneumonia, esophageal stricture, Barrett's metaplasia, and failure to thrive. Small infants and children with complicated GERD or any individuals refractory to medical therapy will require antireflux surgery. Preoperative evaluation of GERD usually includes 24-hour pH monitoring, endoscopic evaluation, an upper gastrointestinal contrast study, and a gastric emptying radionucleotide study. Most children requiring fundoplication are neurologically impaired and also require a gastrostomy tube for feeding.

Laparoscopic antireflux surgery (LARS) in children is similar to that for the adult patient (see Chapter 24). Several types of antireflux operations (Nissen, Thal, Toupet) have been described in children and are dependent upon the presence of a primary esophageal motility disorder. Care must be taken when placing the upper abdominal trocars because of the relatively large liver in children. A 26 or 28 Fr bougie is used during the procedure in small infants, a 40 Fr in young children, and a 50–60 Fr in adolescents. After the fundoplication is completed, a gastrostomy can be created using the percutaneous endoscopic (PEG) technique or by the use of vascular dilators through the abdominal wall under direct laparoscopic vision.

The advantage of the laparoscopic approach in children is that a significant upper abdominal incision is avoided. This is especially important in neurologically impaired children in whom the incision may impair pulmonary function and predispose to atelectasis and pneumonia. In addition, when compared to the standard open procedure, LARS is associated with earlier initiation of feeding and shorter hospital stays.

G. Ovarian Pathology

Laparoscopy is ideal for the evaluation of lower abdominal pain in children, many of whom are adolescent girls. Ovarian pathology can cause abdominal pain as a result of rupture of a cyst, hemorrhage, or torsion.

Initial exploration is carried out through an umbilical camera port. Adnexal torsion is easily identified by the dark blue congested appearance of the adnexa. An additional 5 mm trocar may be inserted suprapubically on the ipsilateral side to aid in detorsion of the adnexa. The lesion may be untwisted and observed. If the ovary is not salvageable or if a neoplastic lesion is suspected, a laparotomy is performed, typically via a Pfannensteil incision. Ovarian cystectomy can also be performed laparoscopically using two 5 mm trocars in the lower abdomen, with preservation of normal ovarian tissue. The harmonic scalpel is a useful tool for ovary-sparing surgery.

H. Thoracoscopy

Video-assisted thoracoscopic surgery (VATS) has been used for the diagnosis and treatment of pleural, pericardial, and parenchymal lung disease in children, as in adults. Indications include evaluation for trauma, mediastinal masses, empyema, or recurrent pneumothoraces, as well as lung biopsies for interstitial lung disease, cavitary lesions, and parenchymal lesions of unknown or presumed malignant cause.

Thoracoscopic treatment can be done safely and effectively in children. Rothenberg et al. recommend the use of a three 5 mm port system in children weighing under 10 kg and two 5 mm ports and one 12 mm port in larger children to allow for the use of the endoscopic stapler. We often place the camera through a 5 or 10 mm port and pass instruments directly through the chest wall without an associated port. This is possible in the chest because it is a rigid cavity and insufflation is not necessary. At the conclusion of the biopsy or resection, a chest tube may be placed through one of the trocar sites.

IV. TECHNIQUES PRINCIPALLY PERFORMED IN CHILDREN

A. Pectus Excavatum

Pectus excavatum (PE) has an incidence of 1 in 300 live births and accounts for approximately 90% of congenital chest wall deformities. Cardiac, pulmonary, and psychosocial function and development can all be adversely affected. Surgical corrective repair has evolved over the past decades. In 1949 Ravitch proposed resection of all involved costal cartilages and sternal osteotomy with various forms of internal bracing. This operative approach involves a large inframammary incision. Within the past decade, Nuss has reported a minimally invasive repair of pectus excavatum (MIRPE). This procedure involves the insertion of a stainless steel bar across the anterior mediastinum under thoracoscopic guidance in order to elevate the sternum. Small incisions on each lateral chest wall are used, as well as a separate 5 mm port site to insufflate the right hemithorax. The chest then conforms to the anatomically normal shape as the child grows. The bar is removed as an outpatient procedure 2 years after the initial operation. Follow-up data have shown satisfactory results in over 90% of patients, with minimal intraoperative blood loss and better cosmetic outcomes. Overall, MIRPE is shown to be less expensive, less morbid, and better tolerated than traditional open procedures. It has become the procedure of choice for pectus excavatum repair.

B. Exploration for Contralateral Inguinal Hernia

Although controversial in children with unilateral inguinal hernia, laparoscopy can be used to determine the presence or absence of a contralateral patent processus vaginalis. In a meta-analysis of 964 children, 39% had evidence of a contralateral patent processus vaginalis by laparoscopic examination. One alternative to standard exploration of the asymptomatic side is laparoscopic visualization of the internal inguinal ring to detect the presence of a patent processus vaginalis. Although originally described using a small umbilical incision, reports have demonstrated excellent visualization by placing a 90 or 120 degree scope through the hernia sac on the symptomatic side (Fig. 3).

After induction of general anesthesia, the patient's abdomen is prepared in the usual fashion. A standard approach to hernia repair is performed on the symptomatic side. The hernia sac is dissected free from the cord structures and up to the level of the internal ring. The sac is then opened and hemostats are placed circumferentially. Dilators can be passed through the hernia sac to gently dilate the internal ring. A 2.7 mm camera inside a 5 mm cannula is passed into the peritoneal cavity through the hernia sac. The abdomen is insufflated to a pressure of 8–10 mmHg, and laparoscopic examination of the contralateral groin is performed. If a patent processus vaginalis is found, the other side is explored and the hernia is repaired in the standard fashion.

C. Cryptorchidism

An undescended testicle that is not palpable on physical examination usually lies in the abdomen or high in the inguinal canal. These testes become less spermatogenic if left in place and should be brought into the scrotum when the patient is approximately 1 year old. An undescended testicle also carries an increased risk of testicular cancer, even after an

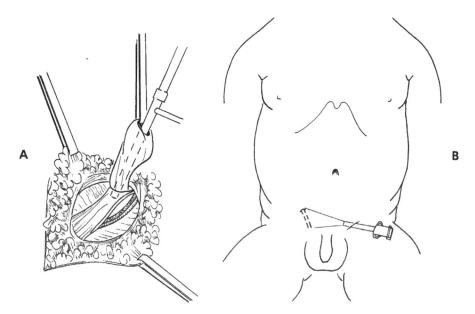

Figure 3 Laparoscopic examination of the contralateral internal inguinal ring by passing the scope through the symptomatic hernia sac.

orchiopexy has been performed. Because of this risk, the testicle needs to be surgically placed into the scrotum so that it may be examined on a regular basis. Initial evaluation using ultrasonography may reveal the location of the testis. If not, laparoscopy may be useful. Exploration in these patients is done using a 5 mm scope at the umbilicus. The patient is placed in the Trendelenburg position, and usually no additional trocars are necessary.

On laparoscopy, one of three situations may be present (Fig. 4): an intra-abdominal testis, testicular agenesis, or a vas deferens and vessels that exit through the internal inguinal ring, ending either at a testis in the inguinal canal or blindly as a result of in utero torsion and testicular atrophy. If an intra-abdominal testis is found, the first stage of a Fowler-Stephens orchiopexy, in which the gonadal vessels are ligated laparoscopically to allow collaterals to develop along the vas deferens, can be done. If cord structures are seen entering the internal ring, the laparoscope is removed and a groin exploration is performed.

D. Meckel's Diverticulectomy

Meckel's diverticulum usually presents in a child with massive, painless lower gastrointestinal bleeding, although intussusception or abdominal pain can also be seen. The diagnosis is often made preoperatively using a ^{99m}TC "Meckel's" scan. Laparoscopy can be useful in the evaluation and treatment of these patients. The abdomen is explored through a 5 mm umbilical port. A 5 mm port is placed in the right upper quadrant and a 10 mm port in the left lower quadrant. The ileocecal junction is identified and the small bowel is followed retrograde using blunt grasping forceps. Curved dissecting forceps are used to isolate the vascular supply to the diverticulum, which is then clipped and divided with laparoscopic scissors. A stapling device is used across the base of the diverticulum, which is then removed through the larger port. Care must be taken not to narrow the lumen of the ileum during stapling, and thus the staple line should be placed perpendicular to the axis of the intestine. The staple line is checked for hemostasis, and the resected specimen is opened on a back table to confirm complete resection of the gastric mucosa. The wounds are then closed in the standard fashion.

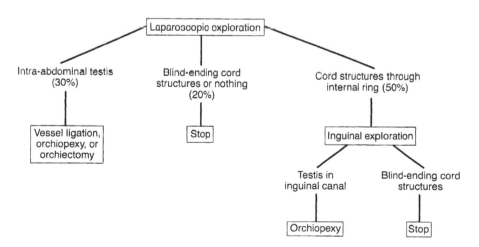

Figure 4   Evaluation of the nonpalpable testis.

E. Pyloromyotomy

Congenital hypertrophic pyloric stenosis is commonly encountered in pediatric surgery. It classically occurs in first-born males and in 1 of every 750 births. The cause is unknown. Patients commonly present in the third or fourth week of life with nonbilious projectile vomiting and may have a hypochloremic, hypokalemic metabolic alkalosis. Once the patient is rehydrated and the electrolyte abnormalities are corrected, the patient is taken to the operating room for surgical correction of the pyloric obstruction.

Open pyloromyotomy can be performed through a right upper quadrant or umbilical incision. The operation takes approximately 15 minutes, and most infants can be discharged within 24 hours. Therefore, few surgeons have been quick to adopt the laparoscopic approach to this procedure.

Laparoscopic extramucosal pyloromyotomy was first described in 1990. The technique involves a 3.5 mm camera port via the umbilicus, through which the pyloric "olive" is located. Another 3.5 mm trocar is inserted through the abdominal wall over the olive. An additional 3.5 mm port is inserted over the duodenal segment, and through this port a grasping forceps is passed to immobilize the segment to be incised. The olive is incised by passing a scalpel through the 3.5 mm port overlying the mass, in the same manner as through the open abdominal approach, leaving the mucosa intact. The incised borders are retracted with spreader forceps. The trocars are then removed and the sites closed with absorbable suture.

F. Hirschsprung's Disease

Hirschsprung's disease is characterized by congenital absence of ganglion cells in the myenteric and submucosal plexuses of the distal colon, resulting in failure of peristalsis in the affected portions of bowel. Hirschsprung's disease always involves the rectum and extends proximally to varying degrees, with no skip areas. Traditional surgical treatment for this disorder includes a colostomy in an area of bowel that has ganglion cells, with a definitive procedure (resection of the aganglionic segment with a "pull-through") several months later. Recently some authors have advocated a single-stage pull-through without colostomy at the time of diagnosis.

Primary laparoscopic endorectal pull-through for Hirschsprung's disease has been described by Georgeson et al. Preoperative bowel preparation in these patients includes either finger dilatation of the rectum or colonic irrigation with saline solution, as well as preoperative fasting and administration of an oral electrolyte solution (Pedialyte), 25 cc/ kg/hr for 4 hours.

The patient is positioned transversely on the end of the operating room table and preoperative intravenous antibiotics are given. CO_2 insufflation of the peritoneum is performed and three 5 mm trocars are placed, two on the right at and just above the level of the umbilicus and one on the left at the level of the umbilicus.

The superior rectal and sigmoid mesenteric vessels are dissected and divided with bipolar cautery or ultrasonic scalpel, while the marginal artery is preserved. The mesentery is mobilized up to the level of the inferior mesenteric artery, which is also divided in patients with high transition zones. Distal pelvic dissection extends to the level of the prostate or cervix anteriorly and to the level of the coccyx posteriorly. Transanal dissection is begun with a circumferential incision in the mucosa 5–10 mm above the pectinate line. Silk traction sutures are placed in the mucosa to facilitate separation from the muscular wall. This submucosal plane dissection is continued to meet the peritoneal dissection. The smooth muscle fibers of the rectal sleeve are divided circumferentially at this level, as well as posteriorly to accommodate the ganglionated colon. The rectum and sigmoid are pulled through the rectal sleeve to a point past the transition zone and a full-thickness biopsy is taken at this site to establish the presence of ganglion cells. If ganglion cells are present, the colon is transected above this point and anastomosed to the rectal mucosa with circumferential absorbable sutures. The peritoneal cavity is inspected laparoscopically to ensure adequate hemostasis. The peritoneum of the pelvis is closed to prevent small bowel herniation.

Oral feeding is begun 1–3 days postoperatively. Rectal dilatations are begun on all patients 3 weeks postoperatively and continued daily by the parents for 6–8 weeks.

The Swenson and Duhamel operations have also been described using laparoscopic techniques.

G. Malrotation

Normal embryonic development of the midgut results from 270° counterclockwise rotation about the superior mesenteric artery. Failure of normal rotation results in classic malrotation or a variety of intestinal rotational abnormalities. Infants usually present with abdominal pain, bilious emesis, and failure to thrive. Diagnostic evaluation usually includes an upper gastrointestinal contrast study to evaluate for a normal duodenal sweep and normal position of the ligament of Treitz. Malrotation with or without midgut volvulus, duodenal stenosis, web or atresia are potential causes of duodenal obstruction. The laparoscopic Ladd's procedure provides a minimally invasive method of treatment for cases of malrotation without midgut volvulus. In any cases of suspected volvulus (i.e., any infant with bilious vomiting) the laparoscopic approach should not be used.

Following insufflation with a Veress needle, a 3.5 mm trocar is placed in the infraumbilical ring. Under direct vision two additional 3.5 mm ports are placed in the right and left mid to lower abdomen. The abdomen is inspected carefully to confirm the diagnosis, and the general tenets of the open Ladd's procedure are performed. The Ladd's bands are divided over the duodenum using sharp dissection and electrocautery followed by widening of the base of the mesentery by incising the peritoneum. The intestine is placed in a state of nonrotation, with the small intestine placed on the patient's right side and the large intestine placed on the patient's left. Finally, an appendectomy is performed.

Advantages to the laparoscopic approach for malrotation without midgut volvulus include minimized postoperative pain, decreased postoperative ileus, and a short hospital stay.

H. Patent Ductus Arteriosus Ligation

Patent ductus arteriosus (PDA) is usually diagnosed in infancy and can be asymptomatic or associated with refractory congestive heart failure. Until 1971 surgical interruption via a left posterolateral thoracotomy was the only available technique. At that time an endovascular nonsurgical closure was described. After numerous modifications and clinical trials it has partially replaced the open thoracotomy, although it is not commonly performed in infants weighing less than 7 or 8 kg. A thoracoscopic approach has been described and has been successfully applied to infants with isolated PDA.

After induction of general anesthesia and intubation, the patient is positioned with the right side down. Two 5 mm trocars are inserted in the leftt hemithorax—one through the posterior part of the third intercostal space for the video and one through the fourth intercostal space on the anterior axillary line for surgical instrumentation. The PDA is identified and the posterior pleura is opened. The aorta is dissected at its junction with the PDA. The pericardium is also dissected on the pulmonary side to identify and protect the recurrent laryngeal nerve. Two titanium clips are then applied across the PDA to obliterate its lumen. The trocars are then removed and the lung is reexpanded. A chest tube is usually not required.

I. Other Procedures

As pediatric surgeons become more comfortable and experienced with laparoscopic techniques, more applications will be seen in the field. Other procedures that hold promise in the treatment of children by minimally invasive means include thoracoscopic or laparoscopic Heller myotomy for achalasia, laparoscopic tracheoesophageal fistula repair, laparoscopic nephrectomy, and exploration for Crohn's disease. Laparoscopic evaluation for cholestasis of the newborn has also been reported. Laparoscopic placement of peritoneal dialysis catheters and laparoscopically assisted insertion or repositioning of ventriculoperitoneal shunts are also presently being performed. Thoracoscopy has been used for resection of mediastinal masses such as teratomas and foregut duplications.

V. POSTOPERATIVE CARE

In general, postoperative care depends on the procedure being performed. Most patients, when fully awake, are started on clear liquids the day of surgery and advanced to a regular diet within 24 hours. Most children who have undergone a laparoscopic procedure have a decreased need for pain medication when compared to children who have undergone a corresponding open procedure. However, many still have a significant amount of abdominal discomfort on the day of surgery and require intravenous or oral narcotics for a short time postoperatively. Their hospital stay may also be decreased, especially with more extensive procedures such as fundoplication and splenectomy.

VI. CURRENT STATUS AND FUTURE INVESTIGATION

As pediatric surgeons become more adept at laparoscopic procedures, there will be more controversy as to which procedure is better for the patient—the open or the laparoscopic version. Although there is a real need for prospective randomized studies to answer this question, the relatively low volume of pediatric cases makes it unlikely that these studies will be done in children. Also, because of the limited number of cases, only those pediatric surgeons most experienced in laparoscopic techniques should undertake these procedures.

More clinical and animal studies are needed to study the effects of pneumo-peritoneum on pediatric patients, as well as studies to evaluate the safety and efficacy of new laparoscopic procedures. We must remember that just because a procedure can be done laparoscopically does not mean that it should be done laparoscopically. The decision must be tailored to the individual patient and should bee based on a careful analysis of the available literature, as well as the experience and skill of the surgeon.

Minimally invasive technology is presently being expanded to treat the fetus as well. Reports have appeared documenting hysteroscopic approaches to managing twin-twin transfusion syndrome and acardiac twins in humans. Animal studies have investigated the possibility of treating urinary tract obstruction, cleft lip, diaphragmatic hernia, and myelomeningocele using hysteroscopic surgery. Future investigations will involve determining the optimal fetal environment for minimally invasive fetal surgery.

VII. TOP TEN SURGICAL TIPS

1. Insufflation pressures should be kept below 10mmHg to avoid complications.
2. Place the Veress needle and trocars carefully, keeping in mind the relative differences between pediatric and adult anatomy.
3. Preoperative placement of a nasogastric tube and a Foley catheter is a necessity in children because of the intra-abdominal position of the stomach and bladder, respectively.
4. Just because a procedure can be done laparoscopically does not mean that it should be done laparoscopically.
5. Right upper quadrant trocars should be placed more inferiorly and laterally in a child because of the relatively large liver.
6. An umbilical hernia does not preclude insufflation by the open approach. In fact, the hernia can be on the site of entry and the defect repaired during closure.
7. Placement of a chest tube is unnecessary after most thoracoscopic procedures.
8. Laparoscopic appendectomy may be of most benefit in adolescent girls who have a pathological condition of uncertain origin.
9. Most children require an intravenous infusion of narcotic medication postoperatively, even after a laparoscopic procedure.
10. Complex laparoscopic procedures should only be performed by those experienced in advanced laparoscopic techniques.

SELECTED READINGS

Bass KD, Rothenberg S, Chang JH. Laparoscopic Ladd's procedure in infants with malrotation. J Pediatr Surg 1998; 33:279–281.

Brooks DC. Current Review of Laparoscopy, 2nd ed. Philadelphia: Current Medicine, 1995.

Estes JM, Szabo Z, Harrison MR. Techniques for in utero endoscopic surgery. Surg Endosc 1992; 6:215–218.

Georgeson KE, Fuenfer MM, Hardin WD. Primary laparoscopic pull-through for Hirschsprung's disease in infants and children. J Pediatr Surg 1995; 30:1017–1022.

Groner JI, Marlow J, Teich S. Groin laparoscopy: a new technique for contralateral groin evaluation in pediatric inguinal hernia repair. J Am Coll Surg 1995; 181:169–170.

Holcomb GW III, Olsen DO, Sharp KW. Laparoscopic cholecystectomy in the pediatric patient. J Pediatr Surg 1991; 26:1186–1190.

Laborde F, Noirhomme P, Karam J, Batisse A, Bourel P, Saint Maurice O. A new video-assisted thoracoscopic surgical technique for interruption of patent ductus arteriosus in infants and children. J Thorac Cardiovasc Surg 1993; 105:278–280.

Lobe TE, Schropp KP. Pediatric Laparoscopy and Thoracoscopy. Philadelphia: WB Saunders, 1994.

Miltenberg DM, Nuchtern JG, Jaksic T, Kozinetiz C, Brandt ML. Laparoscopic evaluation of the pediatric inguinal hernia—meta-analysis. J Pediatr Surg 1998; 33:874–879.

Nuss D, Kelly RE, Croitoru DP, Katz ME. A 10-year review of a minimally invasive technique for the correction of pectus excavatum. J Pediatr Surg 1998; 33:545–552.

Rescorla FJ. Laparoscopic splenectomy. Semin Pediatr Surg 1998; 7:207–212.

Rodgers BM, Ryckman FC, Moazam F, et al. Thoracoscopy for intrathoracic tumors. Ann Thorac Surg 1981; 31:414–420.

Rothenberg S. Experience with 220 consecutive laparoscopic Nissen fundoplications in infants and children. J Pediatr Surg 1998; 33:274–278.

Rothenberg S, Wagener J, Chang J, Fan L. The safety and efficacy of thoracoscopic lung biopsy for diagnosis and treatment in infants and children. J Pediatr Surg 1996; 31:100–104.

Smith BM, Schropp KP, Lobe TE, Rogers DA, Presbury GJ, Wilimas JA, Wong WC. Laparoscopic splenectomy in childhood. J Pediatr Surg 1994; 29:975–977.

Ware R, Filston HC, Schultz WH, Kinney TR. Elective cholecystectomy in children with sickle hemoglobinopathies. Ann Surg 1988; 208:17–22.

39

Video-Assisted Thoracoscopic Surgery

MATTHEW G. BLUM and SUDHIR R. SUNDARESAN

Northwestern Memorial Hospital
Chicago, Illinois, U.S.A.

I. SPECIAL CONSIDERATIONS

The pleural space presents a uniquely convenient cavity for the performance of video-assisted minimally invasive procedures. A rigid bony thorax and collapsible lungs provide an opportunity to visualize the pleural space without requiring positive pressure insufflation. Diagnostic and therapeutic thoracoscopy was reported by the Swedish internist Hans Jacobaeus in 1919. He used a trocar and cystoscope with local anesthesia to drain pleural effusions and perform thoracoscopy. For the next 40 years thoracoscopy was primarily used for lysis of adhesions (pneumolysis) and treatment of tuberculosis. In the 1960s and early 1970s scattered reports of thoracoscopy generally using rigid instruments with distal light sources appeared. Video-assisted thoracoscopy (VATS) developed in the 1980s and 1990s in parallel with the development of video assisted laparoscopy.

VATS procedures are now used for a myriad of pleural and parenchymal processes, both malignant and benign. Well-established indications for VATS include management of pleural and pericardial effusions, pneumothorax management, pulmonary nodule resection, lung biopsy, sympathectomy, esophageal myotomy and anterior approaches for thoracic spinal surgery. More controversial indications include lung and esophageal resections, particularly for malignant processes.

II. INDICATIONS

A. Pleural Effusions

VATS may be used for establishing the diagnosis and treatment of pleural effusions. In 90% of cases, diagnosis can be established using a history and physical with thoracentesis and pleural fluid analysis. If the diagnosis is still unclear, VATS can be utilized to examine and biopsy the pleura and obtain additional pleural fluid. For recurrent effusions and for malignant effusions, pleurodesis can be done at the time of VATS pleural fluid drainage. Technical options for pleurodesis include mechanical abrasion and chemical (doxycycline or talc) pleurodesis. Talc pleurodesis creates substantial adhesions that are difficult to divide. This approach is thus usually reserved for palliation of malignant or end-stage processes where future thoracotomy is unlikely to be necessary.

B. Pericardial Effusions

Pericardial windows using a VATS approach can effectively drain pericardial effusions. Pericardial biopsy can be obtained at the same time if diagnosis is needed. This approach is especially useful for patients who have had recurrent effusion after a subxiphoid pericardial window. Patients with significant pericardial adhesions may not be good candidates for a minimally invasive approach.

C. Pneumothoraces

Patients with pneumothorax are commonly treated by thoracoscopic apical bullectomy/ blebectomy with mechanical pleurodesis (with or without chemical pleurodesis). Patients with recurrent spontaneous pneumothoraces are clearly candidates for surgery due to the very high likelihood of future pneumothorax. Surgical management of first-time pneumothorax is somewhat controversial, but early application of VATS may lessen the length of hospital stay and decrease recurrences. The VATS approach to this clinical problem may be less effective (higher recurrence rate) than open bullectomy/blebectomy with pleurodesis.

D. Lung Nodules

Wedge biopsy of peripheral pulmonary nodules is one of the most commonly performed VATS procedures. Lung nodules of unclear origin should be sent for histology, acid-fast staining, aerobic and anaerobic bacterial culture, and fungal and acid-fast bacillus culture. Patients with solitary pulmonary nodules suspicious for lung cancer may have the nodule removed and frozen section obtained. If lung cancer is confirmed, definitive resection should be performed (usually lobectomy). Some centers have embraced the VATS approach for lobectomy in this circumstance, although the majority of surgeons still convert the VATS to open thoracotomy.

E. Lung Biopsy

Patients with undiagnosed pulmonary infiltrates, often in the setting of immunosuppression, are candidates for VATS lung biopsy. Usually the lung with the worst infiltrates is chosen and biopsies taken from several locations. Patients requiring high levels of oxygen, PEEP, or ventilatory support may not be good candidates for VATS biopsy as they may not tolerate one lung ventilation. Open lung biopsy is recommended in these cases.

F. Sympathectomy

The VATS approach is ideal for dorsal sympathectomy. Sympathectomy for palmar hyperhidrosis is the most common indication. Short stays and a high success rate make treating this condition with VATS highly gratifying. Other less common indications for sympathectomy include Raynaud's phenomenon and disease, causalgia, reflex sympathetic dystrophy, and vascular insufficiency of the upper extremity. Typically resection of the T2–T4 ganglia and the corresponding rami is adequate. Hospital stays of 1–2 days are the norm.

G. Esophageal Myotomy

Myotomy for achalasia, nutcracker esophagus, and diffuse esophageal spasm can be successfully done by VATS. A laparoscopic myotomy for achalasia is probably a better approach because it is easier to add an antireflux procedure, and the myotomy onto the stomach can be more precisely visualized. VATS is more applicable for the long myotomies used to treat diffuse spasm or nutcracker esophagus.

H. Anterior Spinal Approach

Anterior discectomy is easily accomplished using a thoracoscopic approach. Longitudinal port placements 2–3 rib spaces above the desired discectomy spaces in the mid-axillary line are usually used.

I. Lung Resection

Several groups have reported VATS lobectomy, although relatively few surgeons perform this procedure. The VATS approach probably offers slightly better pain control in the early postoperative period. However, the long-term benefits and the late survival following lung cancer resection have yet to be reported and confirmed. VATS wedge resection of small peripheral lung cancers may be a justifiable compromise in patients with marginal pulmonary function.

J. Esophageal Resection

Esophagectomies have been performed in a few centers via the VATS approach. However, this approach has not gained widespread acceptance. Benign esophageal lesions (e.g., leiomyomas, duplication cysts) may be enucleated safely from the wall of the esophagus using VATS technology.

III. PREOPERATIVE CONSIDERATIONS

Just as in conventional thoracotomy, preoperative preparation and evaluation of patients before VATS procedures is important. For patients undergoing evaluation for possible pulmonary resection through a VATS approach, pulmonary function testing, exercise testing (6-minute walk), an appropriate cardiac work-up, and a staging evaluation are critical. There are indirect and nonprospective data that indicate that patients with poorer pulmonary function tolerated a VATS procedure better than they would an open thoracotomy. Nevertheless, careful evaluation of pulmonary function and clinical status will guide the surgeon in judging the safety of conversion to open thoracotomy if it becomes necessary. The only absolute contraindications to VATS procedures are inability to tolerate single lung anesthesia or the patient with complete pleural symphysis.

IV. OPERATIVE PROCEDURE

A. Instrumentation and Equipment

Equipment
Two high-resolution video monitors
Light source
Camera
Thoracoscopes (0 and 30 degree rigid)
Thoracoport trocars
Duval and Pennington lung clamps
Endoscopic fan retractors, grasping forceps, electrocautery
Endo GIA [United States Surgical Corporation (USSC), Norwalk, CT] staplers

---

Video equipment may be purchased from several different manufacturers. Thoracoscopes come in three varieties: rigid 0 degree scopes, rigid angled scopes, and flexible fiberoptic scopes. The 0 degree rigid scope is satisfactory for most VATS applications, but the 30 degree rigid scope may be required for difficult dissections in sulci and inaccessible areas of the mediastinum.

Special thoracoport trocars and cannulas are available for VATS procedures. Compared with the ports for laparoscopy, they are generally shorter and do not have an airtight seal. Alternatively, standard thoracic or endoscopic instruments may be inserted through small (1–2 cm) incisions in the chest wall.

Several types of conventional lung clamps are available in endoscopic form, including Duval and Pennington clamps. These are useful for atraumatically grasping the lung and providing traction to aid in stapling or dissection. Grasping forceps, endoscopic scissors and dissectors are also available. Endoscopic fan-type retractors may be inserted through a port and opened up inside the thorax to provide lung or diaphragm retraction.

The recently developed endoscopic stapling devices are modeled after the conventional GIA (USSC Autosuture, Norwalk, CT) stapler. These stapling devices now have articulating heads, facilitating lung resections at difficult angles. The endoscopic stapler with 3 mm staples is useful for division of pulmonary vessels.

Finally, many surgeons now employ the potassium titanyl phosphate yttrium aluminum garnet (ND-YAG) laser, which allows precise cutting and coagulating of lung tissue. The laser is particularly useful for lesions away from the cut edge of the lung where application of an Endo GIA (USSC Autosuture, Norwalk, CT) stapler is difficult.

B. Operating Room Set-up and Patient Positioning

The operating room setup for a VATS procedure of the left hemithorax is demonstrated in Figure 1. Single lung ventilation is required for all VATS procedures to achieve adequate exposure. Double-lumen tubes or a single lumen tube with a bronchial blocker can be used. Routine cardiopulmonary monitoring includes cardiac electrical activity (ECG), blood pressure (often with a radial arterial line), oxygen saturation, and end-tidal carbon dioxide concentration. A Foley catheter is placed for major procedures or those expected to last longer than 2 hours. Sequential compression stockings may be placed. Preoperative antibiotics (e.g., cefazolin, 1 g intravenously) should be administered. The patient is positioned in the lateral decubitus position with arm positioning appropriate for an open

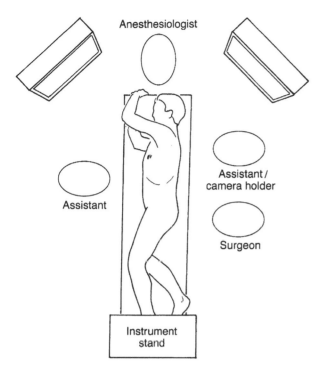

Figure 1 Operating room setup for a VATS procedure on the left hemithorax.

thoracotomy, should one be necessary. Mediastinal evaluation for staging of lung cancers or resection of tumors may be best approached with the patient placed in the supine position.

C. Operative Treatment

1. Surgical Technique—General Considerations

Port Placement. The primary consideration in port placement is arranging them to yield the widest possible triangle centered on the area of interest (Fig. 2). For example, surgery on the apex of the lung might be performed with the camera in the fifth intercostal space in the midaxillary line and the accessory thoracoscopic ports placed in the second or third intercostal spaces anteriorly and posteriorly. Of secondary consideration is the placement of port sites such that they can be utilized as part of a potential thoracotomy or for a chest tube. Placement of the first incision is normally in the midaxillary line between the fourth and ninth intercostal spaces. This incision and the port inserted through it should be positioned to provide the widest possible view of the planned surgical field. Technique for port incisions and placement is similar to that for placing a chest tube. The ipsilateral lung is allowed to collapse for 10 minutes before the incision to allow the lung to fall away from the parietal pleura; 0.25% bupivacaine is injected in the skin and subcutaneous tissues. A 1.5–2 cm skin incision is made, and a Kelly clamp is used to dissect the subcutaneous tissue and intercostal muscle on top of a rib. Electrocautery under direct vision or blunt dissection is used to dissect through the intercostal muscles and pleura. A finger is used to

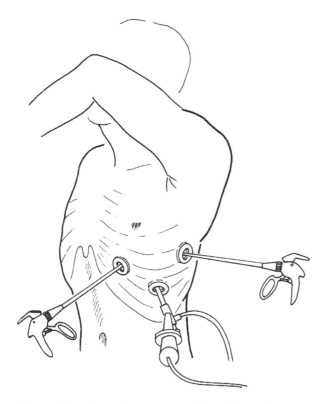

Figure 2 The ports are placed in a triangular arrangement to facilitate exposure and dissection and to avoid the "dueling swords" phenomenon when ports are placed too close together.

feel for adhesions between the lung and the parietal pleura, and a short plastic trocar is placed through the incision. The thoracoscope (with camera mounted) is inserted through this port. Subsequent incisions and ports should complete triangulation of the operative field. Intrathoracic visualization of the chest wall using the camera facilitates accurate placement of additional ports. The surgeon presses on the skin overlying the proposed new port site, and the internal location is noted. If necessary, a 22 gauge needle may be passed through this site and identified from within the thorax to verify that the proposed site is away from adhesions or vital structures. Each additional port site is made as described previously. The cutting edges and sharp points of port placement devices for laparoscopy are not recommended for thoracoscopy as they unnecessarily place the intercostal neurovascular bundle and intrathoracic structures at risk of injury.

Exposure.   The entire thoracic cavity is explored systematically. Adhesions that might interfere with the subsequent dissection must be identified. The rigid thorax and a completely collapsed (atelectatic) lung provide exposure without requiring carbon dioxide insufflation. Insufflation is generally contraindicated, as this could produce a tension pneumothorax. Complete collapse of the ipsilateral lung is required for satisfactory exposure. Extra PEEP on the contralateral lung (commonly used to bring the mediastinum toward the operative field in open thoracic procedures) may reduce the intrapleural space and reduce exposure. The oscillatory motion of thoracic structures caused by the beating heart may unavoidably complicate exposure in thoracoscopic cases.

After introducing the camera and additional ports, a grasping instrument is introduced through one of the accessory ports. The lung is grasped and retracted to visualize the operative field. Adhesions between visceral and parietal pleura are taken down. Operating room table positioning can be used to help gravity position the lung and facilitate exposure.

Dissection. Most procedures performed with the VATS approach (e.g., wedge resections) do not require extensive dissection. The pleura and chest wall may be dissected with endoscopic electrocautery, standard electrocautery using an extended tip through ports, or scissors. The ND-YAG laser may be used to dissect lung parenchyma. Lung resections or blebectomies are performed with the Endo (USSC Autosuture, Norwalk, CT) stapler.

2. Specific VATS Procedures

Pulmonary Wedge Resection for Lung Nodules. The camera is inserted through a port in the midaxillary line, the level depending on the location of the nodule in the lung. Additional operative ports are placed to form an operative triangle. A high-quality CT scan is an important prerequisite to VATS wedge excision of a pulmonary nodule. Small lesions less than 1 cm in size and more than 2 cm from the pleural surface may be quite difficult to find with the VATS approach because digital palpation can be limited. If the nodule is not apparent by visual inspection of the lung, a lung clamp may be brushed gently over the lung parenchyma to collapse the lung surrounding the lesion. A finger inserted through a port site while the lung is manipulated with an instrument may also facilitate palpation of the mass. Finally, if the lesion cannot be located by these techniques, a small access thoracotomy can be performed, and the lung is palpated to determine the site of the lesion. If difficulty locating the nodule is anticipated, a small hook wire may be inserted into the nodule preoperatively using CT guidance.

Once the nodule is located, the surrounding lung edge is grasped with a lung clamp passed through the anterior or posterior port (Fig. 3). The Endo (USSC Autosuture, Norwalk, CT) stapler is passed through the other port and fired sequentially to "wedge" the portion of lung containing the lesion. The ND-YAG laser may be used to cut portions of the lung that are difficult to resect with the Endo GIA (USSC Autosuture, Norwalk, CT) stapler, but with the advent of the articulating head, there are few areas that are not accessible by the stapler. After resection of the nodule, bleeding areas on the cut surface of lung are controlled with cautery. Large air leaks are controlled by additional applications of the Endo GIA (USSC Autosuture, Norwalk, CT) stapler or by oversewing the affected lung through an access thoracotomy. At the conclusion of the procedure, a chest tube is placed through the inferior incision and satisfactory positioning is verified by direct vision with the camera. For small trocar sites, only the skin overlying the site need be closed. Larger incisions require a formal multilayered closure.

Apical Blebectomy and Pleurodesis. The operative triangle is placed superiorly with the camera placed in the fifth intercostal space in the midaxillary line and the anterior and posterior ports placed in the second or third intercostal space. Extensive adhesions

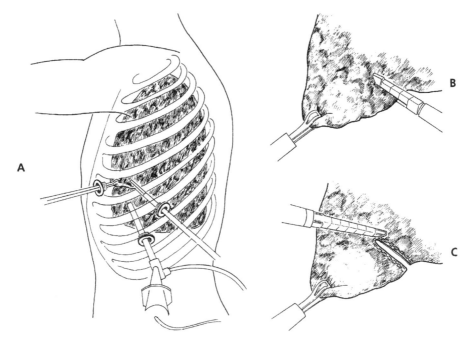

Figure 3 A. Thoracoscopic identification of lung lesion. B. Thoracoscopic wedge resection using the Endo GIA stapler. C. The Endo GIA stapler is fired repeatedly, "wedging" out the affected lung parenchyma.

between blebs and the parietal pleura may exist at the apex of the chest cavity. These adhesions are often quite vascular. Clips or stapling across these adhesions can control bleeding during division. Wedge resection of apical blebs is performed after taking down adhesions. Mechanical pleurodesis is created by abrading the parietal pleura with abrasive gauze roll or bovie scratch pad on a ring clamp. Small, type 1 bullae may be resected with VATS techniques. However, larger or type 2 bullae associated with diffusely emphysematous lung should be handled with open thoracotomy to facilitate precise stapling around the base of the bulla.

Mediastinal Nodal Staging of Intrathoracic Malignancy.   Lesions in the left upper lobe may metastasize to the aortopulmonary window nodes, which are inaccessible by cervical mediastinoscopy. VATS mediastinal lymph node sampling is an alternative to Chamberlain procedure for obtaining aortopulmonary nodal tissue. The camera is inserted through the fifth intercostal space in the posterior axillary line. An additional port is placed in the seventh intercostal space in the midaxillary line. Instruments to retract the lung are introduced through this port. Additional dissection ports are placed superiorly in the auscultatory triangle and anteriorly in the fourth intercostal space. The lymph nodes are dissected by grasping the lymph nodes with one hand and using electrocautery, scissors, and hemoclips in the other hand. Specimens should be removed using a retrieval bag to avoid port-site tumor implants.

Pericardial Window.   The patient is placed in the left lateral decubitus position. The camera is inserted in the fifth intercostal space in the midaxillary line. Additional ports are placed in the third and fifth intercostal spaces approximately 4 cm lateral to the sternum. The position of the internal thoracic arteries must be identified with the camera before placement of these ports. The pericardium is grasped through one port and electrocautery is employed through the other port to incise the pericardium anterior to the phrenic nerve. The pericardium is opened widely. Fluid is sent for cytology and culture, and a chest tube is placed.

Pleural Effusions. Typically only one port site is needed for pleural effusion management, especially if the diagnosis is already known. A single port site in the sixth or seventh intercostal space in the anterior axillary line is created. The camera is inserted through the port site. Effusion is evacuated using a pool-tipped suction. Care should be taken to provide a path for air ingress as the fluid is removed to avoid creating high negative intrathoracic pressure and mediastinal shift. High negative transpleural pressures may also contribute to development of reexpansion pulmonary edema. After fluid removal, the pleural space is thoroughly inspected. Placement of an endo-Kittner through the camera port site alongside the camera can be used to manipulate the lung. Similarly, an extended tip electrocautery can be passed through the camera port to take down adhesions. If talc pleurodesis is desired, the talc insufflater is passed alongside the scope and 4 g of talc insufflated. A single 28 Fr chest tube is placed in a posterior position extending to the apex. Absorbable sutures are used to "snug" the muscle layers and subcutaneous tissues around the chest tube to minimize air and fluid leaks. Pleural biopsies or extensive adhesions may require the addition of one or more working ports.

V. POSTOPERATIVE CARE

The patient is transferred to a thoracic observation unit or intensive care unit post-operatively. Diet is advanced as tolerated on the first postoperative night. Ambulation is initiated the first postoperative day. Antibiotics are administered for 24 hours postoperatively. Oral pain medication, occasionally supplemented with ketorolac or IM/IV narcotic, is usually sufficient. Intravenous fluids are discontinued once diet is adequate. Many patients undergoing VATS procedures have pulmonary disease that renders them sensitive to fluid overload. Intravenous fluids should be administered sparingly. The chest tube is left at 20 cm of water suction until there is no air leak. A chest radiograph is obtained daily. Patients should remain with their chest tube on suction for the radiograph if their chest tube is on suction. When the air leak has resolved and chest tube output is less than 150–200 mL/day, the tube is removed. Usually a patient who has undergone a VATS resection can have the chest tube removed on postoperative day 1 or 2 and be discharged after a radiograph confirms a lack of complicating factors.

VI. MANAGEMENT OF COMPLICATIONS

VATS complications can be divided into two categories: those that are possible with any thoracic procedure and those specific to VATS.

A. Complications Common to any Thoracic Procedure

Air leaks may occur after any thoracic procedure, especially lung resections. The incidence may be slightly higher after VATS procedures. The reason for increased incidence is twofold: unrecognized trocar or clamping injuries may be caused by a surgeon or assistant less experienced with VATS procedures than open thoracotomy, and patients with more severe bullous emphysema are undergoing VATS procedures for bullectomy or resection of lung cancer. Air leaks are managed by maintaining the chest tube on suction. Prolonged air leaks may require discharge with a Heimlich valve, an additional chest tube, higher suction, a repeat VATS procedure, or even open thoracotomy for repair. Minor wound infections are uncommon after VATS procedures; probably the incidence is no higher than after conventional thoracotomy. Other common complications such as atrial arrhythmias, respiratory problems, and deep venous thrombosis appear to occur at a rate equal to or less than after standard thoracotomy.

B. Complications Specific to VATS

1. Tumor Seeding

Individual reports have demonstrated tumor seeding in the chest wall trocar sites. All lung nodules and potentially malignant tissue should be removed in a retrieval sack through the trocar site to minimize this possibility.

2. Uncontrolled Bleeding

Most surgeons reporting moderate to large series of lobectomies or major thoracic resections have encountered a few cases of uncontrolled hemorrhage. No reported deaths have occurred; however, the potential for death or serious morbidity is always present because of the limited exposure. Removing the knife blade from the Endo GIA (USSC Autosuture, Norwalk, CT) stapler before applying it to a pulmonary vessel may help reduce major pulmonary vascular injury. Instruments for an open thoracotomy should be in the room ready for use on a back table. If major vascular injury occurs, the vessel should be tamponaded with a sponge stick and urgent thoracotomy performed.

3. Intercostal Neuralgia

Neuralgia after a VATS procedure is caused by point pressure on an adjacent intercostal nerve by a trocar. The pain is often quite disabling. The problem may be reduced by using the smallest trocar possible. Short-term measures for treating neuralgia include intercostal nerve block with bupivacaine and oral or intramuscular anti-inflammatory agents (indomethacin, ketorolac). Long-term neuralgia is a difficult problem. Management by a chronic pain specialist is recommended.

VII. CURRENT STATUS AND FUTURE INVESTIGATION

VATS technology is being used to manage a wide range of benign and malignant chest diseases. For certain thoracic processes such as diagnosis of pleural disease, open lung biopsy, and resection of solitary pulmonary nodules, VATS procedures have replaced open thoracotomy as the procedure of choice. This transition has occurred without direct prospective randomized comparison between the newer VATS approach and the conventional approach by thoracotomy. For many procedures it is unlikely that such efficacy trials will ever be conducted because VATS provides shorter hospitalization and less postoperative pain and patients increasingly demand minimally invasive procedures. Nonrandomized trials have demonstrated the safety and efficacy of VATS procedures in a broad range of patients. Applications of minimally invasive thoracoscopic procedures for resection of major intrathoracic malignancies await the results of ongoing clinical trials.

As with any surgical technique, the appropriate application of VATS ultimately depends on choosing patients with appropriate pathology and anatomy combined with adequate surgical skill.

SELECTED READINGS

DeKamp MM, Jaklitsch MT, Mentzer SJ, Harpole DH, Sugarbaker DJ. The safety and versatility of video-thoracoscopy: prospective analysis of 895 consecutive cases. J Am Coll Surg 1995; 181:165–167.

Hazelrigg SR, Nunchuck SK, LoCicero J 3rd. Video Assisted Thoracic Surgery Study Group data. Ann Thorac Surg 1993; 56(5):1039–1043.

Kaiser LR, Bavaria JE. Complications of thoracoscopy. Ann Thorac Surg 1993; 56:796–798.

Lewis RJ. Perspectives in the evolution of video assisted thoracic surgery. Chest Surg Clin North Am 1993; 3(2):207–213.

Velasco FT, Rusch VW, Ginsberg RJ. Thoracoscopic management of chest neoplasms. Semin Laparosc Surg 1994; 1:43–51.

40

Esophagectomy

NINH T. NGUYEN

University of California, Irvine, Medical Center
Irvine, California, U.S.A.

PHILIP R. SCHAUER and JAMES D. LUKETICH

University of Pittsburgh Medical Center
Pittsburgh, Pennsylvania, U.S.A.

The two most frequently performed operations for esophageal resection are transthoracic esophagectomy and blunt transhiatal esophagectomy. The transthoracic approach allows the surgeon to mobilize the thoracic esophagus under direct visualization and perform a wide mediastinal lymphadenectomy, which often cannot be performed by a transhiatal approach. In contrast, the transhiatal approach avoids a thoracotomy and therefore possibly reduces associated pulmonary complications. Both techniques, however, can be associated with significant morbidity and mortality.

A minimally invasive surgical approach to esophagectomy was developed in the early 1990s in an attempt to reduce the morbidity associated with open esophagectomy. The initial approach involved thoracoscopic mobilization of the esophagus combined with a standard upper midline laparotomy for the creation of the gastric conduit. In 1994, DePaula and colleagues described the first total laparoscopic transhiatal esophagectomy. Their approach was similar to that of the blunt transhiatal approach but was performed through five to six abdominal trocars. Subsequently, we reported the combined thoracoscopic and laparoscopic approach to esophagectomy. This chapter discusses the preoperative evaluation of patients with esophageal cancer, our technique of thoracoscopic and laparoscopic esophagectomy, and the outcome of minimally invasive esophagectomy.

I. CLINICAL PRESENTATION

The estimated number of new esophageal cancer cases in the United States in 2001 was 13,200, and the majority of these patients will likely die from their disease. The primary symptom of the disease at presentation is progressive dysphagia. Other symptoms include odynophagia, weight loss, regurgitation, gastrointestinal bleeding, and aspiration pneumonia.

II. DIAGNOSTIC TESTS

Diagnostic studies for evaluation of patients with esophageal cancer include upper endoscopy with biopsy, upper gastrointestinal contrast study, computed tomography (CT) of the chest and abdomen, esophageal endoscopic ultrasound, and positron emission tomography (PET). Esophagoscopy is performed to evaluate the proximal and distal extent of tumor involvement, and biopsy is performed to confirm the diagnosis of cancer. An esophagram is performed to provide a "road map" of the esophagus and give information on the site of luminal narrowing, the degree of obstruction, and the presence of concomitant tracheoesophageal fistula. A CT of the chest and abdomen is performed to provide an overall survey for distant metastasis to the liver and lung and local-regional involvement of the cancer. Endoscopic esophageal ultrasound provides information on the depth of tumor penetration through the esophageal wall, the presence of T4 disease (involvement of aorta, trachea, or pericardium), and the presence of lymphadenopathy. PET is used to image biochemical pathways by using short-lived positron-emitting radiopharmaceuticals. A common PET radiophamaceutical is 18-FDG, a glucose analog used to image glucose metabolism. PET evaluates for uptake and retention of radionuclides in the primary tumor, lymph nodes, and distant metastatic sites. Other preoperative work-ups include a pulmonary function test, a 2D echocardiogram, and cardiac stress tests, as appropriate.

If after completion of the above diagnostic tests the patient is considered to be a candidate for an operation, then he or she should undergo laparoscopic staging. Laparoscopic staging consists of diagnostic laparoscopy, placement of a jejunostomy tube, and laparoscopic ultrasound evaluation of the liver. The primary aim of laparoscopic staging is to identify patients with stage IV cancer. These patients would not benefit from an operative resection. In addition, laparoscopic staging provides an accurate staging of the cancer before the initiation of neoadjuvant therapy.

III. INDICATIONS FOR ESOPHAGECTOMY

Indications for esophagectomy include both benign and malignant esophageal diseases. Benign pathology of the esophagus requiring esophagectomy includes severe recalcitrant esophageal stricture from complications of gastroesophageal reflux or lye ingestion. Esophagectomy for malignant disease includes esophageal cancer or a premalignant condition such as Barrett's esophagus with high-grade dysplasia.

IV. NONOPERATIVE TREATMENT

Nonoperative treatment for esophageal cancer should be reserved for the following: patients who refuse surgical intervention, patients who are poor surgical candidates, and patients with stage IV disease. Surgery is rarely performed for palliation because of the high morbidity and mortality associated with esophagectomy. Nonsurgical modalities for palliation of dysphagia include balloon dilation, Nd : YAG laser therapy, photodynamic therapy (PDT), and an expandable metal stent. Balloon dilation is simple, but the duration of palliation may be as short as a few days. Nd : YAG laser utilizes thermal energy for ablation of obstructing esophageal cancer. In contrast, PDT utilizes nonthermal energy to activate a photosensitizing agent that has been taken up by the tumor. The excited photosensitizing agent activates oxygen to produce oxygen radicals and cause vascular occlusion and eventual tumor necrosis. An esophageal stent is another modality for palliation of dysphagia and can be placed endoscopically under fluoroscopic guidance.

V. OPERATIVE TREATMENT

A. Preoperative Preparation

The risks and benefits of the surgical procedure are explained to the patient. Written informed consent is obtained. Patients are informed of the potential need for conversion to both thoracotomy and laparotomy. On the day before the operation, a clear liquid diet is instituted and a bowel preparation regimen is given. The patient is admitted on the day of operation after an overnight fast.

B. Operating Room and Patient Setup

The patient is placed in a supine position. A double-lumen endotracheal tube is placed in preparation for single lung ventilation. Fiberoptic bronchoscopy is performed to confirm the correct position of the double-lumen tube. Standard cardiorespiratory monitoring is employed. In addition, central venous and radial arterial catheters are placed for invasive monitoring. The surgeon performs an esophagoscopy to evaluate the proximal and distal extent of the tumor involvement. At the completion of esophagoscopy, a nasogastric tube and Foley catheter are inserted. Antibiotic prophylaxis is administered (cephalosporin and Flagyl). The equipment for thoracoscopy and laparoscopy are listed below.

C. Equipment for Thoracoscopy

Four thoracic trocars: two 5 mm, one 10 mm, and one 12 mm
A 10 mm angled scope (30°)
Clip applier
Penrose drain
Endoscopic linear stapler
Ultrasonic dissector

D. Equipment for Laparoscopy

Five trocars: three 5 mm, one 11 mm, and one 12 mm
A 10 mm angled scope (45°)
Endoscopic linear stapler
Endoscopic liver retractor
Ultrasonic dissector
Needle catheter jejunostomy
Endoscopic suturing instruments

E. Surgical Technique

Thoracoscopic and laparoscopic esophagectomy is performed in three stages. In the first stage, the patient is positioned in the left lateral decubitus position for thoracoscopic dissection of the thoracic esophagus. In the second stage, the patient is placed in a supine position for creation of the gastric conduit. The third stage consists of mobilization of the cervical esophagus, removal of the surgical specimen, and the creation of the esophagogastric anastomosis.

1. Thoracoscopic Mobilization of the Esophagus

The patient is positioned in a left lateral decubitus position on a bean bag cushion. The surgeon stands facing the patient's back (Fig. 1). Single lung ventilation is initiated by occluding ventilation to the right lung. Four thoracic trocars are introduced in the right chest (Fig. 2). The first trocar is placed at the eighth intercostal space below the tip of the scapula and used for the camera. A 5 mm port is placed immediately posterior to the scapula and used by the surgeon. A 12 mm trocar is placed at the ninth intercostal space and 2 cm behind the posterior axillary line. The last trocar (5 mm) is placed at the sixth intercostal space at the anterior axillary line. Carbon dioxide insufflation is not used during thoracoscopy. The 30° angled scope is used to inspect the pleural cavity and the surface of the lung for any suspicious lesion. The lung lobes are retracted laterally to expose the mediastinal esophagus. The inferior pulmonary ligament is divided with the ultrasonic dissector. The pleura, overlying the esophagus, are divided to expose the intrathoracic esophagus. The azygous vein is isolated and divided with the endoscopic linear stapler (Fig. 3). The esophagus is circumferentially mobilized at a portion below the azygous vein, and a Penrose drain is placed around the esophagus to facilitate esophageal retraction. The esophagus is circumferentially mobilized from the esophageal hiatus up to the thoracic inlet. A paraesophageal lymph node dissection is also performed to remain en-bloc with the surgical specimen. At the completion of the thoracoscopic mobilization of the esophagus, the Penrose drain is left in the chest at the level of the cervical esophagus. This Penrose drain will be retrieved during the cervical dissection of the esophagus. A 28 F chest tube is inserted through the camera port for postoperative chest drainage.

2. Laparoscopic Creation of the Gastric Conduit

The patient is changed to the supine position and sterilely prepped and draped from the neck to the pubic symphysis. The surgeon stands on the patient's right side and the assistant stands on the patient's left side. Abdominal insufflation is achieved using the Veress needle, and pneumoperitoneum is maintained at 15 mmHg. Five abdominal trocars are placed (Fig. 4). The first trocar (11 mm) is placed at the left midclavicular line at the level of the umbilicus. A 5 mm trocar is placed at the left anterior axillary line below the costal margin and used by the assistant surgeon. A 5 mm trocar is placed at the right anterior axillary line below the costal margin and used for retraction of the liver. Another 5 mm trocar is placed at the right midclavicular line below the costal margin. The fifth trocar (12 mm) is placed close to the midline above the umbilicus and used by the surgeon. A needle catheter jejunostomy is placed in the proximal aspect of the jejunum. The patient is placed in reverse Trendelenburg position to help with exposure by displacing the stomach and colon caudally. The greater curvature of the stomach is mobilized carefully to avoid injury to the right gastroepiploic vessels. Adhesions in the posterior aspect of the stomach are divided. Attachments in the first portion of the duodenum also are divided.

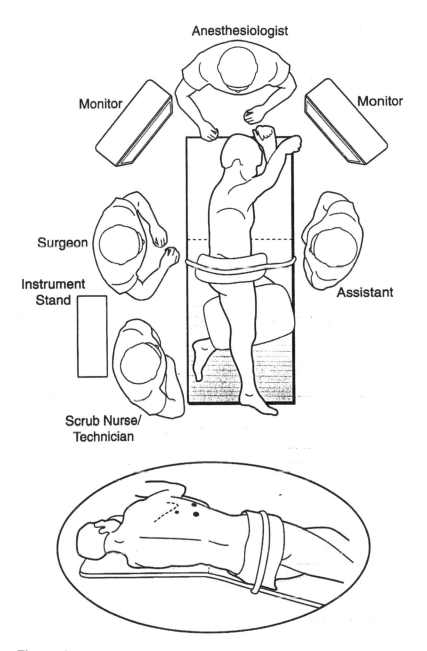

Figure 1 Operative set-up for thoracoscopy.

The gastric fundus is mobilized by dividing the short gastric vessels. The hepatogastric ligament is divided to enter the lesser sac. The left gastric vessel is isolated and divided with the endoscopic linear stapler. In our early experience, we performed either laparoscopic pyloroplasty or pyloromyotomy for gastric drainage. Currently neither pyloroplasty nor pyloromyotomy are being performed. Endoscopic linear staplers are used to create the gastric conduit starting at the distal aspect of the lesser curverature of the

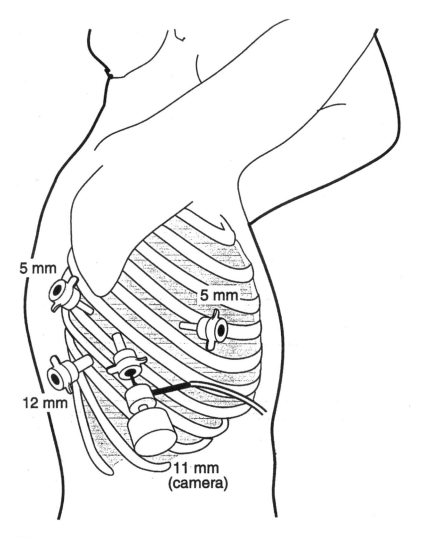

Figure 2   Trocar placement for thoracoscopic esophageal mobilization.

stomach. A small gastric conduit (3 cm diameter) is created based on the greater curvature of the stomach and separated from the surgical specimen near the angle of His (Fig. 5). The gastric conduit is sutured to the surgical specimen (Fig. 6). The last portion of the abdominal dissection is mobilization of the esophageal hiatus to connect with the thoracic dissection. Once the pleural cavity is entered from the abdomen, the surgical dissection must be performed expeditiously to limit the amount of carbon dioxide absorption and the pressure effects of pneumoperitoneum on the heart and the cava. If needed, a portion of the crus of the diaphragm is divided to enlarge the esophageal hiatus to facilitate delivery of the surgical specimen and gastric conduit.

3.   Cervical Anastomosis

A horizontal neck incision is performed above the suprasternal notch. The sternocleidomastoid muscle is retracted laterally. The cervical esophagus is mobilized

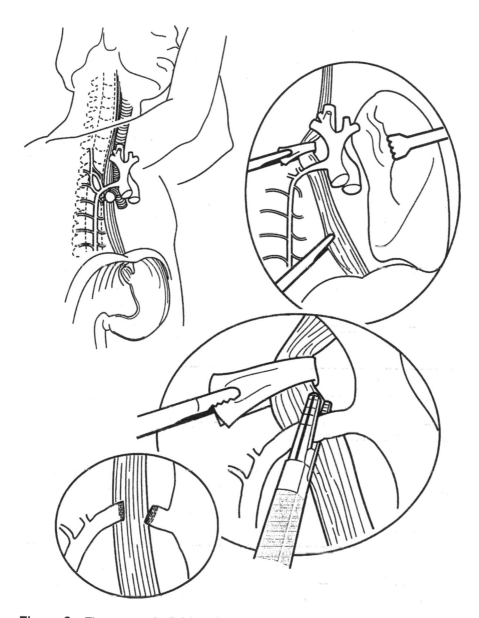

Figure 3 Thoracoscopic division of the azygous vein.

until the dissection plane in the neck is connected with the dissection plane achieved in the right chest. The Penrose drain left during the thoracoscopic dissection is retrieved through the neck incision. Under laparoscopic guidance, the surgical specimen is removed through the neck incision and the gastric conduit is pulled along with it (Fig. 7). The cervical esophagus is divided from the surgical specimen. The nasogastric tube is passed into the gastric conduit, and a two-layer hand-sewn esophagogastric anastomosis is performed (Fig. 8). Antibiotic irrigation solution is used to irrigate the neck wound. The platysma is approximated with interrupted sutures and the skin incision is approximated with staples.

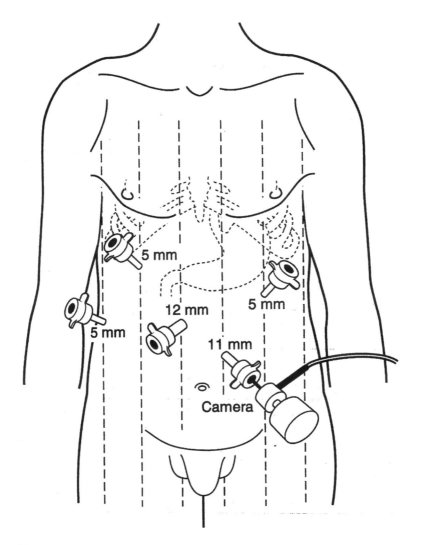

Figure 4 Trocar placement for laparoscopy.

4. Closure

The laparoscope is reinserted to inspect the abdominal cavity for adequate hemostasis. The gastric conduit is sutured to the left and right crus of the diaphragm with interrupted sutures. The fascia layer of the 11 mm and 12 mm trocar sites is closed with 1-0 Vicryl sutures, and skin edges are approximated with subcuticular sutures.

VI. POSTOPERATIVE CARE

All patients are transferred to the intensive care unit for observation on the operative night. The chest tube and nasogastric tube are placed to wall suction. Postoperative analgesia is provided with intravenous morphine using patient-controlled analgesia. The patient

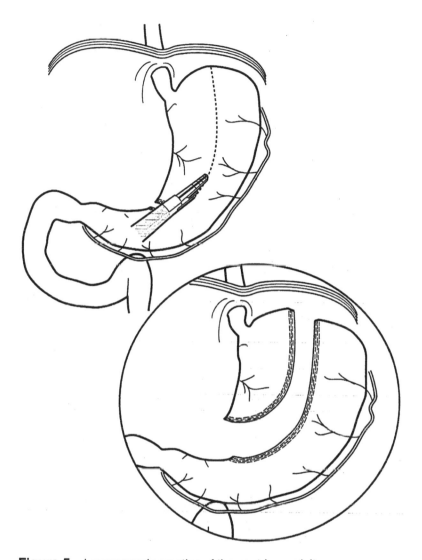

Figure 5 Laparoscopic creation of the gastric conduit.

is transferred to the ward on the first postoperative day. Early ambulation and deep breathing are encouraged. A gastrograffin contrast study is performed on the fourth to sixth postoperative day. The chest tube is removed and clear liquid diet is started when the contrast study demonstrates no anastomotic leak. Supplemental jejunal feeding is administered if needed.

VII. MANAGEMENT OF COMPLICATIONS

Complications of thoracoscopic and laparoscopic esophagectomy are similar to those of conventional open esophagectomy. Intraoperative complications include potential injury

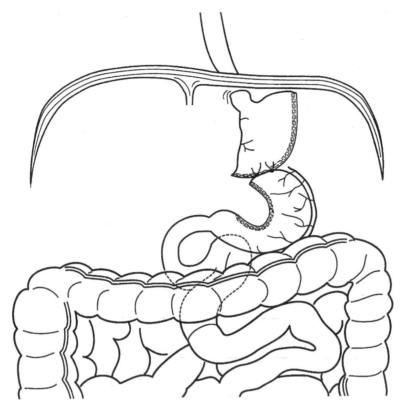

Figure 6   The gastric conduit is sutured to the surgical specimen.

to the pulmonary parenchyma, pulmonary hilum, pericardium, and spleen. Early and late postoperative complications are listed below.

Hematological: bleeding
Pulmonary: atelectasis, respiratory failure, chest tube air leak, pneumonia, chylothorax
Cardiac: arrhythmia, myocardial infarction
Gastrointestinal: anastomotic leak, anastomotic stricture, delayed gastric emptying
Wound: infection
Other: deep venous thrombosis, recurrent laryngeal nerve injury, urinary retention

Anastomotic leak is potentially one of the most serious complications after esophagectomy. Neck anastomotic leak can be treated easily by opening the neck incision, draining the abscess, and applying local wound care. Staple line breakdown of the gastric conduit can result in an empyema and requires more complicated treatments. A small leak can be treated with primary closure at the leak site or T-tube drainage of the gastric conduit and wide drainage of the pleural cavity. A large leak will require returning the gastric conduit back into the abdominal cavity and the creation of a temporary diverting esophagostomy.

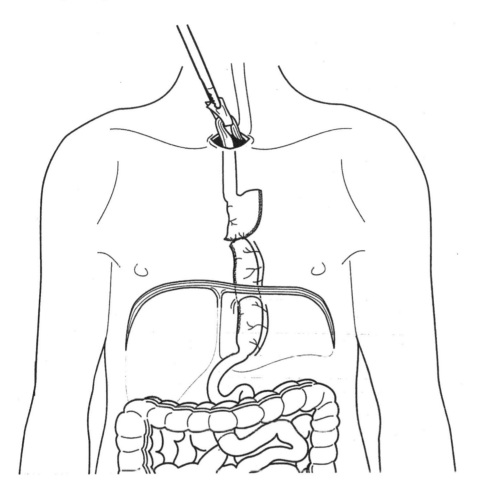

Figure 7 Removal of the surgical specimen and delivery of the gastric conduit to the cervical incision.

VIII. OUTCOMES

Luketich and colleagues reported the largest series of 77 patients who underwent combined thoracoscopic and laparoscopic esophagectomy. Median operative time was 7.5 hours. Median intensive care unit stay was 1 day, and the median length of stay was 7 days. There was no hospital mortality. Major complication rates were 27% and minor complication rates were 55%. Nguyen and colleagues compared outcomes of patients who underwent thoracoscopic and laparoscopic esophagectomy with patients who underwent transhiatal or transthoracic esophagectomy. Thoracoscopic and laparoscopic esophagectomy was associated with shorter operative times, less blood loss, fewer transfusions, and shortened intensive care unit and hospital stays than transthoracic or blunt transhiatal esophagectomy.

As with other laparoscopic operations for cancer, concern has been raised about port site cancer recurrence, the adequacy of surgical margins, and the number of lymph nodes removed. Nguyen and colleagues reported that the mean number of lymph nodes retrieved

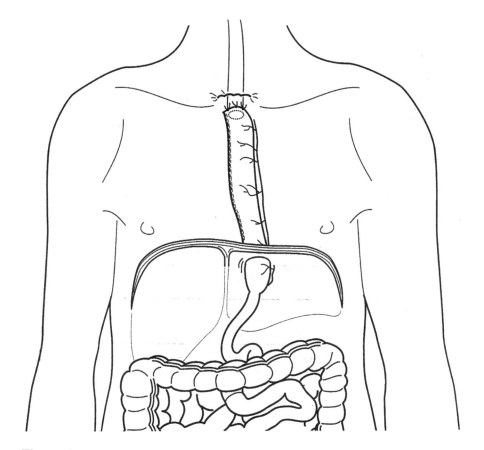

Figure 8 A cervical esophagogastric anastomosis is performed.

during thoracoscopic and laparoscopic esophagectomy was similar to that obtained after transthoracic and blunt transhiatal esophagectomy; all surgical margins were clear of tumor involvement, and in their short follow-up there had not been any port site recurrence.

IX. CURRENT STATUS AND FUTURE INVESTIGATION

Thoracoscopic and laparoscopic esophagectomy can be performed as safely as conventional esophagectomy. Compared with open esophagectomy, applications of thoracoscopy and laparoscopy to esophagectomy eliminate both the thoracotomy and laparotomy incision and therefore further reduce operative trauma and enhance postoperative recovery. Long-term results, however, are not yet available. Prospective clinical investigations of thoracoscopic and laparoscopic esophagectomy in tertiary centers will be required to answer other questions such as the impact of minimally invasive esophagectomy on cancer recurrence and survival.

We advocate that minimally invasive esophagectomy should be performed only in dedicated centers experienced in esophagectomy and esophageal surgery and performed only by surgeons with experience in open esophagectomy and other advanced laparoscopic and thoracoscopic operations. A prospective, randomized trial comparing open and minimally invasive esophagectomy is needed to evaluate outcomes, quality of life, and costs. Future investigations should concentrate on determining the best minimally invasive surgical approach to esophagectomy (total laparoscopic transhiatal, minimally Ivor Lewis resection, or thoracoscopic and laparoscopic esophagectomy), training and credentialing issues, and accumulation of long-term outcome data.

X. TOP TEN SURGICAL TIPS

1. Complete collapse of the right lung is important for obtaining adequate exposure of the thoracic esophagus.
2. The inferior pulmonary ligament is divided to retract the lower lobe of the lung for exposure of the distal third esophagus.
3. A Penrose drain is placed around the esophagus to facilitate retraction. The drain is left at the level of the cervical esophagus during thoracoscopic dissection and recovered later during dissection of the cervical esophagus.
4. The azygous vein is divided to facilitate exposure and dissection of the proximal and middle third esophagus.
5. Care must be taken during dissection of the gastrocolonic omentum to preserve the major blood supply to the gastric conduit (right gastroepiploic vessels).
6. Laparoscopic pyloroplasty or pyloromyotomy is not important for gastric emptying if a narrow gastric conduit (3 cm in diameter) is constructed.
7. Care must be taken during delivery of the gastric conduit to the neck to prevent twisting the conduit.
8. The dissection of the esophageal hiatus should be performed as the last part of the abdominal dissection to prevent leak of carbon dioxide gas into the thoracic cavity.
9. The gastric conduit is sutured to the crus of the diaphragm to obliterate the esophageal hiatus and thus avoid potential postoperative bowel herniation into the chest cavity.
10. Only surgeons with experience in open esophagectomy and other advanced laparoscopic operations should perform thoracoscopic and laparoscopic esophagectomy.

SELECTED READINGS

DePaula AL, Hashiba K, Ferreira EA, de Paula RA, Grecco E. Laparoscopic transhiatal esophagectomy with esophagogastroplasty. Surg Laparosc Endosc 1995; 5:1–5.

Luketich JD, Schauer PR, Christie NA, Weigel TL, Raja S, Fernando HC, Keenan RJ, Nguyen NT. Minimally invasive esophagectomy. Ann Thorac Surg 2000; 70:906–911.

Nguyen NT, Follette DM, Roberts P, Goodnight JE Jr. Thoracoscopic management of postoperative esophageal leak. J Thorac Cardiovasc Surg 2001; 121:391–392.

Nguyen NT, Follette DM, Wolfe BM, Schneider PD, Roberts P, Goodnight JE Jr. Comparison of minimally invasive esophagectomy with transthoracic and transhiatal esophagectomy. Arch Surg 2000; 135:920–925.

Nguyen NT, Schauer PR, Luketich JD. Combined laparoscopic and thoracoscopic approach to esophagectomy. J Am Coll Surg 1999; 188:328–332.

Orringer MB, Marshall B, Stirling MC. Transhiatal esophagectomy for benign and malignant disease. J Thorac Cardiovasc Surg 1993; 105:265–276.

Swanstrom L, Hansen P. Laparoscopic total esophagectomy. Arch Surg 1997; 132:943–947.

41

Obesity Surgery: Roux-en-Y and Gastric Band Procedures

BENJAMIN E. SCHNEIDER AND DANIEL B. JONES

Beth Israel Deaconess Medical Center
Harvard Medical School
Boston, Massachusetts, U.S.A.

DAVID A. PROVOST

University of Texas Southwestern Medical Center
Dallas, Texas, U.S.A.

I. INTRODUCTION

Mason and Ito introduced the original concept of the gastric bypass for weight reduction in 1967. Subsequent refinements led from the open loop gastric bypass to ultimately the development of the laparoscopic Roux-en-Y gastric bypass reported by Wittgrove. Advantages of the laparoscopic approach as compared to open include diminished rates of wound infection, hernia, and pulmonary complications. Other advantages include shorter length of stay and return to activity.

II. CLINICAL PRESENTATION

Obesity is a major health problem in the twenty-first century. In the United States nearly two thirds of adults are considered overweight as defined by a body mass index (BMI) of $> 25 \, \text{kg/m}^2$. The obese (BMI $> 30 \, \text{kg/m}^2$) constitute 30.5% of the population. The cost of obesity to the patient and society are immense. It is estimated that more than \$100 billion are spent annually in treating the direct and indirect cost of obesity. To the individual patient the risk translates to an increased incidence of coronary artery disease, diabetes, hypertension, pulmonary dysfunction, hyperlipidemia, and death. Pharmacological treatments directed at weight reduction do improve results over diet, exercise, and behavioral therapy. However, in the majority of morbidly obese patients, medical therapy is inadequate and ephemeral.

III. OPERATIVE TREATMENT

A number of surgical approaches to obesity have been developed with varying degrees of success. Procedures are classified into gastric restrictive and malabsorptive. The Roux-en-Y gastric bypass, a hybrid of restrictive and malabsorptive procedures, has been demonstrated to be superior in terms of durable weight loss and complications. Described here are the most common laparoscopic procedures performed: gastric bypass and the laparoscopic gastric band. The National Institutes of Health Consensus Development Panel outlined indications for surgical intervention. Potential candidates for surgical intervention should have a BMI $> 40 kg/m^2$ or $> 35 kg/m^2$ with associated obesity-induced high-risk comorbidity. An experienced surgeon in a clinical setting should perform procedures where there exists the capacity for management of these patients, their attendant medical risks, and potential complications.

Absolute contraindications to laparoscopic obesity procedures include an inability to tolerate a general anesthesia, ongoing infection, or the presence of uncorrectable coagulopathy. Previous surgery, particularly gastric surgery, may represent a relative contraindication to laparoscopic bypass. Patients with large ventral hernias may not be readily amenable to laparoscopic approach. Although there is increasing experience with laparoscopic gastric bypass in the superobese (BMI > 50), there are technical constraints in patients who weigh more than 160 kg or have an excessive truncal fat distribution.

IV. SURGICAL TECHNIQUE: ROUX-EN-Y GASTRIC BYPASS

A. Preoperative Preparation

Patients are admitted the day of surgery after an overnight fast. In the operating room, the patient is placed on a beanbag cushion in the supine position. Once general anesthesia is established, the bladder is emptied with a Foley catheter and the stomach decompressed with a nasogastric tube. Sequential compression devices and subcutaneous heparin are used for prophylaxis against deep venous thrombosis. A first-generation cephalosporin is administered prophylactically. A footboard is placed on the table and the patient appropriately padded. The arms are abducted and secured on cushioned boards. The abdomen is prepared and draped in a sterile fashion.

B. Operating Room and Patient Setup

The surgeon and camera operator are situated on the patient's right with the assistant surgeon on the patient's left (Fig. 1). The video monitors are placed on either side of the head of the table. Irrigation, suction, ultrasonic dissector, and videoscopic cables come off the head of the table on the patient's right side.

C. Surgical Technique

1. Port Placement

Pneumoperitoneum to 15–17 mmHg is established via a Veress needle inserted at the midline port site. A second insufflator used to ensure adequate pneumoperitoneum is maintained despite potential port site leaks. A total of six ports are placed including three 5 mm and three 12 mm ports (Fig. 2). Port placement in addition to the 12 mm midline

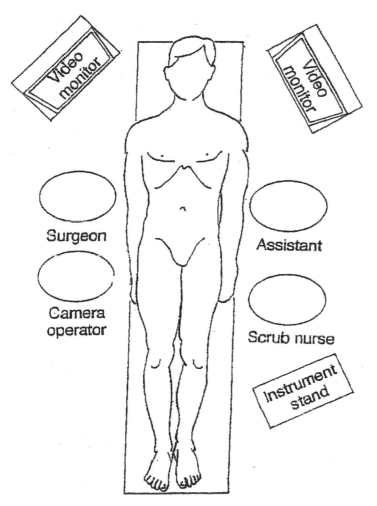

Figure 1 Operating room layout for laparoscopic gastric bypass.

camera port include: a 5 mm right subcostal for placement of a grasper; a 5 mm right port for the liver retractor; a 12 mm right midclavicular port used for stapling and suturing; a left subcostal 5 mm port is used for placement of a grasper; a 12 mm left lateral port placed for dissection and stapling.

D.   Dissection

The falciform ligament is detached from the anterior abdominal wall using the ultrasonic dissector. This maneuver affords improved access to the upper abdomen. The left lateral liver is elevated using a liver retractor placed throughout the right lateral inferior port.

The gastrocolic omentum is divided to identify the superior aspect of the transverse mesocolon. With the colon elevated a mesocolic window is made lateral to the ligament of Treitz (Fig. 3).

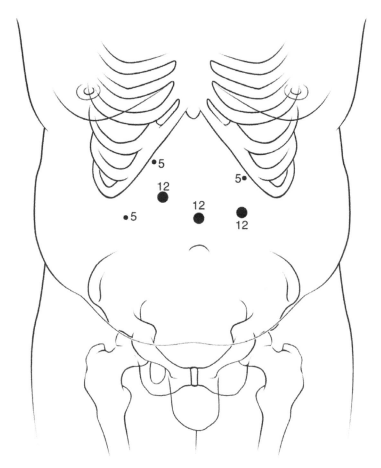

Figure 2 Port placement for laparoscopic gastric bypass.

E. Roux-en-Y

The ligament of Treitz is identified. A 50 cm length of jejunum is measured using Babcock clamps. The bowel is marked at this point with a suture on the proximal bowel (afferent limb). The jejunum is divided with a 60 mm Endo-GIA (2.5 mm staples); its mesentery is divided with a 45 mm Endo-GIA stapler (2.0 mm staples). The distal jejunum is measured for a distance of 75 cm (150 cm in the superobese patient) for use as the Roux limb. Care is taken to avoid twisting of the mesentery. The Roux and afferent limbs are then sutured together with a long traction suture, which is brought out without tying through the right 12 mm port for use as a handle during stapling. Enterotomies are fashioned in both the efferent and afferent limbs. A side-to-side jejunojejunostomy is created using a single firing of an Endo-GIA stapler (2.5 mm × 60 mm stapler). Once hemostasis is confirmed at the anastamosis, the enterostomy is closed. Closure is accomplished by first placing several interrupted stay sutures to approximate the edges. Next, a 2.5 mm Endo-GIA is applied transversely. The mesenteric defect between the leaves of the jejunal mesentery is approximated with interrupted suture. An "antiobstruction stitch" is placed to approximate the divided end of the proximal jejunum to adjacent Roux limb. Next, the Roux limb is

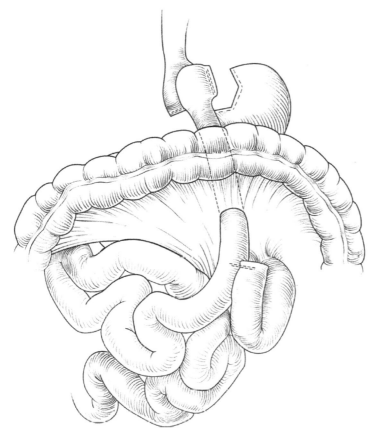

Figure 3   Configuration of the Roux-en-Y gastric bypass.

advanced through the mesenteric defect in a retrocolic antegastric fashion (Fig. 4). Again care is taken to avoid twisting the mesentery.

F.   Gastric Pouch and Gastrojejunostomy

The gastric pouch is sized by inflating the gastric balloon to 20 mL at the level of the GE junction (Fig. 5). The gastro-hepatic ligament is opened extending to the right crus. A retrogastric window is created along the lesser curvature using blunt and ultrasonic dissection preserving the vagus nerve and left gastric artery. The balloon is then deflated and the tube removed. A gastrotomy is performed on the anterior wall of the stomach 5 cm distal to the intended site of gastric division. A looped suture is tied to the anvil of a 21 mm circular stapler and placed within the abdomen. A pointed Flamingo grasper is used to advance the suture through the gastrotomy and to penetrate the anterior gastric wall at the site of the intended gastrojejunostomy (Fig. 6). The suture is pulled with another grasper, thus bringing the anvil through the gastric wall. The anvil suture is cut. At this point it is important to confirm that all tubes are removed from the stomach and esophagus to avoid inadvertent transection during formation of the gastric pouch. Three applications of a 60 mm Endo-GIA (3.5 mm staples) divide the gastric pouch (Fig. 7). It is important to

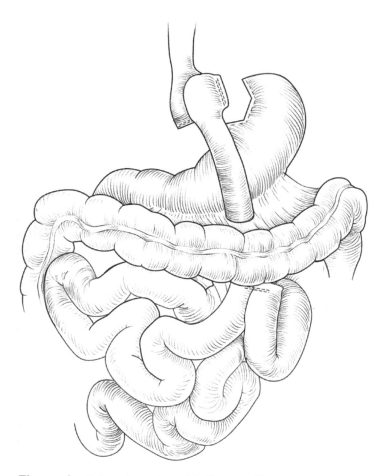

Figure 4   Retrocolic, antegastric Roux-en-Y.

avoid excessive traction on the proximal stomach in order to prevent injury to the splenic capsule. The gastrotomy used for introduction of the anvil is then closed with an Endo-GIA (3.5 mm).

The left inferior port is removed and a 21 mm EEA stapler is placed through the site. The gastrojejunostomy is constructed by first opening and dilating the stapled end of the Roux limb to allow for insertion of the circular stapling device. The anvil spike is deployed through the wall of the jejunum, and then removed. The anvil and stapler are mated, care is taken to maintain proper alignment of the mesentery, and the stapler is fired (Fig. 8). The end of the Roux limb is then divided adjacent to the gastric pouch using an Endo-GIA (2.5 mm staples). The anastamosis is bolstered with interrupted horizontal mattress sutures. A leak test is performed by instilling 60 mL of saline or dilute methylene blue via a nasogastric tube while occluding the Roux limb with a grasper; additional sutures are placed as needed to assure a watertight anastamosis. The nasogastric tube may be left in place once the absence of leak is demonstrated.

The window in the transverse mesocolon and the Peterson's defect closed by approximating the base of the jejunal mesentary, transverse mesocolon, and roux limb

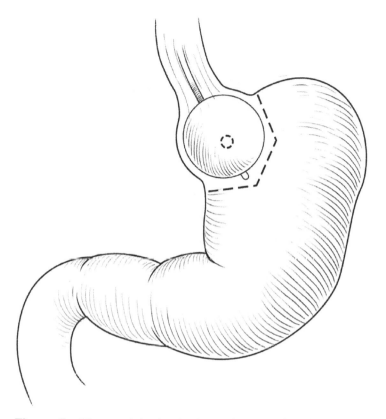

Figure 5 The pouch is sized using an intragastric balloon.

using running sutures in order to prevent internal hernias. The abdomen is irrigated, and hemostasis is confirmed. Pneumoperitoneum is evacuated and the fascia at the 12 mm port sites is closed with absorbable suture. The incisions are irrigated and infiltrated with 0.25% bupivacaine. The skin is approximated with a subcuticular sutures.

G. Postoperative Care

Pneumatic compression devices and heparin are continued postoperatively. A gastrograffin swallow study is obtained on postoperative day 1. In the absence of leak the patient is given liquids orally. By postoperative day 2, the patients may take 30 mL of liquid every 15 minutes. Patients are also started on high-protein supplements, multivitamins, and iron. Patients who have not undergone cholecystectomy are begun on a 6-month course of Ursodiol to prevent gallstone formation. By the sixth week the patient can be advanced to a solid diet. At the 6-month follow-up vitamin B_{12}, folate, ferritin, and iron levels are checked. Patients will continue to require lifelong follow-up.

H. Management of Complications

One must be particularly vigilant for signs of early complications following gastric bypass surgery as delay in diagnosis can lead to disastrous consequences. Hemorrhage may occur

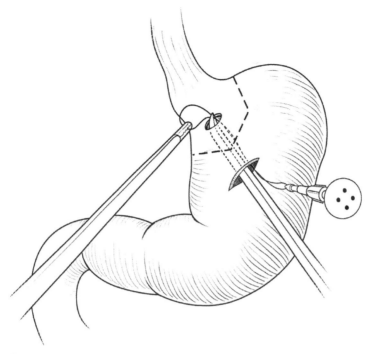

Figure 6   The circular stapler anvil is placed via a distal gastrotomy.

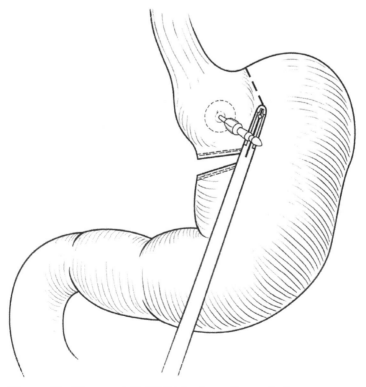

Figure 7   The pouch is created using a linear stapler.

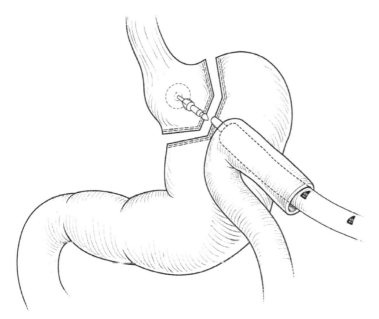

Figure 8 The gastrojejunostomy accomplished by placing the circular stapler through the end of the Roux limb.

particularly along the gastric staple lines. Leak or staple line disruption may present in any number of fashions, but unexplained tachycardia, fluid requirement, pain, pulmonary dysfunction, or fever should be worked up with a gastrograffin study as physical exam in notoriously unreliable. A leak at the jejunojejunostomy is unlikely to be diagnosed with gastrograffin; when leak is suspected early reexploration is the requisite. If a leak is discovered, an attempt should be made at repair with placement of closed suction drains and also a gastrostomy tube within the defunctionalized portion of stomach. Other complications include wound infection, hernia, deep venous thrombosis, pulmonary embolus, gastric distention, anastamotic stenosis, and late micronutrient deficiencies.

I. Outcomes

Early excess weight loss with gastric bypass may be 60–82% with a durable excess weight loss of 50–60%. Operative times range from 1 to 6 hours depending on the patient's habitus as well as the surgeon's experience. Mean hospitalization varies from 1.5 to 4 days. Laparoscopic gastric bypass favorably compares to the open procedure in terms of overall cost, excess weight loss, and safety. It is superior when comparing early quality of life scale, length of hospital stay, incidence of hernia, and wound infection.

V. SURGICAL TECHNIQUE: LAP-BAND

A. Preoperative Preparation

The patient is admitted the day of surgery, having fasted overnight. After induction of general anesthesia the stomach is decompressed with an orogastric tube. The patient is positioned in the lithotomy position on a beanbag cushion (Fig. 9). The arms are secured

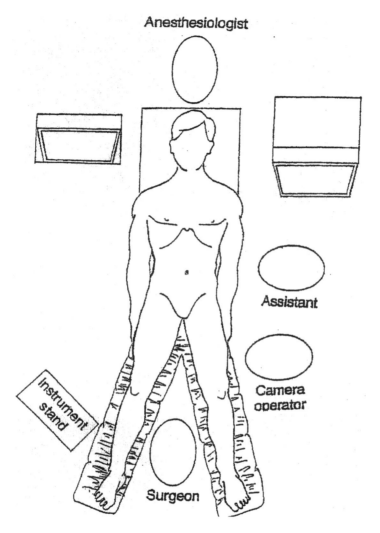

Figure 9   Operating room layout for placement of the laparoscopic gastric band.

on cushioned boards; sequential compression devices and heparin are used for prophylaxis against deep venous thrombosis. A first-generation cephalosporin is administered. The abdomen is prepared and draped sterilely.

B.   Operating Room and Patient Setup

The room is arranged such that the surgeon is situated between the patient's legs with the assistant on the patient's right and the camera operator on the left. The video monitors are placed at both sides of the patient's head. The video cord, insuflator tubing, irrigation, and cautery are passed off to the left of patient's head.

C.   Port Placement

Pneumoperitoneum may be established via either the Veress needle at the umbilicus or left upper quadrant. Next, a 12 mm trocar is placed in the left midrectus 15 cm below the

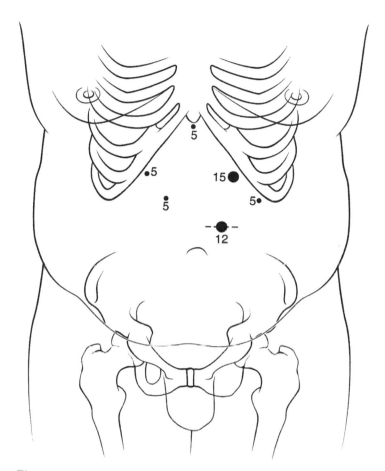

Figure 10 Port placement for laparoscopic gastric band.

xiphoid process. The abdomen is inspected with an angled laparoscope. Additional trocar placement may vary in accordance with the patient's body habitus. A 15 mm subcostal trocar is placed in the left mid-clavicular line (Fig. 10). Right-sided 5 mm ports are placed: subcostal, 15 cm from the xiphoid process; in the midrectus between the levels of the first two ports; and the right subxiphoid.

D. Exposure

With trocar placement complete, perigastric exposure is afforded by placing the patient in reverse Trendelenburg position using gravity to retract the bowel and omentum caudally. The liver is elevated with a retractor placed through the right subcostal port. Retraction on the stomach inferiorly using a Babcock grasper allows for dissection of the lesser curvature.

E. Dissection and Band Placement

An intragastric balloon is placed and inflated with 20 cc of saline in order to size the gastric pouch. Dissection begins high on the lesser curvature at the avascular space of the

Pars Flacida (at the equator of the intragastric balloon). The caudate lobe of the liver is visualized and dissection is continued with identification of the right crus of the diaphragm. The retrogastric tunnel is bluntly dissected along the posterior gastric wall to the angle of His. The band is placed into the abdomen via the 15 mm port. The gastric band is advanced from the angle of His to the peri-gastric opening (Fig. 11). Next, the band tubing is inserted into the band's buckle until the locking system is engaged (Fig. 12).

In order to prevent gastric herniation about the band, three to four interrupted sutures are placed plicating the anterior stomach proximal and distal to the device (Fig. 13). Care is taken to avoid needle injury to the band's balloon during suturing. The abdomen is irrigated and hemostasis confirmed. The distal catheter is retrieved through the left paramedian incision (12 mm port site); the tubing is inspected and placed to avoid kinking. The 15 mm port site is closed with absorbable fascial suture; the remaining trocars removed. The access port and tubing are engaged and excess tubing is placed within the abdomen. The port is then tacked to the anterior rectus sheath with four 2-0 nonabsorbable sutures. In order to secure the access port to the abdominal wall the skin incision at the site is enlarged to afford exposure. The wounds are irrigated and the closed with 4-0 absorbable subcuticular sutures. Steristrips are applied, 0.25% bupivicaine is injected at the port sites, and the orogastric tube removed.

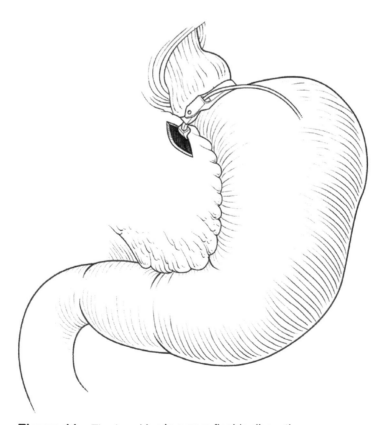

Figure 11   The band is via a pars flacida dissection.

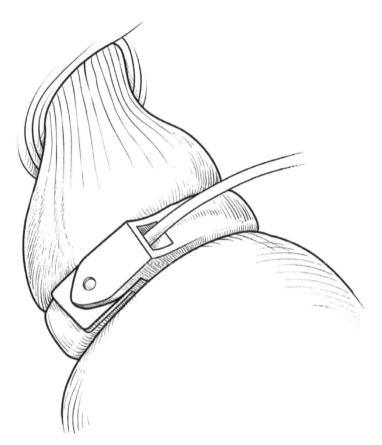

Figure 12   The band correctly oriented.

F.   Postoperative Care

Pneumatic compression devices and subcutaneous heparin are continued postoperatively. A gastrograffin swallow is obtained on postoperative day 1 to confirm band position and to rule out leak or gastric outlet obstruction. If the contrast exam is normal, the patient given a liquid diet. Postoperative adjustment of the band is withheld for 4–6 weeks in order to prevent band slippage or gastric herniation.

G.   Management of Complications

Problems may arise from band slippage, gastric dilation, gastric outlet obstruction, band erosion, or gastric herniation, which require operative revision. Injury to the esophagus or gastric perforation may occur as a result of improper handling of tissues. These potentially devastating complications require exploration, repair, and band removal. Removing an infected port may allow salvage if the band is uninvolved. At a later date a new port may be attached to the remaining band tubing. Dysfunction of the port or tubing is a common complication requiring revision. Reflux, nausea, vomiting, and food intolerance are not uncommon and may require hospitalization.

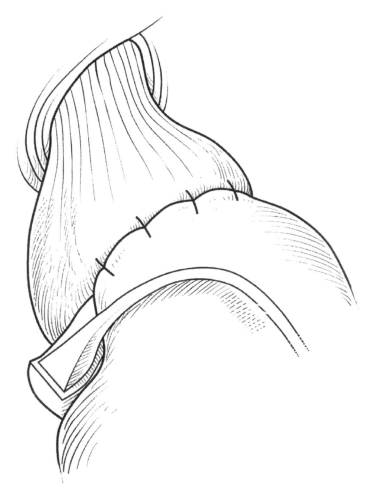

Figure 13 Anterior plication.

H. Outcomes

Excess weight loss following laparoscopic gastric banding is 30–60%. An operative time of 35–90 minutes and hospital stay of 1–3 days makes this an attractive alternative in appropriately selected patients.

VI. TOP TEN TIPS

1. Laparoscopic obesity surgery requires not only advanced technical skills but also knowledge of bariatric fundamentals.
2. Preoperative counseling and patient selection are crucial.
3. In patients undergoing gastric bypass, a cholecystectomy should be performed if gallstones are present.
4. All tubes excluding the endotracheal tube should be removed from the patient's mouth and nose prior to division of the stomach. Failure to do so may result in tube transection or pouch leak.

5. All potential internal hernia defects should be closed.
6. Avoid undo tension at the gastrojejunostomy as this may result in anastamotic leak or stricture.
7. Prevent twisting of the bowel mesentery.
8. Any redundancy in the Roux limb above the mesocolic defect should be reduced to prevent kinking and potential obstruction.
9. Close follow-up is requisite to ensure compliance and to prevent metabolic complications.
10. Port placement is critical to ensure an unobstructed operative field.

VII. CURRENT STATUS AND FUTURE INVESTIGATION

Laparoscopic gastric bypass has demonstrated advantages over the open approach, but it requires a significant degree of experience and skill to perform safely. Despite this the technique is emerging as the gold standard among operations for obesity. In terms of weight loss, comparison between gastric bypass and other malabsorptive procedures may lead to improved limb length criteria.

The gastric band affords a relatively simple laparoscopic approach to the morbidly obese patient. However, long-term weight loss, resolution of comorbid conditions, and outcome analysis are needed.

SELECTED READINGS

DeMaria EJ, Sugerman HJ, et al. High failure rate after adjustable silicon gastric banding for the treatment of morbid obesity. Ann Surg 2001; 233:809–818.

Favretti F, Cadière GB, et al. Laparoscopic banding:selection and technique in 830 patients. Obesity Surg 2002; 12:385–390.

Higa KD, Boone KB, et al. Laparoscopic Rou-en-Y gastric bypass for morbid obesity. Arch Surg 2000; 135:1029–1034.

Jones DB, Nguyen N, Lopez JA, O'Brien P, Provost D. Gastric bypass and adjustable band surgery for obesity. Contemporary Surgery 2003; 59:403–410.

Jones DB, DeMaria E, Provost DA, Smith CD, Morgenstern L, Schirmer B. Treatment of the morbidly obese: SAGES appropriateness statement. Surg Endoscopy, in press.

National Institutes of Health Consensus Development Conference: Gastrointestinal surgery for severe obesity. Ann Intern Med 1991; 115:956–961.

Nguyen NT, Goldman C, et al. Laparoscopic verses open gastric bypass: a randomized study of outcomes, quality of life, and costs. Ann Surg 2001; 234:279–291.

O'Brien PE, Brown WA, et al. Prospective study of laparoscopically placed, adjustable gastric band in the treatment of morbid obesity. Br J Surg 1999; 86:113–118.

Schauer PR, Ikramuddin S, et al. Outcomes after laparoscopic Roux-en-Y gastric bypass for morbid obesity. Ann Surg 2000; 232:515–529.

Schneider B, Villegas L, Blackburn GL, Mun EC, Critchlow JF, Jones DB. Laparoscopic gastric bypass surgery: outcomes. J Lapar Endosc Adv Surg Tech. 2003; 13(4):247–255.

Scott DJ, Provost DA, Jones DB. Laparoscopic Roux-en-Y gastric bypass for morbid obesity. Surg Rounds 2000:177–189.

Wittgrove AC, Clark GW. Laparoscopic gastric bypass, Roux-en-Y-500 patients: technique and results, with 3–60 month follow-up. Obesity Surg 2000; 10:233–239.

42

Minimally Invasive Orthopedic and Spinal Surgery: A Brief Overview

MICHAEL J. BOLESTA

University of Texas Southwestern Medical Center
Dallas, Texas, U.S.A.

I. INTRODUCTION

The musculoskeletal system is finely balanced to serve its many roles, including locomotion and other movements, support, and protection of internal organs. Trauma and disease impair these; in some cases surgery may restore function. It would seem axiomatic that any orthopedic procedure should seek to minimize damage to normal structures and tissues without compromising the correction of pathology. This is the primary principle of orthopedic minimally invasive surgery. By preserving anatomy, morbidity is reduced. There is potentially less pain, less time lost from work and social activities, and less need for acute care and rehabilitative services. Hence, there could be less cost to individuals and society in some cases; the savings may be consumed by the cost of new technologies. Another attraction of minimally invasive surgery is cosmetic. The scars are smaller, and preservation of normal anatomy will minimize soft tissue atrophy. Patients are attracted to these procedures and often will choose physicians based on ability to provide these services.

II. MINIMALLY INVASIVE ORTHOPEDICS: THE PRESENT

The concept of minimally invasive surgery is not new to orthopedic surgeons. Various tools have evolved and contributed to less invasive musculoskeletal management (Table 1). These have led to a large number of less invasive procedures (Table 2).

Trauma has engendered a number of techniques, such as percutaneous pinning, external skeletal fixation, and closed intramedullary nailing. Many degenerative joint and spinal conditions have spawned percutaneous injection therapies of variable efficacy. For example, intradiscal chymopapain can reduce radiculopathy in select cases of lumbar disc herniation, but it can rarely cause transverse myelitis and anaphylaxis, so it is not widely

Table 1   Tools for Minimally Invasive Orthopedic Surgery

Endoscopes, including arthroscope, laparoscope, and thoracoscope
Fluoroscopy
Operative microscope
Frameless stereotaxy
Computer-enhanced fluoroscopy
Procedure specific instrumentation and implants

---

used today. More recently, intradiscal electrothermal therapy (IDET) has been popular, but is still being assessed for long-term efficacy. Another percutaneous technique is vertebroplasty. Osteoporotic vertebral body fractures are injected, usually with polymethylmethacrylate (though other substances are being investigated) to reduce pain, and in some cases to correct kyphotic deformity. Inflatable balloons inserted into the body reduce the fracture and create a cavity for the injectant.

Perhaps the most popular minimally invasive technique is arthroscopy. It was initially a diagnostic tool for knee pathology, but over the past two decades it has become the primary method of treatment for many joint conditions and an important adjuvant in others. Fiber optics, high-density illumination, video technology, and the evolution of operative tools facilitated this branch of orthopedic surgery.

These technical advances also facilitated the evolution of microsurgery. The operative microscope gave surgeons magnification, intense illumination, and stereoscopic vision, even in a confined field. Within orthopedics, microscopy has been embraced by hand and upper extremity surgeons and spinal specialists. Spine surgeons took advantage of this technology to reduce soft tissue dissection needed to perform cervical and lumbar discectomy, for decompression of lumbar stenosis (limited to one or two levels), and to manage cervical spondylosis. For at least 10 years, lumbar microdiscectomy has been the

Table 2   Minimally Invasive Orthopedic Surgery

Percutaneous pinning of extremity fractures
Closed intramedullary nailing of long bone fractures
External skeletal fixators for fractures, extremity deformity, and limb lengthening
Arthroscopic surgery for diagnosis and management
Microscopic lumbar discectomy
Microscopic lumbar decompression
Microscopic cervical discectomy, with and without fusion
Microscopic cervical corpectomy and fusion
Thoracoscopic (VATS) anterior spinal release
Thoracoscopic (VATS) discectomy, with and without fusion
Thoracoscopic (VATS) anterior spinal fusion, with and without instrumentation
Laparoscopic (transperitoneal) anterior lumbar discectomy and fusion
Endoscopic (retroperitoneal) anterior lumbar discectomy and fusion
Endoscopic (retroperitoneal) anterior thoracolumbar and lumbar release
Endoscopic (retroperitoneal) transforaminal discectomy
Endoscopic (posterior) translaminar discectomy
Vertebroplasty

---

standard procedure for herniations that fail nonoperative care. The morbidity has been reduced to the point that many surgeons perform these cases as an outpatient procedure or overnight stay.

Endoscopy has enjoyed burgeoning success within general, thoracic, urological, and gynecological surgery. Historically, the spinal surgeon has teamed with thoracic and general surgeons to approach the anterior thoracic and lumbar spine. It was natural for the spine specialist to observe the developments within other surgical disciplines and seek applications for their patients. Spine surgeons are now treating selected traumatic, degenerative, infectious, neoplastic, and deforming conditions with thoracoscopic and laparoscopic assistance [1,2].

III. MINIMALLY INVASIVE ORTHOPEDICS: THE FUTURES

Materials science has produced new and better substances for prostheses. Many new devices are being applied to orthopedic disorders. Perhaps even more exciting are the developments within molecular biology. The discovery and production of growth factors may allow manipulation fracture and fusion healing, or promote joint cartilage and disk regeneration. Pluripotential stem cells, present even in adults, may be coaxed to restore tissues and structures. All this is speculative, but may be within the realm of possibility. Many of these ideas may take decades to become practical. Detailed discussion of such applications is beyond the purview of this chapter. Tables 3–4 summarize the present, the evolving, and the possible future minimally invasive strategies as applied within orthopedic surgery.

IV. MINIMALLY INVASIVE SURGERY FOR LUMBAR DISK DEGENERATION

Lumbar pain vexes physicians of many specialties. In the United States alone it is estimated to cost society $100 billion every year. It afflicts 50–80% of adults at some time during their lives. Etiology is complex and multifactorial, including physical, social, and

Table 3 Evolving Minimally Invasive Orthopedic Surgery

Endoscopic posterolateral fusion, with and without instrumentation
Nuclear prostheses for early disc degeneration
Total disc prostheses for more advanced disc disease
Growth factors
Bone substitutes
Intradiscal therapies
Less invasive plate fixation of long bone fractures
Meniscal repair and replacement

Table 4 Future Possibilities for Minimally Invasive Orthopedic Surgery

Autogenous stem cells engineered to produce healthy replacement tissues and structures (e.g., joint cartilage, meniscal, and disc regeneration)

psychological components. For most, it is a nuisance. The more severe and recurrent cases account for the bulk of the cost. In select cases, surgery may be appropriate.

The traditional approach has generally involved fusion. Posteriorly this requires a relatively extensive dissection, disrupting the soft tissues. It also requires harvest of pelvic bone, which is always attended by morbidity. Anterior approaches (anterior lumbar interbody fusion) are less painful, but iliac bone does not withstand the loads of the lumbar spine well. Allograft cortical bone (femur) is stronger, but still problematic. In the 1980s the procedure favored by several surgeons was circumferential fusion, the so-called 360. Allograft was placed anteriorly, and pedicle screw instrumentation inserted posteriorly. This had modest success but is a large open procedure requiring a lengthy recovery period. Other surgeons developed posterior lumbar interbody techniques, but they are technically demanding and associated with dural and neural injuries.

In the 1990s interbody cages were introduced. Various designs were employed. All were constructed of material that could sustain the physiological forces seen in the lumbar spine, but were hollow, filled with cancellous bone graft. As stand-alone devices, they had a measure of success in single-level fusion. Clinical outcomes and fusion rates have not been as good with multilevel fusions. There are designs for both anterior and posterior placement.

The anterior approach lends itself well to minimally invasive techniques. Spine surgeons noted the burgeoning field of laparoscopic surgery and recruited their colleagues to help them fuse the lumbar spine [3].

The patient is placed in the supine position in Trendelenburg, shifting the bowels cephalad. The most common level to be approached in this fashion is L5-S1. Anatomically this disc is usually below the bifurcation of the aorta and vena cava, so the spine surgeon can work between the iliac vessels [4]. The access surgeon must ligate the middle sacral artery, but this is not difficult. Generally the iliac vessels do not require much mobilization. A transperitoneal approach is more common, but retroperitoneal technique has also been used. The access surgeon exposes L5-S1, and the spine surgeon uses specially adopted laparoscopic instruments to remove disc material and to insert hollow threaded titanium cylinders packed with bone or other bone-stimulating substance. The U.S. FDA has recently approved the marketing of recombinant BMP-7 for use with anterior cages. The IDE studies showed clinical success and fusion rates comparable to cages filled with autogenous bone graft.

L4-5 and L3-4 can also be approached with similar techniques, but demands more of the access surgeon [4]. The aorta and venal cava are mobilized, sacrificing small branches, much as they would during traditional open technique. The access surgeon must be able to do this laparoscopically, but also be prepared to convert to an open exposure quickly if there is hemorrhage that he cannot control with laparoscopic instruments.

L1-2, L2-3, and L3-4 can be approached laterally using a retroperitoneal approach [5]. Cages have been designed specifically for this type of exposure. The vessels are avoided, but the psoas muscle has to be mobilized, which will cause some hemorrhage.

These techniques have been popular at some centers, but not uniformly adopted for a variety of reasons [6]. They demand two surgeons. With open techniques, the spine surgeon may or may not require such assistance, depending upon training and experience. Endoscopic techniques always involve investment in expensive equipment, though most of it is also used extensively for other types of procedures. The disposable endoscopic equipment adds expense that is not offset in this way. Early in the experience of the surgeons, more operative time is needed. While experience will shorten this, the most disappointing aspect of this particular laparsoscopic procedure is the lack of clear cost effectiveness. Open anterior interbody fusion, with cages or allograft, has very similar perioperative morbidity and length of stay [7]. Furthermore, the cylindrical cages that are so amenable to laparoscopic insertion have proven to be imperfect, whether inserted open or endoscopically. They are good for single-level disease, but not as useful in multi-level degeneration. It is difficult to assess fusion using the metallic devices. Finally, as alternative disc-replacement devices are developed, the need for fusion may diminish. Hence laparoscopic lumbar fusion is limited to centers with surgeons committed to endoscopic techniques.

REFERENCES

1. Crawford AH, Wall EJ, Wolf R. Video-assisted thoracoscopy. Orthop Clin North Am 1999; 30:367–385, viii.
2. Hovorka I, de Peretti F, Damon F, Arcamone II, Argenson C. Five years' experience of the retroperitoneal lumbar and thoracolumbar surgery. Eur Spine J 2000; 9:S30–S34.
3. McAfee PC, Regan JJ, Geis WP, Fedder IL. Minimally invasive anterior retroperitoneal approach to the lumbar spine. Emphasis on the lateral BAK. Spine 1998; 23:1476–1484.
4. Vraney RT, Phillips FM, Wetzel FT, Brustein M. Peridiscal vascular anatomy of the lower lumbar spine. An endoscopic perspective. Spine 1999; 24:2183–2187.
5. Dezawa A, Yamane T, Mikami H, Miki H. Retroperitoneal laparoscopic lateral approach to the lumbar spine: a new approach, technique, and clinical trial. J Spinal Disord 2000; 13:138–143.
6. Cowles RA, Taheri PA, Sweeney JF, Graziano GP. Efficacy of the laparoscopic approach for anterior lumbar spinal fusion. Surgery 2000; 128:589–596.
7. Zdeblick TA, David SM. A prospective comparison of surgical approach for anterior L4–L5 fusion: laparoscopic versus mini anterior lumbar interbody fusion. Spine 2000; 25:2682–2687.

Index

Milton Keynes UK
Ingram Content Group UK Ltd.
UKHW050308111024
449327UK00044B/2484